Skin Infections: Assessment and Management

Skin Infections: Assessment and Management

Edited by Joanne Perry

hayle medical

New York

Hayle Medical,
750 Third Avenue, 9th Floor,
New York, NY 10017, USA

Visit us on the World Wide Web at:
www.haylemedical.com

ISBN: 978-1-63241-576-9

The publisher's policy is to use permanent paper from mills that operate a sustainable forestry policy. Furthermore, the publisher ensures that the text paper and cover boards used have met acceptable environmental accreditation standards.

Printed in China.

Cataloging-in-Publication Data

Skin infections : assessment and management / edited by Joanne Perry.
p. cm.
Includes bibliographical references and index.
ISBN 978-1-63241-576-9
1. Skin--Infections. 2. Skin--Diseases. 3. Skin--Diseases--Diagnosis.
4. Skin--Diseases--Treatment. 5. Dermatology. I. Perry, Joanne.
RL201 .S55 2019
616.5--dc23

Contents

Preface

The purpose of the book is to provide a glimpse into the dynamics and to present opinions and studies of some of the scientists engaged in the development of new ideas in the field from very different standpoints. This book will prove useful to students and researchers owing to its high content quality.

Infection refers to the invasion of an organism's body tissues by disease-causing agents and their multiplication inside the body. Infections of the skin caused due to bacteria, fungi, virus, and parasitic infestations, stings, and bites are called skin infections. They can cause inflammation in the skin. Some of the common examples of bacterial skin infections are cellulitis, erysipelas, impetigo, and folliculitis. Fungal skin infections usually affect the skin, hair, and nails. Parasitic infections are generally caused by protozoa, cnidaria, arthropoda, echinodermata, bryozoa, annelida, platyhelminthes, and cyanobacteria. Viral infections include Butcher's wart, cowpox, Eczema vaccinatum, Condylomata acuminate, Chikungunya fever, etc. The topics included in this book on skin infections are of utmost significance and bound to provide incredible insights to readers. It includes some of the vital pieces of work being conducted across the world, on various topics related to the assessment and management of skin infections. This book attempts to assist those with a goal of delving into dermatology.

At the end, I would like to appreciate all the efforts made by the authors in completing their chapters professionally. I express my deepest gratitude to all of them for contributing to this book by sharing their valuable works. A special thanks to my family and friends for their constant support in this journey.

Editor

Innate Immune Dysfunctions in Aged Mice Facilitate the Systemic Dissemination of Methicillin-Resistant *S. aureus*

Ching Wen Tseng[1,2,3]*, Pierre A. Kyme[1,2,3], Andrea Arruda[1,2,3], V. Krishnan Ramanujan[4], Wafa Tawackoli[4], George Y. Liu[1,2,3]*

1 Division of Pediatric Infectious Diseases, Cedars-Sinai Medical Center, Los Angeles, California, United States of America, **2** Department of Pediatrics, David Geffen School of Medicine, University of California Los Angeles, Los Angeles, California, United States of America, **3** The Immunobiology Research Institute, Cedars-Sinai Medical Center, Los Angeles, California, United States of America, **4** Department of Surgery & Department of Biomedical Sciences, Cedars-Sinai Medical Center, Los Angeles, California, United States of America

Abstract

Elderly humans show increased susceptibility to invasive staphylococcal disease after skin and soft tissue infection. However, it is not understood how host immunity changes with aging, and how that predisposes to invasive disease. In a model of severe skin infection, we showed that aged mice (16- to 20-month-old) exhibit dramatic bacterial dissemination compared with young adult mice (2-month-old). Bacterial dissemination was associated with significant reductions of CXCL1 (KC), polymorphonuclear cells (PMNs), and extracellular DNA traps (NETs) at the infection site. PMNs and primary skin fibroblasts isolated from aged mice showed decreased secretion of CXCL2 (MIP-2) and KC in response to MRSA, and *in vitro* analyses of mitochondrial functions revealed that the mitochondrial electron transport chain complex I plays a significant role in induction of chemokines in the cells isolated from young but not old mice. Additionally, PMNs isolated from aged mice have reduced ability to form NETs and to kill MRSA. Expression of nuclease by *S. aureus* led to increased bacterial systemic dissemination in young but not old mice, suggesting that defective NETs formation in elderly mice permitted nuclease and non-nuclease expressing *S. aureus* to disseminate equally well. Overall, these findings suggest that gross impairment of both skin barrier function and innate immunity contributes to the propensity for MRSA to disseminate in aged mice. Furthermore, the study indicates that contribution of bacterial factors to pathogenicity may vary with host age.

Editor: Malcolm James Horsburgh, University of Liverpool, United Kingdom

Funding: This work is supported by the Telemedicine and Advanced Technology Research Center (TATRC) at the U.S. Army Medical Research and Materiel Command (USAMRMC) under Award No. W81XWH-09-1-0644. The funders had no role in study design, data collection and analysis, decision to publish, or preparation of the manuscript.

Competing Interests: The authors have declared that no competing interests exist.

* E-mail: tsengcw@cshs.org (CWT); george.liu@cshs.org (GYL)

Introduction

Staphylococcus aureus is an important pathogen that causes a wide variety of infections, ranging from skin and soft tissue infections to severe invasive diseases, such as sepsis and endocarditis. Approximately 35% of skin and soft tissue infection cases occur in people over 65 years of age, and 25% of these subjects later present with invasive staphylococcal diseases [1,2,3,4]. Hence, for elderly people, skin and soft-tissue staphylococcal infections are an important risk factor for the development of serious invasive staphylococcal diseases. However, how old age contributes to invasive staphylococcal diseases is not fully understood.

Prior studies have demonstrated that immune cells from elderly subjects, compared to cells isolated from young subjects, exhibit reduced chemotaxis, phagocytosis, and respiratory burst activity in response to bacterial infection [5,6,7]. An *in vitro* study of murine peritoneal macrophages attributes the decreased level of inflammation in elderly to lower levels of Toll-like receptors (TLR) expression on cell surfaces [8], suggesting that innate immune activation decreases with aging. Furthermore, decline in cellular and inflammatory responses has been shown to be associated with dysfunction of mitochondria in cells isolated from aged hosts [9]. Therefore, decreased cellular functions and immune responses may result in ineffective clearance of bacteria and facilitate systemic infection.

To prevent the systemic spread of pathogens, polymorphonuclear cells (PMNs) form neutrophil extracellular DNA traps (NETs) containing DNA, histone, granule enzymes, and antimicrobial components [10,11,12]. NETs promote killing of microorganisms and trap microbes locally [13], thereby preventing dissemination of the pathogens. Several host factors have been shown to contribute to the formation of NETs, including TLR and interleukin (IL)-8 [11,14]. Although NETs have been shown to interact with *S. aureus* and facilitate their killing [10], the effectiveness of NETs in aged mice against *S. aureus* has not been studied.

To investigate whether aging affects the outcome of MRSA infection, we utilized a murine skin infection model and studied host innate immune response to MRSA infection in young and aged mice. We showed that, compared to aged (16- to 22- month-old), mice young (2- month-old) mice exhibit reduced levels of MIP-2, KC, PMN recruitment, and NETs formation, and enhanced systemic dissemination of MRSA in response to infection. Furthermore, we demonstrated that mitochondrial electron transporter chain complex I could have a differential effect on chemokine response to *S. aureus* infection in young and aged mice. The importance of defective NETs in promoting systemic dissemination in elderly mice is suggested by the ability of *S. aureus* nuclease to support *S. aureus* dissemination in young but not old mice.

Results

Aged Mice are More Susceptible to MRSA Dissemination and Persistence Compared to Young Mice

Older people with MRSA skin and soft tissue infection have an increased risk of developing invasive MRSA disease [3], suggesting that age is a significant contributing factor for invasive staphylococcal infection. Macrophages isolated from aged mice show reduced TLR expression on cell surfaces, which may contribute to reduced inflammation in elderly individuals [8]. Because of these findings, we hypothesized that reduced inflammatory response in aged mice could lead to more invasive MRSA infection. In a murine skin infection model, we observed no significant difference of skin lesion size and bacterial burden between young and aged mice on day 3 post-infection (**Fig. 1A and B**). However, older mice showed a dramatic increase in systemic bacterial burden compared to young mice (**Fig. 1C**). At the site of bacterial inoculation, approximately 1.5 fold lower levels of MIP-2 and 2-fold lower KC were observed at 3 hours post-infection in aged mice compared with young mice (**Fig. 1D and 1E**). Because of the lower chemokine levels (MIP-2 and KC), we investigated PMN recruitment to the infection site using a MPO assay. As shown in **Fig. 1F**, significant fewer PMNs were found at the infection site in the aged mice at 3 hours post-infection. These results suggest that impaired chemokine response in aged hosts contributes to the defective immune cell recruitment.

Using a Xenogen imaging system and an isogenic MRSA harboring Tn4001::*luxABCDE* Km^R [15], we examined the invasiveness and persistence of MRSA infection over a period of 14 days in both young and aged mice (**File S1** and **Fig. S1A**). On day 1 post-infection, dense bioluminescence was observed at the infection site in both young and aged mice. However, in aged mice, diffuse bioluminescence was also notable throughout deeper tissues. By day 14 post-infection, the young mice exhibited dense bioluminescence only at the skin infection site, whereas the aged mice continued to display both skin and systemic bioluminescence. Enumeration of CFU showed a significantly higher bacterial burden in the skin and kidneys of aged mice compared to young mice (**File S1**, **Fig. S1B and S1C**). Taken together, these results suggest that the aged mice may develop more invasive and persistent MRSA infection after skin infection.

PMNs Isolated from Aged Mice have Reduced Chemokine Responses to MRSA

Next, we asked whether immune cells or stromal cells play a role in the reduced chemokine responses. Since PMNs contribute to the induction of inflammation at the infection site [16], PMNs and primary skin fibroblasts were isolated from different age groups of mice. PMNs isolated from young and aged mice were infected with MRSA across a range of MOIs. At 18 h post inoculation, PMNs from aged mice showed lower levels of MIP-2 (**Fig. 2A**) and KC (**Fig. 2B**), compared to PMNs from young mice. Similar MIP-2 response to MRSA was observed in peritoneal macrophages isolated from young and aged mice (**File S1** and **Fig. S2A**). Skin fibroblasts isolated from aged mice also revealed a reduced MIP-2 response compared to fibroblasts isolated from young mice (**File S1** and **Fig. S2B**). Additionally, LPS stimulation revealed reduced responses in aged hosts, which is in agreement with previously published work that cells isolated from aged hosts have reduced immune responses to LPS resulting from reduced levels of TLR expression on cell surfaces [8]. Taken together, we showed that select primary cells from the aged mice secrete lower levels of chemokines when challenged with MRSA.

Mitochondrial Electron Chain Transport Complex I (Complex I) Plays a Significant Role in Host Chemokine Responses to MRSA in Young Mice

Mitochondrial activities are critical to many cellular functions and to host inflammatory pathways activated in response to infection [17]. Mitochondrial functions decrease with advanced age and contribute to cellular dysfunctions observed in elderly hosts [18]. Therefore, dysfunction of mitochondria could be intrinsically linked to the decline of chemokine response in aged mice. To test this hypothesis, we first examined whether PMNs isolated from young and aged mice have different levels of mitochondrial membrane potential using tetramethylrhodamine methyl ester (TMRM). TMRM is a mitochondrial membrane potential sensitive dye which is used to track the mitochondrial membrane potential [19]. As shown in **Fig. 2C and 2D**, at 3 and 18 hours post-infection, PMNs isolated from young mice show significantly higher levels of fluorescence intensity than PMNs from aged mice, suggesting that greater depolarization occurred in the mitochondrial membrane of PMNs from the aged animals.

Since the function of complex I is primarily associated with the mitochondrial membrane potential and is affected by aging [20], we next asked whether inhibition of complex I using rotenone (complex I specific blocker) has an impact on chemokine secretion by PMNs. Because high concentrations of rotenone treatment induces apoptosis, a dose titration of rotenone was performed to determine the concentration required to collapse the mitochondrial membrane potential without inducing apoptosis of the cells (data not shown). As shown in **Fig. 2E and 2F**, control PMNs isolated from aged mice showed lower levels of MIP-2 and KC in the culture supernatant at 18 hours post-infection, compared to PMNs from young mice. When treated with 20 nM rotenone, PMNs from young mice revealed significant reductions of MIP-2 and KC in the culture supernatant. By contrast, rotenone treatment had a minimal effect on PMNs from aged mice. Under certain conditions, rotenone treatment resulted in increased levels of MIP-2 in the aged cells, suggesting mitochondrial complex I may have differential effect on inflammatory responses in young and aged hosts. The underlying cause of this differential effect is unclear. Similar assays were also performed using skin fibroblasts isolated from young and aged mice. Consistent with the results obtained with PMNs, skin fibroblasts from aged animals secrete a lower level of MIP-2 (**Fig. 2G**) and KC (**File S1** and **Fig. S3A and S3B**) when infected with MRSA, and were less responsive to rotenone repression of Complex I functions, compared to skin fibroblasts from young mice. These results are consistent with a prior report that cells isolated from aged animals are less responsive to rotenone treatment [21]. However, no significant difference in KC was observed when infected skin fibroblasts were treated with antimycin A (Complex III inhibitor) or oligomycin (Complex V inhibitor) (**File S1** and **Fig. S3**). Overall, these results suggest that functional complex I plays a significant role in KC and MIP-2 responses to MRSA infection in young but not aged mice.

PMNs Isolated from Aged Mice have Reduced Anti-MRSA Activity and Reduced NETs Formation

Prior studies have shown that PMNs isolated from aged hosts have reduced ability to generate oxygen metabolite and to

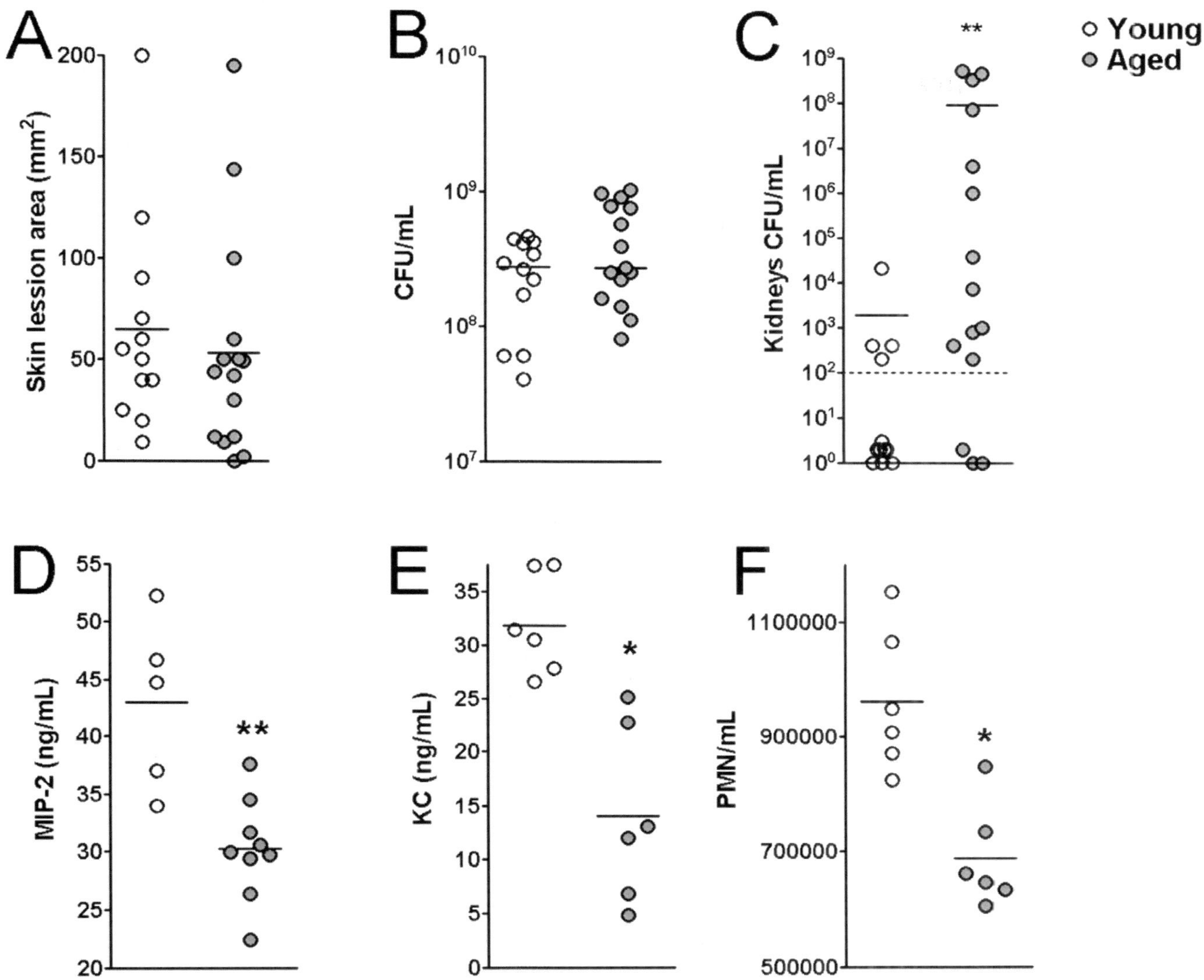

Figure 1. MRSA infection induces lower KC and PMNs at the infection site in aged mice. Age- and gender- matched mice were infected subcutaneously (s.c.) with 10^9 CFUs of CST9. On day 3 post-infection, the mice were sacrificed, and (A) skin lesion size, (B) skin CFUs and (C) kidney CFUs were determined. (D) MIP-2, (E) KC, and (F) PMNs from the lesions were quantitated at 3 hours post-infection. At least 3 mice were infected for each time point for IVIS analysis. At least 3 mice in each age group were infected for the chemokine, cytokine, and PMN analyses. $^*p<0.05$, $^{**}p<0.01$ for comparisons of young and aged mice.

phagocytose *S. aureus*, compared with young mice [6]. To examine whether PMNs from aged mice have reduced ability to kill MRSA, an *in vitro* PMN killing assay was performed. As shown in **Fig. 3A**, PMNs from aged mice were ineffective at clearing MRSA in the suspension, consistent with a previous report that PMNs from elderly people have reduced ability to kill bacteria [22].

During acute inflammation, formation of neutrophil extracellular traps (NETs) by PMNs is a critical host strategy that kills invading organisms and prevents them from systemic dissemination [10]. To examine the possibility that young and aged mice have different ability to form NETs, PMNs were isolated from young and aged mice and assessed for NETs formation. As shown in **Fig. 3B and C**, following treatment with PMA or infection with MRSA, PMNs from young mice exhibited ~2.5 fold higher concentration of NETs compared to PMNs from aged mice. To correlate to *in vivo* findings, infected tissues procured from young and aged mice were stained for DNA. DNase treatment has been shown to eliminate NETs formation [23]. Therefore, to examine whether DNase treatment would abrogate the NETs *in vitro*, PMNs were isolated from mice of different age groups and treated with or without DNase I during induction of NETs by PMA and *S. aureus*. As shown in **Fig. 3D**, reduced amount of the extracellular DNA fibers were observed in the DNase treated samples. Additionally, reduced numbers of PMNs were positive for the NETs formation with DNase treatment for PMNs derived from young mice. This is in contrast to PMNs isolated from aged hosts for which no significant difference in NETs was observed with or without DNase treatment (**Fig. 3E**). *In vivo* (**Fig. 3F**), infected skin tissues from young mice revealed meshed networks of extracellular DNA stain at the edge of the infection site, with very few bacteria notable beyond the extracellular DNA meshes. By contrast, this extracellular DNA network was not observed in the aged mice. To examine whether the increased levels of the extracellular DNA networks in the infected tissue of young mice are NETs, we stained

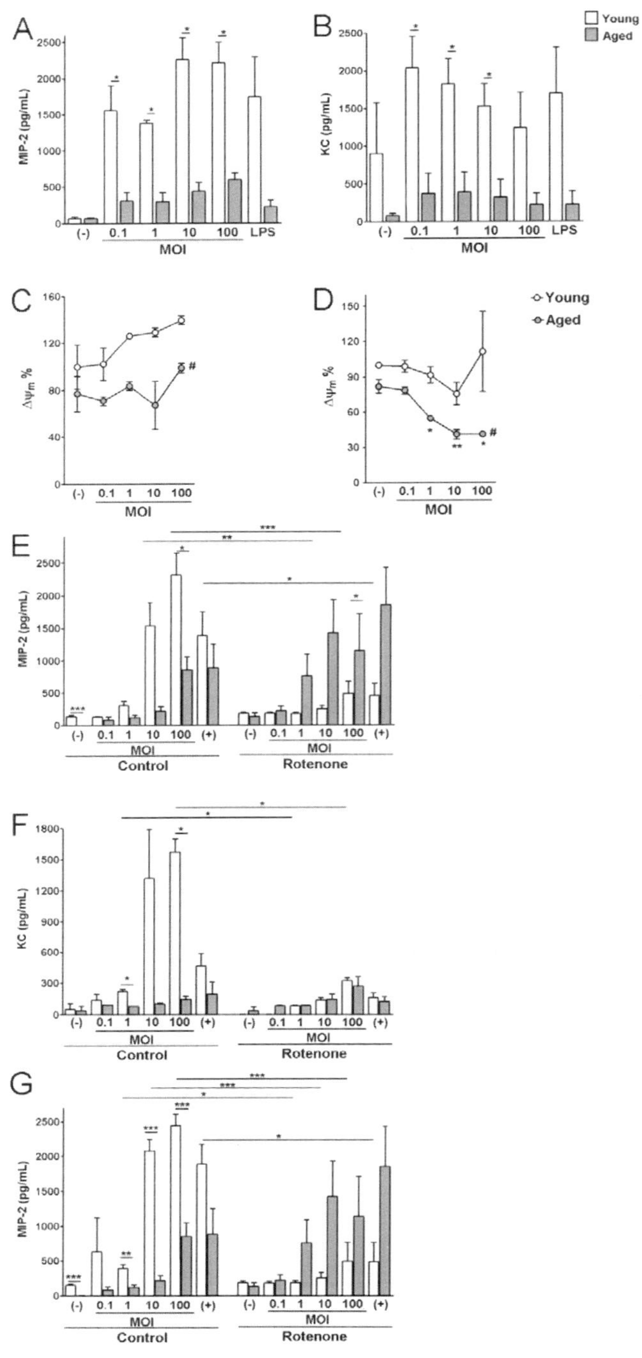

Figure 2. Mitochondrial electron transporter chain complex I plays an important role in the induction of MIP-2 in primary cells isolated from young but not old mice. (A) PMN KC at 18 h post-infection; (B) PMN MIP-2 at 18 h post-infection. (C) PMN membrane potential at 3 hours post-infection. (D) PMN membrane potential at 18 hours post-infection. The fluorescence of uninfected PMNs isolated from young mice is arbitrary set as 100%. (E–G) Primary cells were infected for 18 h with MRSA in the presence or absence of rotenone, and culture supernatants were collected for chemokine analyses. (E) PMN MIP-2, (F) PMN KC, and (G) skin fibroblast MIP-2. *$p<0.05$, **$p<0.01$, ***$p<0.005$. #$p<0.05$ for membrane potentials of young versus aged PMNs after infection with MRSA across a range of MOIs.

the infected tissue collected from both young and aged mice with elastase (**Fig. 3G**). In the tissue section of the infected young mice, increased levels of cellular debris, extracellular elastase, and DNA fibers positive of elastase were observed, which is in contrast to tissue sections collected from infected aged mice. Furthermore, we examined whether the increased levels of DNA fibers in young could be degraded by DNase. To avoid destruction of DNA fibers by the nuclease expressed by *S. aureus*, young mice were infected with 10^9 CFU of nuclease-negative (Nuc$^-$) *S. aureus* with or without daily treatment with 1 μg of DNase I. On day 3 post-infection, the mice that received the DNase I treatment showed reduced amount of DNA fiber at the infection site while the mice that received Nuc$^-$ *S. aureus* infection had increased amount of DNA fibers at the infection site (**Fig. S4**). Similar reductions in DNA fibers were observed in all DNase I treated mice. Thus, the impairment of PMN recruitment and reduced NETs formation in aged hosts, among others, may lead to more invasive MRSA infection in aged hosts.

Nuclease is a Virulence Factor in Young but not Aged Mice

Prior studies have shown that nuclease expression by pathogens leads to destruction of NETs and facilitates systemic dissemination of the bacteria [13,24,25,26]. We have shown in this study that the increased NETs formation occurs at the infection site of young mice (**Fig. 3G**). To test the hypothesis that deficiency of NETs formation in aged hosts leads to systemic dissemination of *S. aureus*, we infected young and aged mice with an *S. aureus* nuclease knockout and its isogenic nuclease expressing strain. As shown in **Fig. 4A**, nuclease expression did not have a significant effect on skin lesion size in each age group. Consistent with previous skin CFU findings from the MRSA infection (**Fig. 1B**), young and old mice infected with either strain of *S. aureus* show no difference in skin CFUs (**Fig. 4B**). However, nuclease expression in *S. aureus* contributed to an approximately 5 fold higher bacterial burden in the kidney in young mice but not in old mice (**Fig. 4C**). Additionally, young and old mice show an approximately 100 fold difference in kidney CFUs after infection with either strain of *S. aureus*. These results demonstrate that nuclease is important for the dissemination of *S. aureus* in young mice but not in aged host. Furthermore, the data suggest that defective NETs formation contribute, at least in part, to the increased dissemination of *S. aureus* in aged hosts.

Discussion

With an aging global population, there is an increasing need to understand why elderly individuals are more susceptible to infection. Age-dependent immune changes are likely to contribute to the increased incidence of severe infections [2], and based on epidemiologic studies, the elderly population is more prone to invasive MRSA disease [3]. Aging impacts a number of innate immune functions, impairing the host's ability to clear invading pathogens [27]. Epidemiologic studies reported an increased incidence of soft-tissue infections in the elderly population [28], and increased susceptibility to invasive disease after a cutaneous infection [4]. Results from our murine model closely mimic the human clinical features in that we do not find a difference in skin lesion size, but observe a dramatic difference in MRSA dissemination into the bloodstream between young and aged mice.

Based on our finding that PMNs from aged mice are impaired in their ability to kill MRSA, we initially hypothesized that aged mice would exhibit a high CFU burden in the subcutaneous tissues, and this would lead to bacterial dissemination into deep

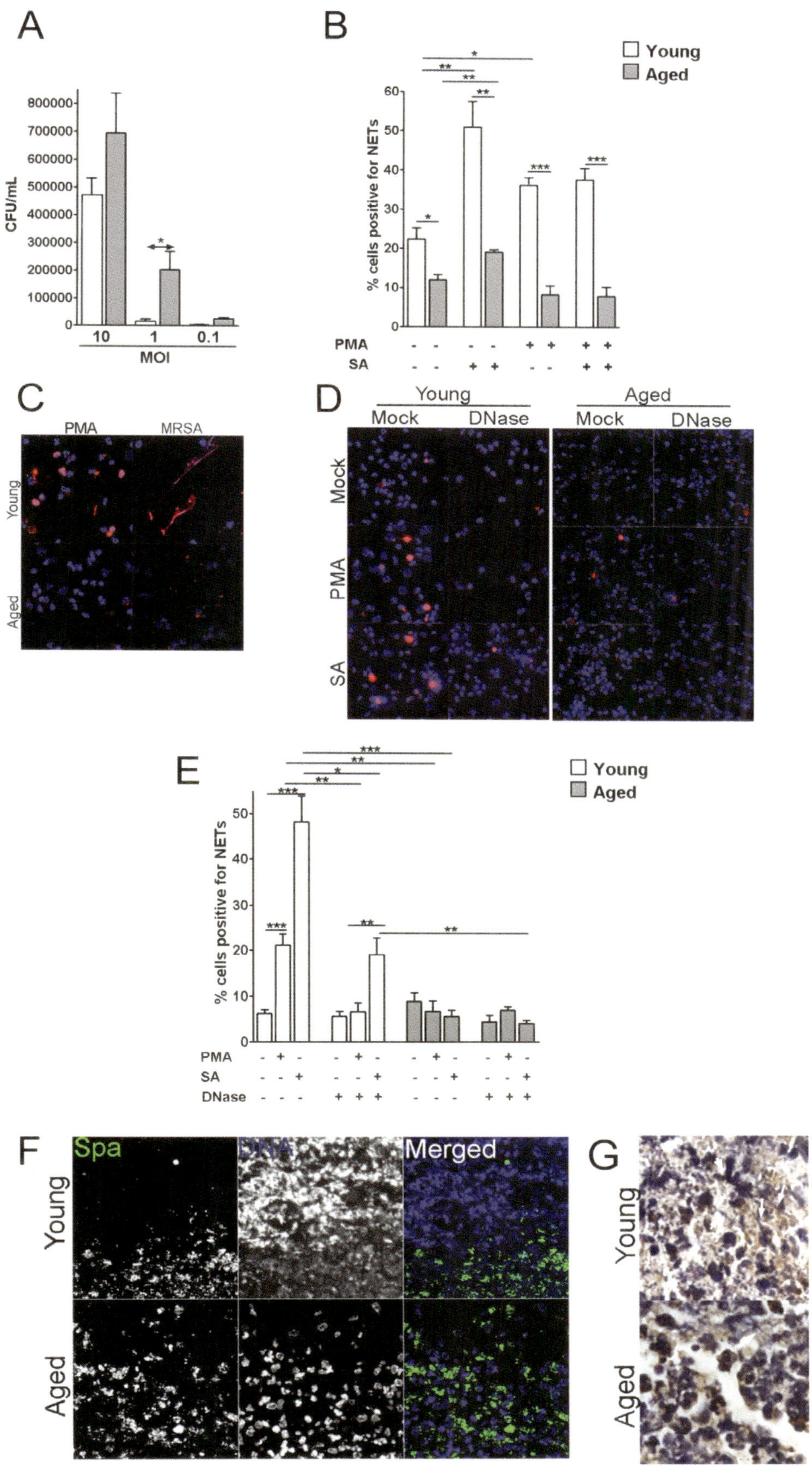
A
CFU/mL
MOI
10
1
0.1
B
Young
Aged
% cells positive for NETs
PMA
SA
C
PMA
MRSA
Young
Aged
D
Young
Aged
Mock
DNase
Mock
PMA
SA
E
Young
Aged
% cells positive for NETs
PMA
SA
DNase
F
Spa
DNA
Merged
Young
Aged
G
Young
Aged

Figure 3. Aged mice show defective NETs formation in response to MRSA. (A) PMNs show reduced bactericidal activities against MRSA at 1 hours post infection, *in vitro* (n = 3). (B–C) PMNs from young and aged mice were incubated with or without 20 nM PMA for 1 h, and then with either MRSA at MOI of 10 or PBS for another 2 h. (B) Quantitative analysis of percentage of cells that is NETs positive (n = 3). (C) Representative image of *in vitro* NETs formation. Cells were stained for histone (Red) and DNA (Blue). (D–E) PMNs from young and aged mice were incubated with 20 nM PMA or MRSA at MOI of 10 with or without 100 ng of DNase I for 2 h. (D) Representative images of *in vitro* NETs formation with or without DNase treatment. Cells were stained for histone (Red) and DNA (Blue). (E) Quantitative analysis of percentage of cells that are NETs positive (n = 3). (F) NETs formation within skin lesions on day 3 post-infection. Infected tissues were stained for staphylococcal protein A (Spa) (green) and DNA (blue) (400×). (G) Immunochemical stain of elastase within skin lesions on day 3 post-infection. Infected tissues were stained for elastase and counter stained with hematoxylin (1000×). **p*<0.05, ***p*<0.01, ****p*<0.005.

tissues by sheer spill over effect. Though a dramatic difference in dissemination of MRSA was observed, unexpectedly, there was no difference in bacterial burden between young and aged animals under the skin. We interpreted these data as evidence of a prominent defect in skin barrier function in aged mice.

Current understanding of mechanisms that limit bacterial dissemination is incomplete. However, a critical factor that has been implicated is the formation of NETs by PMNs which facilitate trapping and killing of pathogens during infection [10,25]. Published studies have shown that pathogens that have an ability to evade NETs entrapment have a greater predilection to disseminate [26,29]. We showed in aged mice that both PMN recruitment and NETs formation are severely impaired. Reduced PMNs could be explained at the cellular level by the inability of primary cells from aged mice to produce chemokines (KC and MIP-2) to recruit PMNs. Reduced PMNs in turn would lead to reduced NETs formation. Additionally, we demonstrated that aged PMNs have an inherent defect in NETs formation. Previous studies have shown that nuclease expression allows pathogens to escape NETs and promote systemic dissemination of the pathogen [24,25,26]. Consistent with the hypothesis that deficiency of NETs in aged mice promotes systemic dissemination of MRSA, we showed that nuclease expression by *S. aureus* leads to enhanced bacterial dissemination in young but not old mice. Taken together, the result suggests that defective NETs formation plays a role in the increased *S. aureus* dissemination in aged mice, but it does not exclude the possibility that other factors, such as defective skin structural barrier functions, are also involved in the increased invasiveness of *S. aureus* in aged hosts. Further investigations are necessary to tease out the detailed mechanisms.

The finding that nuclease promotes bacterial growth in young but not old mice point to a concept that virulence could be age specific. It is well appreciated from studies of mutant mice or mice of different backgrounds that bacterial virulence is sometimes dependent on host expression of factors that interact with the bacterial factor. For example, pathogenicity associated with LPS requires host expression of TLR4 [30]. Likewise, the concept that virulence is frequently tissue specific is also important because it informs on the effectiveness of anti-virulence strategies including vaccine development. However, the effect of host age on virulence of microbial factors is not well studied. Our demonstration that virulence is age specific points to the role of host immunity as a critical determinant of whether a virulence factor induces pathology. This concept could be important in the context that vaccines against specific virulence determinants could be effective against one age group but not another.

While many immune defects (e.g. phagocytosis, reactive oxygen section) are associated with aging, the fundamental age-dependent cellular changes that are responsible for these defects are not known. However, it is well appreciated that cells from aged individuals have altered mitochondrial functions which could impact their ability to respond to external stimuli, including pathogens. In our model, we showed that both skin fibroblasts and PMNs isolated from aged mice have reduced ability to secrete chemokines in response to MRSA, compared to young mice. Blocking of the mitochondrial electron chain complex I, but not complexes III or V, revealed a significant contribution of complex

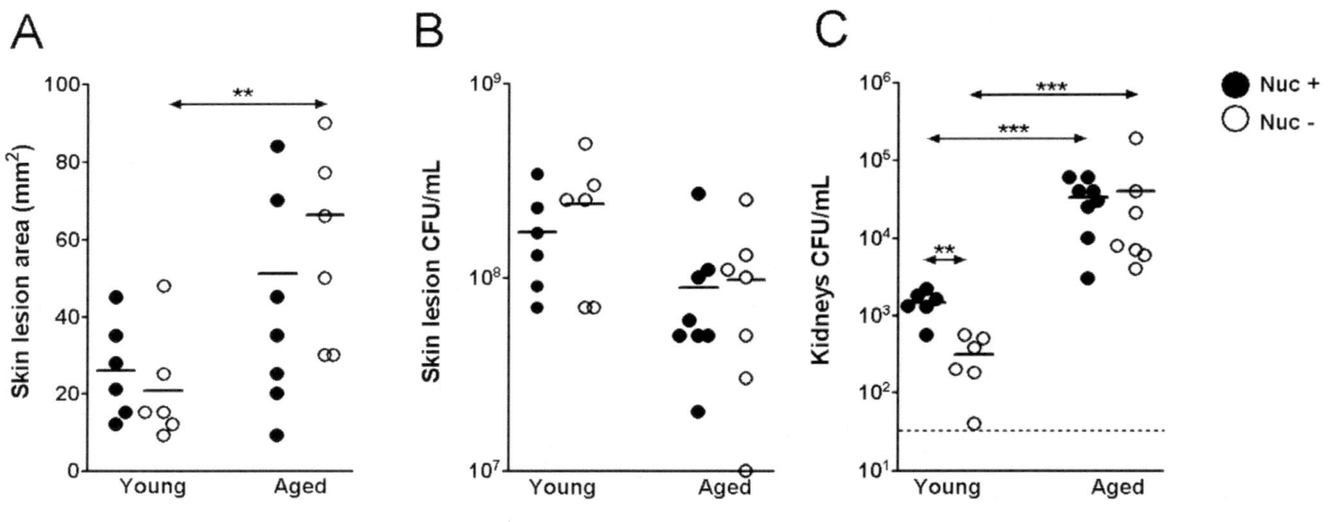

Figure 4. Expression of *S. aureus* Nuclease increases *S. aureus* burden in the kidneys of young, but not aged mice. Gender- and age-matched mice were infected subcutaneously (s.c.) with 10^9 CFUs of a nuclease expressing *S. aureus* (UAMS 1552) (Nuc+) and an isogenic nuclease non-expressing *S. aureus* (UAMS 1472) (Nuc–). On day 3 post-infection, the mice were sacrificed, and (A) skin lesion size, (B) skin CFUs, and (C) kidney CFUs were measured. **p*<0.05.

I function to chemokine responses in cells derived from young mice but not aged mice. Interestingly, blocking of mitochondrial complexes did not have the same effect on NETs formation (unpublished results). Therefore, age-dependent changes in mitochondrial functions could differentially account for changes in immune functions between young and older hosts. The exact role of mitochondrial function in *S. aureus* induced chemokine responses is not clear. Complex I function has been shown to play a role in lipopolysaccharide (LPS) induced inflammatory responses by modulating NF-κB activation [17], suggesting that TLR4-dependent immune activation pathway is dependent on the mitochondrial function. Pertinently, Sweeney *et. al.* reported that the up-regulation of mitochondrial biogenesis transcription factors in *S. aureus* sepsis is TLR2- and TLR4-dependent, which further suggests an interplay between mitochondrial functions and TLR-dependent innate immune activation [31]. Additional studies are required to elucidate how mitochondrial functions modulate *S. aureus*-induced inflammation in our model.

Overall, we have generated a murine model of MRSA infection in aged mice that captures the hallmark clinical finding that elderly individuals are more susceptible to invasive disease after skin infection, which may result from the grossly leaky barrier function and declined innate immunity in the aged mice. We have demonstrated defective chemokine response, PMN recruitment, NETs formation, and bacterial clearance in the aged mice that could explain these findings. Furthermore, we have shown that deficiency of NETs formation likely plays a role in promoting the dissemination of MRSA in aged hosts. To the best of our knowledge, the defective NETs formation in aged mice has not been described previously. Further experiments will be required to address the detailed mechanism of NETs dysfunctions in aged hosts, which could lead to specific immune boosting strategies.

Materials and Methods

Bacterial Strains and Growth Conditions

A clinical MRSA isolate from a skin infection (CST9) was used for this study. Nuclease positive *S. aureus* strain (UAMS 1552) and Nuclease negative isogenic strain (UAMS 1471) were generous gifts from Dr. Mark Smeltzer [32]. MRSA strains were routinely cultured on sheep blood agar plates, and colonies with comparable hemolytic phenotype were used for each experiment. Bacteria were also cultured in Todd-Hewitt broth at 37°C with shaking at 250 rpm.

Murine Skin Infection Model

Two- and 6-month-old male and female CD1 mice were purchased from Charles River Laboratories. Six-month-old mice were maintained in the animal facility in Cedars-Sinai Medical Center until they reached 16- to 22-month-old. Infection of mice was performed using previously established protocols [33]. Briefly, an overnight bacterial culture was diluted 1:200 in pre-warmed media and incubated at 37°C with shaking at 250 rpm until an A_{540} reached ~2.5. Bacteria were harvested by centrifugation at 4000 rpm for 10 min at 4°C, and then washed twice with equal volume of Dulbecco's PBS (DPBS) (Mediatech). The bacteria were resuspended in DPBS to a concentration of approximately 10^{10} CFU/mL. One hundred microliters of suspension was injected subcutaneously in each flank. Injections were performed with careful visualization of the needle to assure that the injection site was not intramuscular.

All animal experiments were approved by the Cedars-Sinai Committee on the Use and Care of Animals and performed using accepted veterinary standards.

Determination of Lesion Size and Tissue Bacterial CFUs

Following euthanization, lesions were measured, then were excised and homogenized in 1 mL of DPBS for CFUs determination following previously established protocols [33]. Lesions defined by darkened area of necrosis were measured using previously established methods [34].

Immunofluorescent Assays (IFA) and Immunochemical Analysis

Infected tissues were excised and fixed in 10% formalin (Medical Chemical Corporation) overnight. Paraffin embedding was performed by the Department of Pathology at Cedars-Sinai Medical Center. Tissue sections were deparaffinized and blocked with PBS with 0.05% Tween 20 (ISC Biosciences) and 0.5% BSA (blocking buffer) for 1 hour at room temperature. For *in vitro* assays, tissue samples were fixed with 10% formalin at room temperature for 30 min. The samples were blocked with PBS-0.05% Triton-X 100 and 0.5% BSA at room temperature for 1 hour. After incubation of samples with rabbit anti-staphylococcal protein A antibody (Sigma) at room temperature for 1 hour, slides were washed for 5 min with PBS 3 times Then, the slides were incubated with corresponding FITC- conjugated secondary antibody (Jackson ImmunoResearch Laboratory), and hoechst (at a final concentration of 1 μg/mL) in PBS-0.5% BSA. After a final wash, the tissue sections were mounted with Prolong AntiFade (Invitrogen). The stained slides were examined using an Olympus BX51 fluorescent microscope.

For immunochemical analysis of elastase, the tissue sections were deparaffinized and processed for antigen retrieval using 10 mM sodium citrate buffer (pH 6.0) at 95°C for 10 min. The tissue section slides were washed for 5 min with PBST 3 times, and then incubated with 1:100 diluted rabbit anti-elastase antibody (Abcam) at room temperature for 2 hours. After 3 washes for 5 min with PBST, 100 μL of the broad spectrum antibody detection solution was added to each sample following the manufacture protocol (Invitrogen). The slides were visualized by DAB solution (BD Biosciences) and counter stained by hematoxylin. After mounting using histomount (Invitrogen), the stained slides were analyzed using a BX51 microscope.

Enzyme Linked Immunosorbent Assay (ELISA), and Myeloperoxidase (MPO) Assay

Animals were euthanized at 3 and 72 h post-infection, and the skin and muscle lesions were homogenized in 1 mL of PBS-Triton X-100 (0.05%) with protease inhibitor cocktails (Roche). The homogenized suspension was centrifuged at 15,000×*g* for 10 min, and supernatants were collected and examined using ELISAs and MPO assay. Mouse IL-10, MIP-2, and KC (R & D Systems) specific ELISAs were performed according to the manufacturer's instructions. MPO activity (Invitrogen) was determined according to the manufacturer's instructions. and isolated murine PMNs were used as standard to convert the MPO activity to PMN number.

In vitro Infection of Primary Cells

Macrophages, PMNs [35,36], and skin fibroblasts [37] were isolated from mice of different age groups using modified established protocols. For PMN isolation, 4% thioglycollate was injected into the peritoneal cavity of mice. After 4 hours, 7 mL of DPBS was injected into the peritoneal cavity to collect peritoneal cells. Isolated PMNs were washed with DPBS twice, and red blood cells were lysed using ddH_2O. The cells were collected using centrifugation at 500×*g* for 10 min at 4°C. Cell viability was determined using trypan blue assay. Skin biopsy samples were digested in a Petri dish with 0.25% of trypsin (Invitrogen) for approximately 1 hour. The dermis layer was removed and minced into small pieces using sterile razor blades. The minced sample was transferred into a 50 mL conical tube and 10 mL of 0.25% trypsin was added to the sample and incubated at 37°C for 1 hour with gentle agitation. After the incubation, the suspension was filtered using a 70 µm tissue strainer, and the cells were collected by centrifugation at 700×*g* for 10 min. The cells were washed twice with DMEM and cultured in 20% FBS-DMEM with 1% penicillin and streptomycin in a 5% CO_2 incubator. Passages 4 to 7 of cultured skin fibroblasts were used for *in vitro* experiments.

To assess the impact of mitochondrial electron chain complexes on specific cellular functions, isolated cells were incubated with or without 20 nM of rotenone (Complex I specific inhibitor) for 18 hours in DMEM-5% FBS in a 37°C 5% CO_2 incubator. For PMNs, after rotenone treatment, cells were collected by centrifugation at 700×*g* for 10 min and washed with HBSS twice. PMNs were stained with trypan blue to verify viability before plating and infection with MRSA. The PMNs were resuspended in DMEM with 5% FBS with or without 20 nM of rotenone, and 1×10^4 viable cells were plated in each well of 96 well plates for infection. For skin fibroblast, media were removed and cells were washed twice with HBSS, and 400 µL of DMEM with 5% FBS with or without 20 nM of rotenone was added to each well. Diluted MRSA were added to each well to a final MOI of 0.1 to 100. To facilitate the interaction of cells and MRSA, the tissue culture plates containing isolated cells and MRSA were centrifuged at 700×*g* for 10 min at room temperature. After centrifugation, the cells were incubated at 37°C with 5% CO_2 for 3 and 18 hours. After incubation, the culture supernatants were collected and assayed using ELISAs.

Assay for Mitochondrial Membrane Potential

Mitochondrial membrane potential was measured using a previously established tetramethylrhodamine methyl ester (TMRM) method [19]. Briefly, PMNs isolated from young and aged mice were washed with DPBS three times before resuspended in DMEM-5% FBS. Ten thousand viable PMNs were plated in each well in a 96 well tissue culture plate. Cells were infected with MRSA at MOIs ranging from 0 to 100. At 3 and 18 hours post-infection, the cells were centrifuged at 700×*g* for 10 min, and culture supernatants were carefully removed. The cells were then resuspended in DMEM containing 20 nM TMRM. After incubation at 37°C with 5% CO_2 for 20 min, fluorescence was measured using a microtiter plate reader at excitation 540 nm and emission 570 nm.

NETs Formation

NETs were visualized using a modified established protocol [38]. One hundred thousand viable PMNs isolated from different age groups of mice were seeded in each well, in tissue culture plates. The cells were treated with or without 20 nM of phorbol myristate acetate (PMA) for 1 hour before infection. Diluted bacterial suspensions were added to each well to a final multiplicity of infection (MOI) of 10. After addition of the bacterial suspension, the tissue culture plates were centrifuged at 700×*g* for 10 min at room temperature to facilitate interaction of the cells and the bacteria. After centrifugation, the plates were incubated at 37°C with 5% CO_2 for 2 hours, fixed with 4% formalin at room temperature for 30 min. For DNase I treatment, 10^5 viable PMNs isolated from mice of different age groups were seeded in each well in tissue culture plates. The cells were treated with or without 100 ng of DNase I (Sigma) plus PMA (20 nM) or MRSA at MOI of 10. After addition of the stimuli, the tissue culture plates were centrifuged at 700×*g* for 10 min at room temperature, incubated at 37°C with 5% CO_2 for 2 hours, and fixed with 4% formalin at room temperature for 30 min. The samples were blocked with PBS-0.05% Triton-X 100 and 1% BSA (blocking buffer) at room temperature for 1 hour. After incubation of samples with rabbit anti-histone H3 body (AbCam) in blocking buffer at room temperature for 1 hour, slides were washed for 5 min with PBS 3 times. Then, the slides were incubated with corresponding Texas Red-conjugated secondary antibody (Jackson ImmunoResearch Laboratory) and hoechst (at a final concentration of 1 µg/mL) in PBS-0.5% BSA. After a final wash, the tissue sections were mounted with Prolong AntiFade (Invitrogen). The stained slides were examined using an Olympus BX51 fluorescent microscope. The total number of PMNs and the number of NETs-positive PMNs were counted from five random fields of each sample. The percentage of NETs-positive cells was determined as the number of histone-positive cells divided by the total number of cells multiplied by 100%.

Statistical Analysis

Data were analyzed using unpaired *t* – test unless otherwise indicated (Prism 4.03, Graphpad Software, Inc.). *p* values less than 0.05 were considered significant, and were noted in the figures. In bar graphs, results were presented as mean ± SEM (n≥3).

Ethics Statement

This study was performed under strict accordance with the recommendations in the Guide for the Care and Use of Laboratory Animals. CSMC is accredited by the Association for Assessment and Accreditation of Laboratory Animal Care International (AAALAC), and in compliance with NIH guideline of laboratory animal care and use. The protocol was approved by the institutional animal use and care committee of the Cedars-Sinai Medical Center (IACUC 3402). All procedures were performed under isoflurane anesthesia, and all efforts were made to minimize suffering.

Supporting Information

Figure S1 Examination of invasiveness and persistence of subcutaneously injected MRSA. Young and aged mice were infected s.c. with 10^9 CFUs of CST9 and followed for 14 days. (A) Visualization of MRSA dissemination. CST9 harboring Tn4001::*luxABCDE* Km^R was used for infection of mice. Bioluminescence at the infection site and deep tissues was followed over a period of 14 days using an IVIS system. At least 3 mice in each age group were infected for each time point for IVIS analysis. b: back of mice; d: dorsa of mice. (B) Skin lesion CFU (n = 6); (C) CFU in Kidneys (n = 6).

Figure S2 Macrophages and skin fibroblasts isolated from aged mice show reduced MIP-2 response to MRSA infection. (A) Macrophage MIP-2 at 18 h post-infection; (B) skin fibroblast MIP-2 at 18 h post-infection. *$p<0.05$, compared between young and aged mice.

Figure S3 Mitochondrial electron chain complex III and V have limited effect on KC levels in skin fibroblasts isolated from both young and aged mice when responding to MRSA infection. (A) Young; (B) Aged.

Figure S4 *In vivo* DNase administration reduced DNA fibers at the site of infection. Young mice were infected with 10^9 CFU of Nuc$^-$ *S. aureus* and half were treated daily with 1 μg DNase I. On day 3 post-infection, the mice were sacrificed and the infected tissues were excised. After embedding, the tissue slices were analyzed for the presence of elastase by immunohistochemistry.

File S1 Supporting methods and materials.

Acknowledgments

We thank Dr. George Stewart and Dr. Meredith Gregory-Ksander for critical reading.

Author Contributions

Conceived and designed the experiments: CWT GYL. Performed the experiments: CWT PAK AA WT. Analyzed the data: CWT VKR GYL. Contributed reagents/materials/analysis tools: WT GYL. Wrote the paper: CWT GYL.

References

1. Demling RH, Waterhouse B (2007) The increasing problem of wound bacterial burden and infection in acute and chronic soft-tissue wounds caused by methicillin-resistant Staphylococcus aureus. J Burns Wounds 7: e8.
2. Klevens RM, Morrison MA, Nadle J, Petit S, Gershman K, et al. (2007) Invasive methicillin-resistant Staphylococcus aureus infections in the United States. JAMA 298: 1763–1771.
3. Kuehnert MJ, Hill HA, Kupronis BA, Tokars JI, Solomon SL, et al. (2005) Methicillin-resistant-Staphylococcus aureus hospitalizations, United States. Emerg Infect Dis 11: 868–872.
4. Laupland KB, Church DL, Mucenski M, Sutherland LR, Davies HD (2003) Population-based study of the epidemiology of and the risk factors for invasive Staphylococcus aureus infections. J Infect Dis 187: 1452–1459.
5. Goldstein E, Bartlema HC, van der Ploeg M, van Duijn P, van der Stap JG, et al. (1978) Effect of ozone on lysosomal enzymes of alveolar macrophages engaged in phagocytosis and killing of inhaled Staphylococcus aureus. J Infect Dis 138: 299–311.
6. Lipschitz DA, Udupa KB (1986) Influence of aging and protein deficiency on neutrophil function. J Gerontol 41: 690–694.
7. Wenisch C, Patruta S, Daxbock F, Krause R, Horl W (2000) Effect of age on human neutrophil function. J Leukoc Biol 67: 40–45.
8. Renshaw M, Rockwell J, Engleman C, Gewirtz A, Katz J, et al. (2002) Cutting edge: impaired Toll-like receptor expression and function in aging. J Immunol 169: 4697–4701.
9. Csiszar A, Wang M, Lakatta EG, Ungvari Z (2008) Inflammation and endothelial dysfunction during aging: role of NF-kappaB. J Appl Physiol 105: 1333–1341.
10. Brinkmann V, Reichard U, Goosmann C, Fauler B, Uhlemann Y, et al. (2004) Neutrophil extracellular traps kill bacteria. Science 303: 1532–1535.
11. Clark SR, Ma AC, Tavener SA, McDonald B, Goodarzi Z, et al. (2007) Platelet TLR4 activates neutrophil extracellular traps to ensnare bacteria in septic blood. Nat Med 13: 463–469.
12. Ermert D, Urban CF, Laube B, Goosmann C, Zychlinsky A, et al. (2009) Mouse neutrophil extracellular traps in microbial infections. J Innate Immun 1: 181–193.
13. Wartha F, Beiter K, Normark S, Henriques-Normark B (2007) Neutrophil extracellular traps: casting the NET over pathogenesis. Curr Opin Microbiol 10: 52–56.
14. Gupta AK, Hasler P, Holzgreve W, Gebhardt S, Hahn S (2005) Induction of neutrophil extracellular DNA lattices by placental microparticles and IL-8 and their presence in preeclampsia. Hum Immunol 66: 1146–1154.
15. Francis KP, Joh D, Bellinger-Kawahara C, Hawkinson MJ, Purchio TF, et al. (2000) Monitoring bioluminescent Staphylococcus aureus infections in living mice using a novel luxABCDE construct. Infect Immun 68: 3594–3600.
16. Wagner C, Iking-Konert C, Hug F, Stegmaier S, Heppert V, et al. (2006) Cellular inflammatory response to persistent localized Staphylococcus aureus infection: phenotypical and functional characterization of polymorphonuclear neutrophils (PMN). Clin Exp Immunol 143: 70–77.
17. Zmijewski JW, Lorne E, Zhao X, Tsuruta Y, Sha Y, et al. (2008) Mitochondrial respiratory complex I regulates neutrophil activation and severity of lung injury. Am J Respir Crit Care Med 178: 168–179.
18. Kriete A, Mayo KL (2009) Atypical pathways of NF-kappaB activation and aging. Exp Gerontol 44: 250–255.
19. Floryk D, Houstek J (1999) Tetramethyl rhodamine methyl ester (TMRM) is suitable for cytofluorometric measurements of mitochondrial membrane potential in cells treated with digitonin. Biosci Rep 19: 27–34.
20. Petrosillo G, Matera M, Moro N, Ruggiero FM, Paradies G (2009) Mitochondrial complex I dysfunction in rat heart with aging: critical role of reactive oxygen species and cardiolipin. Free Radic Biol Med 46: 88–94.
21. Genova ML, Bovina C, Marchetti M, Pallotti F, Tietz C, et al. (1997) Decrease of rotenone inhibition is a sensitive parameter of complex I damage in brain non-synaptic mitochondria of aged rats. FEBS Lett 410: 467–469.
22. Fu YK, Arkins S, Li YM, Dantzer R, Kelley KW (1994) Reduction in superoxide anion secretion and bactericidal activity of neutrophils from aged rats: reversal by the combination of gamma interferon and growth hormone. Infect Immun 62: 1–8.
23. Meng W, Paunel-Gorgulu A, Flohe S, Witte I, Schadel-Hopfner M, et al.(2012) Deoxyribonuclease is a potential counter regulator of aberrant neutrophil extracellular traps formation after major trauma. Mediators Inflamm 2012: 149560.
24. Berends ET, Horswill AR, Haste NM, Monestier M, Nizet V, et al. (2010) Nuclease expression by Staphylococcus aureus facilitates escape from neutrophil extracellular traps. J Innate Immun 2: 576–586.
25. Sumby P, Barbian KD, Gardner DJ, Whitney AR, Welty DM, et al. (2005) Extracellular deoxyribonuclease made by group A Streptococcus assists pathogenesis by enhancing evasion of the innate immune response. Proc Natl Acad Sci U S A 102: 1679–1684.
26. Walker MJ, Hollands A, Sanderson-Smith ML, Cole JN, Kirk JK, et al. (2007) DNase Sda1 provides selection pressure for a switch to invasive group A streptococcal infection. Nat Med 13: 981–985.
27. Niwa Y, Kasama T, Miyachi Y, Kanoh T (1989) Neutrophil chemotaxis, phagocytosis and parameters of reactive oxygen species in human aging: cross-sectional and longitudinal studies. Life Sci 44: 1655–1664.
28. Young LM, Price CS (2008) Community-acquired methicillin-resistant Staphylococcus aureus emerging as an important cause of necrotizing fasciitis. Surg Infect (Larchmt) 9: 469–474.
29. Bianchi M, Niemiec MJ, Siler U, Urban CF, Reichenbach J (2011) Restoration of anti-Aspergillus defense by neutrophil extracellular traps in human chronic granulomatous disease after gene therapy is calprotectin-dependent. J Allergy Clin Immunol.
30. Poltorak A, He X, Smirnova I, Liu MY, Van Huffel C, et al. (1998) Defective LPS signaling in C3H/HeJ and C57BL/10 ScCr mice: mutations in Tlr4 gene. Science 282: 2085–2088.
31. Sweeney TE, Suliman HB, Hollingsworth JW, Piantadosi CA (2010) Differential regulation of the PGC family of genes in a mouse model of Staphylococcus aureus sepsis. PLoS One 5: e11606.
32. Tsang LH, Cassat JE, Shaw LN, Beenken KE, Smeltzer MS (2008) Factors contributing to the biofilm-deficient phenotype of Staphylococcus aureus sarA mutants. PLoS One 3: e3361.
33. Tseng CW, Kyme P, Low J, Rocha MA, Alsabeh R, et al. (2009) Staphylococcus aureus Panton-Valentine leukocidin contributes to inflammation and muscle tissue injury. PLoS One 4: e6387.
34. Bunce C, Wheeler L, Reed G, Musser J, Barg N (1992) Murine model of cutaneous infection with gram-positive cocci. Infect Immun 60: 2636–2640.
35. Itou T, Collins LV, Thoren FB, Dahlgren C, Karlsson A (2006) Changes in activation states of murine polymorphonuclear leukocytes (PMN) during inflammation: a comparison of bone marrow and peritoneal exudate PMN. Clin Vaccine Immunol 13: 575–583.
36. Kim SY, Nguyen AD, Gao JL, Murphy PM, Mansfield BC, et al. (2006) Bone marrow-derived cells require a functional glucose 6-phosphate transporter for normal myeloid functions. J Biol Chem 281: 28794–28801.
37. Rittie L, Fisher GJ (2005) Isolation and culture of skin fibroblasts. Methods Mol Med 117: 83–98.
38. Fuchs TA, Brill A, Duerschmied D, Schatzberg D, Monestier M, et al. (2010) Extracellular DNA traps promote thrombosis. Proc Natl Acad Sci U S A 107: 15880–15885.

2

Differential Effects of *Bartonella henselae* on Human and Feline Macro- and Micro-Vascular Endothelial Cells

Moez Berrich[1], Claudine Kieda[2], Catherine Grillon[2], Martine Monteil[1], Nathalie Lamerant[2], Julie Gavard[3], Henri Jean Boulouis[1]*, Nadia Haddad[1]

1 Unité Mixte de Recherche de Biologie Moléculaire et Immunologie Parasitaires et Fongiques, Ecole Nationale Vétérinaire d'Alfort, Université Paris-Est, Maisons-Alfort, France, **2** Unité Propre de Recherche 4301, Centre de Biophysique Moléculaire, Centre National de la Recherche Scientifique, Orléans, France, **3** Unité 1016 Inserm, Institut Cochin, CNRS, Université Paris Descartes, Paris, France

Abstract

Bartonella henselae, a zoonotic agent, induces tumors of endothelial cells (ECs), namely bacillary angiomatosis and peliosis in immunosuppressed humans but not in cats. *In vitro* studies on ECs represent to date the only way to explore the interactions between *Bartonella henselae* and vascular endothelium. However, no comparative study of the interactions between *Bartonella henselae* and human (incidental host) ECs *vs* feline (reservoir host) ECs has been carried out because of the absence of any available feline endothelial cell lines.

To this purpose, we have developed nine feline EC lines which allowed comparing the effects of *Bartonella* strains on human and feline micro-vascular ECs representative of the infection development sites such as skin, *versus* macro-vascular ECs, such as umbilical vein.

Our model revealed intrinsic differences between human (Human Skin Microvascular ECs –HSkMEC and Human Umbilical Vein ECs – iHUVEC) and feline ECs susceptibility to *Bartonella henselae* infection.
While no effect was observed on the feline ECs upon *Bartonella henselae* infection, the human ones displayed accelerated angiogenesis and wound healing.

Noticeable differences were demonstrated between human micro- and macro-vasculature derived ECs both in terms of pseudo-tube formation and healing. Interestingly, *Bartonella henselae* effects on human ECs were also elicited by soluble factors.

Neither *Bartonella henselae*-infected Human Skin Microvascular ECs clinically involved in bacillary angiomatosis, nor feline ECs increased cAMP production, as opposed to HUVEC.

Bartonella henselae could stimulate the activation of Vascular Endothelial Growth Factor Receptor-2 (VEGFR-2) in homologous cellular systems and trigger VEGF production by HSkMECs only, but not iHUVEC or any feline ECs tested.

These results may explain the decreased pathogenic potential of *Bartonella henselae* infection for cats as compared to humans and strongly suggest that an autocrine secretion of VEGF by human skin endothelial cells might induce their growth and ultimately lead to bacillary angiomatosis formation.

Editor: Holger Bruggemann, Max Planck Institute for Infection Biology, Germany

Funding: The authors gratefully acknowledge financial support from the CNRS, the Conseil Régional du Centre, the Canceropole GO, the Ligue Contre le Cancer (call Ile-de-France) and the Direction Générale de l'Enseignement et de la Recherche (Ministère de l'Agriculture, de l'Alimentation, de la Pêche et des Affaires rurales). The funders had no role in study design, data collection and analysis, decision to publish, or preparation of the manuscript.

Competing Interests: The authors have declared that no competing interests exist.

* E-mail: hjboulouis@vet-alfort.fr

Introduction

Since its discovery in 1992 [1], *Bartonella henselae* (*B. henselae*) is considered as the main agent of cat scratch disease (CSD) in humans and is also responsible for a growing number of diseases in patients [2]. This facultative intracellular bacterium is now known to be responsible for more serious diseases in both immunocompetent patients,*e.g.* endocarditis, and immunosuppressed patients, such as bacillary angiomatosis and peliosis [3], characterized by pseudotumoral proliferation of endothelial cells (ECs). These unusual vascular lesions occur mainly or exclusively in the skin, liver and spleen [3]. Cats are the main reservoir of this zoonotic bacterium [4]. However, as compared to humans, normal or immunosuppressed cats display high rates of sub-clinical infections and remain usually healthy, with only chronic bacteraemia [4,5,6]. In addition, in cats, *B. henselae* infection has not yet been associated with bacillary angiomatosis or peliosis [7,8].

Two genotypes (I and II) of *B. henselae* have been described on the basis of 16S rRNA sequence analysis [9]. Epidemiological studies strongly suggest that genotype I is more virulent in humans than genotype II [9,10,11,12,13]. In particular, only genotype I has been found associated to date to bacillary angiomatosis and peliosis [14], but this observation has to be confirmed by further studies.

The presence of *B. henselae* micro-colonies adjacent to proliferating endothelial cells has been histologically demonstrated, and suggested that *Bartonella*/ECs interactions might trigger a proangiogenic process, potentially leading to vascular lesions [15]. Due to the lack of any appropriate animal model, cultured ECs provide tools to study the interactions between *B. henselae* and the vascular endothelium.

These approaches have been useful for identifying *B. henselae* virulence factors. *B. henselae* adhesin A (BadA) (originally described as "pilus") [16] is important for pathogenicity [17], being involved in the adhesion to extracellular-matrix proteins and to ECs. It activates hypoxia-inducible factor-1 and pro-angiogenic cytokines secretion [18]. Recently, the VirB/VirD4 type IV secretion system and subsets of its translocated *B. henselae* effector proteins (BepA and BepG) were found to modulate the angiogenic activity of *B. henselae* [19,20]. Other studies have suggested that the process through which *B. henselae* triggers ECs proliferation involved released or secreted bacterial factors [21,22,23,24].

Host factors have also been found *in vitro* to play a role in *B. henselae* driven angiogenesis. VEGF (Vascular Endothelial Growth Factor) is known as the main angiogenic factor, which positively regulates migration, proliferation and survival of endothelial cells and has been shown to be over-secreted in the tumor micro-environment [25]. According to McCord et *al* [26], ECs infected by *B. henselae* Houston I may upregulate expression and production of pro-angiogenic proteins. Studies of VEGF expression in clinical samples [27] or *in vitro* [22,27,28], suggest a paracrine loop type of VEGF activity. Moreover, the anti-apoptotic activity of *B. henselae* BepA, in human umbilical vein endothelial cells (HUVEC), correlates with an important elevation of intracellular adenosine 3′, 5′-cyclic monophosphate (cAMP) level [29]. A more recent study demonstrated that *B. henselae* infection involves the intrinsic apoptotic pathway [30].

ECs are morphologically and functionally heterogeneous with major differences between those from the macro- *versus* micro-circulation as documented for a variety of tissues [31,32,33]. Except rare cases where ECs of the microvasculature have been included in *Bartonella* infection *in vitro* experiments [26,28,30,34], studies are mostly based on the use of primary HUVEC or other macrovasculature-derived cells like the hybrid EA.Hy.926. These cells originate from a large vessel of the placenta and are very different from microvasculature-derived ECs [31,32,33,35] clinically involved in bacillary angiomatosis and peliosis.

In addition, primary ECs will not allow providing repeatable and reproducible data, as these cultures lead to highly activated cells, in limited amounts and for a short term. Cell lines, established in a controlled identical manner, represent the best alternative to overcome these problems.

No comparative studies on the interactions between *B. henselae* and human (incidental host) ECs *versus* feline (reservoir host) ECs have ever been undertaken, because of the absence of any available feline ECs. Hence, feline ECs lines were developed and the *in vitro* effects of infection by distinct *Bartonella* species/strains (*B. henselae* genotype I/II and *B. tribocorum*) on human *versus* feline ECs derived from the macro- and micro-vasculature were compared. By studying various parameters as *in vitro* angiogenesis, stimulation of wound-healing, induction of cAMP, production of VEGF and activation of VEGF Receptor-2 (VEGFR-2), we demonstrated the crucial significance of the tissue origin of ECs and the specificity of the relationship between various strains of *B. henselae* with human *versus* feline cell lines. Our work contributes to the understanding of the differential outcomes of *B. henselae* infection in humans *versus* cats.

Materials and Methods

Human endothelial cell lines

Two immortalized lines of human organospecific ECs previously developed [31] were used in this study: one isolated from macrovasculature (immortalized Human Umbilical Vein Endothelial Cells: iHUVEC) and one isolated from the skin microvasculature (Human Skin Microvascular Endothelial Cells: HSkMEC) [36].

Feline endothelial cell lines

Establishment. Four immature and not viable embryos were aseptically removed at the School of Veterinary Medicine, Alfort, France, in the reproductive diseases service by therapeutic caesarean from queen after 45 days of gestation, and organs or tissues biopsies were taken from each embryo. Tissues and organs were placed in RPMI medium (Gibco, BRL, Cergy Pontoise France) without fetal bovine serum (FBS), supplemented by antibiotics and stored at 4°C.

Isolation of macrovascular (from umbilical vein FOmEC) or microvascular (from Skin FSkMEC, Peripheral Lymph Node FPLNMEC, Lung FLuMEC, Brain FBrMEC, Liver FLiMEC, Peyer's patches FPPMEC, Intestine FIntMEC, Heart FHeMEC) ECs was performed [31,37,38]. Immortalization was realized as already described for human endothelial cells [31]. Lines were characterized, patented (CNRS-ENVA, French patent N° 10/00094) and deposited at the Collection Nationale de Cultures de Microorganismes (Institut Pasteur, Paris, France).

The feline ECs lines were cultured in OptiMEM medium (Gibco BRL,Cergy Pontoise, France) +2% of FBS+0.2% of fungizone+0.4% of gentamicin (Gibco BRL) and were maintained in a humidified atmosphere containing 5% carbon dioxide (CO_2) at 37°C.

Characterization

a- Intracellular von Willebrand factor (vWF) and Angiotensin -Converting Enzyme (ACE) detection. Established cell lines were grown on twelve-well microscope slides (ICN Bio-medicals, Aurora, OH, USA) for 48 h. Monolayers were fixed for 10 min with paraformaldehyde (PFA, 2%) and permeabilized, for 30 min at 37°C, with Triton X100 (0,05%) (Sigma, France).

For intracellular vWF detection, a rabbit polyclonal anti-human vWF antibody (A0082-Dako) (20 µg/ml), was applied to the cells for 2 h at RT and washed twice with c-PBS containing 1% bovine serum albumin (c-PBS-BSA). The second antibody was a goat Fluorescein IsoThioCyanate (FITC)-anti-rabbit immunoglobulin antibody (20 µg/ml) (SBE, CliniSciences, Montrouge, France), and cells were further incubated for overnight at 4°C.

For ACE detection, polyclonal rabbit anti-human ACE antibody (sc 20791- Santa Cruz Biotechnology) and, further, a secondary goat Fluorescein IsoThioCyanate (FITC)-anti-rabbit immunoglobulin antibody (SBE, CliniSciences, Montrouge, France) was used. Cells were examined by fluorescence microscopy (Leica DMI 4000 B).

b- Angiogenesis assays. A 96-well plate (Falcon, BD Biosciences, Grenoble, France) was coated with Matrigel^{TM} (BD Biosciences) mimicking the extracellular matrix (40 µl by well). The Matrigel^{TM} was allowed to polymerize for 1 h at 37°C before cell seeding (8×10^3 cells/well). ECs rearrangements and capillary-like structure formation were observed each hour until the 24th hour and then every day until the 7th day. It was photographed regularly under a microscope (Nikon TMS, Japan)

Monkey kidney epithelial cells (Vero line, ATCC, CCL-81) were used as a non endothelial cell control.

Bacterial strains

Four strains of *B. henselae* were used, based on their species origin (human or feline) and genotype (I or II). The two strains isolated from human patients were the reference strain Houston-1 (genotype I (H1) / ATCC 49882) [1] and the genotype II Marseille strain (H2) kindly supplied by Jean Marc Rolain (Unité des rickettsies, Marseille, France). The two strains isolated from cats were a genotype I strain (F1/ Strain 297172) kindly supplied by Bruno Chomel (University of California, Davis, USA) and a genotype II *B. henselae* strain initially isolated in our laboratory (F2). *B. tribocorum* (Bt) (CIP 105476 T), isolated from rat and without known pathogenicity for human and cats was also used.

All *Bartonella* strains were cultured on sheep blood agar medium (BioMerieux, Craponne, France) for 5 to 7 days in humidified atmosphere at 35°C and 5% CO_2.

To investigate the specificity of *Bartonella*-triggered angiogenesis, we used *Escherichia coli* (*DH5α*) (Invitrogen, France) as a negative control. This bacterium was grown at 37°C on Luria-Bertani (LB) agar or in LB broth (Sigma, France). Heat-inactivated *B. henselae* were used in order to check if dead bacteria were still able to stimulate ECs angiogenesis. The inactivation of heat-treated bacteria (56°C, 30 min) was checked on sheep blood agar medium.

Generation of *Bartonella* culture supernatants

B. henselae strains and *B. tribocorum* were harvested from blood agar plates and suspended in Schneider medium 1x (Gibco, France). The bacterial cultures were gently shaken in Schneider medium for 18 h at 200 rpm and 37°C on an orbital shaker (Innova 4230, New Brunswick Scientific, Edison, NJ, USA). After 18 h of incubation, the suspensions were removed from the flasks and spun at 1000 g and 4°C for 10 minutes to form a soft pellet. The supernatants were removed and passed through a 0.22 μm filter to remove all bacteria. The bacteria-free supernatants were dialyzed with OptiMEM and concentrated in a Centrifugal filter (Amicon ® Ultra-15 Millipore, France). Culture supernatant control medium was also generated through similar methods. Protein concentrations were determined by bicinchoninic acid assay (BC Assay Kit, Uptima, Interchim, France).

In vitro induction of angiogenesis

Twenty-four hours before infection of ECs (iHUVEC - immortalized Human Umbilical Vein Endothelial Cells-, HSkMEC -Human Skin Microvascular Endothelial Cells-, FOmEC-Feline Umbilical vein Macrovascular Endothelial Cells and FSkMEC-Feline Skin Microvascular Endothelial Cells), antibiotics were removed from the culture medium. ECs (8×10^3 cells/well) were infected with *Bartonella* at a multiplicity of infection (M.O.I.) of 50, 100 and 150 bacteria per cell or treated with bacteria culture supernatant (protein concentration: 250 μg/ml) and then were seeded on 96 well plates previously coated with Matrigel™ (BD Biosciences, Grenoble, France). Videos for ECs rearrangement and capillary-like structure formation were acquired and registered for image analysis (Zeiss axiovision program). The Zeiss axiovert 200 M, videomicroscope equipped for temperature, gas and humidity controls was used to acquire images in time lapse conditions and reconstitute the kinetics of the angiogenesis dynamic process. The pseudo-vessel formation was monitored continuously during the first 24 hours and then observed every day during the following 7 days.

Capillary-like structure formation was quantified by measuring the length of tubes and counting the branching points [39].

Healing test

iHUVEC, HSkMEC, FOmEC and FSkMEC were seeded in 24-well plates at a density of 10^5 cells/well and allowed to attach overnight in OptiMEM medium without antibiotics. When cells came to confluence, a wound was made in the center of the well using the extremity of a sterile pipette tip. Then, ECs were infected with bacteria (100 M.O.I.) for 24 h. The healing was observed and photographed under a Nikon TMS microscope. Healing distances (in μm) were measured at time 0 and 24 h after the wound.

Determination of intracellular cAMP level

After infection of ECs (iHUVEC, HSkMEC, FOmEC and FSkMEC) by *Bartonella* strains with 150 M.O.I.for 30 h in 24 well plates, cells were washed with PBS and lysed. Intracellular cAMP levels were determined by the EIA system (Biotrak, Amersham, Biosciences, France) as described by the manufacturer.

Measurement of VEGF levels in conditioned medium (ELISA)

VEGF concentration in culture medium was measured using a commercially available human VEGF ELISA Kit (R&D Systems, Minneapolis, MN, USA) according to the manufacturer's instructions. Briefly, cells were plated at a density of 5×10^4 cells/0,5 ml/well in a 24 well plate and 12 h later cells were infected with *Bartonella* at a M.O.I. of 100. Conditioned medium was collected 72 h after infection, cellular debris and extracellular bacteria removed by centrifugation, and the medium was kept at −80°C until VEGF quantitation was undertaken. Cell number was determined immediately after medium recovery.

Western blot analysis of VEGF-R2

24 h after infection (M.O.I.of 100), iHUVEC, HSkMEC, FOmEC and FSkMEC were lysed in TNT lysis buffer (10 mM Tris-HCL pH 7.5; 150 mM NaCL; 1% Nonidet P-40; 1% Triton X100 and 2 mM EDTA) supplemented with protease and phosphatase inhibitors (10 μg/ml leupeptin and apropotin; 1 mM phenylmethylsulfonyl fluoride; 25 mM NaF and 300 μM vanadate) for 15 min at 4°C. Equal amounts of samples were subjected to SDS-polyacrylamide gel electrophoresis and transferred onto a polyvinylidene difluoride membrane. Membranes were incubated with either anti-VEGFR-2 or anti-phosphorylated Y1175 VEGFR-2 (Cell signaling, Ozyme, Saint-Quentin-en-Yvelines, France). Daylight680 fluorescent dye-conjugated secondary antibody was used for revelation and membranes were scanned using the Odyssey Infra-Red Imaging System (Li-Cor BioSciences, EuroSep, Cergy-Pontoise, France).

Statistical analysis

All experiments were performed at least three times (except VEGF production: twice) and gave comparable results. Differences between mean values of experimental and control groups were analyzed by Student's t-test. *P*-values less than 0.05 were considered to be statistically significant. The data were expressed as mean ± standard deviation (SD).

Results

Establishment of new feline endothelial cell lines

In order to compare the feline ECs with their human counterparts (i.e HSkMEC – Human Skin Microvascular EC - and iHUVEC – immortalized Human Umbilical Vein EC -), two feline cell lines (FSkMEC - Feline Skin Microvascular EC - and FOmEC- Feline Umbilical Macrovascular EC -) were selected among the nine established feline ECs lines which have been characterized for EC markers as vWf and ACE (data not shown).

Moreover, because ECs can retain *in vitro* their ability to undergo angiogenesis, feline ECs lines were tested for their potentiality to form capillary-like structures in the classical Matrigel™ assay. All feline ECs were capable of performing

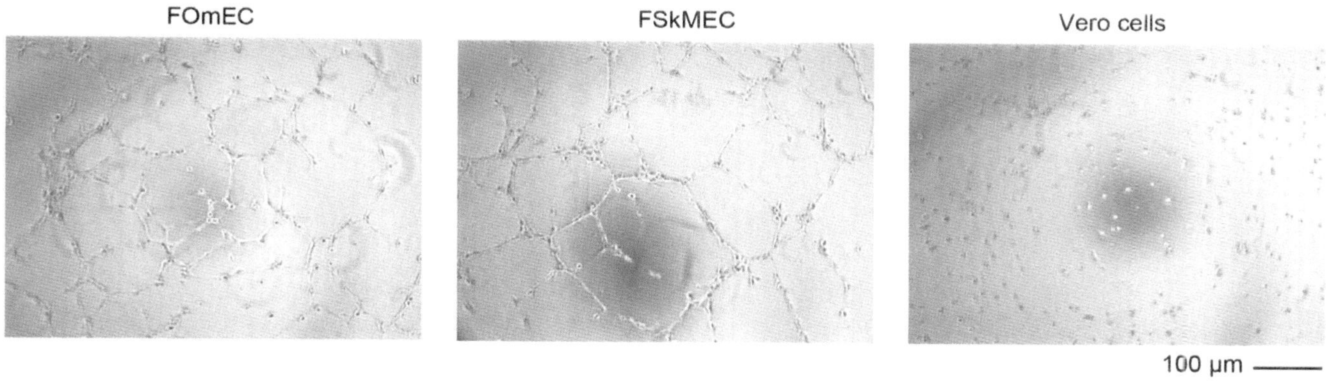

Figure 1. *In vitro* angiogenesis of feline ECs 10 h after seeding on Matrigel™. Feline ECs are able to form pseudovessels. FOmEC: Feline Umbilical Vein Endothelial Cells; FSkMEC: Feline Skin Microvascular Endothelial Cells. Vero cells: Monkey kidney epithelial cells used as non-endothelial control cells. Original magnification: 50x.

angiogenesis on Matrigel™. Figure 1 shows angiogenesis observed with FSkMEC and FOmEC.

Angiogenic response of ECs to *Bartonella* infection

Capillary-like structures of uninfected feline ECs (Fig. 1) began to form within two hours after seeding on Matrigel™ as compared to uninfected human ECs, while occurring within approximately five hours for macrovasculature derived ECs (iHUVEC) and within 10 hours for microvasculature ECs (HSkMEC) (table 1). The network of pseudo-vessels persisted in human ECs, until 24 hours for macro-vasculature derived ECs and until 7 days for microvascular ECs. Of note this network disappeared only after 20 hours with feline ECs (table 1).

In parallel, we monitored the effects of *Bartonella* (*B. henselae* genotype I/II and *B. tribocorum*) infection on the four cell lines. Irrespective of the species of origin and genotypes of *Bartonella*, infected HSkMEC efficiently achieved angiogenesis in terms of tube formation, extended projections morphology, branching points and number of cells as compared to uninfected cells (Fig. 2 A). The influence of *Bartonella* infection on the formation of the capillary-like network by HSkMEC was dose-dependent (data not shown). Infection accelerated angiogenesis by few hours in Human Skin Microvascular cells (table 1).

Importantly, kinetics of angiogenesis of the FSkMEC was not changed upon *Bartonella* infection whatever strain used (Fig. 2B, Fig. 3B and table 1). Angiogenesis of FSkMEC and FOmEC started 2 h after seeding on Matrigel™. The destruction of the network was slightly faster in the infected feline cell lines (18 hours) as compared to uninfected cells (20 hours) (table 1). No effect was observed upon infection on the structure of the newly formed vessels (Fig. 2B and Fig. 3B). Importantly, as a negative control, no pro-angiogenic effect was observed, both on human and feline ECs with *E. coli* or with heat-inactivated *B. henselae* (data not shown).

The observed effects were quantified. As shown on Fig. 3A, *Bartonella*-infection increased capillary-like formation by HSkMEC by a factor 1.8 to 2.6 as compared to uninfected ECs ($p<0.05$) and the number of branching points by a factor of 1.78 to 3 ($p<0.05$) (Fig. 3 A). This network was observed until 7 days with these cells, and then disappeared (table 1).

Capillary-like formation was increased in iHUVEC by a 2 fold upon infection such as in HSkMEC. However, as opposed to HSkMEC, *B. henselae* infection did not speed this effect (table 1). The network was observed only until 24 hours, before resorbing (table 1).

Thus, the effect of *Bartonella*-induced angiogenesis was more potent in human ECs than feline ECs (where infection even accelerated network destruction). Moreover, capillary-like structures were markedly more durable in micro- *versus* macro-vasculature ECs.

Table 1. Effect of *Bartonella* on ECs angiogenesis kinetics.

		Feline EC		Human EC	
		unifected	**infected**	**uninfected**	**infected**
Beginning of angiogenesis	Macrovascular	2 h	2 h	5 h	5 h
	Microvascular	2 h	2 h	10 h	8 h
End of angiogenesis	Macrovascular	20 h	18 h	24 h	24 h
	Microvascular	20 h	18 h	7days	7 days

Acceleration of the pseudovessel rearrangement induced by infection with *B. henselae* strains or their supernatants was observed only with human microvasculature-derived ECs (HSkMEC). In feline cells, bacterial infection accelerates the network destruction. Noticeably, uninfected human ECs from micro- and macro-vasculature display differences in the angiogenesis kinetics.
Similar results were obtained when ECs were treated by corresponding *B. henselae* supernatants.
Results from one out of four independent experiments are shown.
Human Macrovascular EC: immortalized Human Umbilical Vein Endothelial Cells (iHUVEC); Human Microvascular EC: Human Skin Microvascular Endothelial Cells (HSkMEC); Feline Macrovascular EC: Feline Umbilical Vein Endothelial Cells (FOmEC); Feline Microvascular EC: Feline Skin Microvascular Endothelial Cells (FSkMEC).

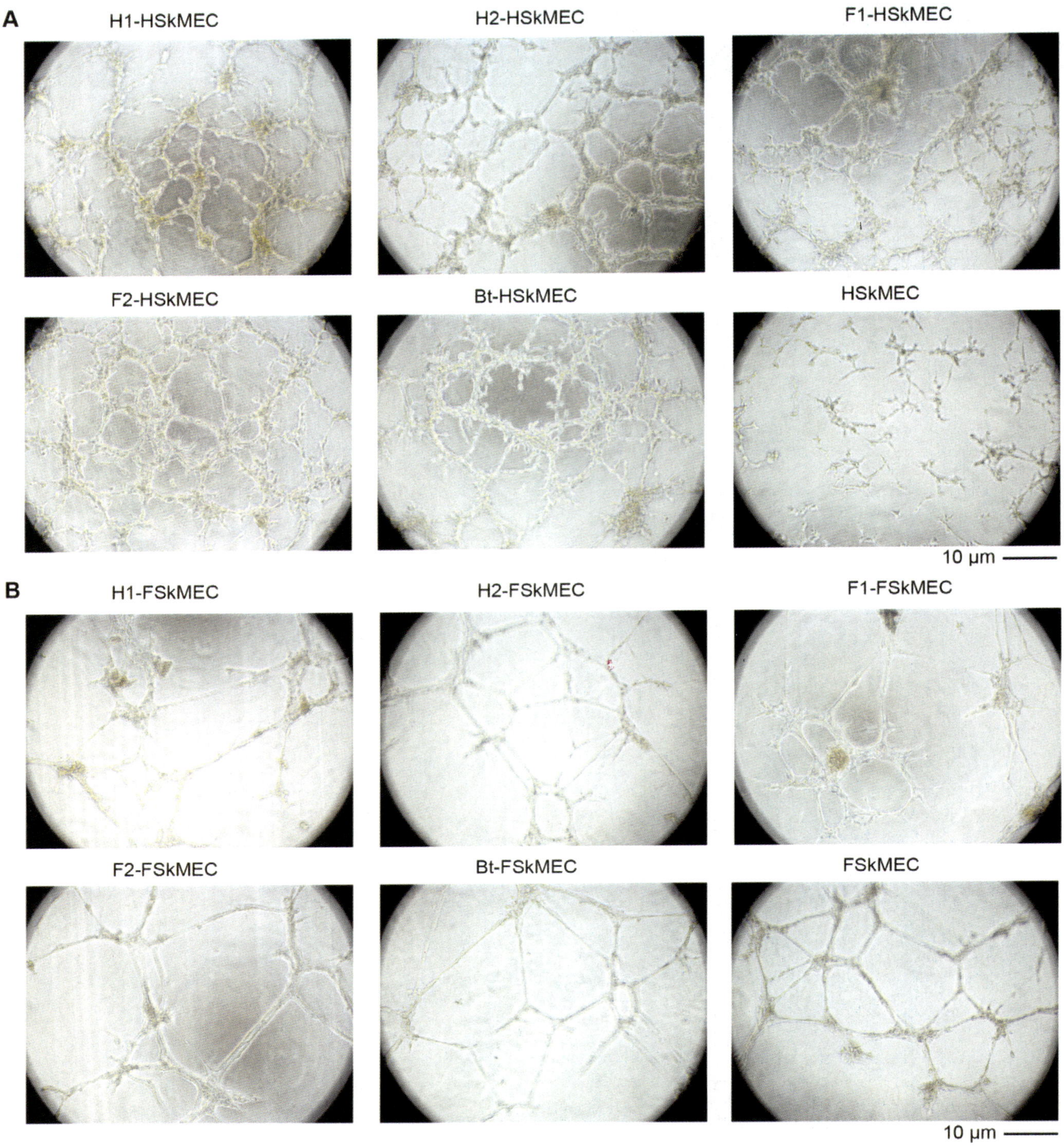

Figure 2. Effect of various *Bartonella* strains on human and feline ECs capillary-like structure formation on Matrigel^{TM}. HSkMEC (Human Skin Microvascular Endothelial Cells) infection by *B. henselae* (multiplicity of infection: 100 bacteria/cell) increases capillary-like structure formation as compared to uninfected cells (A). In contrast, *B. henselae* infection has no visible effect on FSkMEC (Feline Skin Microvascular Endothelial Cells) (B). Pictures have been taken 10 h and 20 h after seeding of FSkMEC and HSkMEC, respectively. Original magnification: 50x. H1: *B. henselae* human type I strain (reference strain Houston-1 ATCC 49882); H2: *B.henselae* human type II strain (Marseille); F1: *B. henselae* feline type I strain (F1 297172); F2: *B. henselae* feline type II strain; Bt: *B. tribocorum*.

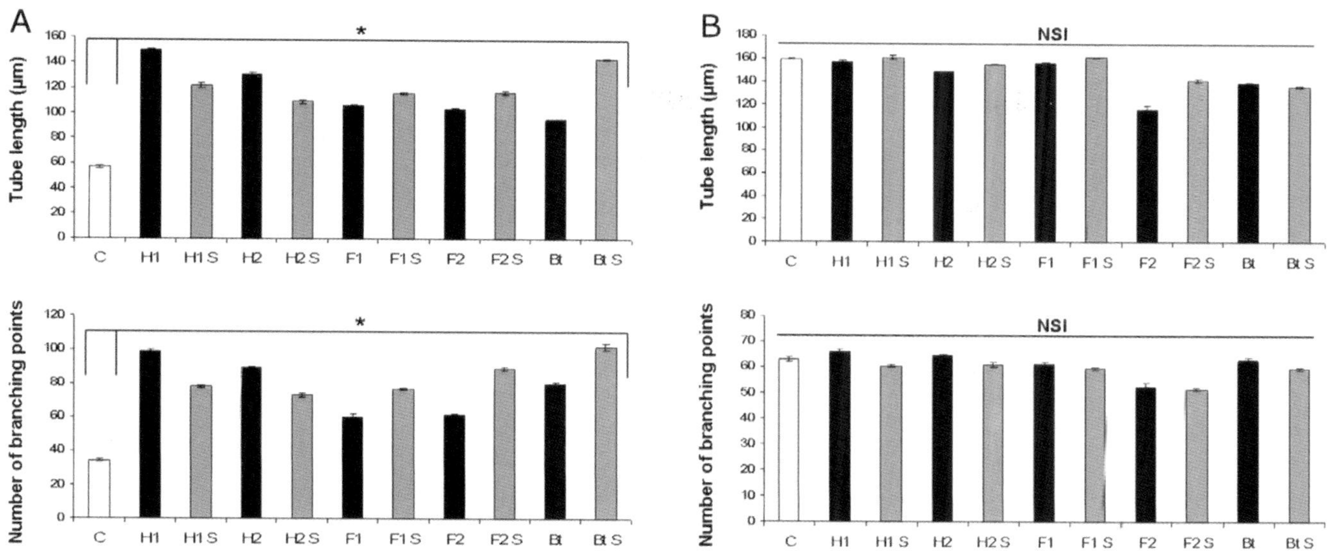

Figure 3. Quantitative analysis of capillary-like structure formation by cell projection length and branching point number determination. Human Skin Microvascular ECs (HSkMEC) infection by *B. henselae* strains (M.O.I.of 100, black bars) or treatment by their culture supernatants (250 µg/ml, grey bars) increases angiogenesis assessed by cell projection length and branching point number when compared to uninfected cells (white bars) (measures performed 20 hours p.i.) (A). In contrast, Feline Skin Microvascular ECs (FSkMEC) infection by *B. henselae* or treatment by their culture supernatants has no such effect (measures performed 10 hours p.i.) (B). Data from four independent experiments are shown as mean ± standard deviation (*$p<0.05$ *versus* uninfected or untreated controls). NSI: No Significant Increase. C: uninfected or untreated controls cell; S: *Bartonella* culture supernatant; H1: *B. henselae* human type I strain (reference strain Houston-1 ATCC 49882); H2: *B. henselae* human type II strain (Marseille); F1: *B. henselae* feline type I strain (F1 297172); F2: *B. henselae* feline type II strain; Bt: *B. tribocorum*.

Angiogenic response of ECs to *Bartonella* culture supernatants

In order to investigate the effects of *Bartonella* secretome, different *Bartonella* culture supernatants were generated and tested for their ability to induce angiogenesis in human and feline ECs. *Bartonella* culture supernatants did induce tube formation in human ECs. The pro-angiogenic responses obtained with *Bartonella* culture supernatants were accelerated by a factor 1.9 to 2.5 ($p<0.05$), as in *Bartonella*-infected human ECs (Fig. 3A). The resulting effect of *Bartonella* or their culture supernatants on the morphology of human ECs was similar, *i.e.* ECs appeared elongated with long membrane projections (data not shown).

In the system of feline endothelial cells, *Bartonella* culture supernatants, as bacteria themselves, did not influence angiogenesis (Fig. 2B and Fig. 3B).

Wound-induced migration of human ECs by *Bartonella* infection

As ECs migration is an essential step for angiogenesis, the significance of the site of infection in term of endothelium susceptibility was examined. The endothelial cell reaction according to their tissue origin was followed upon *Bartonella* infection by measuring their migration speed to heal a mechanical wound (Fig. 4A and 4B). In uninfected cells (at 24 h), wound-healing was at least twice faster in iHUVEC than in HSkMEC (4.5±0.7 and 1.25±0.35 µm within 24 h, respectively with $p=0.015$) (Fig. 4C). Infection speeded the wound-healing for both iHUVEC and HSkMEC. Remarkably, in iHUVEC, healing speed was approximately doubled, whereas in HSkMEC, it was increased by a factor of 4.3 up to 7.8 ($p<0.05$) (Fig. 4).

In feline ECs (FOmEC and FSkMEC) wound-induced migration was recorded and no stimulation by *Bartonella* infection was observed (Fig. 4A and Fig. 4C).

Effect of *Bartonella* infection on human and feline ECs on cAMP production

It was shown in the HUVEC model that *B. henselae* genotype I (reference strain Houston-1) triggered the production of cAMP [29]. As, according to these authors, anti apoptosis was mediated through increased cAMP levels, this induction was assessed in ECs upon infection by distinct *Bartonella* strains. In uninfected ECs of the macro- or the micro-vasculature, the levels of cAMP produced by the feline ECs (FOmEC [12.06±7.13 fmol] and FSkMEC [19.38±4.11 fmol]) were significantly weaker than in human ECs (iHUVEC [203.57±57.66 fmol] and HSkMEC [32.68±1.80 fmol]) ($p<0.05$) (Fig. 5). Moreover, cAMP production by human ECs of the macrovasculature (iHUVEC) was higher than microvasculature-derived ECs (HSkMEC) by a factor of 6.2 (203.57±57.66 *vs* 32.68±1.80 fmol respectively with $p=0.0004$). In feline ECs, the low levels of production did not allow to detect any significant difference between ECs of the macro- and the micro-vasculatures (Fig. 5).

Upon infection, cAMP increased only in human macrovasculature ECs (iHUVEC) infected by strain H1 by a factor of 2.2 (reaching 405.16±6.72 fmol) ($p<0.05$). Strains F1, F2 and Bt did not induce any change. Human Skin Microvasculature ECs were not affected by any of the strains.

Feline ECs from micro- or macro-vasculature ECs did not react to the bacterial infection (Fig. 5).

Bartonella increases VEGF production in human microvascular ECs

The involvement of VEGF in *B. henselae* effect on angiogenesis was investigated. We took into account: a) the origin of the bacterial strains (human *versus* feline); b) the bacterial genotype (I *versus* II); c) the ECs species (human *versus* feline), and d) their type (macro *versus* micro vessels derived-ECs).

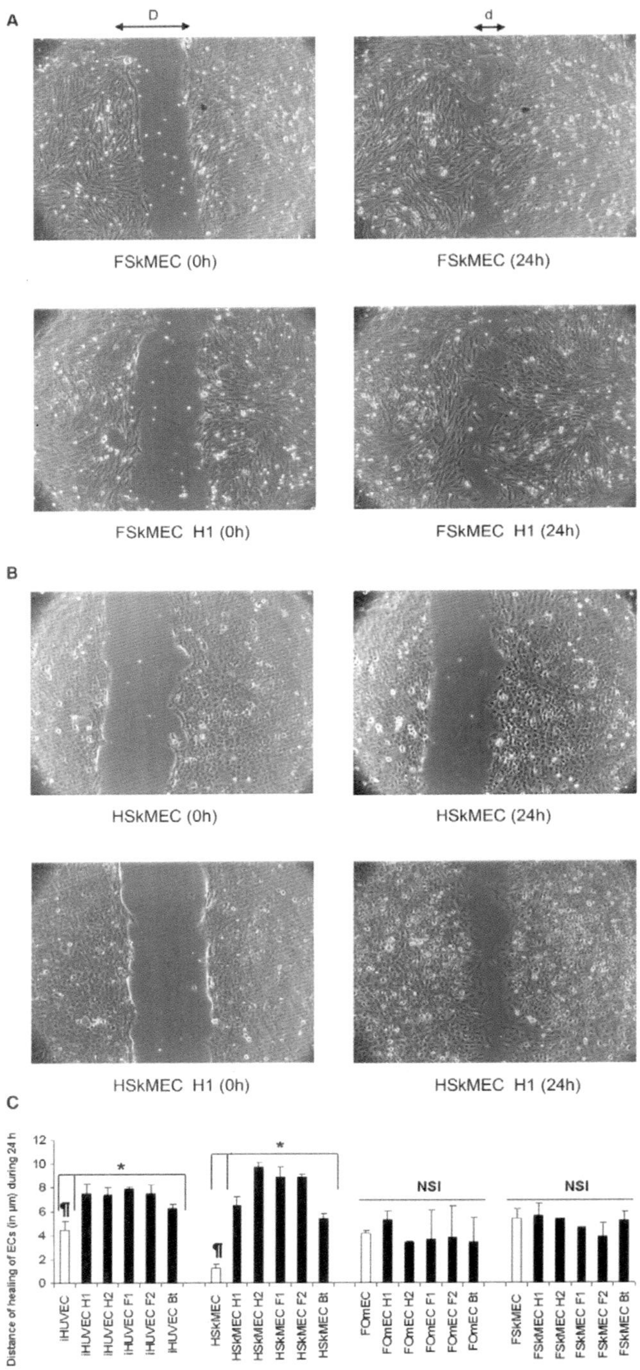

Figure 4. Effect of human and feline ECs *Bartonella* infection on cell migration assessed in wound healing assay. A: Healing test (FSkMEC and FSkMEC-H1) Healing distance = D − d. B: Healing test (HSkMEC and HSkMEC-H1) C: Quantification of the effect of *Bartonella* infection on wound healing *B. henselae* infection increased strongly human Skin Microvascular ECs (HSkMEC) migration, in a less extent human macrovascular ECs (iHUVEC) migration but did not affect feline ECs (FOmEC and FSkMEC). Results show mean ± standard deviation from three independent experiments. (iHUVEC *versus* HSkMEC controls: ¶p = .015; infected cells *versus* uninfected cells: *p<0.05). NSI: No Significant Increase. H1: *B. henselae* human type I strain (reference strain Houston-1 ATCC 49882); H2: *B. henselae* human type II strain (Marseille); F1: *B. henselae* feline type I strain (F1 297172); F2: *B. henselae* feline type II strain; Bt: *B. tribocorum*.

A differential production of VEGF was measured between non infected microvascular and macrovascular ECs both of human and feline origin as shown on Fig. 6. Human and feline microvascular ECs produced high levels of VEGF [717.88±32.50 and 1623.19±72.81 pg/ml respectively] as compared to human and feline macrovascular ECs [3.75±3.12 and 6.88±5.0 pg/ml respectively, p = 0.001] (Fig. 6).

An increase in VEGF production by *B. henselae* infection was induced only in human microvascular skin-derived cells (HSkMEC) (Fig. 6).

Interestingly, the four *B. henselae* strains significantly increased VEGF production by HSkMEC by a factor of 2.1 to 2.4 while *B. tribocorum* was less effective (factor of 1.3) ($p<0.05$). Feline microvascular cells production of VEGF was not significantly affected by the various strains.

Effects of *B. henselae* infection on VEGFR-2 activation

The level of activation of the VEGF receptor VEGFR-2 was estimated by monitoring VEGFR-2 phosphorylation in Western-blot. Figure 7 indicates that ECs (iHUVEC, HSkMEC, FOmEC and FSkMEC) infection by *Bartonella* was associated with an increased phosphorylation of VEGFR-2.

In addition, the level of the VEGFR-2 phosphorylated form was significantly higher by a 2 fold when ECs were infected by a strain originating from a homologous host (*i.e.* when human ECs were infected by *B. henselae* strains originating from humans and when feline ECs were infected by *B. henselae* strains originating from cats). In particular, VEGFR-2 phosphorylation induced in human ECs (HSkMEC and iHUVEC) by strain H1 was respectively 2.2 to 3.3 higher than that induced by F1. Conversely, VEGFR-2 phosphorylation induced in Feline ECs (FSkMEC and FOmEC) by H1 was lower than that induced by F1 respectively 0.95 to 0.6 (Fig. 7A and 7B). *B. tribocorum* induced a comparable activation of VEGFR-2, whatever the origin of cell lines (Fig. 7A).

Discussion

B. henselae is a facultative intracellular pathogen associated with the induction of vasoproliferative tumors in humans (bacillary angiomatosis and peliosis) that are not observed in cats (host reservoir) [4,6,7,8].

Our original cellular models allowed us to reveal intrinsic differences in the angiogenesis kinetics and the wound-healing process between human micro- and macro-vasculature-derived ECs. Importantly, our results strongly suggest that effects of *B. henselae* on microvasculature-derived cells strongly differ from macrovasculature ones.

In human cells, *Bartonella* infection affected the angiogenic process at two different levels: a) a slight acceleration of the pseudovessel rearrangement was observed, only with microvasculature-derived ECs (Table 1) and b) the number of pseudo-vessels was increased in both micro- and macro-vasculature-derived ECs (figure 3).

One key point of our findings concerns feline ECs from both micro- and macro-vasculatures. Indeed, not only *B. henselae* had no visible pro-angiogenic effect *in vitro*, but the infection seemed to accelerate the network destruction of the feline cells. These results might recapitulate the clinical situation, *i.e.* the absence of bacillary angiomatosis in cats (even in FIV and/or FeLV infected cats) *versus* bacillary angiomatosis in humans and even in dogs as recently described [40].

Hence, our cellular models are relevant to understand the cellular and molecular bases of the pro-angiogenic potential of *B.*

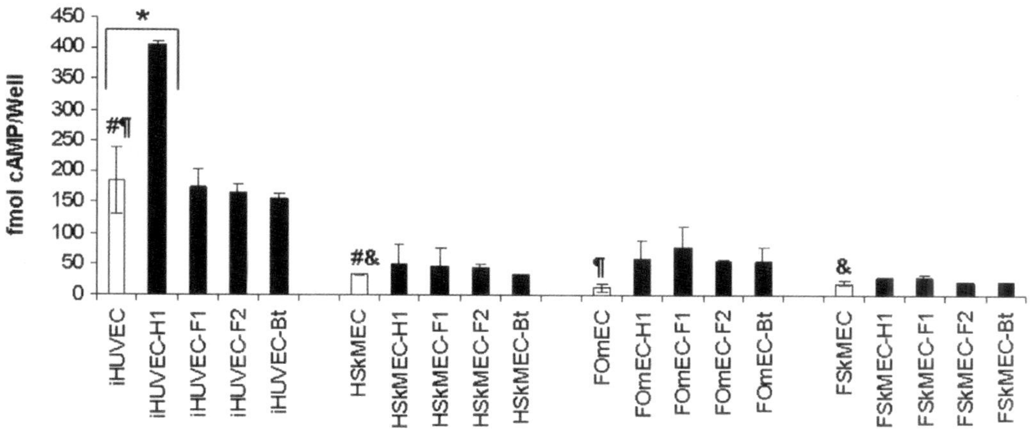

Figure 5. Effect of *B. henselae* infection on intracellular cAMP production in human and feline EC lines. *B. henselae* infection did not significantly increase cAMP production by ECs, except for iHUVEC infected by H1 strain. Results were monitored 30 h post infection with bacteria (M.O.I. of 150) and expressed in fmol/well as mean ± standard deviation (*$p<0.05$ for the differences between infected cells *versus* uninfected cells; #, ¶ and & $p<0.05$, for the differences between uninfected cells). H1: *B. henselae* human type I strain (reference strain Houston-1 ATCC 49882); F1: *B. henselae* feline type I strain (F1 297172); F2: *B. henselae* feline type II strain; Bt: *B. tribocorum*. iHUVEC: immortalized Human Umbilical Vein Endothelial Cells; HSkMEC: Human Skin Microvascular Endothelial Cells; FOmEC: Feline Umbilical Vein Endothelial Cells; FSkMEC: Feline Skin Microvascular Endothelial Cells.

henselae and to explore the mechanisms underlying bacillary angiomatosis/peliosis.

This model of infection shows that, independently of the bacterial species (*B. henselae vs B. tribocorum*), or of the *B. henselae* genotype (I or II), *Bartonella* tested here can induce *in vitro* angiogenesis. Interestingly, *B. tribocorum* has no known pro-angiogenic potential *in vivo*. Moreover we did not detect any obvious difference of activity between the different strains of *Bartonella* tested contrary to the work of Chang et *al*[30].

Furthermore, the stimulatory effect of *B. henselae* is not dependent upon attachment or penetration in the target cell suggesting that *B. henselae* may produce and secrete endothelial cell-stimulatory factor(s).

In addition, the inactivation of *B. henselae* by heat treatment abolished its vasoproliferative activity, suggesting that the angiogenic effect of *B. henselae* on ECs require live bacteria.

Previous studies dedicated to understand the interactions between primary HUVEC and *B. henselae* Houston 1 (genotype I) have suggested a correlation between the anti-apoptotic activity of *B. henselae* and an increased cAMP production [29]. Remarkably, in our study, the stimulation of cAMP production was observed only when *B. henselae* Houston 1 was inoculated to

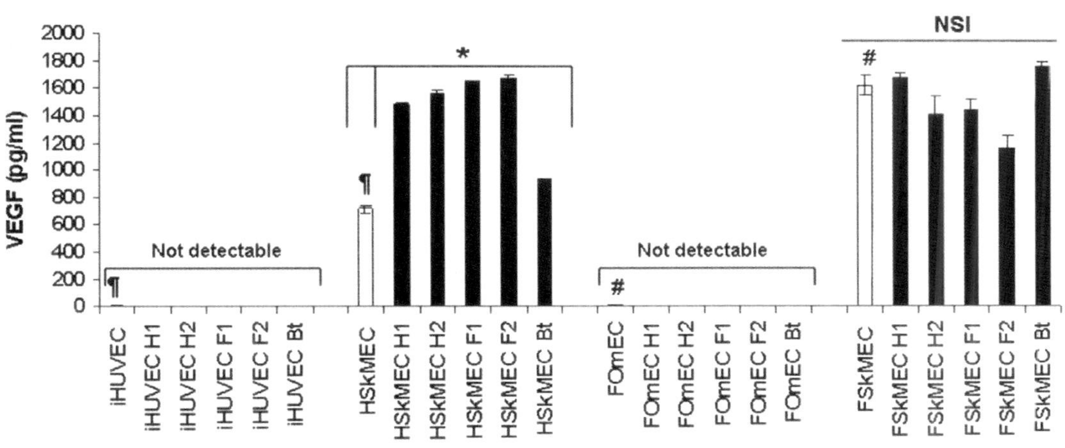

Figure 6. VEGF production in human and feline macro- and micro-vascular ECs upon infection with *Bartonella* strains. *B. henselae* triggers VEGF production in Human Skin Microvascular ECs (HSkMEC) but not in human macrovascular ECs (iHUVEC) or in feline macro- (FOmEC: Feline Umbilical vein Endothelial Cells) or micro- (FSkMEC: Feline Skin Microvascular Endothelial Cells) vascular ECs. In addition, a clear differential production of VEGF between micro- and macro-vascular ECs is shown both in human and in cat. VEGF level was determined by ELISA after 72 h of infection and data shown as mean ± standard deviation (*$p<0.05$ infected *versus* uninfected cells; ¶ and #$p<0.0015$ for the differences between uninfected cells). NSI: No Significant Increase. iHUVEC: immortalized Human Umbilical Vein Endothelial Cells; HSkMEC: Human Skin Microvascular Endothelial Cells; FOmEC: Feline Umbilical Vein Endothelial Cells; FSkMEC: Feline Skin Microvascular Endothelial Cells. H1: *B. henselae* human type I strain (reference strain Houston-1 ATCC 49882); H2: *B. henselae* human type II strain (Marseille); F1: *B. henselae* feline type I strain (F1 297172); F2: *B. henselae* feline type II strain; Bt: *B. tribocorum*.

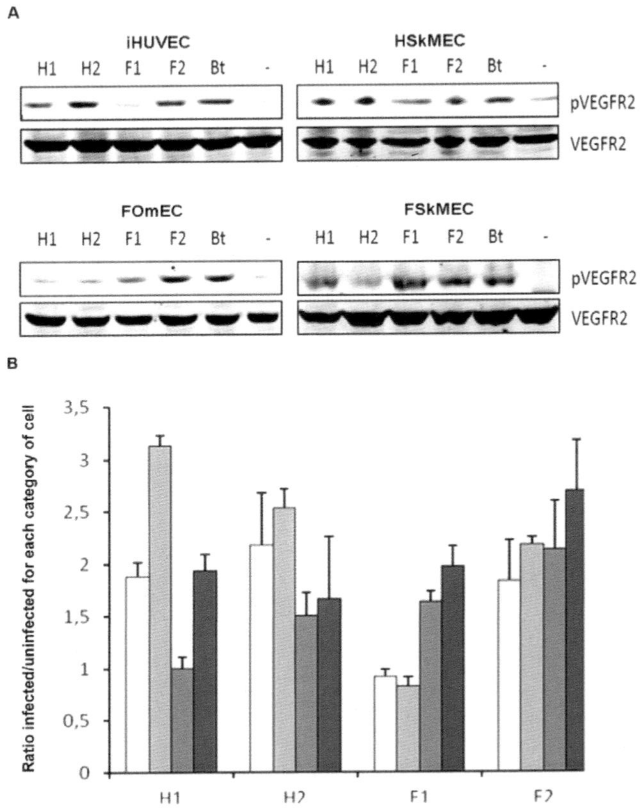

Figure 7. *B. henselae* -mediated VEGFR-2 activation on ECs. A: Homologous type of *B. henselae* -mediated VEGFR-2 activation on ECs. *B. henselae* strains from human origin (H1 and H2) mostly stimulated VEGFR-2 phosphorylation in human ECs (HUVEC an HSkMEC) and the strains from feline origin (F1 and F2) stimulated VEGFR-2 phosphorylation in feline ECs (FOmEC and FSkMEC). Western blot analysis of VEGFR-2 and phosphorylated VEGFR-2 (pVEGFR-2) following a 24 hours infection of ECs by *B. henselae* were shown as one representative experiment out of three. iHUVEC: immortalized Human Umbilical Vein Endothelial Cells; HSkMEC: Human Skin Microvascular Endothelial Cells; FOmEC: Feline Umbilical Vein Endothelial Cells; FSkMEC: Feline Skin Microvascular Endothelial Cells. H1: *B. henselae* human type I strain (reference strain Houston-1 ATCC 1 49882); H2: *B. henselae* human type II strain (Marseille); F1: *B. henselae* feline type I strain (F1 297172); F2: *B. henselae* feline type II strain; Bt: *B. tribocorum*; - : Uninfected cells. **B:** Quantitative analysis of *Bartonella*-mediated VEGFR-2 activation on ECs. *Bartonella* strains effect on VEGFR-2 activation expressed as levels increase over uninfected controls. ECs (iHUVEC, HSkMEC, FOmEC and FSkMEC) infection by *Bartonella* was associated with an increased phosphorylation of VEGFR-2. Serie 1 (White bar): iHUVEC: immortalized Human Umbilical Vein Endothelial Cells. Serie 2 (Light grey bar): HSkMEC: Human Skin Microvascular Endothelial Cells. Serie 3 (Dark grey bar): FOmEC: Feline Umbilical Vein Endothelial Cells. Serie 4 (Black bar): FSkMEC: Feline Skin Microvascular Endothelial Cells. H1: *B. henselae* human type I strain (reference strain Houston-1 ATCC 49882); H2: *B. henselae* human type II strain (Marseille); F1: *B. henselae* feline type I strain (F1 297172); F2: *B. henselae* feline type II strain.

iHUVEC. Such effect was never obtained when skin-derived EC - HSkMEC –, which are directly involved in bacillary angiomatosis, were used, even when they were infected by Houston 1. This points to the fact that macrovasculature-derived ECs (iHUVEC/HUVEC) deeply differ from microvasculature ECs [31,32,33,41,42]. Remarkably, in our study, cAMP production does not reflect ECs proliferation in the case of infected microvascular ECs. According to these results, microvascular skin endothelial cells- HSkMEC, clearly represent a better model for clinical bacillary angiomatosis.

Feline macro- and/or micro-vasculature ECs cAMP production was weak and not related to infection.

Such low level of cAMP production by human microvasculature ECs (HSkMEC) does not corroborate the pro-angiogenic effect of *B. henselae* interaction with human ECs. Nishihara et *al* [43], have shown that the effects of cAMP are highly cell type-specific. cAMP either promotes or antagonizes apoptosis in a cell type, environment- and stimulus- related manner. These, together with our results, illustrate that the model based on HUVEC which is not the clinical cell target, does not allow any definitive conclusion about the role of cAMP during *B. henselae*-anti-apoptotic activity.

VEGF, one of the main pro-angiogenic factors, plays a critical role in blood vessel formation [44] and pathological angiogenesis [45]. This factor seems also to be involved in *Bartonella*-induced angiogenesis. For instance, in *verruga peruana* (induced by *B. baciliformis*), the primary source of vascular endothelial growth factor (VEGF) is the epidermis [46] and endothelium of verruga peruana expresses VEGF receptors (VEGFR1 and VEGFR2) [46].

In addition, while HUVEC did not produce VEGF in response to *B. henselae*, infection promotes their proliferation [22]. Further study by Kempf et *al* showed the importance of VEGF in *B. henselae*-mediated ECs proliferation although it appeared not to be produced by ECs only. Overall, this strongly suggests that a paracrine loop could be involved in *B. henselae* VEGF action [27,28]. However, up to now, the majority of these studies have been carried out on macrovascular ECs (i.e. HUVEC). Interestingly, using our species- and organ-specific ECs model, we showed that *B. henselae* increased VEGF production by Human Skin Microvascular ECs but not by iHUVEC or feline macro- or micro-vascular ECs. These results, which might explain the decreased pathogenic potential of *B. henselae* infection for cat as compared to human, strongly suggests the involvement of an autocrine secretion of VEGF by skin ECs. This finding points out that the mechanism of *B. henselae*-mediated angiogenesis induction implies autocrine VEGF production and stimulation of the infected endothelium.

In parallel to VEGF production, the phosphorylation of VEGFR-2 was observed in ECs upon infection, mostly by homologous strains. This phenomenon is of high interest in the context of epidemiological human infection. As *B. henselae* isolates infecting a human have always a feline origin, it is tempting to speculate that an adaptive switch is taking place upon cat scratch in humans. Altogether, our results raise the hypothesis of host-dependent signaling in ECs upon bacterial infection as VEGFR-2 activation is more prominent in human ECs exposed to homologous strains. The same holds true for feline ECs. Because bacillary angiomatosis is not detected in cats infected by homologous strains, alternate mechanisms are likely taking place, Our results support the fact that VEGF signaling might be increased in human ECs through an autocrine production, which does not occur in feline ECs. Paracrine VEGF activation cannot be excluded; therefore, it will be interesting to further investigate whether VEGF can be released in the perivascular microenvironment by other cells, such as macrophages and polymorphonuclear cells. Our results on VEGF and VEGFR-2 are in apparent contradiction with those obtained by Scheidegger et *al* [47]. However, the concentration ranges and source of VEGF were far for being comparable.

Our study highlights the ECs organo- and species- specificity in their interactions with *B. henselae*. Indeed, our model further demonstrates the difference of reactivity displayed by human *vs* feline ECs on the one hand and by the macro- *vs* the micro-vasculature on the other hand. Additionally, local physiological microenvironment is most likely to play an important role. In this context, our cellular systems will allow studying the process of specific ECs infection by *B. henselae*. They will offer new possibilities to investigate bacterial and cellular factors which determine human *vs* cat reactivity, as well as the mechanisms involved in anti-apoptotic and/or pro-angiogenic effects, ultimately resulting to bacillary angiomatosis and peliosis only in humans.

In conclusion, according to the validated hypothesis stating the organospecificity of the endothelium [31,36,37,38], our work extends this concept to the species-specific endothelial cell phenotypes. In this scenario, ECs could act as a major reservoir for infectious pathogens. Moreover, at a second level the ECs from the same tissue but from different species display similar organospecificity but distinct responses to infection. This is clearly illustrated by the reactivity of the human skin-derived ECs compared to the feline skin-derived ECs. It will further be necessary to evidence the molecular mechanism by which feline ECs are recognized but not activated upon binding of *B henselae*, while human ECs are activated to grow and proceed to tumor-like state. The co-activation signaling should indicate differential gene induction and regulation processes.

Such information will provide new insights into the mechanisms of species-specific tolerance *versus* pathologic infections as observed in AIDS malignancies.

Acknowledgments

We thank Bruno Allouche (Ecole Nationale Vétérinaire d'Alfort), David Gosset, (CNRS Orléans) and Michèle Mitterrand (CNRS Orléans) for skilful technical help.

Author Contributions

Conceived and designed the experiments: MB MM NH HJB CK CG. Performed the experiments: MB MM CG JG. Analyzed the data: MB MM CK CG NH HJB. Contributed reagents/materials/analysis tools: MB CK CG MM NL JG HJB NH. Wrote the paper: MB CK CG MM NL JG HJB NH. Revised/edited the manuscript: MB CK CG MM NL JG HJB NH. Contributed to discussion: MB CK CG MM NL JG HJB NH.

References

1. Regnery RL, Anderson BE, Clarridge JE 3rd, Rodriguez-Barradas MC, Jones DC, et al. (1992) Characterization of a novel Rochalimaea species, R. henselae sp. nov., isolated from blood of a febrile, human immunodeficiency virus-positive patient. J Clin Microbiol 30: 265–274.
2. Chomel BB, Boulouis HJ, Breitschwerdt EB, Kasten RW, Vayssier-Taussat M, et al. (2009) Ecological fitness and strategies of adaptation of Bartonella species to their hosts and vectors. Vet Res 40: 29.
3. Koehler JE, Sanchez MA, Garrido CS, Whitfeld MJ, Chen FM, et al. (1997) Molecular epidemiology of bartonella infections in patients with bacillary angiomatosis-peliosis. N Engl J Med 337: 1876–1883.
4. Boulouis HJ, Chang CC, Henn JB, Kasten RW, Chomel BB (2005) Factors associated with the rapid emergence of zoonotic Bartonella infections. Vet Res 36: 383–410.
5. Guptill L (2010) Feline bartonellosis. Vet Clin North Am Small Anim Pract 40: 1073–1090.
6. Breitschwerdt EB (2008) Feline bartonellosis and cat scratch disease. Vet Immunol Immunopathol 123: 167–171.
7. Buchmann AU, Kempf VA, Kershaw O, Gruber AD (2010) Peliosis hepatis in cats is not associated with Bartonella henselae infections. Vet Pathol 47: 163–166.
8. Buchmann AU, Kershaw O, Kempf VA, Gruber AD (2010) Does a feline leukemia virus infection pave the way for Bartonella henselae infection in cats? J Clin Microbiol 48: 3295–3300.
9. Bergmans AM, Schellekens JF, van Embden JD, Schouls LM (1996) Predominance of two Bartonella henselae variants among cat-scratch disease patients in the Netherlands. J Clin Microbiol 34: 254–260.
10. Bouchouicha R, Durand B, Monteil M, Chomel BB, Berrich M, et al. (2009) Molecular epidemiology of feline and human Bartonella henselae isolates. Emerg Infect Dis 15: 813–816.
11. Fournier PE, Robson J, Zeaiter Z, McDougall R, Byrne S, et al. (2002) Improved culture from lymph nodes of patients with cat scratch disease and genotypic characterization of Bartonella henselae isolates in Australia. J Clin Microbiol 40: 3620–3624.
12. Sander A, Ruess M, Deichmann K, Bohm N, Bredt W (1998) Two different genotypes of Bartonella henselae in children with cat-scratch disease and their pet cats. Scand J Infect Dis 30: 387–391.
13. Woestyn S, Olive N, Bigaignon G, Avesani V, Delmee M (2004) Study of genotypes and virB4 secretion gene of Bartonella henselae strains from patients with clinically defined cat scratch disease. J Clin Microbiol 42: 1420–1427.
14. Chang CC, Chomel BB, Kasten RW, Tappero JW, Sanchez MA, et al. (2002) Molecular epidemiology of Bartonella henselae infection in human immunodeficiency virus-infected patients and their cat contacts, using pulsed-field gel electrophoresis and genotyping. J Infect Dis 186: 1733–1739.
15. LeBoit PE, Berger TG, Egbert BM, Beckstead JH, Yen TS, et al. (1989) Bacillary angiomatosis. The histopathology and differential diagnosis of a pseudoneoplastic infection in patients with human immunodeficiency virus disease. Am J Surg Pathol 13: 909–920.
16. Batterman HJ, Peek JA, Loutit JS, Falkow S, Tompkins LS (1995) Bartonella henselae and Bartonella quintana adherence to and entry into cultured human epithelial cells. Infect Immun 63: 4553–4556.
17. Riess T, Raddatz G, Linke D, Schafer A, Kempf VA (2007) Analysis of Bartonella adhesin A expression reveals differences between various B. henselae strains. Infect Immun 75: 35–43.
18. Riess T, Andersson SG, Lupas A, Schaller M, Schafer A, et al. (2004) Bartonella adhesin a mediates a proangiogenic host cell response. J Exp Med 200: 1267–1278.
19. Pulliainen AT, Dehio C (2009) Bartonella henselae: subversion of vascular endothelial cell functions by translocated bacterial effector proteins. Int J Biochem Cell Biol 41: 507–510.
20. Scheidegger F, Ellner Y, Guye P, Rhomberg TA, Weber H, et al. (2009) Distinct activities of Bartonella henselae type IV secretion effector proteins modulate capillary-like sprout formation. Cell Microbiol 11: 1088–1101.
21. Conley T, Slater L, Hamilton K (1994) Rochalimaea species stimulate human endothelial cell proliferation and migration in vitro. J Lab Clin Med 124: 521–528.
22. Maeno N, Oda H, Yoshiie K, Wahid MR, Fujimura T, et al. (1999) Live Bartonella henselae enhances endothelial cell proliferation without direct contact. Microb Pathog 27: 419–427.
23. McCord AM, Cuevas J, Anderson BE (2007) Bartonella-induced endothelial cell proliferation is mediated by release of calcium from intracellular stores. DNA Cell Biol 26: 657–663.
24. Palmari J, Teysseire N, Dussert C, Raoult D (1996) Image cytometry and topographical analysis of proliferation of endothelial cells in vitro during Bartonella (Rochalimaea) infection. Anal Cell Pathol 11: 13–30.
25. Red-Horse K, Ferrara N (2006) Imaging tumor angiogenesis. J Clin Invest 116: 2585–2587.
26. McCord AM, Burgess AW, Whaley MJ, Anderson BE (2005) Interaction of Bartonella henselae with endothelial cells promotes monocyte/macrophage chemoattractant protein 1 gene expression and protein production and triggers monocyte migration. Infect Immun 73: 5735–5742.
27. Kempf VA, Volkmann B, Schaller M, Sander CA, Alitalo K, et al. (2001) Evidence of a leading role for VEGF in Bartonella henselae-induced endothelial cell proliferations. Cell Microbiol 3: 623–632.
28. Resto-Ruiz SI, Schmiederer M, Sweger D, Newton C, Klein TW, et al. (2002) Induction of a potential paracrine angiogenic loop between human THP-1 macrophages and human microvascular endothelial cells during Bartonella henselae infection. Infect Immun 70: 4564–4570.
29. Schmid MC, Scheidegger F, Dehio M, Balmelle-Devaux N, Schulein R, et al. (2006) A translocated bacterial protein protects vascular endothelial cells from apoptosis. PLoS Pathog 2: e115.
30. Chang CC, Chen YJ, Tseng CS, Lai WL, Hsu KY, et al. (2010) A comparative study of the interaction of Bartonella henselae strains with human endothelial cells. Vet Microbiol.
31. Kieda C, Paprocka M, Krawczenko A, Zalecki P, Dupuis P, et al. (2002) New human microvascular endothelial cell lines with specific adhesion molecules phenotypes. Endothelium 9: 247–261.
32. Chi JT, Chang HY, Haraldsen G, Jahnsen FL, Troyanskaya OG, et al. (2003) Endothelial cell diversity revealed by global expression profiling. Proc Natl Acad Sci U S A 100: 10623–10628.
33. Lang I, Pabst MA, Hiden U, Blaschitz A, Dohr G et al. (2003) Heterogeneity of microvascular endothelial cells isolated from human term placenta and macrovascular umbilical vein endothelial cells. Eur J Cell Biol 82: 163–173.
34. McCord AM, Resto-Ruiz SI, Anderson BE (2006) Autocrine role for interleukin-8 in Bartonella henselae-induced angiogenesis. Infect Immun 74: 5185–5190.
35. Kumar S, West DC, Ager A (1987) Heterogeneity in endothelial cells from large vessels and microvessels. Differentiation 36: 57–70.

36. Carreau A, El Hafny-Rahbi B, Matejuk A, Grillon C, Kieda C (2011) Why is the partial oxygen pressure of human tissues a crucial parameter?:Small molecules and hypoxia. J Cell Mol Med.
37. Bizouarne N, Denis V, Legrand A, Monsigny M, Kieda C (1993) A SV-40 immortalized murine endothelial cell line from peripheral lymph node high endothelium expresses a new alpha-L-fucose binding protein. Biol Cell 79: 209–218.
38. Bizouarne N, Mitterrand M, Monsigny M, Kieda C (1993) Characterization of membrane sugar-specific receptors in cultured high endothelial cells from mouse peripheral lymph nodes. Biol Cell 79: 27–35.
39. Tan W, Palmby TR, Gavard J, Amornphimoltham P, Zheng Y, et al. (2008) An essential role for Rac1 in endothelial cell function and vascular development. FASEB J 22: 1829–1838.
40. Yager JA, Best SJ, Maggi RG, Varanat M, Znajda N, et al. (2010) Bacillary angiomatosis in an immunosuppressed dog. Vet Dermatol.
41. Conway EM, Carmeliet P (2004) The diversity of endothelial cells: a challenge for therapeutic angiogenesis. Genome Biol 5: 207.
42. Pries AR, Kuebler WM (2006) Normal endothelium. Handb Exp Pharmacol. pp 1–40.
43. Nishihara H, Kizaka-Kondoh S, Insel PA, Eckmann L (2003) Inhibition of apoptosis in normal and transformed intestinal epithelial cells by cAMP through induction of inhibitor of apoptosis protein (IAP)-2. Proc Natl Acad Sci U S A 100: 8921–8926.
44. Yancopoulos GD, Davis S, Gale NW, Rudge JS, Wiegand SJ, et al. (2000) Vascular-specific growth factors and blood vessel formation. Nature 407: 242–248.
45. Leung DW, Cachianes G, Kuang WJ, Goeddel DV, Ferrara N (1989) Vascular endothelial growth factor is a secreted angiogenic mitogen. Science 246: 1306–1309.
46. Cerimele F, Brown LF, Bravo F, Ihler GM, Kouadio P, et al. (2003) Infectious angiogenesis: Bartonella bacilliformis infection results in endothelial production of angiopoetin-2 and epidermal production of vascular endothelial growth factor. Am J Pathol 163: 1321–1327.
47. Scheidegger F, Quebatte M, Mistl C, Dehio C (2010) The Bartonella henselae VirB/Bep System Interferes with Vascular Endothelial Cell Growth Factor (VEGF) Signalling in Human Vascular Endothelial Cells. Cell Microbiol.

The Dominant Australian Community-Acquired Methicillin-Resistant *Staphylococcus aureus* Clone ST93-IV [2B] Is Highly Virulent and Genetically Distinct

Kyra Y. L. Chua[1,2,4], Torsten Seemann[3], Paul F. Harrison[3], Shaun Monagle[6], Tony M. Korman[7], Paul D. R. Johnson[4], Geoffrey W. Coombs[8], Brian O. Howden[9], John K. Davies[1], Benjamin P. Howden[1,2,4,5*¶], Timothy P. Stinear[1,2*¶]

1 Department of Microbiology, Monash University, Clayton, Australia, **2** Department of Microbiology and Immunology, University of Melbourne, Parkville, Australia, **3** Victorian Bioinformatics Consortium, Monash University, Clayton, Australia, **4** Department of Infectious Diseases, Austin Centre for Infection Research, Austin Health, Heidelberg, Australia, **5** Department of Microbiology, Austin Health, Heidelberg, Australia, **6** Department of Anatomical Pathology, Eastern Health, Box Hill, Australia, **7** Department of Infectious Diseases, Monash Medical Centre, Clayton, Australia, **8** Department of Microbiology and Infectious Diseases, PathWest Laboratory Medicine WA, Royal Perth Hospital, Perth, Australia, **9** Microsurgical Consultants, Blackburn, Australia

Abstract

Community-associated methicillin-resistant *Staphylococcus aureus* (CA-MRSA) USA300 has spread rapidly across North America, and CA-MRSA is also increasing in Australia. However, the dominant Australian CA-MRSA strain, ST93-IV [2B] appears distantly related to USA300 despite strikingly similar clinical and epidemiological profiles. Here, we compared the virulence of a recent Australian ST93 isolate (JKD6159) to other MRSA, including USA300, and found that JKD6159 was the most virulent in a mouse skin infection model. We fully sequenced the genome of JKD6159 and confirmed that JKD6159 is a distinct clone with 7616 single nucleotide polymorphisms (SNPs) distinguishing this strain from all other *S. aureus* genomes. Despite its high virulence there were surprisingly few virulence determinants. However, genes encoding α-hemolysin, Panton-Valentine leukocidin (PVL) and α-type phenol soluble modulins were present. Genome comparisons revealed 32 additional CDS in JKD6159 but none appeared to encode new virulence factors, suggesting that this clone's enhanced pathogenicity could lie within subtler genome changes, such as SNPs within regulatory genes. To investigate the role of accessory genome elements in CA-MRSA epidemiology, we next sequenced three additional Australian non-ST93 CA-MRSA strains and compared them with JKD6159, 19 completed *S. aureus* genomes and 59 additional *S. aureus* genomes for which unassembled genome sequence data was publicly available (82 genomes in total). These comparisons showed that despite its distinctive genotype, JKD6159 and other CA-MRSA clones (including USA300) share a conserved repertoire of three notable accessory elements (SSC*mec*IV, PVL prophage, and pMW2). This study demonstrates that the genetically distinct ST93 CA-MRSA from Australia is highly virulent. Our comparisons of geographically and genetically diverse CA-MRSA genomes suggest that apparent convergent evolution in CA-MRSA may be better explained by the rapid dissemination of a highly conserved accessory genome from a common source.

Editor: Malcolm James Horsburgh, University of Liverpool, United Kingdom

Funding: This research was supported by the National Health and Medical Research Council of Australia Project Grant 1008556, the CASS Foundation and the Austin Hospital Medical Research Foundation. The funders had no role in study design, data collection and analysis, decision to publish, or preparation of the manuscript.

Competing Interests: The authors have declared that no competing interests exist.

* E-mail: tstinear@unimelb.edu.au (TPS); Benjamin.Howden@austin.org.au (BPH)

¶ These authors contributed equally to this work.

Introduction

Infections with community-associated methicillin-resistant *Staphylococcus aureus* (CA-MRSA) in patients with no contact with the hospital environment are now well described worldwide [1]. In some regions such as North America, the CA-MRSA phenomenon has become particularly well defined. Here, the epidemic CA-MRSA strain USA300 is the most common cause of skin infections in patients presenting to the emergency department [2]. Much of the work performed thus far to understand the CA-MRSA phenomenon has focused on USA300 and these studies have demonstrated the importance of virulence determinants in both the staphylococcal accessory and core genome such as Panton-Valentine leukocidin (PVL), α-hemolysin (Hla) and α-type phenol soluble modulins (PSMs) [3,4,5,6,7,8,9,10].

In contrast to healthcare-associated MRSA where a limited number of clones are prevalent, CA-MRSA strains are polyclonal with an epidemiological association between clone type and geographic origin [1,11]. Furthermore, minor genetic differences between CA-MRSA strains, even to a single nucleotide, may result in significant differences in the observed virulence of a strain [12]. Hence, while the genomic mediators of virulence have been well defined in USA300, these may not be applicable to other CA-MRSA clones. Therefore, a detailed understanding of the virulence phenotype and virulence determinants in other global clones of CA-MRSA has the potential to provide new and important insights into staphylococcal pathogenesis.

In Australia, *S. aureus* ST93-IV [2B] has recently emerged to become the dominant CA-MRSA clone. First described in the early 2000s, it is colloquially known as the "Queensland" clone [13]. However, since this initial description, ST93-IV [2B] has been reported across Australia and is responsible for the increasing prevalence of all CA-MRSA nationwide [14]. ST93 is associated with skin infection and severe invasive infection including necrotizing pneumonia, deep-seated abscesses, and septicemia [14,15]. This PVL positive clone is a singleton by MLST eBURST analysis and is therefore distinct to other *S. aureus* clones, including previously sequenced strains [16]. While predominantly an Australian strain, it has recently also been reported in the United Kingdom, with many cases having epidemiological links to Australia [16,17]. Other less frequent clones of CA-MRSA in Australia include PVL negative ST1-IV [2B] (WA-1) and PVL positive ST30-IV [2B] (SouthWest Pacific, SWP) [14]. The dominant health-care associated clone of MRSA in Australia is multi-resistant ST239-III [3A] [14].

To investigate the apparent enhanced clinical virulence of ST93-IV [2B], we examined a recent clinical isolate (JKD6159) that caused an outbreak of both severe and minor staphylococcal infections within a household, representative of the typical spectrum of disease associated with this clone. We compared the virulence of JKD6159 to three other well-characterized and representative Australian MRSA strains and the epidemic North American strain, USA300 and found that JKD6159 was the most virulent clone in two *in vivo* models.

We next sequenced, fully assembled and annotated the genome of *S. aureus* ST93-IV [2B] (JKD6159) and then sequenced three non-ST93 Australian CA-MRSA clones. We employed comparative genomics against these strains, the 19 published, complete *S. aureus* genomes and 59 unassembled, publically available *S. aureus* genomes to try and identify genetic factors that might explain the recent emergence, and increased virulence of ST93-IV [2B].

Materials and Methods

Bacterial strains and culture

The bacterial strains used in this study are described in Table 1. For all experiments, bacteria were grown in brain heart infusion broth (BHI, Oxoid). For growth kinetic experiments, overnight cultures of *S. aureus* were diluted 1:100 and incubated at 37°C with shaking (180 rpm). Optical density at 600 nm (OD_{600}) and viable counts were performed hourly until stationary phase was achieved and at 24 hours after commencement of the experiment. These experiments were performed in triplicate. For the *Galleria mellonella* killing assay and the mouse skin infection assay, *S. aureus* were harvested at the stationary phase of growth after 18 hours incubation (OD_{600} approx. 2.0), washed, diluted and resuspended in PBS. The bacterial inoculum (CFU) and viable counts were determined by plating onto BHI agar and colony enumeration.

DNA Manipulation and Molecular Typing

DNA was extracted using the GenElute kit according to the manufacturer's instructions (Sigma-Aldrich). Detection of *lukSF-PV* was performed as described by Lina *et al.* [18]. MLST was performed as described by Enright *et al.* [19], and Pulsed Field Gel Electrophoresis (PFGE) performed as previously described [20]. SCC*mec* typing was performed as previously described [21]. SCC*mec* nomenclature was used as proposed by the International Working Group on the Classification of Staphylococcal Cassette Chromosome Elements (IWG-SCC) [22]. A Roman numeral indicates the SCC*mec* type with a lowercase letter indicating the subtype. The *ccr* complex and the *mec* complex are indicated by an Arabic numeral and an uppercase letter respectively.

Wax Moth (*Galleria mellonella*) virulence assay

Final stage instar *G. mellonella* larvae were infected with *S. aureus* and time to death measured as described previously [23]. Approximately 10^6 CFU of *S. aureus* suspended in 10 μL of PBS was injected into the first left proleg of each larva. Each experimental group consisted of at least 16 larvae. All experiments included biological triplicates. The larvae were incubated at 37°C and assessed daily for six days. Larvae were considered dead when there was no movement in response to stimuli. The control groups were PBS injected and non-injected larvae.

Mouse skin infection assay

Mice were housed in individually ventilated cages and received food and water ad libitum. Six-week-old female BALB/c mice were anesthetized with intraperitoneal ketamine/xylazine, and inoculated in the right flank by intradermal injection, with 10^8 CFU of *S. aureus* (in 50 μL of PBS suspension). This dose of *S. aureus* was determined in preliminary experiments as the lower limit of inoculum, which produced consistent dermonecrosis for all strains of *S. aureus* tested. Mice were assessed and weighed daily for five days. On the 5th day, the mice were culled. The infected area of skin and muscle was harvested and these tissues were homogenized and CFU measured by plating onto BHI and colony enumeration. Skin lesion area was quantitated by obtaining a digital image of the lesion and processed using ImageJ [24]. For each *S. aureus* strain, at least 15 mice were assessed – the tissues for four of these mice were used for histological analysis and data for these mice were not available for CFU enumeration.

Table 1. Bacterial strains used in this study.

S. aureus strain	Type	Date of Isolate Recovery	Place of Isolate Recovery	Relevant Characteristics	*lukSF-PV*	Reference
JKD6159	ST93-IV [2B]	2004	Melbourne, Australia	Dominant Australian CA-MRSA clone	+	This work
JKD6272	ST1-IV [2B]	2002	Melbourne, Australia	Australian CA-MRSA clone	−	This work
JKD6260	ST1-IV [2B]	2008	Port Hedland, Australia	Australian CA-MRSA clone	+	This work
JKD6177	ST30-IV [2B]	2003	Melbourne, Australia	Australian CA-MRSA clone	+	This work
FPR3757 USA300	ST8-IV [2B]	NA	San Francisco, USA	Dominant North American CA-MRSA clone	+	[38]
JKD6009	ST239-III [3A]	2002	New Zealand	Dominant Australian hospital-associated MRSA clone, AUS2/3	−	[47]

NA: not available.

Ethics Statement

All studies were reviewed and approved by the Animal Ethics Committee at the University of Melbourne approval number 0911248.2.

Whole Genome sequencing of Australian CA-MRSA strains JKD6159 (ST93-IV [2B]), JKD6272 (ST1-IV [2B]), JKD6260 (ST1-IV [2B]) and JKD6177 (ST30-IV [2B])

We have previously described the sequencing, complete assembly and annotation of the genome of JKD6159, however the comparative genomics have not previously been reported [25]. Here, we also sequenced and partially assembled the genomes of three Australian CA-MRSA strains, using Illumina GAIIx 36 bp paired-end chemistry, yielding an average of 555 Mbp of reads per strain (~200× coverage). These genomes were *de novo* assembled to draft form using Velvet 1.0 [26]. The reads from whole genome sequencing of these strains were also included in defining the core and accessory genome of JKD6159. The sequences are accessible from the NCBI Sequence Read Archive under accession SRA026511.1.

Analysis of the JKD6159 genome sequence

A read mapping approach was developed to define a *S. aureus* core genome and the accessory genome for a given strain. Sequence reads from each *S. aureus* strain were aligned separately to the completed JKD6159 reference genome using SHRiMP 2.0 [27]. Publically available completed genomes (Table 2) were shredded into 75 bp reads at 25× coverage to produce a set of synthetic sequence reads. Those positions in JKD6159 that were covered by at least one read from each and every genome defined a *S. aureus* core genome. Reads from JKD6159 that did not map to any S. *aureus* genome (Table 2) were used to define JKD6159 regions of difference. Reads from any strain that did not map to the core genome represented that strain's accessory genome. SNPs were identified using Nesoni v0.35, which used the sequence reads for each genome aligned to the above-defined core genome to construct a tally of putative differences at each nucleotide position, including substitutions, insertions, and deletions (www.bioinformatics.net.au). This tally was then employed in a simple Bayesian model to decide whether a base (or deletion) could be called for the position, and if so, whether it differed from the reference sequence. A similar procedure was used to determine the presence or absence of insertions between positions in the reference. NCBI BLASTn+, Artemis and BRIG were also used for comparisons of JKD6159 with selected *S. aureus* genomes [28] (http://sourceforge.net/projects/brig/). SNPs were identified in the accessory genome elements pMW2, ϕSA2, and SCC*mec*IV for strains carrying them by read mapping using Nesoni v0.35 against reference sequences of each element taken from *S. aureus* MW2. Phylogenetic analyses were performed using a distance method, based on pairwise nucleotide sequence alignments for the *S. aureus* core genome among all strains or selected accessory elements among some strains. Split decomposition analysis was employed using uncorrected p distances with bootstrapping as implemented in SplitsTree4 [29].

Statistical analysis

Kaplan Meier plots of *G. mellonella* killing results were analysed using the log rank test. Percentage mouse weight change at day 5, viable counts of *S. aureus* in mouse tissues and skin lesion area of each isolate versus JKD6159 were analyzed using the Mann Whitney test. All analyses were performed using Prism 5 for Macintosh v5.0b (GraphPad Software Inc.).

Table 2. *Staphylococcus aureus* completed genomes used in this study.

	Genome	Multilocus Sequence Type (Clonal Complex)	Reference
1	NCTC8325	8 (8)	[48]
2	N315	5 (5)	[49]
3	Mu50	5 (5)	[49]
4	Mu3	5 (5)	[50]
5	MW2	1 (1)	[37]
6	USA300 FPR3757	8 (8)	[38]
7	USA300 TCH1516	8 (8)	[39]
8	MRSA252	36 (30)	[51]
9	MSSA476	1 (1)	[51]
10	RF122	151	[52]
11	Newman	8 (8)	[53]
12	COL	250 (8)	[54]
13	JH1	105 (5)	[55]
14	JH9	105 (5)	[55]
15	ED98	5 (5)	[56]
16	TW20	239 (8)	[57]
17	04-02981	225 (5)	[58]
18	S0385	398	[59]
19	JKD6008	239 (8)	[60]

Results

Clinical Details

Staphylococcus aureus JKD6159 was isolated from the blood of a young male intravenous drug user with no prior health care exposure, who presented with a severe sepsis syndrome in 2004. He had cavitating pulmonary lesions, polyarticular septic arthritis and multiple deep-seated muscle abscesses. The isolate was resistant to methicillin, but susceptible to erythromycin, clindamycin, tetracycline, ciprofloxacin, rifampicin, fusidic acid and vancomycin. The patient required extensive surgical debridement and prolonged antimicrobial therapy with vancomycin and subsequently, linezolid, but eventually made a full recovery. In addition, the patient reported multiple household family members with recurrent skin infections. The *SmaI* PFGE pattern was identical between JKD6159 and the *S. aureus* isolates from three other family members, indicating an intra-familial outbreak with the same clone (Figure 1). Further typing demonstrated that JKD6159 was ST93-IV [2B]. This isolate was representative of the Australian CA-MRSA Queensland clone.

S. aureus strain JKD6272 was isolated from the blood of a woman with pneumonia and septic shock who had no prior hospitalizations. The isolate was resistant to methicillin and fusidic acid but susceptible to erythromycin, clindamycin, tetracycline, ciprofloxacin, rifampicin, trimethoprim and vancomycin. Further typing demonstrated that JKD6272 was ST1-IV [2B], and PVL negative. This isolate was representative of the Australian CA-MRSA clone WA-1.

S. aureus strain JKD6260 was isolated from a wound swab from a patient with a skin infection. The isolate was resistant to methicillin, fusidic acid and ciprofloxacin, but susceptible to erythromycin, clindamycin, tetracycline, rifampicin, mupirocin,

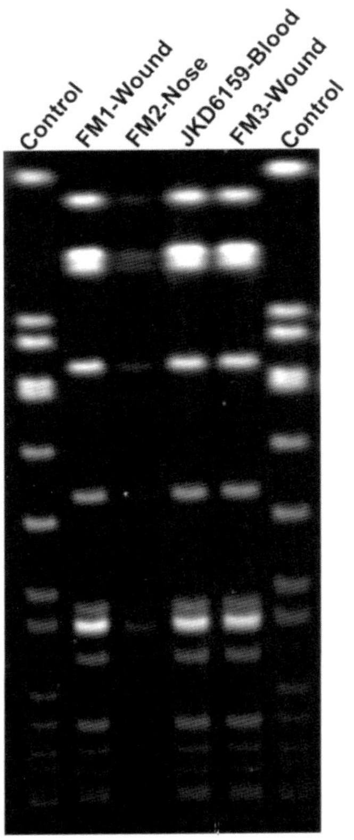

Figure 1. *Sma*I pulsed field gel electrophoresis analysis. PFGE of index isolate, *S. aureus* JKD6159 and isolates from three family members, FM1, FM2, FM3.

trimethoprim and vancomycin. Typing demonstrated that JKD6272 was ST1-IV [2B], and PVL positive.

S. aureus strain JKD6177 was isolated from the blood of a patient with mitral valve endocarditis. He had recurrent skin infections with MRSA prior to presentation. The isolate was resistant to methicillin, but susceptible to erythromycin, clindamycin, tetracycline, ciprofloxacin, rifampicin, fusidic acid and vancomycin. Typing demonstrated that JKD6177 was ST30-IV [2B], and PVL positive. This isolate was representative of the SouthWest Pacific clone of CA-MRSA.

JKD6159 exhibits high virulence in two animal models

The reports of severe infections associated with ST93-IV [2B], and the severity of disease in our patient led us to compare the virulence of JKD6159 with other well-characterized clones of *S. aureus* (Table 1). All *S. aureus* strains tested had the same growth curve characteristics, indicating that any differences in virulence were not due to differential growth kinetics (Figure S1). However, JKD6159 was significantly more virulent than other community and healthcare-associated MRSA strains, including the USA300 strain FPR3757, in both an invertebrate and mouse infection model of *S. aureus* infection. In the *Galleria mellonella* larvae assay, JKD6159 caused significantly more rapid time-to-death than all other *S. aureus* strains ($p<0.001$, Fig. 2A). The differential virulence seen in the larvae assay was mirrored by the results of a mouse skin infection assay. Mice infected with JKD6159 developed large skin lesions and lost significantly more weight over a 5-day experimental period than mice infected with the other strains ($p<0.05$, Figure 2B-C). In line with these findings, the bacterial load in mouse tissues was highest in JKD6159-infected mice ($p<0.05$, Figure 2D). Histopathological analysis of mouse tissues showed that all CA-MRSA strains caused extensive epidermal and fat necrosis with myositis including in some cases myonecrosis, whilst infection with the hospital-associated MRSA strain JKD6009 caused less severe inflammatory changes with only mild myositis. Representative sections are shown in Figure 2E-I.

Comparative genome analysis of JKD6159

To gain insight into the high virulence of *S. aureus* ST93 strain JKD6159 we fully sequenced, assembled and annotated its genome and used it as a reference genome for comprehensive comparative genomics [25]. The JKD6159 genome consisted of a single 2,811,434 bp circular chromosome and a 20,730 bp circular, pMW2-like plasmid. For comparison, we also sequenced the genomes of three other Australian CA-MRSA isolates (JKD6272, JKD6260 & JKD6177) that were representative of the commonly occurring ST1 and ST30 clones (Table 1, Table S1, Figure 3A). Whole genome DNA:DNA comparisons showed that the architecture of the JKD6159 chromosome was conserved compared to other *S. aureus* strains (Figure 3B). Using a read-mapping approach to objectively and comprehensively define the core and accessory genome of JKD6159, we found that 2,302,644 bp of JKD6159 (81.9%) was absolutely conserved amongst all 20 *S. aureus* strains with fully assembled genomes and 62 strains for which only unassembled sequence data was available (Table 2, Table S1, Figure 3). Pairwise comparisons of the concatenated 2,302,644 bp JKD6159 core genome with the core genomes of other *S. aureus* strains uncovered 78,967 variable nucleotide positions among all strains and permitted the construction of a high-resolution phylogeny by split decomposition analysis that confirmed the divergent genotype of ST93 (Figure 4A). ST93 was clearly divergent from other *S. aureus* strains with 7616 single nucleotide polymorphisms (SNPs) distinguishing this strain from other genomes. In comparison, the USA300 genome contained only 167 SNPs that varied from other strains. The JKD6159 core genome, like other *S. aureus* genomes, contained the genes encoding the important virulence factors Hla and α-type PSMs. The genes encoding gamma-hemolysin were also present.

Using the read mapping approach, we determined that 18.1% of the JKD6159 chromosome constituted its accessory genome (Figure 3A), a proportion that is consistent across all *S. aureus* genomes (range 13.2% [RF122]−18.1% [JH1]) and is also consistent with previous assessments based on microarray analyses [30,31]. For a strain associated with severe clinical disease and high virulence in animal models, the accessory genome of JKD6159 was notable for the absence of common virulence-associated factors such as toxic shock syndrome toxin, exfoliative toxins and most of the staphylococcal enterotoxins; a finding consistent with an earlier report [32]. There were no recognized pathogenicity islands in JKD6159 although it contained the *S. aureus* genomic islands, νSAα, νSAβ and νSAγ (Figure 4B). Within νSAα there was a complement of tandem lipoprotein genes and eleven staphylococcal superantigen-like (*ssl*) genes, however *ssl9* appeared to be a pseudogene. Two of the 11 *ssl* CDS, *ssl3* (SAA6159_00377) and *ssl4* (SAA6159_00378), encoded proteins with predicted N-terminal sequences that demonstrated significant variation from orthologs in other strains. Although the exact role of SSLs is still being defined, they play a role in modulating the host immune system; in particular neutrophil and complement activation, both of which are key to human defense against *S. aureus* [33]. SSLs have been shown to be upregulated in some CA-MRSA strains [34]. We postulate that these variant SSLs may in part contribute to the strain's increased virulence.

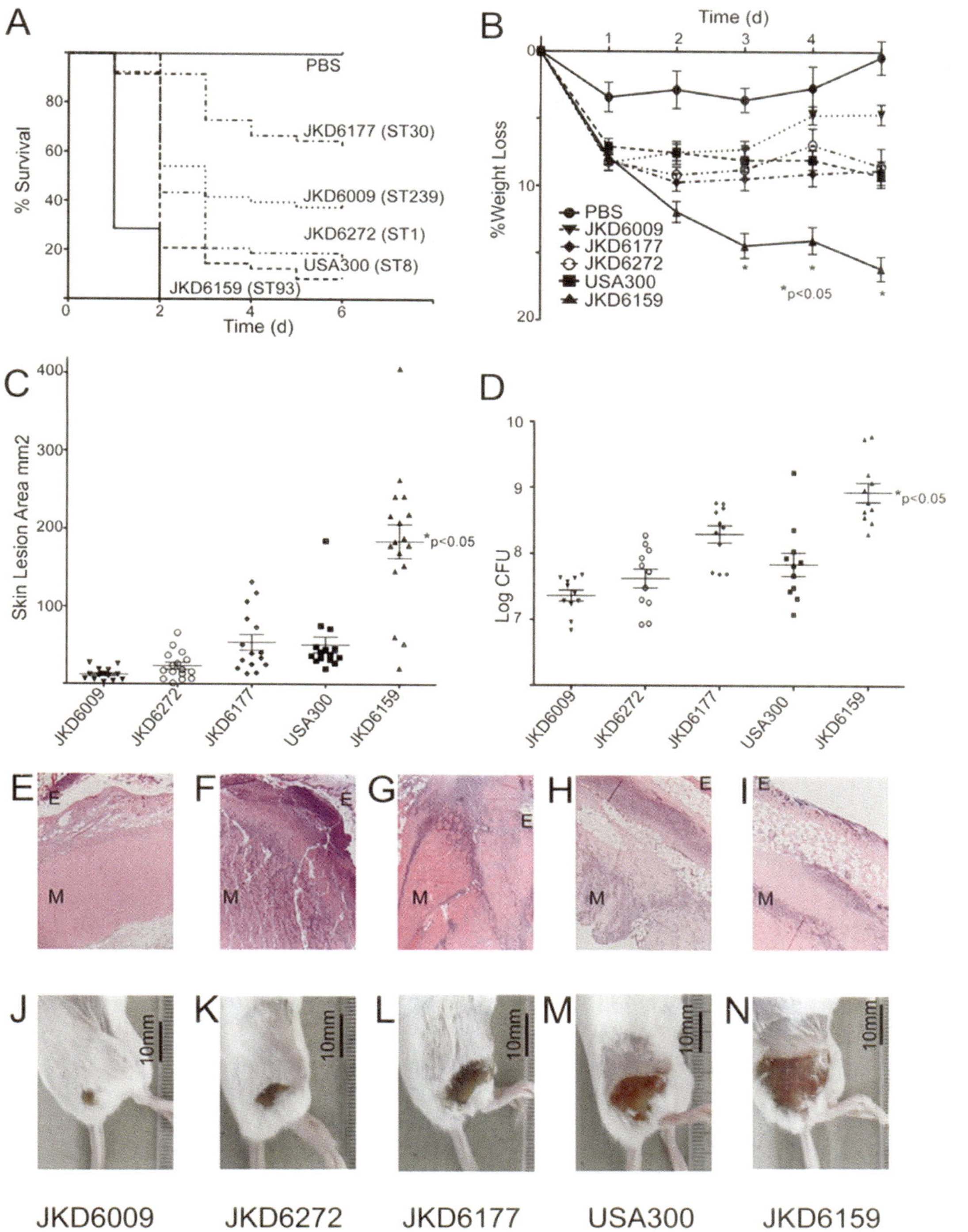

Figure 2. Virulence characteristics of *S. aureus* isolates. *S. aureus* JKD6159 (ST93-IV [2B], CA-MRSA) compared to four other MRSA strains. (A) *Galleria mellonella* virulence assay. Kaplan-Meier plot showing the percent survival of larvae injected with *S. aureus* strains JKD6159, JKD6009 (ST239-III [3A], hospital-associated MRSA), JKD6272 (ST1-IV [2B], CA-MRSA), JKD6177 (ST30-IV [2B], CA-MRSA), FPR3757 USA300 (ST8-IV [2B], CA-MRSA) up to 6 days post injection. The reduced survival time for larvae infected with JKD6159 compared to all other strains was significant ($p<0.0001$). (B) BALB/c mouse skin infection assay. Weight loss induced by intradermal infection with *S. aureus* strains is demonstrated as percentage loss of weight over 5 days. The difference in percentage weight loss between JKD6159 and all other strains was significant ($p<0.05$). At least 15 mice were used for each bacterial strain. Data shown are mean weight loss and SEM. (C) BALB/c mouse skin infection assay. Skin lesion area (mm^2) at 5 days after infection was greatest with JKD6159 infected mice ($p<0.05$). Data shown are mean area and SEM. (D) BALB/c mouse skin infection assay. Recovery of *S. aureus* (log CFU) from infected tissues at 5 days after infection was greatest with JKD6159 infected mice ($p<0.05$). Data shown are mean CFU and SEM. (E-I) BALB/c mouse skin infection assay. Representative H&E stained histology sections from infected tissues at 100× magnification from JKD6009, JKD6272, JKD6177, USA300 and JKD6159 respectively. There was no significant difference in degree of inflammation observed in the CA-MRSA strain infections. However, mice infected with JKD6009, the hospital-associated MRSA strain had less marked inflammation and only mild myositis. (J-N) BALB/c mouse skin infection assay with representative macroscopic appearance of lesions resulting from infection with JKD6009, JKD6272, JKD6177, USA300 and JKD6159 respectively.

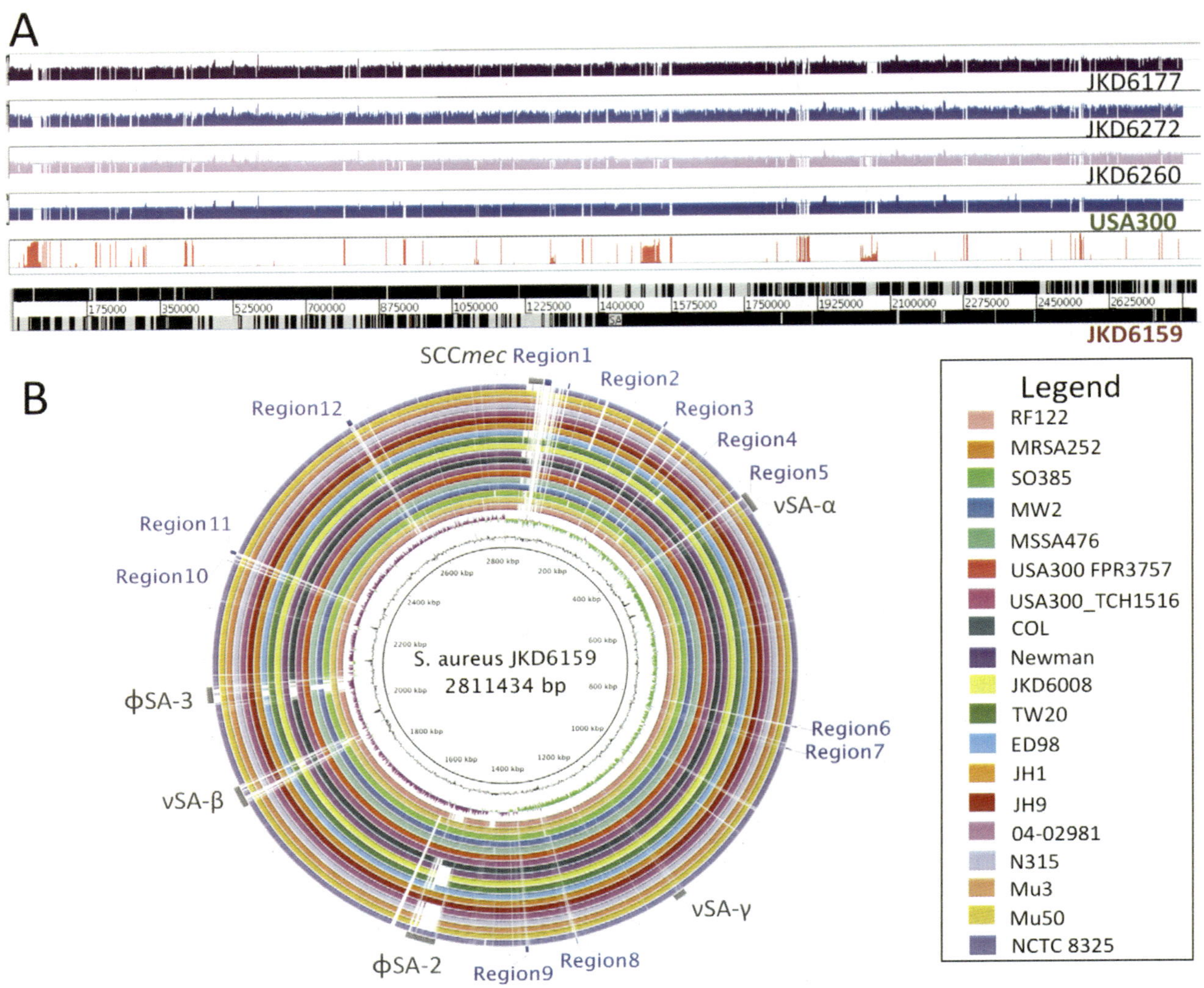

Figure 3. Whole genome sequence analysis and comparison of JKD6159 with other *S. aureus* strains. (A) Artemis linear view of JKD6159 chromosome, with vertical red bars identifying the position of accessory genome elements as determined by read mapping against 19 publicly available completed genomes and 62 unpublished, partially assembled genome sequences. Increasing height of vertical red lines indicates increasing specificity for JKD6159. Shown above the accessory genome analysis are the mapped positions of the short-reads obtained from Illumina sequencing CA-MRSA strains JKD6177, JKD6272 and JKD6260. Depicted also is an example of the synthetic reads obtained from completed whole genome sequences (USA300 shown here) to facilitate the comprehensive read mapping approach described in the methods. (B) Circular diagram of the JKD6159 chromosome showing (from inner to outer), % G+C, GC skew and the homology based on BLASTn+ analysis of JKD6159 to 19 completed *S. aureus* genomes (refer color-coded legend). Outer circle shows the location of accessory elements (grey) and the 12 regions of difference (blue) not present in the other *S. aureus* genomes examined.

In vSAβ, like other *S. aureus* genomes, JKD6159 had a cluster of serine protease genes and *lukDE*. However, unlike MW2 and FPR3757 USA300, the bacteriocin gene cluster was located elsewhere. In each of vSAα and vSAβ there were loci harboring distinctive type I restriction-modification systems. Restriction-modification systems attack foreign DNA, restricting DNA transfer [35,36]. Type I systems consists of enzyme subunits which are encoded by the genes *hsdR, hsdM and hsdS*. The HsdS (specificity) subunit contains target recognition domains (TRD1 and TRD2) that allow for target sequence specificity. In JKD6159 the *hsdS* genes in each of these regions (SAA6159_00387 and SAA6159_01737) contained previously unreported TDR1 and TDR2 domains. Additionally, there was a third restriction modification system with a distinct *hsdS* gene (SAA6159_00055) in a novel 10 kb locus adjacent to SCC*mec* (Table S2). These differences in the restriction-modification system of JKD6159 may explain its relative resistance to the uptake of foreign DNA that we have observed during laboratory manipulation of this strain (unpublished observations).

JKD6159 contained two prophages ϕSA2 and ϕSA3. As in the other major CA-MRSA clones, ϕSA2 habours *lukSF-PV* [1], the genes that encode the two component pore-forming Panton-Valentine leukocidin (PVL). JKD6159 also contained ϕSA3, which is present in many other *S. aureus* genomes including MW2 (Figure 3B). This bacteriophage inserts into and disrupts the beta-hemolysin gene. In JKD6159, ϕSA3 contained genes encoding staphylokinase, and chemotaxis inhibitory protein but unlike MW2, did not harbor enterotoxin genes. A gene encoding an enterotoxin-like protein similar to that in RF122 (SAB0026) was also present in JKD6159.

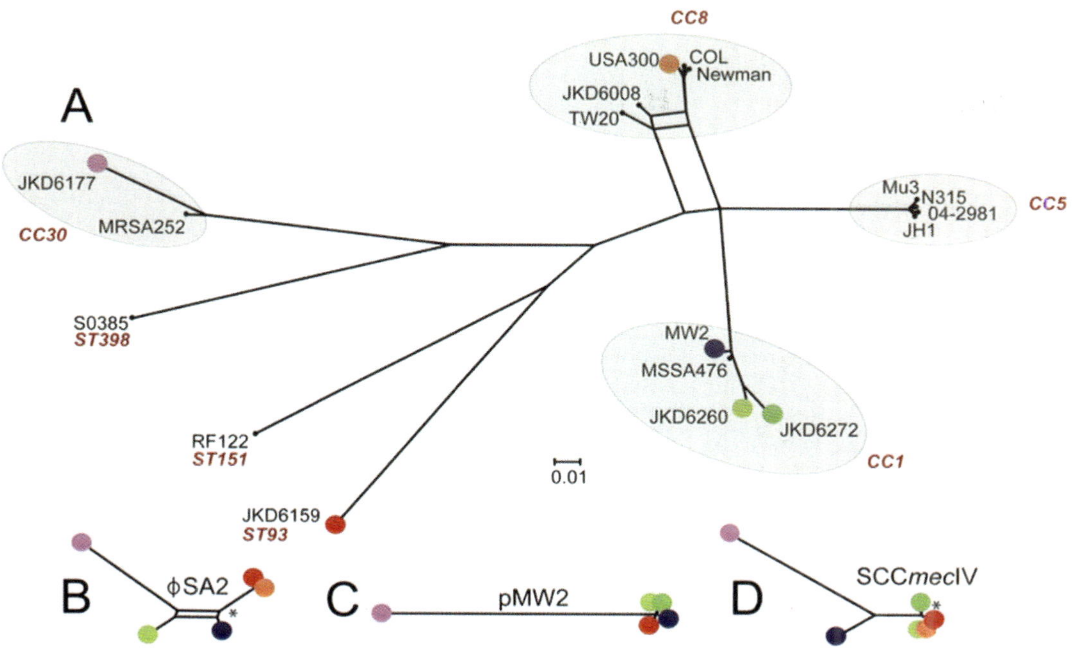

Figure 4. Phylogenetic analysis of *S. aureus* strains. Phylogenetic analysis based on the core genomes of *S. aureus* strains and selected accessory elements from CA-MRSA strains. (A) *S. aureus* phylogeny inferred by split decomposition analysis from pairwise comparisons of the 78,967 variable nucleotide positions identified from the core chromosome sequences of 20 completed *S. aureus* chromosomes and the 62 *S. aureus* strains for which unassembled reads were available, including the CA-MRSA strains sequenced in this study, JKD6177, JKD6260, JKD6272. CA-MRSA strains are indicated in colour (red JKD6159, pink JKD6177, orange FPR3757 USA300, blue MW2, light green JKD6260, dark green JKD6272) (B-D), Phylogenetic relationship of ϕSA2, pMW2 and SCC*mec*IV inferred by split decomposition analysis of nucleotide differences for each of these accessory elements between CA-MRSA strains. Scale bar indicates the number of nucleotide substitutions per site. All nodes have 100% bootstrap support except those indicated by asterisk (*) which have >60% support (1000 replicates). CC: clonal complex. ST: sequence type.

The accessory genome of JKD6159 also contained 12 regions not present in the 19 other published, complete *S. aureus* genomes. These regions spanned 40,776 bp of the chromosome. The 32 CDS contained therein are listed in Table S2 and lie within segments identified as Regions 1–12 (Figure 3B, Table S2). JKD6159 also contained two copies of a Group II intron (Regions 6 & 11) that to our knowledge is the first example of this type of mobile DNA element in *S. aureus*.

As expected from its antibiotic phenotype, JKD6159 had few antibiotic resistance elements. It contained the SCC*mec*IV element found in other CA-MRSA strains but it did not have the adjacent arginine catabolic mobile element (ACME) seen in USA300. JKD6159 contained a *bla* operon located on a plasmid. This plasmid was identical to pMW2 and pSAS (from MSSA476). This plasmid was also highly similar to that carried on other community *S. aureus* strains including pWBG757 (NCBI Accession GQ900397.1), pSAP073A (NCBI Accession GQ900425.1), pWBG763 (NCBI Accession GQ900467.1), and pWBG750 (NCBI Accession GQ900392.1). Other mobile DNA present in JKD6159 included six intact copies and four partial copies of the insertion sequence element IS*Sau*3.

Comparison of JKD6159 with other CA-MRSA

Comparisons of JKD6159 with the three other complete, publicly available genomes of CA-MRSA (MW2, USA300 FPR3757, USA300 TCH1516) [37,38,39], and the unassembled sequences for CA-MRSA strains JKD6272, JKD6260 & JKD6177, highlighted ϕSA2, pMW2 and SCC*mec*IV as elements common to these CA-MRSA strains, although JKD6272 did not contain ϕSA2, the phage bearing *lukSF-PV* required for expression of Panton Valentine Leukocidin (PVL). While high-resolution phylogenomic analysis based on SNP comparisons of the 2,302,644 bp *S. aureus* core genome demonstrated that some of these strains were distantly related to each other (Figure 4A), the same analysis based on SNP comparisons of only the accessory elements identified more limited sequence differences and produced individual tree topologies that suggested all strains except JKD6177 had recently acquired these elements (Figure 4B-C). Most striking was the limited sequence diversity among SCC*mec*, with 0.4 SNPs/100 bp for all CA-MRSA strains compared with 3.4 SNPs/100 bp across the entire chromosome for the same set of strains. These data are consistent with the contemporary acquisition of SSC*mec* by these diverse strains from a common source and the recent emergence of the global CA-MRSA phenomenon.

Discussion

ST93 MRSA is now the most common CA-MRSA clone in Australia [14]. The reasons for its recent emergence are unknown but this increase is consistent with a worldwide spread of other global CA-MRSA clones. ST93 MRSA causes severe clinical disease that appears to mimic USA300. Little is known about ST93 although MLST and other typing methods have shown that ST93 is distinct to other *S. aureus* clones [16]. To understand the genetic basis for its recent emergence, we have compared both the virulence and genome of a recent clinical ST93 MRSA isolate (JKD6159) with other CA-MRSA including USA300.

We have demonstrated that ST93-IV [2B] was highly virulent in both the *Galleria* larvae virulence assay and mouse skin infection model. We used the *Galleria* model as a screening assay and validated our results in the mouse skin infection model. The *Galleria* killing assay has been previously used to assess the virulence of *S. aureus* [23,40]. *Galleria mellonella* larvae are easily reared to large numbers, they can be maintained at 37°C and the assay gives consistently reproducible results. Furthermore, whilst the precise mechanisms by which *S. aureus* kills *Galleria* larvae remain uncertain, our *Galleria* assay time-to-death rates were comparable to the more conventional BALB/c mouse skin infection results. The skin infection assay was chosen because it approximates the most common disease presentation associated with the ST93 clone. The mouse skin infection model is a well-validated model and the histological lesions that result from staphylococcal infection are comparable to human staphylococcal skin infection [3,4,7,8,9]. The murine model for staphylococcal infections has some limitations in that mouse neutrophils are less susceptible to the effects of PVL than human and rabbit neutrophils [5,10,41]. Nonetheless, the pathology of murine skin infection caused by *S. aureus* is similar to that seen in rabbit staphylococcal skin infection [42].

While the whole genome sequence of JKD6159 demonstrated a relative paucity of recognizable virulence determinants, this ST93 strain did contain genes encoding the three most important CA-MRSA virulence factors, namely Hla, PVL and α-type PSMs [4,5,6,7,8,10]. Given that we found few novel genes and no apparent candidates within these to explain the observed heightened virulence of JKD6159, it is possible that there are small genetic changes such as SNPs which lead to regulatory changes and therefore altered gene expression that are the reason for the observed increased virulence of JKD6159 compared to other CA-MRSA including USA300. These subtle mutations could impact known global regulators such as *agr*, or even other regulatory systems including sRNAs. The importance of SNPs that alter gene expression has been previously demonstrated in USA300 [12]. Investigations are underway to determine the relative contribution of SNPs to the enhanced virulence of JKD6159 using large-scale comparative genomics and virulence assessment approaches. Experiments are also in progress to determine the relative expression of Hla, PVL and α-type PSMs in ST93 compared to other CA-MRSA clones.

Because recent studies by others using *spa* gene high-resolution melt curve profiles have demonstrated genetic diversity within ST93 [43], we are currently examining additional methicillin-susceptible and methicillin-resistant ST93 isolates to determine whether the observations reported here in JKD6159 are representative of ST93 as a whole. In addition to assessing the generalizability of our findings, these studies will also be used to exploit any phenotypic differences we find through more extensive comparative and functional genomics to further enhance our understanding of the molecular basis for the emergence and enhanced virulence of ST93 CA-MRSA.

Our implementation of DNA sequence read mapping enabled us to accurately define at the nucleotide level, the core and accessory genome of *S. aureus* JKD6159. This approach is not biased by decisions based on orthology of protein coding sequences (CDS) and enables more precise quantification of differences and similarities between genomes. In this manner we demonstrated that the accessory genome constitutes between 13.2% [RF122] to 18.1% [JH1 and JKD6159] of the *S. aureus* chromosome. Read mapping also uncovered that JKD6159 shared elements with other CA-MRSA namely the PVL phage ϕSA2, pMW2 and SCC*mec*IV.

Comparative genomics supports the association previously reported between PVL and genetically disparate CA-MRSA *S. aureus* clones, and hence suggests a possible role for the PVL-containing phage in the emergence of community *S. aureus* infections. The PVL toxin has been associated epidemiologically with severe clinical presentations such as necrotizing pneumonia [44]. The laboratory evidence for its importance has focused on its role in staphylococcal virulence and the results of these studies are seemingly contradictory [3,4,5,9,45,46]. We found that JKD6159 (PVL positive) showed the highest comparative virulence in both animal models (Figure 2). Interestingly, the PVL negative clone JKD6272 was as virulent as the other non-ST93 PVL strains including USA300, suggesting that the enhanced virulence of JKD6159 in our animal models may be PVL independent. The role of PVL and other genes encoded on ϕSA2 in dissemination and spread of *S. aureus* remains frustratingly uncertain.

Overall, the close relationship among distinct accessory genome elements including ϕSA2, pMW2 and SCC*mec*IV, in otherwise distantly related global *S. aureus* strains (which are separated by large distances in space and time) is an intriguing finding, and indicates the very recent acquisition of these elements from a common source by horizontal gene transfer. This association infers, but does not prove, a possible role for these elements in the fitness-for-spread and virulence of these strains in the community. These observations also suggest there are common strong selective pressures acting on genetically diverse *S. aureus* populations that are driving these specific gene acquisition events. These factors merit further investigation as they may hold clues for control of this global public health problem.

Supporting Information

Figure S1 Growth rates of *S. aureus* strains. Comparative growth rates of *S. aureus* strains used in this study, showing no significant differences in growth characteristics between the strains.

Table S1 Published, incomplete *S. aureus* genome sequences used in this study and mean read coverage against *S. aureus* JKD6159.

Table S2 Genomic Regions of Difference (1) - (12) in *S. aureus* strain ST93 JKD6159 compared to other non-ST93 *S. aureus* strains.

Acknowledgments

Aspects of this research were reported at the 14th International Symposium on Staphylococci and Staphylococcal Infections, Bath, UK, September 2010. We thank Elizabeth Grabsch, Daniel Martin and Russell Goodman for technical assistance in the preparation of this manuscript.

Author Contributions

Conceived and designed the experiments: TPS BPH. Performed the experiments: KYLC TPS TS PFH SM. Analyzed the data: KYLC BPH TPS TS PFH. Contributed reagents/materials/analysis tools: TMK PDRJ GWC BOH JKD. Wrote the paper: KYLC BPH TPS TS JKD GWC.

References

1. David MZ, Daum RS (2010) Community-associated methicillin-resistant *Staphylococcus aureus*: epidemiology and clinical consequences of an emerging epidemic. Clin Microbiol Rev 23: 616–687.

2. Moran GJ, Krishnadasan A, Gorwitz RJ, Fosheim GE, McDougal LK, et al. (2006) Methicillin-resistant *S. aureus* infections among patients in the emergency department. N Engl J Med 355: 666–674.

3. Voyich JM, Otto M, Mathema B, Braughton KR, Whitney AR, et al. (2006) Is Panton-Valentine leukocidin the major virulence determinant in community-associated methicillin-resistant *Staphylococcus aureus* disease? J Infect Dis 194: 1761–1770.
4. Labandeira-Rey M, Couzon F, Boisset S, Brown EL, Bes M, et al. (2007) *Staphylococcus aureus* Panton-Valentine leukocidin causes necrotizing pneumonia. Science 315: 1130–1133.
5. Diep BA, Chan L, Tattevin P, Kajikawa O, Martin TR, et al. (2010) Polymorphonuclear leukocytes mediate *Staphylococcus aureus* Panton-Valentine leukocidin-induced lung inflammation and injury. Proc Natl Acad Sci U S A 107: 5587–5592.
6. Bubeck Wardenburg J, Bae T, Otto M, Deleo FR, Schneewind O (2007) Poring over pores: alpha-hemolysin and Panton-Valentine leukocidin in *Staphylococcus aureus* pneumonia. Nat Med 13: 1405–1406.
7. Wang R, Braughton KR, Kretschmer D, Bach TH, Queck SY, et al. (2007) Identification of novel cytolytic peptides as key virulence determinants for community-associated MRSA. Nat Med 13: 1510–1514.
8. Li M, Diep BA, Villaruz AE, Braughton KR, Jiang X, et al. (2009) Evolution of virulence in epidemic community-associated methicillin-resistant *Staphylococcus aureus*. Proc Natl Acad Sci U S A 106: 5883–5888.
9. Brown EL, Dumitrescu O, Thomas D, Badiou C, Koers EM, et al. (2009) The Panton-Valentine leukocidin vaccine protects mice against lung and skin infections caused by *Staphylococcus aureus* USA300. Clin Microbiol Infect 15: 156–164.
10. Li M, Cheung GY, Hu J, Wang D, Joo HS, et al. (2010) Comparative analysis of virulence and toxin expression of global community-associated methicillin-resistant *Staphylococcus aureus* strains. J Infect Dis 202: 1866–1876.
11. Chambers HF, Deleo F (2009) Waves of resistance: *Staphylococcus aureus* in the antibiotic era. Nat Rev Micro 7: 629–641.
12. Kennedy AD, Otto M, Braughton KR, Whitney AR, Chen L, et al. (2008) Epidemic community-associated methicillin-resistant *Staphylococcus aureus:* recent clonal expansion and diversification. Proc Natl Acad Sci U S A 105: 1327–1332.
13. Munckhof WJ, Schooneveldt J, Coombs GW, Hoare J, Nimmo GR (2003) Emergence of community-acquired methicillin-resistant *Staphylococcus aureus* (MRSA) infection in Queensland, Australia. Int J Infect Dis 7: 259–264.
14. Coombs GW, Nimmo GR, Pearson JC, Christiansen KJ, Bell JM, et al. (2009) Prevalence of MRSA strains among *Staphylococcus aureus* isolated from outpatients, 2006. Commun Dis Intell 33: 10–20.
15. Peleg AY, Munckhof WJ, Kleinschmidt SL, Stephens AJ, Huygens F (2005) Life-threatening community-acquired methicillin-resistant *Staphylococcus aureus* infection in Australia. Eur J Clin Microbiol Infect Dis 24: 384–387.
16. Coombs GW, Nimmo GR, Bell JM, Huygens F, O'Brien FG, et al. (2004) Genetic diversity among community methicillin-resistant *Staphylococcus aureus* strains causing outpatient infections in Australia. J Clin Microbiol 42: 4735–4743.
17. Ellington MJ, Ganner M, Warner M, Boakes E, Cookson BD, et al. (2010) First international spread and dissemination of the virulent Queensland community-associated methicillin-resistant *Staphylococcus aureus* strain. Clin Microbiol Infect 16: 1009–1012.
18. Lina G, Piemont Y, Godail-Gamot F, Bes M, Peter MO, et al. (1999) Involvement of Panton-Valentine leukocidin-producing *Staphylococcus aureus* in primary skin infections and pneumonia. Clin Infect Dis 29: 1128–1132.
19. Enright MC, Day NP, Davies CE, Peacock SJ, Spratt BG (2000) Multilocus sequence typing for characterization of methicillin-resistant and methicillin-susceptible clones of *Staphylococcus aureus*. Journal of Clinical Microbiology 38: 1008–1015.
20. Horne KC, Howden BP, Grabsch EA, Graham M, Ward PB, et al. (2009) Prospective comparison of the clinical impacts of heterogeneous vancomycin-intermediate methicillin-resistant *Staphylococcus aureus* (MRSA) and vancomycin-susceptible MRSA. Antimicrob Agents Chemother 53: 3447–3452.
21. Coombs GW, Monecke S, Ehricht R, Slickers P, Pearson JC, et al. (2010) Differentiation of clonal complex 59 community-associated methicillin-resistant *Staphylococcus aureus* in Western Australia. Antimicrob Agents Chemother 54: 1914–1921.
22. International Working Group on the Classification of Staphylococcal Cassette Chromosome Elements (IWG-SCC) (2009) Classification of staphylococcal cassette chromosome *mec* (SCC*mec*): guidelines for reporting novel SCC*mec* elements. Antimicrob Agents Chemother 53: 4961–4967.
23. Gao W, Chua K, Davies JK, Newton HJ, Seemann T, et al. (2010) Two novel point mutations in clinical *Staphylococcus aureus* reduce linezolid susceptibility and switch on the stringent response to promote persistent infection. PLoS Pathog 6: e1000944.
24. Rasband WS (1997–2011) ImageJ. U S National Institutes of Health, Bethesda, Maryland, USA, available at http:/imagejnihgov/ij/, accessed 9 December 2009.
25. Chua K, Seemann T, Harrison PF, Davies JK, Coutts SJ, et al. (2010) Complete genome sequence of *Staphylococcus aureus* strain JKD6159, a unique Australian clone of ST93-IV community methicillin-resistant *Staphylococcus aureus*. J Bacteriol 192: 5556–5557.
26. Zerbino DR, Birney E (2008) Velvet: algorithms for de novo short read assembly using de Bruijn graphs. Genome Res 18: 821–829.
27. Rumble SM, Lacroute P, Dalca AV, Fiume M, Sidow A, et al. (2009) SHRiMP: accurate mapping of short color-space reads. PLoS Comput Biol 5: e1000386.
28. Carver TJ, Rutherford KM, Berriman M, Rajandream MA, Barrell BG, et al. (2005) ACT: the Artemis Comparison Tool. Bioinformatics 21: 3422–3423.
29. Huson DH, Bryant D (2006) Application of phylogenetic networks in evolutionary studies. Mol Biol Evol 23: 254–267.
30. Fitzgerald JR, Sturdevant DE, Mackie SM, Gill SR, Musser JM (2001) Evolutionary genomics of *Staphylococcus aureus*: insights into the origin of methicillin-resistant strains and the toxic shock syndrome epidemic. Proc Natl Acad Sci U S A 98: 8821–8826.
31. Lindsay JA, Holden MT (2004) *Staphylococcus aureus*: superbug, super genome? Trends Microbiol 12: 378–385.
32. Vandenesch F, Naimi T, Enright MC, Lina G, Nimmo GR, et al. (2003) Community-acquired methicillin-resistant *Staphylococcus aureus* carrying Panton-Valentine leukocidin genes: worldwide emergence. Emerg Infect Dis 9: 978–984.
33. Foster TJ (2005) Immune evasion by staphylococci. Nat Rev Microbiol 3: 948–958.
34. Voyich JM, Braughton KR, Sturdevant DE, Whitney AR, Said-Salim B, et al. (2005) Insights into mechanisms used by *Staphylococcus aureus* to avoid destruction by human neutrophils. J Immunol 175: 3907–3919.
35. Murray NE (2000) Type I restriction systems: sophisticated molecular machines (a legacy of Bertani and Weigle). Microbiol Mol Biol Rev 64: 412–434.
36. Corvaglia AR, Francois P, Hernandez D, Perron K, Linder P, et al. (2010) A type III-like restriction endonuclease functions as a major barrier to horizontal gene transfer in clinical *Staphylococcus aureus* strains. Proc Natl Acad Sci U S A 107: 11954–11958.
37. Baba T, Takeuchi F, Kuroda M, Yuzawa H, Aoki K, et al. (2002) Genome and virulence determinants of high virulence community-acquired MRSA. Lancet 359: 1819–1827.
38. Diep BA, Gill SR, Chang RF, Phan TH, Chen JH, et al. (2006) Complete genome sequence of USA300, an epidemic clone of community-acquired meticillin-resistant *Staphylococcus aureus*. Lancet 367: 731–739.
39. Highlander SK, Hulten KG, Qin X, Jiang H, Yerrapragada S, et al. (2007) Subtle genetic changes enhance virulence of methicillin resistant and sensitive *Staphylococcus aureus*. BMC Microbiol 7: 99.
40. Peleg AY, Monga D, Pillai S, Mylonakis E, Moellering RC, Jr., et al. (2009) Reduced susceptibility to vancomycin influences pathogenicity in *Staphylococcus aureus* infection. J Infect Dis 199: 532–536.
41. Loffler B, Hussain M, Grundmeier M, Bruck M, Holzinger D, et al. (2010) *Staphylococcus aureus* panton-valentine leukocidin is a very potent cytotoxic factor for human neutrophils. PLoS Pathog 6: e1000715.
42. Kobayashi SD, Malachowa N, Whitney AR, Braughton KR, Gardner DJ, et al. (2011) Comparative Analysis of USA300 Virulence Determinants in a Rabbit Model of Skin and Soft Tissue Infection. J Infect Dis 204: 937–941.
43. Tong SY, Lilliebridge RA, Holt DC, McDonald MI, Currie BJ, et al. (2009) High-resolution melting analysis of the spa locus reveals significant diversity within sequence type 93 methicillin-resistant *Staphylococcus aureus* from northern Australia. Clin Microbiol Infect 15: 1126–1131.
44. Gillet Y, Issartel B, Vanhems P, Fournet JC, Lina G, et al. (2002) Association between *Staphylococcus aureus* strains carrying gene for Panton-Valentine leukocidin and highly lethal necrotising pneumonia in young immunocompetent patients. Lancet 359: 753–759.
45. Bubeck Wardenburg J, Palazzolo-Ballance AM, Otto M, Schneewind O, DeLeo FR (2008) Panton-Valentine leukocidin is not a virulence determinant in murine models of community-associated methicillin-resistant *Staphylococcus aureus* disease. J Infect Dis 198: 1166–1170.
46. Diep BA, Palazzolo-Ballance AM, Tattevin P, Basuino L, Braughton KR, et al. (2008) Contribution of Panton-Valentine leukocidin in community-associated methicillin-resistant *Staphylococcus aureus* pathogenesis. PLoS One 3: e3198.
47. Howden BP, Stinear TP, Allen DL, Johnson PD, Ward PB, et al. (2008) Genomic analysis reveals a point mutation in the two-component sensor gene *graS* that leads to intermediate vancomycin resistance in clinical *Staphylococcus aureus*. Antimicrob Agents Chemother 52: 3755–3762.
48. Gillaspy AF, Worrell V, Orvis J, Roe BA, Dyer DW, et al. (2006) The *Staphylococcus aureus* NCTC 8325 Genome. In: Fischetti VA, Novick RP, Ferretti JJ, Portnoy DA, Rood JI, eds. Gram Positive Pathogens: ASM Press. pp 381–412.
49. Kuroda M, Ohta T, Uchiyama I, Baba T, Yuzawa H, et al. (2001) Whole genome sequencing of meticillin-resistant *Staphylococcus aureus*. Lancet 357: 1225–1240.
50. Neoh HM, Cui L, Yuzawa H, Takeuchi F, Matsuo M, et al. (2008) Mutated response regulator graR is responsible for phenotypic conversion of *Staphylococcus aureus* from heterogeneous vancomycin-intermediate resistance to vancomycin-intermediate resistance. Antimicrob Agents Chemother 52: 45–53.
51. Holden MT, Feil EJ, Lindsay JA, Peacock SJ, Day NP, et al. (2004) Complete genomes of two clinical *Staphylococcus aureus* strains: evidence for the rapid evolution of virulence and drug resistance. Proc Natl Acad Sci U S A 101: 9786–9791.
52. Herron-Olson L, Fitzgerald JR, Musser JM, Kapur V (2007) Molecular correlates of host specialization in *Staphylococcus aureus*. PLoS One 2: e1120.
53. Baba T, Bae T, Schneewind O, Takeuchi F, Hiramatsu K (2008) Genome sequence of *Staphylococcus aureus* strain Newman and comparative analysis of staphylococcal genomes: polymorphism and evolution of two major pathogenicity islands. J Bacteriol 190: 300–310.
54. Gill SR, Fouts DE, Archer GL, Mongodin EF, Deboy RT, et al. (2005) Insights on evolution of virulence and resistance from the complete genome analysis of

an early methicillin-resistant *Staphylococcus aureus* strain and a biofilm-producing methicillin-resistant *Staphylococcus epidermidis* strain. J Bacteriol 187: 2426–2438.
55. Mwangi MM, Wu SW, Zhou Y, Sieradzki K, de Lencastre H, et al. (2007) Tracking the in vivo evolution of multidrug resistance in *Staphylococcus aureus* by whole-genome sequencing. Proc Natl Acad Sci U S A 104: 9451–9456.
56. Lowder BV, Guinane CM, Ben Zakour NL, Weinert LA, Conway-Morris A, et al. (2009) Recent human-to-poultry host jump, adaptation, and pandemic spread of *Staphylococcus aureus*. Proc Natl Acad Sci U S A 106: 19545–19550.
57. Holden MT, Lindsay JA, Corton C, Quail MA, Cockfield JD, et al. (2010) Genome sequence of a recently emerged, highly transmissible, multi-antibiotic- and antiseptic-resistant variant of methicillin-resistant *Staphylococcus aureus*, sequence type 239 (TW). J Bacteriol 192: 888–892.
58. Nubel U, Dordel J, Kurt K, Strommenger B, Westh H, et al. (2010) A timescale for evolution, population expansion, and spatial spread of an emerging clone of methicillin-resistant *Staphylococcus aureus*. PLoS Pathog 6: e1000855.
59. Schijffelen MJ, Boel CH, van Strijp JA, Fluit AC (2010) Whole genome analysis of a livestock-associated methicillin-resistant *Staphylococcus aureus* ST398 isolate from a case of human endocarditis. BMC Genomics 11: 376.
60. Howden BP, Seemann T, Harrison PF, McEvoy CR, Stanton JA, et al. (2010) Complete genome sequence of *Staphylococcus aureus* strain JKD6008, an ST239 clone of methicillin-resistant *Staphylococcus aureus* with intermediate-level vancomycin resistance. J Bacteriol 192: 5848–5849.

4

Antibacterial Activity and Mechanism of a Scorpion Venom Peptide Derivative *In Vitro* and *In Vivo*

Luyang Cao[9], Chao Dai[9], Zhongjie Li, Zheng Fan, Yu Song, Yingliang Wu, Zhijian Cao*, Wenxin Li*

State Key Laboratory of Virology, College of Life Sciences, Wuhan University, Wuhan, P. R. China

Abstract

BmKn2 is an antimicrobial peptide (AMP) characterized from the venom of scorpion *Mesobuthus martensii* Karsch by our group. In this study, Kn2-7 was derived from BmKn2 to improve the antibacterial activity and decrease hemolytic activity. Kn2-7 showed increased inhibitory activity against both Gram-positive bacteria and Gram-negative bacteria. Moreover, Kn2-7 exhibited higher antibacterial activity against clinical antibiotic-resistant strains such as methicillin-resistant *Staphylococcus aureus* (MRSA). In addition, the topical use of Kn2-7 effectively protected the skin of mice from infection in an *S. aureus* mouse skin infection model. Kn2-7 exerted its antibacterial activity via a bactericidal mechanism. Kn2-7 killed *S. aureus* and *E. coli* rapidly by binding to the lipoteichoic acid (LTA) in the *S. aureus* cell wall and the lipopolysaccharides (LPS) in the *E. coli* cell wall, respectively. Finally, the hemolytic activity of Kn2-7 was significantly decreased, compared to the wild-type peptide BmKn2. Taken together, the Kn2-7 peptide can be developed as a topical therapeutic agent for treating bacterial infections.

Editor: Paulo Lee Ho, Instituto Butantan, Brazil

Funding: This work was supported by grants from Natural Science Foundation of China (NSFC) (No. 31071942), the China Specific Project for Developing New Drugs (Nos. 2009ZX09103-612 and 2011ZX09102-001-32), and the National Basic Research Program of China (Nos. 2010CB529800 and 2010CB530100). The funders had no role in study design, data collection and analysis, decision to publish, or preparation of the manuscript.

Competing Interests: The authors have declared that no competing interests exist.

* E-mail: zjcao@whu.edu.cn (ZC); liwxlab@whu.edu.cn (WL)

9 These authors contributed equally to this work.

Introduction

Drug resistance poses an increasing threat to global public health, and new antibiotic-resistant pathogens have continued to emerge [1,2]. Methicillin-resistant *Staphylococcus aureus* (MRSA) is considered one of the most threatening pathogens due to the high mortality rate and increased medical costs associated with treating it. [3,4]. New types of antimicrobial agents are urgently needed to respond to the threat of pathogens that evolve resistance against conventional antibiotics [5].

AMPs are distributed among a wide range of species, including insects, plants, humans, and even single-celled organisms [6]. The structures of AMPs generally present highly amphiphilic topologies, in which hydrophilic and hydrophobic side chains are located on opposite faces of the molecule [7,8]. These peptides are potent antimicrobial agents against bacteria, fungi, viruses, and parasites, and several AMPs have been reported to inhibit the growth of MRSA [9,10,11]. Their broad spectrum activity and low potential to induce resistance make AMPs an attractive family of compounds with the potential to be developed as therapeutics agents. During the last decade, several antimicrobial peptides have been investigated as therapeutic agents [12,13].

Scorpion venom contains a diversity of bioactive peptides that represent a tremendous resource for use in drug design and development [14,15]. Moreover, several AMPs have been found in scorpion venom, including hadrurin [16], scorpine [17], opistoporins, parabutoporin [18], ISCTs [19], mucroporin [9] and StCT1 [20]. These scorpion venom peptides commonly exhibit cytolysis or microbial inhibition functions.

In a previous study by our group, we characterized an antimicrobial peptide, BmKn2, derived from the venom of the scorpion *Mesobuthus martensii* Karsch [21]. In the present study, a derivative of BmKn2, was designed to increase the antibacterial activity and reduce the hemolytic activity. Kn2-7 showed increased inhibitory activity against both Gram-positive bacteria and Gram-negative bacteria in contrast to BmKn2. Meanwhile, Kn2-7 could inhibit HIV-1 by direct interaction with viral particle [22]. Moreover, the hemolytic activity of Kn2-7 was significantly lower than that of BmKn2. In addition, Kn2-7 exhibited higher antibacterial activity against clinical antibiotic-resistant strains. Topical application of Kn2-7 effectively protected skin from infection in an *S. aureus* mouse skin infection model. Finally, the antibacterial mechanism of Kn2-7 was clarified in this study.

Results

Antimicrobial Screening of BmKn2 Derivatives

Seven BmKn2-derived peptides were designed based on the amino acid sequence of BmKn2 (Figure 1A). The secondary structures of BmKn2 and its mutants were predicted to be 100% α-helical in nature. The helical wheels of BmKn2 and its mutants were divided into two parts, and the hydrophobic face and the hydrophilic face were labeled (Figure 1B).

These peptides were used to determine the inhibitory activities against the representative Gram-positive bacteria *S. aureus* AB94004 and the representative Gram-negative bacteria *E. coli* AB94012. The antimicrobial functional screening results showed

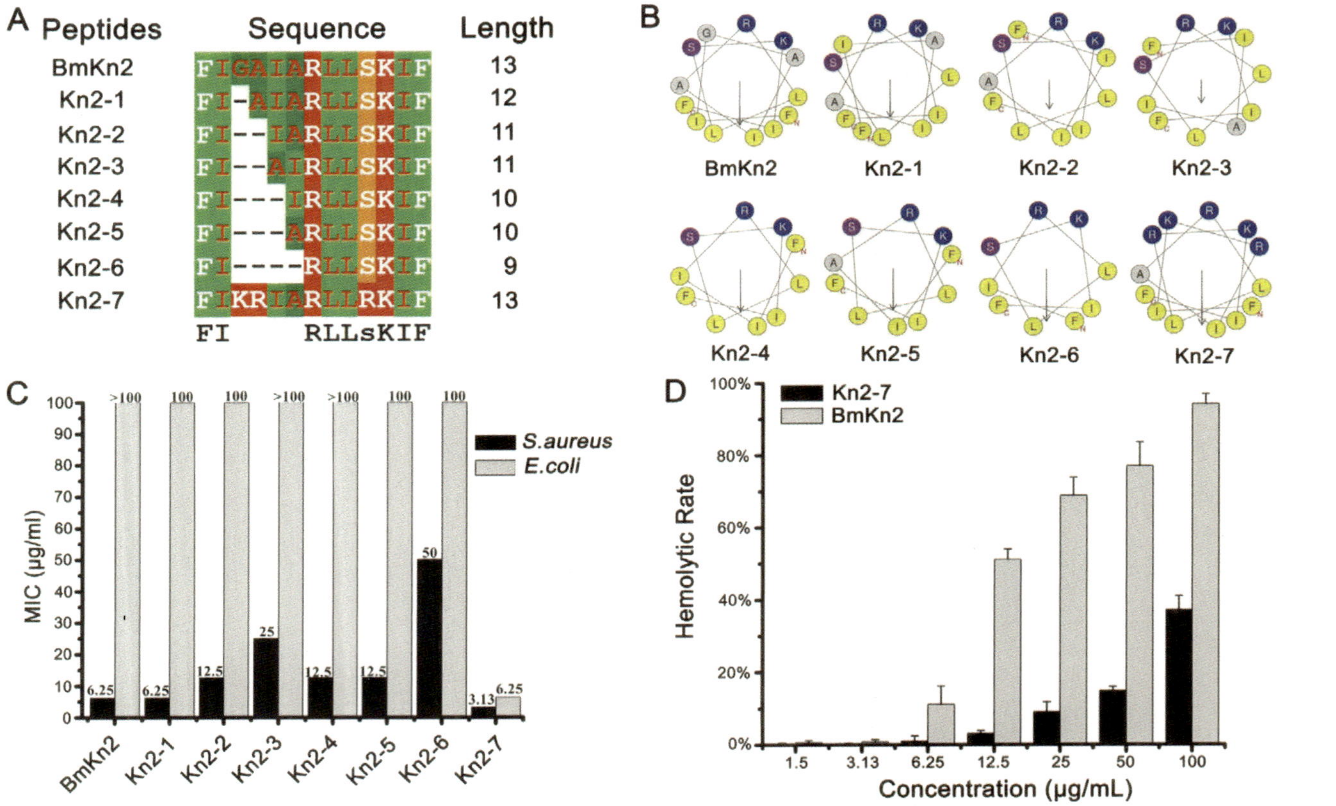

Figure 1. Screening, antimicrobial and hemolytic activities of Kn2-7 *in vitro*. (A) Multiple alignments of Kn2-7 and its seven derivatives. (B) Predicted secondary structure of Kn2-7 and its seven derivatives. (C) Antibacterial activity screening of Kn2-7 and its seven derivative peptides. (D) Hemolytic activity of Kn2-7. The hemolytic activities of the Kn2-7 and BmKn2 peptides were estimated by monitoring the increase in the absorbance at 570 nm after incubating human red blood cells with different peptide concentrations at 37 °C for 1 h. The positive control was 0.1% Triton X-100, and 0.85% saline was used as a blank.

that the Kn2-7 mutant exhibited the strongest inhibitory activity (Figure 1C).

The peptide Kn2-7 had little hemolytic activity at high concentration (Figure 1D). According to the method of Käber modified by Achmarine, the HC_{50} values of the mutant peptide Kn2-7 and the wild-type peptide BmKn2 were 90.27 μg/mL and 17.13 μg/mL, respectively (Figure 1D). Therefore, the hemolytic activity of Kn2-7 was significantly decreased, compared to the wild-type peptide BmKn2.

In Vitro Antibacterial Activity of Kn2-7

In view of the *in vitro* antibacterial activity of Kn2-7, we selected it as the object of further study. Kn2-7 not only exhibited enhanced inhibitory activity against both Gram-positive bacteria and Gram-negative bacteria in contrast to wild-type BmKn2 (Table 1).

The antibiotic-resistant pathogens used in this study were clinical isolates, all of which were tested with corresponding antibiotics to verify their resistance prior to conducting experiments. As shown in Table 2, Kn2-7 was more effective against the antibiotic-resistant pathogens than the wild-type BmKn2.

Kn2-7 was not only able to inhibit the growth of standard strains, but it was also able to effectively inhibit the growth of clinically isolated antibiotic-resistant strains. As shown in Figure 2, at a concentration of MICs, Kn2-7 and BmKn2 both inhibited the growth of *S. aureus* completely. Additionally, Kn2-7 and BmKn2

Table 1. MICs of Kn2-7 against Gram-positive and Gram-negative strains.

Strains	MIC (μg/mL)	
	Kn2-7	BmKn2
Gram-positive bacteria		
S. aureus AB94004	3.13	6.25
S. aureus ATCC 25923	3.13	6.25
B. subtilis AB91021	6.25	12.5
B. thuringiensis AB92037	6.25	12.5
M. luteus AB93113	6.25	6.25
Gram-negative bacteria		
E. coli AB94012	6.25	>100
E. coli ATCC 25922	25	>100
P. aeruginosa AB93066	25	50
P. aeruginosa A092994	50	>100
P. aeruginosa A093052	100	>100
P. aeruginosa A093056	50	>100
P. aeruginosa A093085	50	>100
P. aeruginosa A093115	100	>100

Table 2. MICs of Kn2-7 against clinical isolated antibiotic-resistant bacterial strains.

Strains	MIC (μg/mL)				
	Kn2-7	BmKn2	Vancomycin	Penicillin	Cefotaxime
Penicillin resistant					
P1383	6.25	12.5	6.25	10000	6.25
P1389	6.25	12.5	6.25	10000	3.13
Methicillin resistant					
P1374	3.13	12.5	6.25	5000	400
P1369	3.13	12.5	6.25	20000	400
P1381	6.25	12.5	3.13	5000	400
P1386	6.25	12.5	3.13	10000	100
Penicillin sensitive					
P1111	3.13	6.25	3.13	25	6.25

All strains were clinical isolates obtained from the 302nd Military Hospital, Beijing, China. All data are from experiments that were repeated at least three times with an MIC of no greater than 2 fold.

inhibited the growth of MRSA P1386 completely. At a concentration of 6.25 μg/mL, the mutant peptide Kn2-7 and kanamycin both inhibited the growth of *E. coli* AB94012, while the wild-type BmKn2 peptide had no effect against *E. coli* AB94012.

In Vivo Antibacterial Activity of Kn2-7

To determine the *in vivo* antibacterial activity of Kn2-7, an *S. aureus* mouse skin infection model was established. After infection, the mice were observed daily. As shown in Figure 3A, one day after infection, the skin of the mice in the group treated with Kn2-7 had become scabbed over, while the wounded skin sections of the group treated with placebo were wet and presented with blistering. Additionally, blisters and light tissue fluid leakage could be observed in the wounded skin sections of the group that was not treated. Four days after infection, the skin sections of the group treated with Kn2-7 were healed, and their scabs were desquamated. However, the blisters in the skin sections in the group treated with placebo became larger. Furthermore, the skin sections exhibited a great amount of tissue fluid leakage in the group without treatment.

A group of mice was euthanized 4 hours after infection, and their skin viable counts were measured as a control. Other groups were euthanized 4 days after infection. As shown in Figure 3B, the colony counts in mice treated with the peptide Kn2-7 were clearly lower than those of the placebo-treated mice and the mice that were untreated.

The histological morphology of the skin sections was observed. As shown in Figure 3C, most of the epidermis of the scratched skin sections was defective, while other parts of the skin were normal compared to normal skin with intact structure. Four days after the skin of the mice was scratched, the epidermis recovered, and the biopsy specimens were observed to be normal. Four days after infection, the untreated group and the group treated with placebo lost nearly all of their epidermis, and the dermis was infected to a certain extent. However, the skin sections treated with Kn2-7 recovered almost fully and presented nearly intact structures.

Antibacterial Mechanism

Secondary structure analysis. As shown in Figure 4A and Figure 4B, Kn2-7 and the wild-type peptide BmKn2 displayed

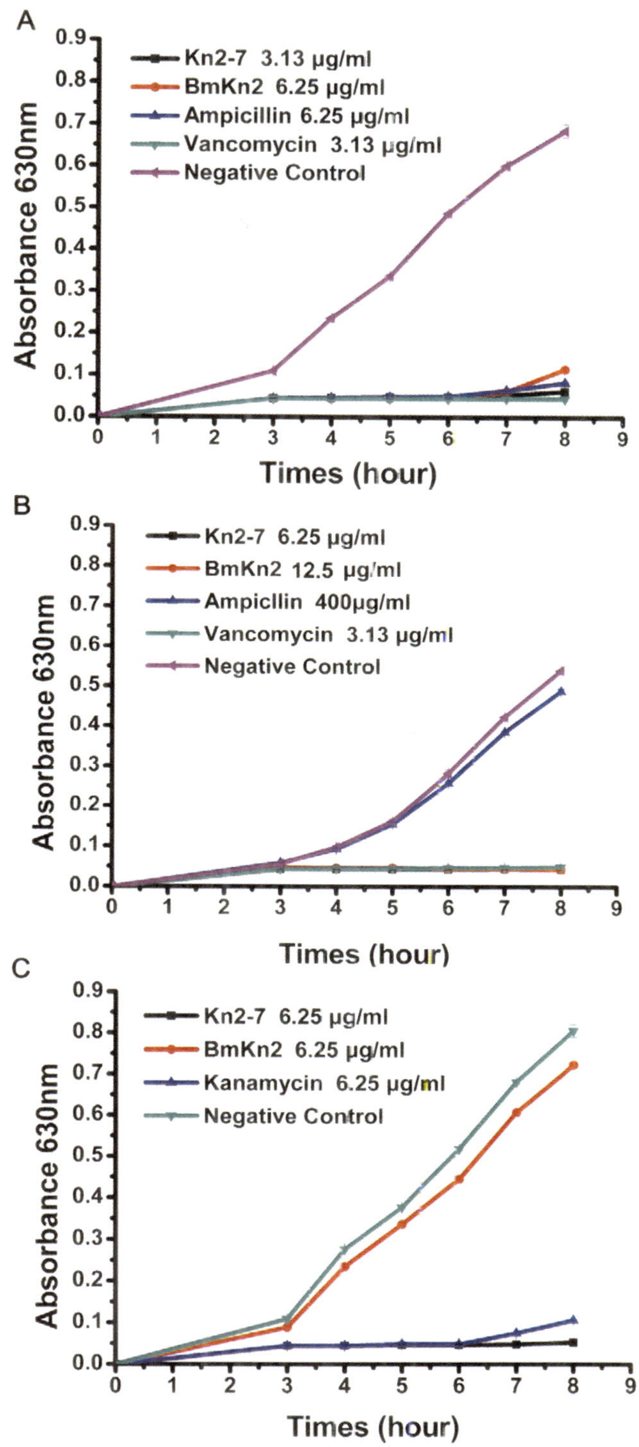

Figure 2. Gowth inhibitory activities of Kn2-7. (A) Growth curves of *S. aureus* AB94004 treated with Kn2-7, BmKn2 or antibiotics. (B) Growth curves of MRSA P1386 treated with Kn2-7, BmKn2 or antibiotics. (C) Growth curves of *E. coli* AB94012 treated with Kn2-7, BmKn2 or antibiotics.

typical α-helical profiles in the structure-promoting solution TFE (30% and 70%). However, both Kn2-7 and BmKn2 displayed random coil profiles in water.

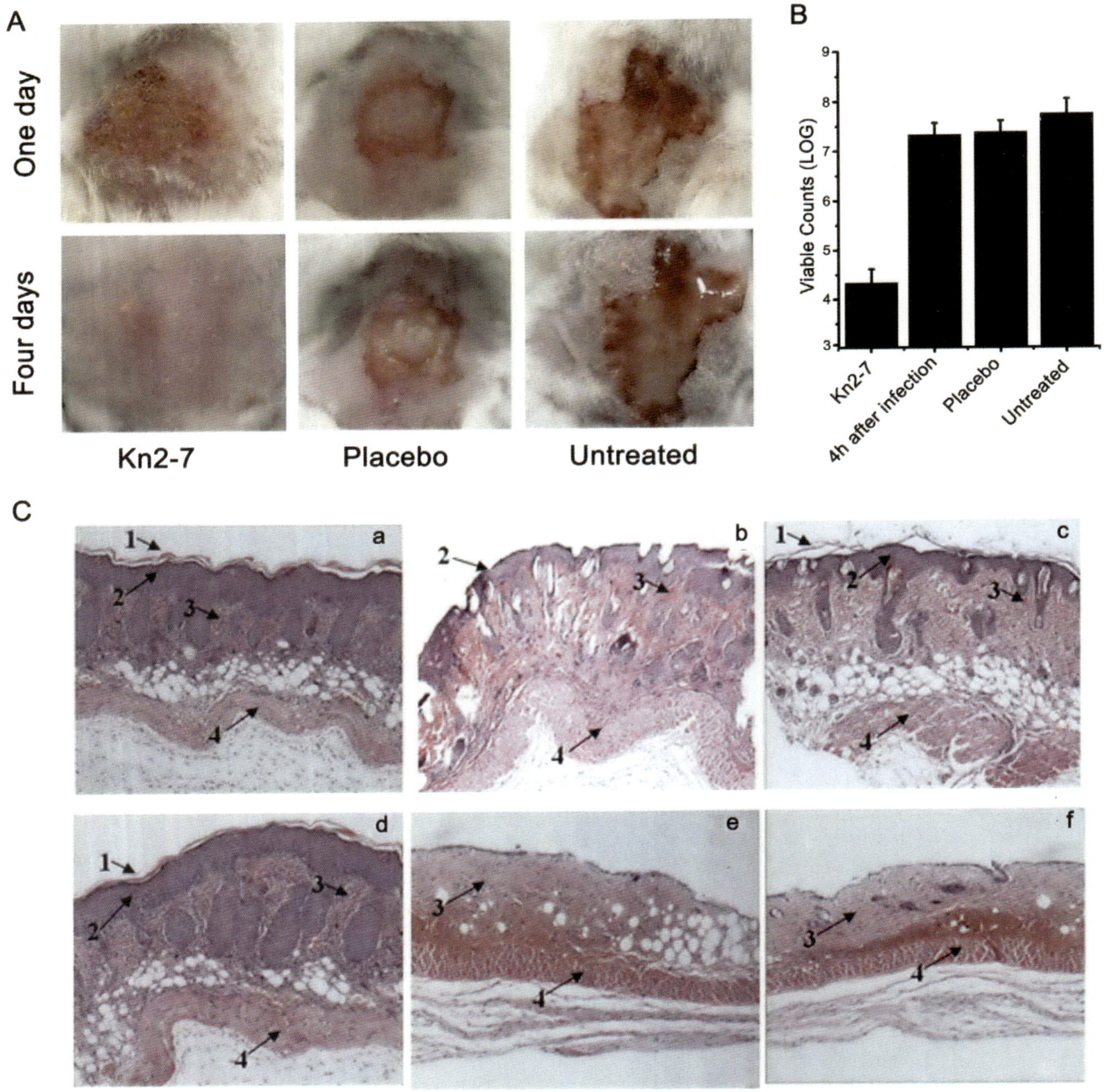

Figure 3. ***In vivo*** **antibacterial activity of Kn2-7.** (A) Mice were observed after being treated with the peptide on days 1 and 4. (B) Cutaneous viable counts in treated mice. Eight mice per group were euthanized, and the viable counts of the surviving *S. aureus* bacteria were then determined. (C) Histological morphologies of the skin in treated mice. (a) Normal dorsal skin of mice. (b) Immediately after the skin was scratched. (c) Four days after the skin was scratched. (d) Four days after *S. aureus* infection in skin treated with Kn2-7. (e) Four days after *S. aureus* infection in skin treated with BmKn2. (f) Four days after *S. aureus* infection in skin treated with a placebo. (g) Four days after *S. aureus* infection in untreated skin. Numbered arrows indicate the following: 1, corneum; 2, epidermis; 3, dermis; and 4, muscular layer.

Enzyme release assay of Kn2-7. The enzymatic activities of the supernatants were measured via an enzyme release assay immediately after treatment with Kn2-7 or BmKn2. As shown in Figure 4C, the supernatant from *S. aureus* AB94004 treated with ampicillin exhibited increasing catalase activity over time. However, the supernatant treated with Kn2-7 or BmKn2 showed almost the same catalase activity at each time point. As shown in Figure 4D, the supernatant from *E. coli* AB94012 treated with kanamycin presented increasing catalase activity over time. However, the supernatant treated with Kn2-7 showed nearly the same high enzymatic activity at each time point. In contrast, the supernatant treated with the wild-type peptide BmKn2 showed low catalase activity at each time point and did not exhibit increasing catalase activity over time.

Bactericidal effect of Kn2-7. Kn2-7 exerted bactericidal effects on both *S. aureus* AB94004 and *E. coli* AB94012. As shown in Figure 5A and Figure 5B, when the peptide concentration increased, the killing rate also increased. Additionally, Kn2-7 was

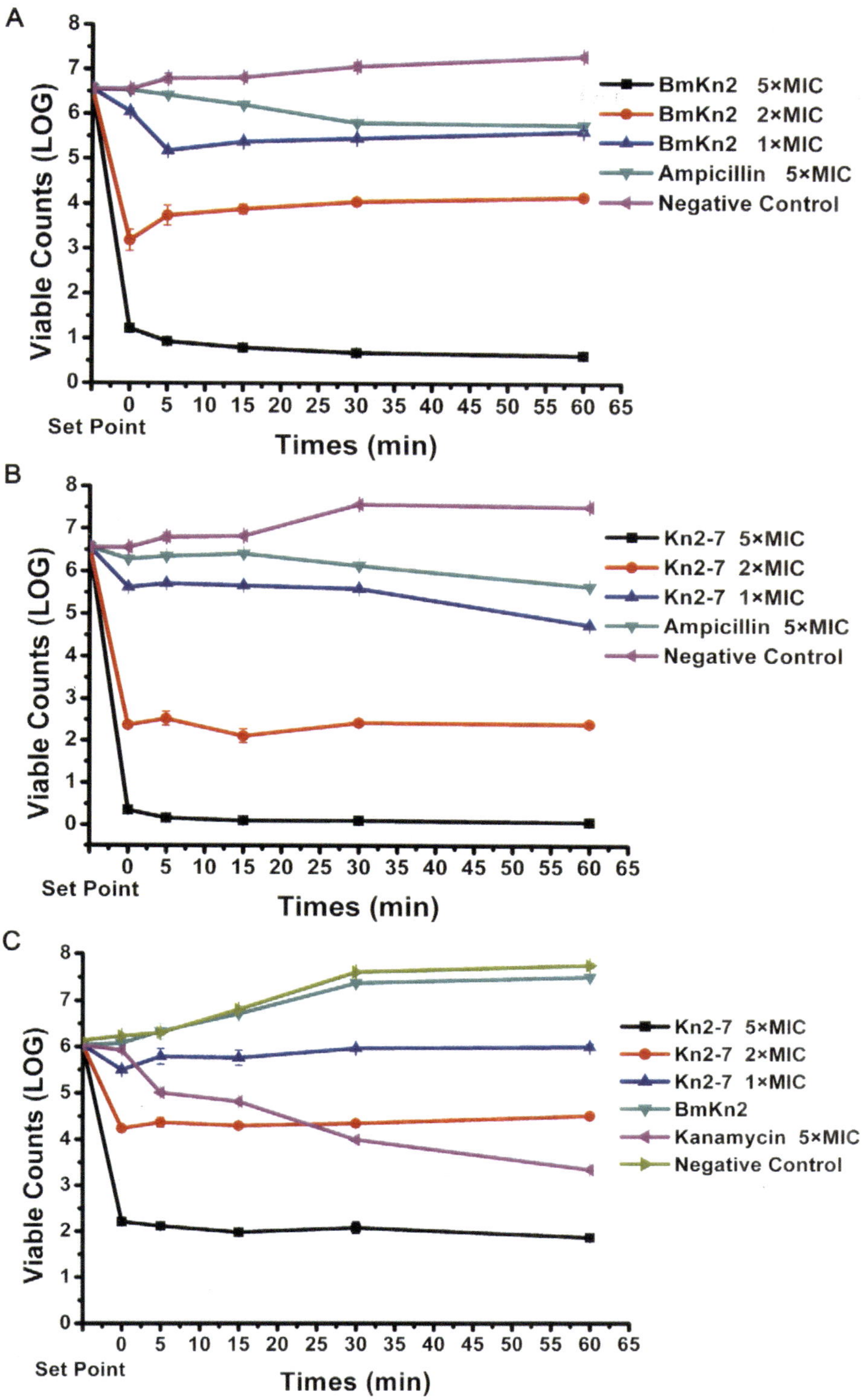

Figure 4. Secondary structure and enzyme release assay of Kn2-7. (A) and (B) Secondary structure analysis of the Kn2-7 and BmKn2 peptides. (A) Circular dichroism spectra of 0.1 mg/mL of Kn2-7 in water, 30% TFE/H_2O or 70% TFE/H_2O. (B) Circular dichroism spectra of 0.1 mg/mL of BmKn2 in water, 30% TFE/H_2O or 70% TFE/H_2O. (C) and (D) Enzyme release assay. (C) *S. aureus* AB94004 treated with Kn2-7 or BmKn2 was harvested, and the catalase activities of the supernatants were measured; 0.9% saline was used as the negative control, and ampicillin sodium was used as the antibiotic control. (D) *E. coli* AB94012 treated with Kn2-7 or BmKn2 was harvested, and the catalase activities in the supernatants were measured; 0.9% saline was used as the negative control, and kanamycin was used as the antibiotic control.

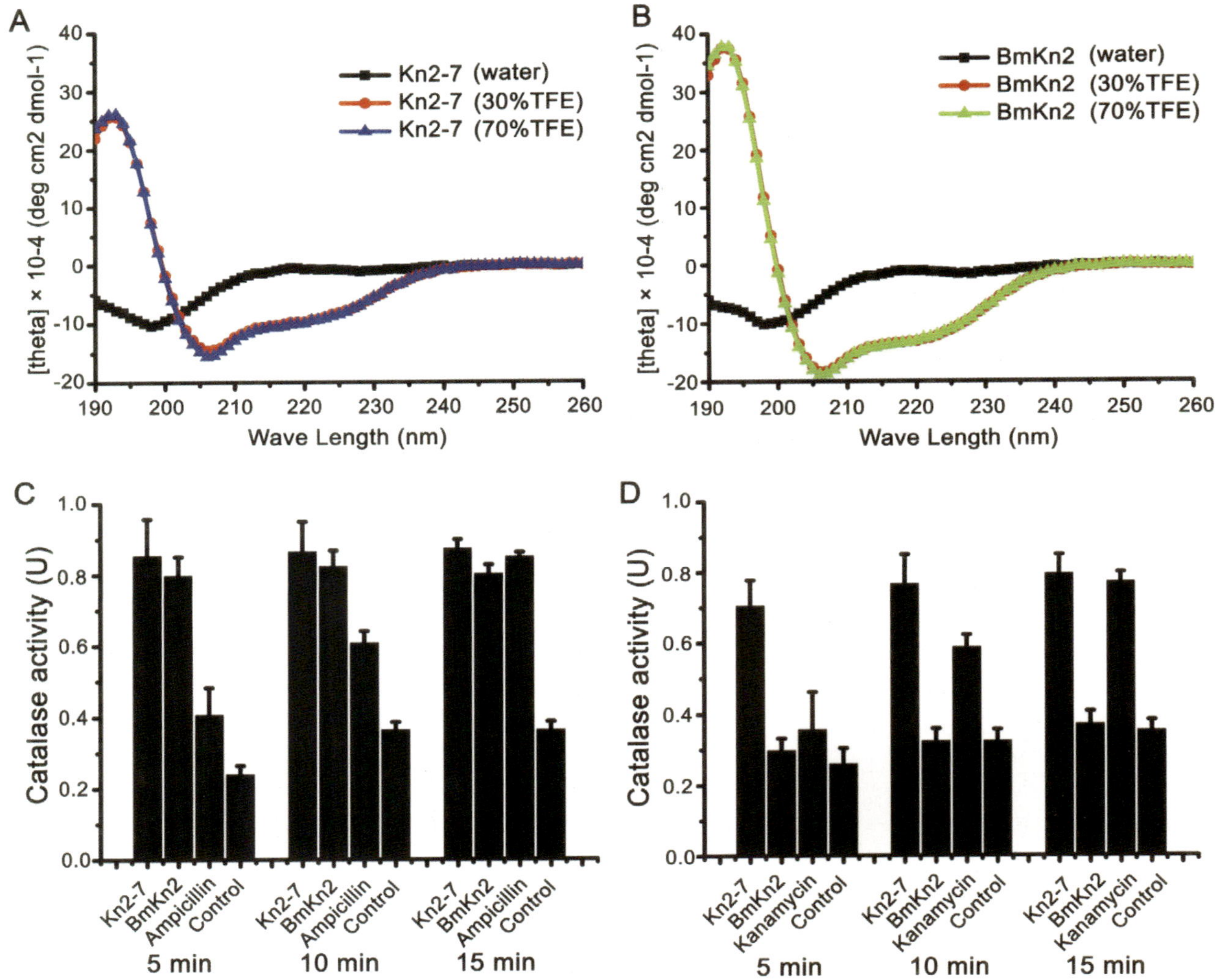

Figure 5. Bactericidal assays of the Kn2-7 and BmKn2 peptides against *S. aureus* and *E. coli* AB94012. Set point indicates untreated bacteria, and 0 minutes was defined as the time of the first sample collection, which was immediately after mixing bacteria and Kn2-7 or BmKn2. The other samples were collected at 5 min, 15 min, 30 min or 60 min. All of the counts were the average of three dishes, and the experiment was repeated at least three times. (A) Time-killing curve of Kn2-7 against *S. aureus* AB94004. (B) Time-killing curve of BmKn2 against *S. aureus* AB94004. (C) Time-killing curve of Kn2-7 against *E. coli* AB94012.

able to kill *E. coli* AB94012 rapidly, whereas the wild-type peptide BmKn2 was not able to kill *E. coli* AB94012 (Figure 5C).

Transmission electron microscopy. Semi-thin sections of *S. aureus* AB94004 and *E. coli* AB94012 treated with Kn2-7 or BmKn2 were prepared to observe the structural changes in the cell walls and membranes of the bacteria (Figure 6). Cracks were observed in the cell walls of the bacteria. Additionally, membrane disruption was observed in the peptide-treated bacteria. Furthermore, semi-thin sections of bacteria treated with Kn2-7 or BmKn2 showed that there was a release of cell content upon cell wall disruption. As shown in Figure 5B, BmKn2 had no effect against *E. coli* AB94012. However, Kn2-7 accumulated on the surface of *E. coli* AB94012, combined with the cell wall and membrane, and then formed microspheres that surrounded the bacteria.

Biolayer interferometry. BLI was performed to identify the target of Kn2-7 in *S. aureus* and *E. coli*. LTA is the main component of the peptidoglycan layer surrounding Gram-positive bacteria, while LPS is the main component of the cell wall surrounding Gram-negative bacteria. As shown in Figure 7A and Figure 7B, curve B3 and curve E3 indicated that the designed peptide Kn2-7 bound strongly to LTA, as did the wild-type peptide BmKn2. Meanwhile, curve A3 and curve D3 indicated that only the Kn2-7 mutant was able to bind to LPS, while wild-type BmKn2 could not. LTA confer a portion of the negative charge associated with the peptidoglycans Gram-positive bacteria, and LPS confer a portion of the negative charge associated with the outer membrane surrounding Gram-negative bacteria, respectively.

LTA and LPS competition binding assay. To confirm the results of the BLI titrations, 250 μg/mL of Kn2-7 or BmKn2 was mixed with an equal volume of 1 mg/mL LTA or LPS. Then, the MICs of Kn2-7 or BmKn2 mixed with LTA against *S. aureus* and *E. coli* were measured. As shown in Figure 7C, the MICs of Kn2-7 and BmKn2 against *S. aureus* AB94004 were 3.13 and 6.25 μg/mL, respectively. The MIC of the Kn2-7 against *E. coli* AB94012 was 6.25 μg/mL. LTA and LPS exhibit no inhibitory activity against *S. aureus* or *E. coli*. The MICs of Kn2-7 and BmKn2 treated

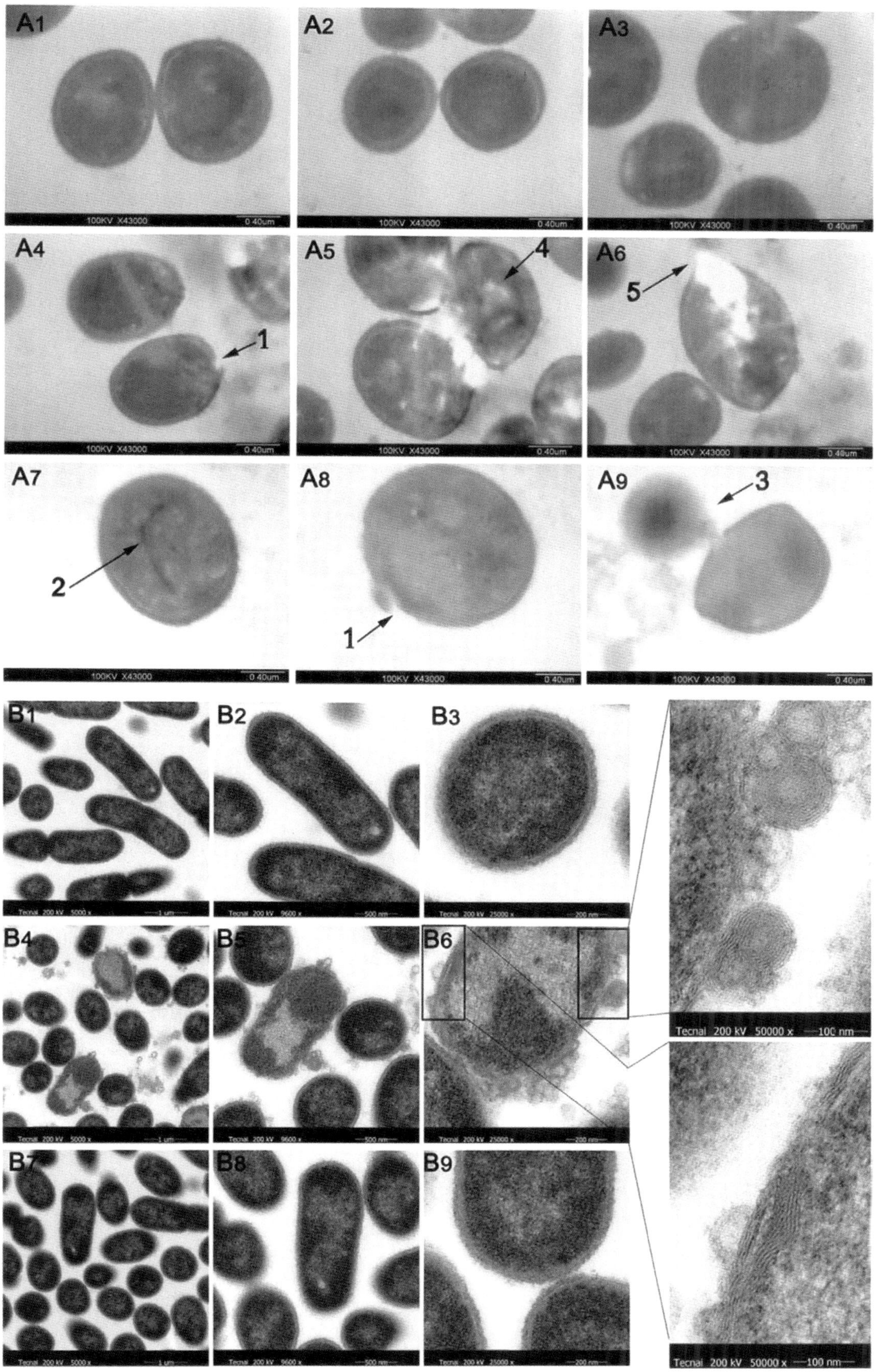
A1
A2
A3
A4
A5
A6
A7
A8
A9
1
4
5
2
1
3
100KV X43000
0.40um
B1
B2
B3
B4
B5
B6
B7
B8
B9
Tecnai 200 kV 50000 x 100 nm

Figure 6. Transmission electron microscopy of *S. aureus* and *E. coli* treated with Kn2-7. (A) Transmission electron microscopy was performed with Kn2-7-treated *S. aureus*. (A1), (A2) and (A3) were negative controls. (A4), (A5) and (A6) show *S. aureus* treated with Kn2-7 for 2 min. (A7), (A8) and (A9) show *S. aureus* treated with BmKn2 for 2 min. (B) Transmission electron microscopy was performed with Kn2-7-treated *E. coli*. (B1), (B2) and (B3) were the negative controls. (B4), (B5) and (B6) show *E. coli* treated with Kn2-7 for 2 min. (B7), (B8) and (B9) show *E. coli* treated with BmKn2 for 2 min.

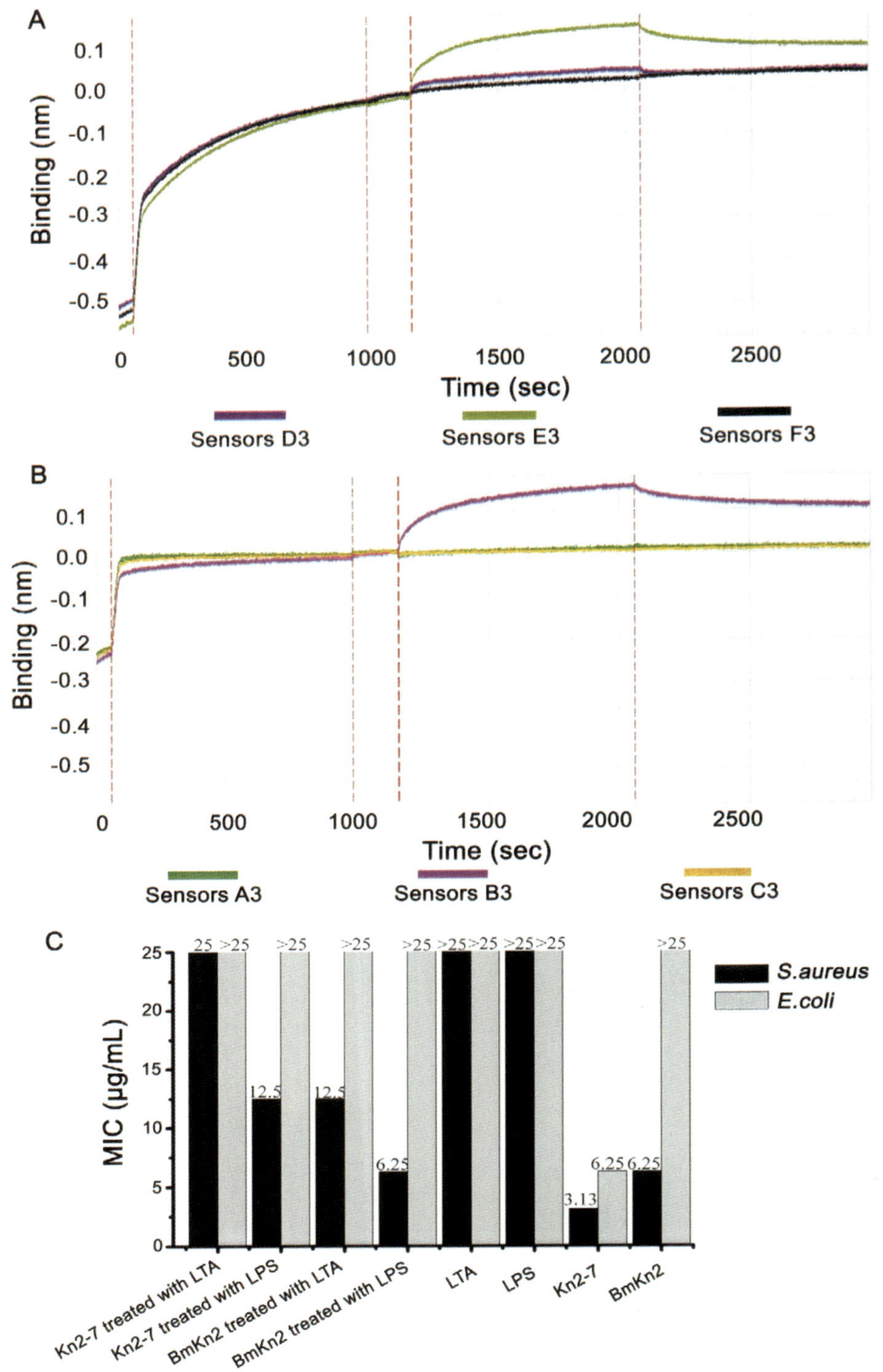

Figure 7. Binding assay of Kn2-7 and LTA or LPS. (A) Interaction of 10 µg/ml of Kn2-7 with 500 µg/ml of LPS or 500 µg/mL of LTA. Curve A3 is LPS, curve B3 is LTA and curve C3 is buffer. (B) Interaction of 10 µg/mL of BmKn2 with 500 µg/mL of LPS or 500 µg/mL of LTA. Curve D3 is LPS, curve E3 is LTA and curve F3 is the buffer. (C) MICs of Kn2-7 and BmKn2 treated with LTA or LPS against *S. aureus* and *E. coli*.

with LTA against *S. aureus* were 25 and 12.5 μg/mL, respectively. The MIC of Kn2-7 treated with LTA against *E. coli* AB94012 was at least 25 μg/mL. Meanwhile, the MICs of the Kn2-7 and BmKn2 treated with LPS against *S. aureus* were 12.5 and 6.25 μg/mL, respectively, and the MIC of the Kn2-7 mutant treated with LPS against *E. coli* was at least 25 μg/mL. All of these results further confirmed that both the Kn2-7 and BmKn2 peptides bind to LTA, but only the mutant Kn2-7 peptide was able to bind to LPS.

Discussion

The structure-function relationship of some antimicrobial peptides has been analyzed to unravel the regular pattern of antibacterial activity, hemolytic activity and toxicity [23]. However, the regular patterns of antibacterial activity, hemolytic activity and toxicity have still need to be clarified. More recently, molecular design of antimicrobial peptides has become an important and attractive strategy for developing new antimicrobial drugs. In this study, six BmKn2-derived peptides were designed with the aim of increasing the proportion of polar residues at first. But the activity of the six deletion mutants did not improve. So Kn2-7 peptide was designed to increase the net positive charge of BmKn2 to improve its affinity for bacteria. The antibacterial activities of Kn2-7 were better than those of BmKn2. Moreover, Kn2-7 showed higher antibacterial activity than the other antimicrobial peptides identified from scorpion venoms to date [9,11,17,18,19,20]. Furthermore, the hemolytic activity of Kn2-7 reduced observably compared to the wild-type peptide BmKn2. High hemolytic activity is always an obstacle to the application of AMPs. Increasing the net positive charge of AMPs may be a good way to improve the high hemolytic activity. Topical application of Kn2-7 cured the skin of mice infected with *S. aureus*. Compared with conventional antibiotics, Kn2-7 has many advantages, such as broad-spectrum activities, rapid killing ability, low levels of induced resistance, and broad anti-inflammatory activities. Kn2-7 may have the therapeutic potential for topical use.

New AMPs have been continuously isolated and identified. Several bilayer interaction and disruption models have been proposed for those AMPs that depend on membrane interference for their antibacterial activity, such as "barrel-stave pore", "carpet mechanism", "toroidal pore" and "disordered toroidal pore" [24]. New molecular models has been proposed to describe the mechanism more accurately, such as "form ion channels" [25] and "internalization into the cytoplasm" [26]. In the present study, the results of secondary structure analysis, bactericidal assays, enzyme release assays provided solid evidence that the inhibitory effect of Kn2-7 on the bacteria was mediated through rapid killing. However, the binding mode of Kn2-7 to the surface of *E. coli* seems different from that of *S. aureus*. The results of biolayer interferometry and competition binding assay proved to be so. The findings of TEM indicated that the bacterial cell wall of *S. aureus* was disrupted immediately upon treatment with Kn2-7. Kn2-7 accumulated on the surface of *E. coli*, combined with the outer membrane, and then formed microspheres surrounded the bacteria. This mode is consistent with the model of carpet mechanism in general. To the best of our knowledge, the structures of the microspheres were first observed in the antibacterial mechanism study and our results provide conclusive evidence for the model of carpet mechanism.

AMPs have both a cationic and amphiphilic nature. Their positive net charge ensures that AMPs can accumulate at the surface of bacteria that contain anionic polymers, such as LTA and LPS. Then, these peptides interact with the membranes of the microbes, resulting in membrane disruption [27]. The results of BLI titrations and competition binding assays showed that Kn2-7 disrupted the cell walls of *S. aureus* and *E. coli* through binding to LTA and LPS, respectively. The question of why the mutant peptide Kn2-7 can bind to both LTA and LPS while the wild-type peptide BmKn2 can bind to only LTA is of particular interest. Kn2-7 has five net positive charges while BmKn2 only has two. Therefore we speculate that increasing the numbers of positively charged residues turned out to have improved the affinity to the bacterial surface.

In conclusion, we described both *in vitro* and *in vivo* antimicrobial activities of Kn2-7, a scorpion venom peptide derivative, against Gram-positive bacteria and Gram-negative bacteria including clinical isolates, MRSA, MRCNS, PRSA and PRSE. The antimicrobial and hemolytic activities of Kn2-7 peptide were notably improved compared to the wild-type peptide BmKn2. The binding mode of Kn2-7 to the surface of *E. coli* was different from that of *S. aureus*. The peptide Kn2-7 disrupted the cell surface structure of *S. aureus* and *E. coli* via binding to LTA and LPS, respectively. Taken together, these data strongly suggest that Kn2-7 peptide can be developed as a topical therapeutic agent for treating bacterial infections.

Materials and Methods

Strains

S. aureus AB94004, *S. aureus* ATCC 25923, *E. coli* AB94012, *E. coli* ATCC 25922, *Pseudomonas aeruginosa* AB93066, *Bacillus thuringiensis* AB92037, *Bacillus subtilis* AB91021, and *Micrococcus luteus* AB93113 were purchased from the China Center of Type Culture Collection (CCTCC).

Clinical isolated *Pseudomonas aeruginosa* strains A092994, A093052, A093056, A093085 and AC93115 were obtained from Hubei Maternal and Child Health Hospital.

Clinical isolates were obtained from the 302nd military hospital of Beijing, China, including penicillin-resistant *S. aureus* (PRSA) P1383, penicillin-resistant *S. epidermidis* (PRSE) P1389, methicillin-resistant *S. aureus* (MRSA) P1381, P1386 and P1374, methicillin-resistant coagulase-negative *Staphylococcus* (MRCNS) P1369, and penicillin-sensitive *S. epidermidis* (PSSE) P1111.

BmKn2 Derivatives and Chemical Synthesis

Six deleted mutants and one point mutant were designed with the aim of enhancing the net positive charge of the hydrophilic side of the peptide while maintaining the amphipathic character of the peptides. BmKn2 and the seven derivatives of this peptide noted above were synthesized with amidated C-termini by More Biotech (Wuhan) Ltd., China.

Hemolytic Activity

The hemolytic activities of Kn2-7 and BmKn2 peptides were tested against human red blood cells [9]. HC_{50} values were obtained according to the method of Käber, modified by Achmarine [28]. Saline solution at a concentration of 0.85% was used as the negative control, and 0.1% Triton X-100 was used as the positive control.

Antimicrobial Assays *in Vitro*

Minimum inhibitory concentration (MIC) analysis. The MIC was determined via a microdilution assay in 96-well microtiter plates according to the broth microdilution guideline of Clinical and Laboratory Standards Institute (CLSI) [29].

Growth inhibitory assay. The time growth curves of *S. aureus* and MRSA treated with BmKn2 or its derivatives were determined based on measurements taken at 630 nm at each time point. Different concentrations of peptide were added to the tested strains, which were cultured in 96-well plates using the same method as was used for determining the MIC.

Antimicrobial assays *in vivo*

Experimental animals. Female BALB/c mice weighing 18–20 g were purchased from the Hubei Research Center of Laboratory Animals. All animal studies were approved by the Institutional Animal Care and Use Committee of Wuhan University.

Gel preparation. Kn2-7 or BmKn2 was prepared in gel form in 0.5% hydroxypropylcellulose to a final concentration of 5 mg/mL.

Mouse skin abrasion and infection model. Mice were injected with 150 mg/kg of cyclophosphamide 4 days prior to infection. Subsequently, the mice were injected with 100 mg/kg of cyclophosphamide 1 day prior to infection. After being anesthetized, the dorsal skin of the mice was shaved, and abrasions were produced in a 1×1 cm^2 area using a blade. These abrasion wounds damaged only the stratum corneum and upper layer of the epidermis, but not the dermis. Five minutes later, the wounds were inoculated with 20 µl of *S. aureus* (10^7–10^8 CFUs) using a micropipettor. A group of mice was killed 4 h after infection to control for the infectious dose. Four hours after infection, the wounds of the other mice were smeared with 20 µl of 5 mg/mL gel or a placebo gel, which was used as a negative control. The treatment lasted for 4 days, with two peptide gel applications being performed daily (morning and evening at 8 h intervals). After 4 days of treatment, the mice were killed, and the wound area of the skin was immediately excised and homogenized. Suitable dilutions of the homogenates were plated on LB plates to determine the number of living bacteria (CFUs).

Histological examination. After the animals were euthanized, biopsy specimens of the excised wound area of the skin were collected and immediately fixed in phosphate-buffered formalin (10%, pH = 7.4). Then, the biopsy specimens were embedded in paraffin and stained with hematoxylin and eosin.

Statistical analysis. In each experiment, the mean CFU was calculated using $\log_{10}$-transformed data. Based on the averages of three experiments, the mean, range, and coefficient of variation were calculated.

Antibacterial Mechanism

Secondary structure analysis. The secondary structures of Kn2-7 and BmKn2 were analyzed using Heliquest (http://heliquest.ipmc.cnrs.fr/cgi-bin/ComputParams.py) and circular dichroism (CD) assays. The CD assay was performed at room temperature in nitrogen-flushed cells using a 2-mm path with a Jasco J-810 spectropolarimeter. Kn2-7 and BmKn2 were measured at concentrations of 0.1 mg/mL in water, 30% TFE/H_2O or 70% TFE/H_2O. The peptide configuration was obtained by analyzing the data with CD deconvolution software.

Enzyme release assay. Bacterial suspensions and serial-diluted peptides were mixed at a ratio of 4:1 in different tubes with a final volume of 2 ml. The mixtures were then incubated at 37°C with continuous shaking. At each time point, 200 µl of the treated bacterial suspension was transferred to sterilized tubes. After centrifugation, the supernatants were transferred to a sterilized 1.5-ml tube, and catalase activity was measured with a Catalase Assay Kit (Beyotime, Jiangsu, China) using the method for measuring peroxidase activity.

Bactericidal assay. Bactericidal curves for Kn2-7 and BmKn2 were determined against *S. aureus* AB94004 and *E. coli* AB94012. A 400 µl aliquot of the peptide solution was added to 1,600 µl of a bacterial suspension. At each time point, 200 µl of the treated bacterial suspension was transferred to a sterilized 1.5-ml tube. After centrifugation at $1{,}000\times g$ for 5 min, the supernatant was removed, and the pellet was resuspended in 200 µl of LB medium. The bacterial suspensions were placed on agar plates and incubated at 37°C until viable colonies could be counted.

Transmission electron microscopy. Overnight-cultured S. aureus AB94004 and E. coli AB94012 were transferred to LB medium and cultured to the exponential phase. A 200 µl aliquot of the peptide solution was added to 800 µl of the bacterial suspensions at the final concentration of 1×MIC. The samples were cut into semi-thin sections. Microscopy was performed using a HITACHI H-8100 Transmission Electron Microscope.

Biolayer Interferometry. Biolayer Interferometry (BLI) experiments were performed on OCT RED (FortéBio, Inc.). A total of 500 µg/mL of lipoteichoic acid from *S. aureus* (LTA, Sigma, L2515), lipopolysaccharides from *E. coli* (LPS, Sigma, L2880) or buffer (10 mM HEPES, pH 7.4 and 0.14 M NaCl) was dispensed into 96-well microtiter plates at a volume of 200 µl per well. The operating temperature was 30°C. Biosensor tips (FortéBio, Inc., Menlo Park, CA) were pre-wetted with the buffer for 60 seconds at baseline. Then, 10 µg/mL Biotin-Kn2-7 or Biotin-BmKn2 was loaded onto the biosensor tips for 900 seconds. Baseline 2 was subsequently established for 300 seconds. Dissociation of Kn2-7 or BmKn2 occurred for 900 seconds in the buffer. Data were generated automatically by the Octet® User Software (version 3.1) and were subsequently analyzed from the resultant text files using Excel 2000.

LTA and LPS competition binding assay. A total of 250 µg/mL of each peptide solution was mixed with an equal volume of 1 mg/mL of the LTA or LPS solution. Then, the MICs of BmKn2 and Kn2-7 treated with LTA or LPS against *S. aureus* AB94004 and *E. coli* AB94012 were measured.

Author Contributions

Conceived and designed the experiments: LC ZC CD. Performed the experiments: LC CD ZL ZF YS. Analyzed the data: LC ZC YW WL. Contributed reagents/materials/analysis tools: LC ZC YW WL. Wrote the paper: LC ZC.

References

1. Allen HK, Donato J, Wang HH, Cloud-Hansen KA, Davies J, et al. (2010) Call of the wild: antibiotic resistance genes in natural environments. Nat Rev Microbiol 8: 251–259.
2. Andersson DI, Hughes D (2010) Antibiotic resistance and its cost: is it possible to reverse resistance? Nat Rev Microbiol 8: 260–271.
3. Hebert C, Weber SG (2011) Common approaches to the control of multidrug-resistant organisms other than methicillin-resistant Staphylococcus aureus (MRSA). Infect Dis Clin North Am 25: 181–200.
4. Ippolito G, Leone S, Lauria FN, Nicastri E, Wenzel RP (2010) Methicillin-resistant Staphylococcus aureus: the superbug. Int J Infect Dis 14 Suppl 4: S7–11.
5. Brogden NK, Brogden KA (2011) Will new generations of modified antimicrobial peptides improve their potential as pharmaceuticals? Int J Antimicrob Agents 38: 217–225.
6. Maroti G, Kereszt A, Kondorosi E, Mergaert P (2011) Natural roles of antimicrobial peptides in microbes, plants and animals. Res Microbiol 162: 363–374.
7. Godballe T, Nilsson LL, Petersen PD, Jenssen H (2011) Antimicrobial beta-peptides and alpha-peptoids. Chem Biol Drug Des 77: 107–116.
8. Zasloff M (2002) Antimicrobial peptides of multicellular organisms. Nature 415: 389–395.

9. Dai C, Ma Y, Zhao Z, Zhao R, Wang Q, et al. (2008) Mucroporin, the first cationic host defense peptide from the venom of Lychas mucronatus. Antimicrob Agents Chemother 52: 3967–3972.
10. Mygind PH, Fischer RL, Schnorr KM, Hansen MT, Sonksen CP, et al. (2005) Plectasin is a peptide antibiotic with therapeutic potential from a saprophytic fungus. Nature 437: 975–980.
11. Zhao Z, Ma Y, Dai C, Zhao R, Li S, et al. (2009) Imcroporin, a new cationic antimicrobial peptide from the venom of the scorpion Isometrus maculates. Antimicrob Agents Chemother 53: 3472–3477.
12. Fjell CD, Hancock RE, Cherkasov A (2007) AMPer: a database and an automated discovery tool for antimicrobial peptides. Bioinformatics 23: 1148–1155.
13. Jenssen H, Hamill P, Hancock RE (2006) Peptide antimicrobial agents. Clin Microbiol Rev 19: 491–511.
14. Fan S, Sun Z, Jiang D, Dai C, Ma Y, et al. (2010) BmKCT toxin inhibits glioma proliferation and tumor metastasis. Cancer Lett 291: 158–166.
15. Ma Y, Zhao R, He Y, Li S, Liu J, et al. (2009) Transcriptome analysis of the venom gland of the scorpion Scorpiops jendeki: implication for the evolution of the scorpion venom arsenal. BMC Genomics 10: 290.
16. Torres-Larios A, Gurrola GB, Zamudio FZ, Possani LD (2000) Hadrurin, a new antimicrobial peptide from the venom of the scorpion Hadrurus aztecus. Eur J Biochem 267: 5023–5031.
17. Conde R, Zamudio FZ, Rodriguez MH, Possani LD (2000) Scorpine, an anti-malaria and anti-bacterial agent purified from scorpion venom. FEBS Lett 471: 165–168.
18. Moerman L, Bosteels S, Noppe W, Willems J, Clynen E, et al. (2002) Antibacterial and antifungal properties of alpha-helical, cationic peptides in the venom of scorpions from southern Africa. Eur J Biochem 269: 4799–4810.
19. Dai L, Yasuda A, Naoki H, Corzo G, Andriantsiferana M, et al. (2001) IsCT, a novel cytotoxic linear peptide from scorpion Opisthacanthus madagascariensis. Biochem Biophys Res Commun 286: 820–825.
20. Yuan W, Cao L, Ma Y, Mao P, Wang W, et al. (2010) Cloning and functional characterization of a new antimicrobial peptide gene StCT1 from the venom of the scorpion Scorpiops tibetanus. Peptides 31: 22–26.
21. Zeng XC, Wang SX, Zhu Y, Zhu SY, Li WX (2004) Identification and functional characterization of novel scorpion venom peptides with no disulfide bridge from Buthus martensii Karsch. Peptides 25: 143–150.
22. Chen Y, Cao L, Zhong M, Zhang Y, Han C, et al. (2012) Anti-HIV-1 Activity of a New Scorpion Venom Peptide Derivative Kn2–7. PLoS One 7: e34947.
23. Fjell CD, Hiss JA, Hancock RE, Schneider G (2012) Designing antimicrobial peptides: form follows function. Nat Rev Drug Discov 11: 37–51.
24. Melo MN, Ferre R, Castanho MA (2009) Antimicrobial peptides: linking partition, activity and high membrane-bound concentrations. Nat Rev Microbiol 7: 245–250.
25. Paulmann M, Arnold T, Linke D, Ozdirekcan S, Kopp A, et al. (2012) Structure-activity analysis of the dermcidin-derived peptide DCD-1L, an anionic antimicrobial peptide present in human sweat. J Biol Chem.
26. Mochon AB, Liu H (2008) The antimicrobial peptide histatin-5 causes a spatially restricted disruption on the Candida albicans surface, allowing rapid entry of the peptide into the cytoplasm. PLoS Pathog 4: e1000190.
27. Brogden KA (2005) Antimicrobial peptides: pore formers or metabolic inhibitors in bacteria? Nat Rev Microbiol 3: 238–250.
28. Kirillov LV (1976) [Method of quantitative determination of vaccine activity against botulism of the mink]. Dev Biol Stand 32: 203–209.
29. Hou Z, Lu J, Fang C, Zhou Y, Bai H, et al. (2011) Underlying mechanism of in vivo and in vitro activity of C-terminal-amidated thanatin against clinical isolates of extended-spectrum beta-lactamase-producing Escherichia coli. J Infect Dis 203: 273–282.

5

Distribution of Staphylococcal Cassette Chromosome mec Types and Correlation with Comorbidity and Infection Type in Patients with MRSA Bacteremia

Jiun-Ling Wang[1,2*¶], Jann-Tay Wang[1¶], Shey-Ying Chen[3], Yee-Chun Chen[1], Shan-Chwen Chang[1*]

1 Department of Internal Medicine, National Taiwan University Hospital, National Taiwan University, Taipei, Taiwan, **2** Department of Internal Medicine, E-Da Hospital/I-Shou University, Kaohsiung County, Taiwan, **3** Department of Emergency Medicine, National Taiwan University Hospital, National Taiwan University, Taipei, Taiwan

Abstract

Background: Molecular epidemiological definitions that are based on staphylococcal cassette chromosome *mec* (SCC*mec*) typing and phylogenetic analysis of methicillin-resistant Staphylococcus aureus (MRSA) isolates are considered a reliable way to distinguish between healthcare-associated MRSA (HA-MRSA) and community-associated MRSA (CA-MRSA). However, there is little information regarding the clinical features and outcomes of bacteremia patients with MRSA carrying different SCC*mec* types.

Methods: From January 1 through December 31, 2006, we recorded the demographic data and outcomes of 159 consecutive adult MRSA bacteremia patients from whom isolates for SCC*mec* analysis were collected. All participants were patients at a tertiary care center in Taiwan.

Principal Findings: The following SCC*mec* types were identified in MRSA isolates: 30 SCC*mec* II (18.9%), 87 SCC*mec* III (54.7%), 22 SCC*mec* IV (13.8%), and 20 SCC*mec* V (12.6%). The time from admission to the first MRSA-positive blood culture for patients infected with isolates with the SCC*mec* III element (mean/median, 50.7/26 days) was significantly longer than for patients infected with isolates carrying SCC*mec* IV or V (mean/median, 6.7/3 days for SCC*mec* IV; 11.1/10.5 days for SCC*mec* V) ($P<0.05$). In univariate analysis, community onset, soft tissue infection, and deep-seated infection were predictors for SCC*mec* IV/V. In multivariate analysis, length of stay before index culture, diabetes mellitus, and being bedridden were independent risk factors associated with SCC*mec* II/III.

Conclusions: These findings are in agreement with previous studies of the genetic characteristics of CA-MRSA. MRSA bacteremia with SCC*mec* II/III isolates occurred more among patients with serious comorbidities and prolonged hospitalization. Community onset, skin and soft tissue infection, and deep-seated infection best predicted SCC*mec* IV/V MRSA bacteremia.

Editor: Frank R. DeLeo, National Institute of Allergy and Infectious Diseases, National Institutes of Health, United States of America

Funding: This study was supported by a grant from the National Science Council (96-2314-B-002-031-)in Taiwan. The funders had no role in study design, data collection and analysis, decision to publish, or preparation of the manuscript.

Competing Interests: The authors have declared that no competing interests exist.

* E-mail: dtmed111wang@ntu.edu.tw (JLW); changsc@ntu.edu.tw (SCC)

¶ These authors contributed equally to this work.

Introduction

Community-associated methicillin-resistant *Staphylococcus aureus* (CA-MRSA) has been isolated mainly from skin or soft tissue infections [1,2], although severe invasive infections caused by CA-MRSA strains, such as pyomyositis, osteomyelitis, necrotizing fasciitis, severe pneumonia, and sepsis, have also been reported [3–7]. CA-MRSA strains share a common pulsed field gel electrophoresis (PFGE) pattern, show greater susceptibility to most non-β-lactam antibiotics, and carry staphylococcal cassette chromosome *mec* (SCC*mec*) type IV or V elements; these characteristics are not typical of healthcare-associated MRSA (HA-MRSA) strains [1].

In recent years, CA-MRSA has emerged as an important cause of healthcare-associated and nosocomial bacteremia in many countries [8–10]. In contrast to the US and Europe, the major CA-MRSA strains in Taiwan are ST59, SCC*mec* IV or ST59, SCC*mec* V_T; the major clone in nosocomial MRSA infections in Taiwan is SCC*mec* III: ST239, followed by SCC*mec* II: ST 5 [11–16]. Molecular epidemiological definitions, based on staphylococcal cassette chromosome *mec* (SCC*mec*) typing and phylogenetic analysis of MRSA isolates, are considered the most reliable way to distinguish between HA-MRSA and CA-MRSA [17]. In a study of MRSA bacteremia by Seybold et al., CA-MRSA strains (as defined by PFGE) were associated with injection drug use and with skin and soft tissue infection [8]. In their study of CA-MRSA strains defined by antibiogram phenotype, Popovich et al. concluded that demographic data and risk factors could not reliably distinguish patients infected with CA-MRSA strains from those infected with HA-MRSA strains [9].

SCC*mec* II and III, which are larger elements, may not be suited to CA-MRSA strains; these elements show a different distribution of antibiotic resistance genes and toxin genes compared to SCC*mec* IV and V [17]. In this study, we compared the demographic characteristics, clinical features, and outcomes of patients with MRSA isolates with different SCC*mec* types.

Materials and Methods

Patient Selection

This study was conducted according to the principles expressed in the Declaration of Helsinki and was approved by the Institutional Review Board (No. 200705068R) of National Taiwan University Hospital (NTUH), Taipei, Taiwan. The Institutional Review Board waived the need for informed consent from participants because the study involved very minimal risk to the subjects, did not include intentional deception, and did not involve sensitive populations or topics; this waiver does not adversely affect the rights and welfare of the subjects.

NTUH is a university hospital with 2500 beds that provides primary and tertiary care in northern Taiwan. From January 1 through December 31, 2006, all patients age >16 years with MRSA bacteremia admitted to NTUH were identified from information in a laboratory database.

Data Collection

All patients were evaluated using a structured form. The clinical course of the infection and the infection foci were evaluated and recorded based on information supplied by primary care physicians and medical records. Diagnosis of the infection focus was based on clinical, bacteriological, and radiological results. The infection was considered "deep-seated" if any of the following were present: infective endocarditis, mycotic aneurysm, osteomyelitis, septic arthritis, pyomyositis, necrotizing pneumonia/empyema, or abscess formation in any deep organ, such as the liver or kidney. Modified Duke criteria were used to evaluate infective endocarditis [18]. Catheter-related bacteremia was defined by a semi-quantitative culture of the vascular catheter tip that yielded more than 15 MRSA colonies in the absence of other sources of bacteremia [19]. The other sites of infection at the onset of bacteremia were defined according to the US Centers for Disease Control and Prevention criteria [20]. If no infection focus could be identified, the bacteremia was classified as primary bacteremia.

The following data were recorded for each patient: age, sex, underlying illness, hospitalization history or outpatient department involvement within the previous year, existence of a percutaneous device catheter, time from admission until a MRSA-positive culture, initial laboratory findings, and outcome.

"Health care–associated" was defined using previously published definitions [8,9], which include hospital-onset infection or the presence of any of the following HA-MRSA risk factors within the year prior to the index culture: (1) residence in a longterm care facility, (2) prior admission to an acute care facility (3) use of central intravenous catheters or longterm venous access devices, (4) use of urinary catheters, (5) use of other longterm percutaneous devices (6) prior surgical procedures, and/or (7) need for any form of dialysis [8,9].

Microbiological Laboratory Procedures

Identification of *S.aureus* was based on colony morphology, Gram staining, a positive catalase reaction, slide agglutination test results (bioMérieux, Marcy l'Etoile, France), and/or results obtained with the Phoenix system (Becton Dickinson, Sparks, MD, USA). Antibiotic susceptibility testing for *S. aureus* in this study included oxacillin, vancomycin, minocycline, levofloxacin, ciprofloxacin, tetracycline, trimethoprim/sulfamethoxazole, gentamicin, clindamycin, and rifampin and was performed according to standard microbiological methods [21]. Resistance to oxacillin was confirmed by PCR for the *mec*A gene. The presence of the PVL gene lukF-lukS was determined by PCR using a primer that was described previously [22], and the presence of 10 staphylococcal enterotoxin virulence genes (sea, seb, sec, sed, see, seg, seh, sei, sej, and tst) was also determined by PCR using the protocol of Jarraud et al. [23]. The presence of the SCC*mec* elements (I–V) and the *mec*A gene was determined by methods described previously [14,24–26]. Analysis of the polymorphic X-region of the protein A gene (spa) and multilocus sequence typing (MLST) for the major pulso type was performed as described previously [27–28]. Analysis of PFGE patterns was performed using GelCompar software (Applied Maths, Austin, TX, USA). We performed spa typing and PFGE typing of all isolates, but only performed MLST on major pulsotypes in different SCC*mec*types.

Statistical Analysis

Mean values and standard deviations were calculated for continuous variables. Percentages were used for categorical variables. For univariate analysis, SCC*mec* types were compared using the chi-square test or Fisher's exact test as indicated for categorical variables and the analysis of variance (ANOVA) test with least-significant-difference post-hoc tests for continuous variables. Due to their similar biological features, we considered SCC*mec* II and III to be one group and SCC*mec* IV and SCC*mec* V to be another group. The associations between potential risk factors and SCC*mec* II/III or SCC*mec* IV/V in patients with MRSA bacteremia were also investigated using univariate and multivariate logistical regression. Crude and adjusted odds ratios (ORs) and the corresponding 95% confidence intervals (CIs) were calculated. Cumulative survival after the day of the first MRSA-positive blood culture was calculated using the Kaplan-Meier method. Differences in cumulative survival for patients with different SCC*mec* types were tested with the log-rank test. The effect of infection with CA-MRSA on outcome was evaluated using a multivariate Cox proportional hazards regression model adjusted for age, sex, and underlying comorbidities. The data were analyzed using SPSS software for Windows (Release 15.0; SPSS, Chicago, IL).

Results

Patients, Risk Factors, and Clinical Features

During the study period, there were 159 consecutive adult patients with MRSA bacteremia from whom isolates were collected for microbiological analysis (101 men, 63.5%; 58 women, 36.5%). Twelve patients from whom isolates were not collected were excluded from the study. There were no differences between the study group and the excluded group in terms of sex, age, and ward distribution. The mean age of the 159 adult patients was 67.3±16.5 years. The MRSA SCC*mec* types were as follows: 30 SCC*mec* II (18.9%), 87 SCC*mec* III (54.7%), 22 SCC*mec* IV (13.3%), and 20 SCC*mec* V (12.6%). All SCC*mec* V isolates belonged to SCC*mec* type V_T [13]. Seven patients matched the criteria for CA-MRSA bacteremia (4.4%), including 4 (57.1%) MRSA isolates with SCC*mec* IV and 3 (42.9%) with SCC*mec* V. In the remaining 152 (95.6%) patients with HA-MRSA bacteremia, 29 (18.2%) patients had community-onset infections and 123 (77.4%) had hospital-onset infections. For 29 patients with community-onset HA-MRSA bacteremia, the SCC*mec* type distribution was as follows: 4

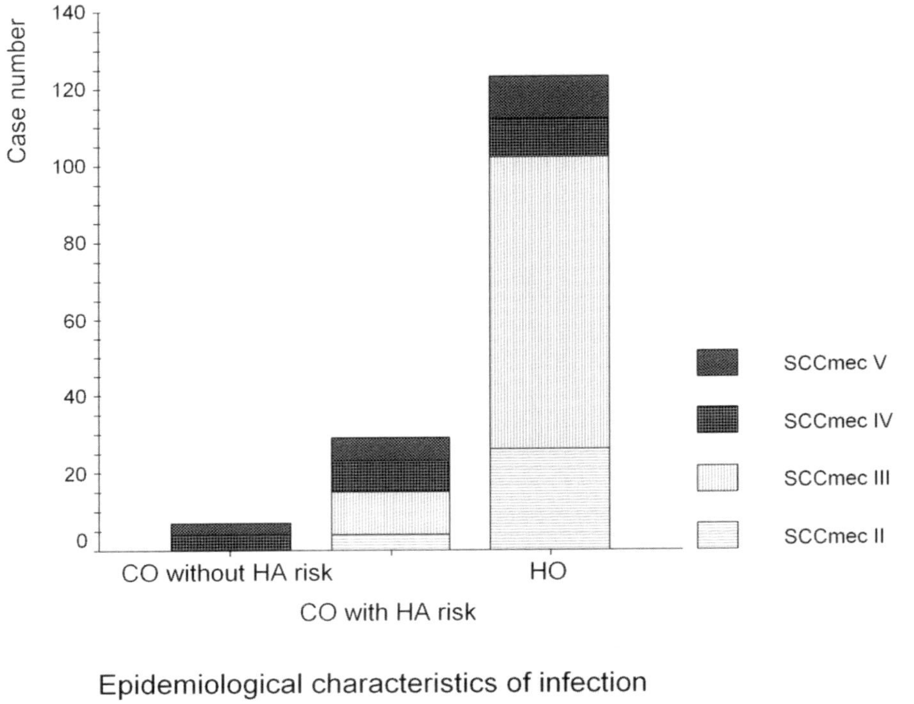

Figure 1. The distribution of SCCmec: community-onset (CO) or hospital-onset (HO) and healthcare-associated (HA) factor.

(13.8%) SCC*mec* II, 11 (37.9%) SCC*mec* III, 8 (27.6%) SCC*mec* IV, and 6 (20.7%) SCC*mec* V. In 123 patients with hospital-onset HA-MRSA bacteremia, the distribution of SCC*mec* types was 26 (21.1%) SCC*mec* II, 76 (61.3%) SCC*mec* III, 10 (8.1%) SCC*mec* IV, and 11 (8.9%) SCC*mec* V. The distribution of each SCC*mec* type in a heathcare setting (either community-onset or hospital-onset, with or without healthcare associated factor) is shown in Figure 1.

MRSA Bacteremia Patient Characteristics Associated with Specific MRSA SCC*mec* Types

Table 1 summarizes the demographic data and comorbidities of all patients. The mean age of patients with MRSA SCC*mec* V (56.9 years) was significantly lower than that of patients with MRSA SCC*mec* II (69.9) and MRSA SCC*mec* III (69.0) ($P<0.05$). MRSA carrying SCC*mec* II/III was more likely to occur in the ICU, and

Table 1. Comparison of demographic data and comorbidities of MRSA bacteremia patients with different SCCmec types.

Characteristic, n (%)	SCC*mec* II n = 30	SCC*mec* III n = 87	SCC*mec* IV n = 22	SCC*mec* V n = 20	Total n = 159	*P*
Sex, male	20 (66.7)	56 (64.4)	12 (54.5)	13 (65.0)	101 (63.5)	0.816
Age, mean years ± SD	69.9±14.9	69.0±15.9	66.6±15.6	57.0±19.4	67.3±16.5	0.02
Community onset	4 (13.3)	11 (12.6)	12 (54.5)	9 (45.0)	36 (22.6)	<0.001
ICU onset	15 (50)	40 (46)	2 (9.1)	0 (0)	57 (35.8)	<0.001
Length of hospital say before index culture mean days ± SD, median (range)	35.9±33.1 28 (0–157)	50.7±71.3 26 (0–360)	6.7±9.0 3 (0–33)	11.1±12.2 10.5 (0–39)	36.8±57.6 19.0 (0–360)	0.001
Comorbid condition						
No underlying disease	0 (0)	0 (0)	1 (4.8)	2 (10)	3 (1.9)	0.017
Diabetes mellitus	7 (23.3)	35 (40.2)	2 (9.1)	6 (30.0)	50 (31.4)	0.027
Cancer	10 (33.3)	25 (28.7)	5 (22.7)	11 (55)	51 (32.1)	0.106
Liver cirrhosis	2 (6.7)	12 (13.8)	1 (4.5)	4 (20)	19 (11.9)	0.375
End-stage renal disease	3 (10)	16 (18.4)	4 (18.2)	1 (5)	24 (15.1)	0.409
Cerebrovascular disease	5 (16.7)	24 (27.6)	3 (13.6)	2 (10)	34 (21.4)	0.242
Charlson comorbidity score ≥3	17 (56.7)	55 (63.2)	10 (45.5)	11 (55)	93 (58.5)	0.490
Bed-ridden status	7 (23.3)	28 (32.2)	3 (13.6)	1 (0.5)	39 (24.5)	0.035
Recent surgery	10 (33.3)	16 (18.4)	0 (0)	2 (10.0)	28 (17.6)	0.009

Table 2. Comparison of clinical characteristics and outcomes of MRSA bacteremia patients with different SCCmec types.

Clinical syndrome,n (%)	SCC*mec* II n=30	SCC*mec* III n=87	SCC*mec* IV n=22	SCC*mec* V n=20	Total n=159	*P*
Infection focus*[1]						
Primary bacteremia	6 (20.0)	15 (17.2)	6 (27.3)	5.(25.0)	32 (20.1)	0.695
Skin and soft tissue	0 (0)	6 (6.9)	5 (22.7)	3.(15.0)	14 (8.8)	0.015
Central catheter related infection	13 (43.3)	35 (40.2)	7 (31.8)	3 (15.0)	58 (36.5)	0.152
Surgical site or prosthetic infection	5 (16.7)	12 (13.8)	1 (4.5)	0 (0)	18 (11.3)	0.187
Pneumonia	11 (36.7)	27 (31.0)	3 (13.6)	6 (30)	47 (29.6)	0.326
Deep-seated infection*[2]	2 (6.7)	3 (3.4)	6 (27.3)	3 (15.0)	14 (8.8)	0.004
Endocarditis	1 (3.3)	2 (2.3)	3 (13.6)	1 (5.0)	7 (4.4)	0.140
Septic arthritis and osteomyelitis	0 (0)	0 (0)	4 (18.2)	1 (5.0)	5 (3.1)	<0.001
Necrotizing pneumonia and empyema	1 (3.3)	2 (2.3)	0 (0)	2 (10)	5 (3.1)	0.256
Outcome						
Persistent bacteremia*[3]	4 (13.3)	5 (5.7)	1 (4.5)	1 (5.0)	11 (6.9)	0.532
7-day mortality	6 (20.0)	8 (9.2)	0 (0)	0 (0)	14 (8.8)	0.002
30-day mortality	12 (40)	26 (29.9)	4 (18.2)	8 (40.0)	50 (31.4)	0.309

*[1]Some patients had more than one focus of infection.
*[2]Deep-seated infection not related to surgery or prosthesis.
*[3]Persistent bacteremia (>7 days).

MRSA carrying SCC*mec* IV/V was more likely to occur in the community ($P<0.05$). The time from admission to the first MRSA-positive blood culture for patients infected with isolates with the SCC*mec* III element (mean/median, 50.7/26 days) was significantly longer than for patients infected with isolates carrying SCC*mec* IV or V (mean/median, 6.7/3 days for SCC*mec* IV; 11.1/10.5 days for SCC*mec* V) ($P<0.05$). Compared to patients with SCC*mec* V isolates, MRSA bacteremia patients with SCC*mec* III isolates were more likely to be bedridden, but their infections were less likely to be associated with underlying disease ($P<0.05$). Patients with SCC*mec* III isolates were also more likely to have diabetes compared to those with MRSA SCC*mec* IV ($P<0.05$). Compared to patients with SCC*mec* IV isolates, those with MRSA carrying SCC*mec* II were more likely to have had surgery within the previous three months ($P<0.05$)

Table 2 shows the clinical characteristics and outcomes of bacteremia patients infected with MRSA with different SCC*mec* types. In terms of infection sites, MRSA with SCC*mec* IV was more often associated with superficial skin and soft tissue infections than MRSA with SCC*mec* II ($P=0.015$). In addition, patients with MRSA carrying SCC*mec* IV were significantly more likely to have non-prosthetic septic arthritis/osteomyelitis ($P<0.001$) and deep-seated infections not related to surgery or prosthesis ($P=0.008$) compared to MRSA bacteremia patients with SCC*mec* II and SCC*mec* III isolates.

SCC*mec* II/III vs. SCC*mec* IV/V

In subsequent analyses, we grouped patients with SCC*mec* II and SCC*mec* III isolates together for comparison with patients with SCC*mec* IV and SCC*mec* V isolates. In univariate analysis, age, ICU onset, length of stay before index culture, diabetes mellitus, bedridden status, recent surgery, and catheter-related infection were associated with recovery of SCC*mec* II/III isolates (Table 3). Community onset, skin and soft tissue infection, and deep-seated infection (not related to surgery/prosthesis) were risk factors associated with isolates carrying SCC*mec* IV/V (Table 3). Multivariate analysis revealed four independent factors associated with patients infected by MRSA carrying SCC*mec* II/III: ICU onset (OR, 16.82; 95% CI, 3.52–80.15), length of stay before index culture (OR 1.07; 95% CI, 1.03–1.10), diabetes mellitus (OR, 4.51; 95% CI, 1.51–13.42), and bedridden status (OR, 5.90; 95% CI, 1.61–21.61) (Table 3).

In univariate analysis, MRSA bacteremia patients with SCC*mec* II/III isolates had more catheter-related infections and had more often had recent surgery, and patients with SCC*mec* IV/V isolates had more skin and soft tissue infections and more deep-seated infections. However, these associations failed to reach significance in multivariate analysis.

Mortality Analysis

Figure 2 shows the Kaplan-Meier survival curves for MRSA bacteremia patients with isolates carrying different SCC*mec* types.

Table 3. Results of univariate and multivariate logistic regression analyses (SCC mec I/III isolates vs. SCCmec IV/V isolates).

	Univariate OR (95% CI)	Multivariate OR (95% CI)
ICU onset	17.74 (4.10–76.84)	16.82 (3.52–80.15)
Recent surgery	5.71 (1.29–25.24)	
Bedridden	4.06 (1.35–12.23)	5.90 (1.61–21.61)
Diabetes	2.38 (1.01–5.61)	4.51 (1.51–13.42)
Catheter-related infection	2.23 (1.00–4.95)	
Length of hospital say before index culture	1.07 (1.04–1.11)	1.07 (1.03–1.10)
Age	1.03 (1.01–1.04)	
Skin and soft tissue infection	0.23 (0.08–0.71)	
Deep-seated infection	0.16 (0.05–0.52)	
Community-onset	0.15 (0.07–0.33)	

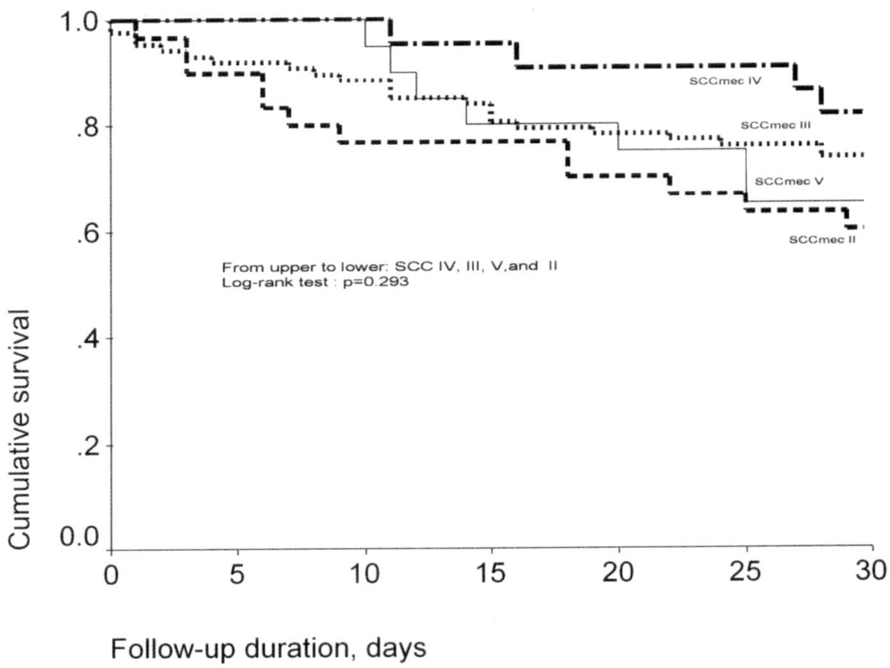

Figure 2. Thirty-day Kaplan-Meier survival curves for MRSA bacteremia patients according to SCCmec type.

The 30-day cumulative survival was 60%, 70.1%, 81.8%, and 60% for patients with SCC*mec* II, III, IV, and V isolates, respectively. There was no significant difference in survival (P= 0.293, log-rank test). The 30-day cumulative survival was 67.5% for patients with SCC*mec* II/III isolates and 71.4% for patients with SCC*mec* IV/V isolates; no significant differences emerged (P= 0. 403, log-rank test)(Figure 3).

To determine whether the SCC*mec* type would independently affect 30-day mortality, we performed Cox-regression analysis by controlling for age, sex, and comorbidity (Charlson score). After

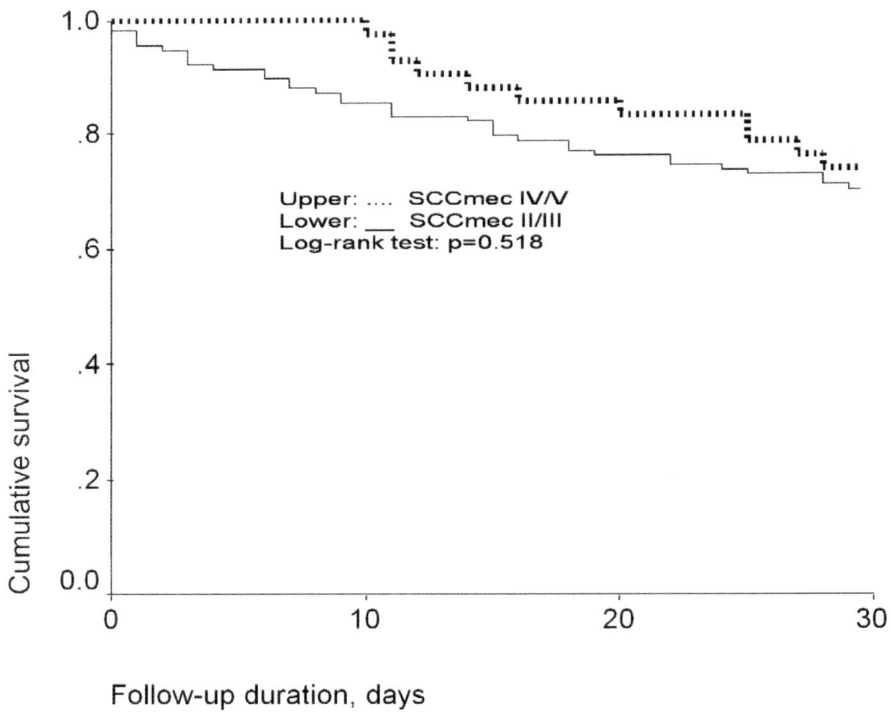

Figure 3. Thirty-day Kaplan-Meier survival curves for MRSA bacteremia patients: SCCmec II/III vs. SCCmec IV/V.

adjustment for age, sex, and comorbidity (Charlson score), the 30-day mortality of patients with SCC*mec* IV/V isolates was not significantly higher than that of patients with SCC*mec* II/III isolates (adjusted hazard ratio, 0.793; 95% CI, 0.406–1.547; $P = .496$).

Genotype, Antimicrobial Susceptibility, and Virulence Gene Profile of the MRSA Isolates

Table 4 shows the genotype, antibiotic susceptibility, and virulence gene profile of isolates with four different SCC*mec* types. The genotypes of the HA-MRSA strains (SCC*mec* II and III) were more homogeneous (the same identical spa type and pulsotypes) than those of the CA-MRSA strains (SCC*mec* IV and V). Figure 4 shows the PFGE of MRSA isolates containing 4 different SCC*mec* types. The main pulsotypes carried with SCC*mec* II were ST5, spa t002, and agr 2 and were positive for the sec, seg, sei, and tst genes. The main strain carrying SCC*mec* IV and V was ST59 and was positive for spa t437, agr 1, and seb. The major differences in virulence gene profiles and antibiotic susceptibility between SCC*mec* IV and SCC*mec* V isolates were the pvl carrier rate (9% vs. 85%) and gentamicin susceptibility (36% vs. 90%), respectively. The major strain carrying SCC*mec* III was spa ST239 and was positive for spa t037, agr1, and sea. Isolates with SCC*mec* III were often multi-drug resistant except for rifampin.

Discussion

We conducted a large one-year retrospective study in a medical center in Taiwan that included 159 consecutive adult patients with MRSA bacteremia. We recorded bacterial genotyping results, antibiotic susceptibility, and virulence gene profiling results for each patient. In this study, the percentage of MRSA bacteremia patients with community-onset, healthcare-associated MRSA with SCC*mec* IV/V was 48%; among patients with hospital-onset, healthcare-associated MRSA, the frequency was 17%. This finding is similar to those of previous studies in US populations that found that CA-MRSA strains (USA 300) are an important cause of healthcare-related infections [8–10,29,30]. We compared the demographic characteristics, risk factors, and outcomes of adult MRSA bacteremia patients from whom strains with different SCC*mec* types were isolated (SCC*mec* II, III, IV, and V). Microbiological study of the isolates showed that the major clones of CA-MRSA strains in Taiwan (SCC*mec* IV/V, spa t437, ST59 with or without the pvl gene) or HA-MRSA strains in Taiwan (SCC*mec* III, spa t037, ST239 and SCC*mec* II, spa t002, and ST5 with the tst gene) differed from those in the United States and Europe. In addition, we found the demographic and clinical characteristics of patients with MRSA bacteremia differed according to specific SCC*mec* subtype.

Two recent studies of MRSA bacteremia used the USA300 PFGE pattern and typical antibiotic phenotype for differentiating CA-MRSA and HA-MRSA strains [8–9]. The association we identified between SCC*mec* II/III and ICU onset and length of stay before index culture was similar to results from previous studies [8–10,30]. Previous studies identified a trend between a longer hospital stay before index culture and greater risk of ICU admission in HA-MRSA bacteremia patients [8,9]. Our cohort also showed longer hospitalization before index culture and more cases of ICU onset. In our study, the number of days the patient was bedridden and diabetes mellitus were other risk factors associated with SCC*mec* II/III isolates. SCC*mec*types IV and V are considerably smaller than

Table 4. Molecular typing, antimicrobial susceptibility, and virulence genes of MRSA isolates with different SCCmec types.

	SCC*mec* II n = 30	SCC*mec* III n = 87	SCC*mec* IV n = 22	SCC*mec* V n = 20
Major *spa* type (%)	t002 (97%)	t037 (93%)	t437 (68%)	t437 (75%)
MLST*	ST5	ST239	ST59	ST59
Major agr type (%)	agr 2 (93%)	agr 1 (98%)	agr 1 (77%)	agr 1 (85%)
Antibiotic susceptibility profile				
Oxacillin MIC≥128 µg/mL (%)	100	99	0	0
Vancomycin MIC = 2 µg/mL (%)	7	30	0	0
Susceptible rate to non-β-lactam (%)				
Erythromycin	0	0	9	10
Clindamycin	0	18	23	15
Gentamicin	0	1	36	90
Levofloxacin	0	0	100	90
Ciprofloxacin	0	0	100	90
Trimethoprim-sufamethoxazole	100	0	100	100
Minocycline	100	62	91	100
Tetracycline	100	0	41	40
Rifampin	53	83	96	80
Virulence gene				
pv l (%)	0	0	9	85
Enterotoxin gene (*sea-sej,tst*)	*sec*: 77% *seg:* 100% *sei:* 100% *tst:* 87%	*sea*: 87% *seb*: 2% *seg*: 1% *sei*: 1%	*seb*: 68% *sec*: 9% *seg*: 23% *sei*: 23%	*seb*: 80% *seg*: 10% *sei*: 10% *sej*: 10%

*We only performed MLST on strains from major pulsotypes for the different SCCmec types.

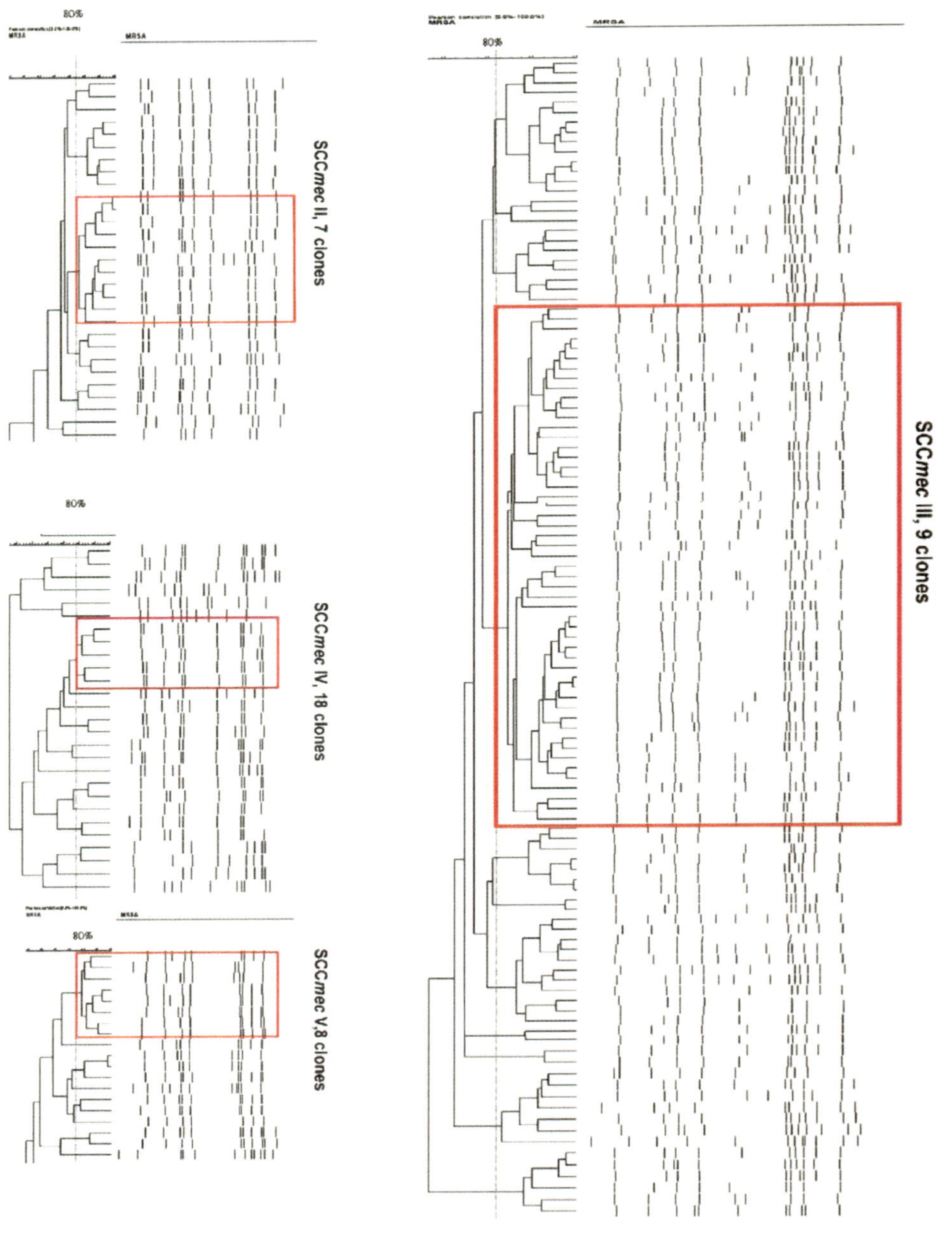

Figure 4. Pulsed-field gel electrophoresis of different SCCmec types; red indicates the major pulsotype.

SCC*mec* elements I–III. Our finding support the idea that HA-MRSA strains do not survive well in the community setting and that antibiotic selective pressure or cross-transmission in the hospital were needed for the survival of HA-MRSA strains [17].

Little has been published regarding the role or association of specific MRSA genotypes with particular presentations. Fowler et al. showed that MRSA ST30 was associated with a significant trend towards higher levels of hematogenous complications [31]. Edgeworth et al. suggested that the ST239 strain was associated with an increased rate of vascular access device-related bacteremia [32]. In univariate analysis in this study, the bacteremia patients with HA-MRSA strains (t002, ST5 and t037, ST239) had more catheter-related infections, and patients with CA-MRSA strains (mainly spa t437 and ST59) showed a trend towards more skin and soft tissue infections and deep-seated infections; however, neither association reached significance in multivariate analysis. Our findings support previous reports that CA-MRSA strains are highly associated with skin and soft tissue infection, osteomyelitis, and necrotizing pneumonia, although the CA-MRSA strain in Taiwan was not USA300 [1–5]. Although our investigation only included patients with MRSA bacteremia, it extended the finding that certain *S. aureus* genotypes are more likely to be associated with some clinical syndromes or with infection severity [31–33]. Several studies suggest that CA-MRSA strains harboring the smaller SCC*mec* type IV element grow faster and achieve higher infection burdens than nosocomial MRSA strains [34–38]. In agreement with this observation, we found that there were more deep-seated infections involving MRSA with SCC*mec* IV/V than other subtypes.

However, in our study MRSA isolates with SCC*mec* IV/V were not more lethal than SCC*mec* II/III isolates. This may be due to more severe comorbidities and more isolates with high vancomycin MIC (MIC = 2) in patients with MRSA carrying SCC*mec* II/III.

Our study had some limitations. First, the SCC*mec* and genotype distribution was different than that reported in other parts of the world, so our results cannot be generalized to populations in which the distribution of CA-MRSA and HA-MRSA strains differs from Taiwan. Second, differences in infection presentation and outcome may be explained by factors other than SCC*mec* genotype, such as virulence genes, antibiotic MIC for the bacterial isolates, adequate infection drainage, and empirical vancomycin therapy. The study size may be too small to address associations between genotype and clinical syndromes or severity.

In conclusion, in this study of 159 adult MRSA bacteremia patients, specific demographic and clinical risk factors were found to predict recovery from bacteremia caused by MRSA with different SCC*mec* types. MRSA isolates carrying SCC*mec* II/III were found more frequently in patients with significant comorbidities and prolonged hospitalization. Community onset, skin and soft tissue infection, and deep-seated infection best predicted MRSA isolates carrying SCC*mec* IV/V.

Author Contributions

Conceived and designed the experiments: JLW JTW SCC. Performed the experiments: JLW JTW. Analyzed the data: JLW JTW SYC YCC. Contributed reagents/materials/analysis tools: JLW JTW. Wrote the paper: JLW JTW.

References

1. Naimi TS, LeDell KH, Como-Sabetti K, Borchardt SM, Boxrud DJ, et al. (2003) Comparison of community- and health care-associated methicillin-resistant Staphylococcus aureus infection. JAMA 290: 2976–2984.
2. King MD, Humphrey BJ, Wang YF, Kourbatova EV, Ray SM, et al. (2006) Emergence of community-acquired methicillin-resistant Staphylococcus aureus USA 300 clone as the predominant cause of skin and soft-tissue infections. Ann Intern Med 144: 309–317.
3. Bocchini CE, Hulten KG, Mason EO, Jr., Gonzalez BE, Hammerman WA, et al. (2006) Panton-Valentine leukocidin genes are associated with enhanced inflammatory response and local disease in acute hematogenous Staphylococcus aureus osteomyelitis in children. Pediatrics 117: 433–440.
4. Pannaraj PS, Hulten KG, Gonzalez BE, Mason EO, Jr., Kaplan SL (2006) Infective pyomyositis and myositis in children in the era of community-acquired, methicillin-resistant Staphylococcus aureus infection. Clin Infect Dis 43: 953–60.
5. Francis JS, Doherty MC, Lopatin U, Johnston CP, Sinha G, et al. (2005) Severe community-onset pneumonia in healthy adults caused by methicillin-resistant Staphylococcus aureus carrying the Panton-Valentine leukocidin genes. Clin Infect Dis 40: 100–107.
6. Miller LG, Perdreau-Remington F, Rieg G, Mehdi S, Perlroth J, et al. (2005) Necrotizing fasciitis caused by community-associated methicillin-resistant Staphylococcus aureus in Los Angeles. N Engl J Med 352: 1445–1453.
7. Adem PV, Montgomery CP, Husain AN, Koogler TK, Arangelovich V, et al. (2005) Staphylococcus aureus sepsis and the Waterhouse-Friderichsen syndrome in children. N Engl J Med 353: 1245–1251.
8. Seybold U, Kourbatova EV, Johnson JG, Halvosa SJ, Wang YF, et al. (2006) Emergence of community-associated methicillin-resistant Staphylococcus aureus USA300 genotype as a major cause of health care-associated blood stream infections. Clin Infect Dis 42: 647–656.
9. Popovich KJ, Weinstein RA, Hota B (2008) Are community-associated methicillin-resistant Staphylococcus aureus (MRSA) strains replacing traditional nosocomial MRSA strains? Clin Infect Dis 46: 787–794.
10. Maree CL, Daum RS, Boyle-Vavra S, Matayoshi K, Miller LG (2007) Community-associated methicillin-resistant Staphylococcus aureus isolates causing healthcare-associated infections. Emerg Infect Dis 13: 236–242.
11. Vandenesch F, Naimi T, Enright MC, Lina G, Nimmo GR, et al. (2003) Community-acquired methicillin-resistant Staphylococcus aureus carrying Panton-Valentine leukocidin genes: worldwide emergence. Emerg Infect Dis 9: 978–984.
12. Boyle-Vavra S, Daum RS (2007) Community-acquired methicillin-resistant Staphylococcus aureus: the role of Panton-Valentine leukocidin. Lab Invest 87: 3–9.
13. Boyle-Vavra S, Ereshefsky B, Wang CC, Daum RS (2005) Successful multiresistant community-associated methicillin-resistant Staphylococcus aureus lineage from Taipei, Taiwan, that carries either the novel Staphylococcal chromosome cassette *mec* (SCC*mec*) type VT or SCCmec type IV. J Clin Microbiol 43: 4719–4730.
14. Wang JL, Chen SY, Wang JT, Wu GH, Chiang WC, et al. (2008) Comparison of both clinical features and mortality risk associated with bacteremia due to community-acquired methicillin-resistant Staphylococcus aureus and methicillin-susceptible S. aureus. Clin Infect Dis 46: 799–806.
15. Chen FJ, Lauderdale TL, Huang IW, Lo HJ, Lai JF, et al. (2005) Methicillin-resistant Staphylococcus aureus in Taiwan. Emerg Infect Dis 11: 1760–1763.
16. Huang YC, Su LH, Wu TL, Lin TY (2006) Changing molecular epidemiology of methicillin-resistant Staphylococcus aureus bloodstream isolates from a teaching hospital in Northern Taiwan. J Clin Microbiol 44: 2268–2270.
17. Kluytmans-Vandenbergh MF, Kluytmans JA (2006) Community-acquired methicillin-resistant Staphylococcus aureus: current perspectives. Clin Microbiol Infect 12 Suppl 1: 9–15.
18. Li JS, Sexton DJ, Mick N, Nettles R, Fowler VG, Jr., et al. (2000) Proposed modifications to the Duke criteria for the diagnosis of infective endocarditis. Clin Infect Dis 30: 633–8.
19. Mermel LA, Farr BM, Sherertz RJ, Raad II, O'Grady N, et al. (2001) Guidelines for the management of intravascular catheter-related infections. Clin Infect Dis 32: 1249–1272.
20. Garner JS, Jarvis WR, Emori TG, Horan TC, Hughes JM (1998) CDC definitions for nosocomial infections, 1988. Am J Infect Control 16: 128–140.
21. Bannerman TL (2003) Staphylococcus, Micrococcus, and other catalase-positive cocci that grow aerobically. In: Murray PR, Baron EJ, Jorgensen JH, Pfaller MA, Yolken RH, eds. Manual of clinical microbiology, 8th ed. Washington, DC: American Society of Microbiology Press. pp 384–404.
22. Lina G, Piemont Y, Godail-Gamot F, Bes M, Peter MO, et al. (1999) Involvement of Panton-Valentine leukocidin-producing Staphylococcus aureus in primary skin infections and pneumonia. Clin Infect Dis 29: 1128–1132.
23. Jarraud S, Mougel C, Thioulouse J, Lina G, Meugnier H, et al. (2002) Relationships between Staphylococcus aureus genetic background, virulence factors, agr groups (alleles), and human disease. Infect Immun 70: 631–641.
24. Ito T, Katayama Y, Asada K, Mori N, Tsutsumimoto K, et al. (2001) Structural comparison of three types of staphylococcal cassette chromosome *mec* integrated in the chromosome in methicillin-resistant *Staphylococcus aureus*. Antimicrob Agents Chemother 45: 1323–36.
25. Ito T, Ma XX, Takeuchi F, Okuma K, Yuzawa H, et al. (2004) Novel type V staphylococcal cassette chromosome mec driven by a novel cassette chromosome recombinase, ccrC. Antimicrob Agents Chemother 48: 2637–2651.
26. Takano T, Higuchi W, Otsuka T, Baranovich T, Enany S, et al. (2008) Novel characteristics of community-acquired methicillin-resistant Staphylococcus aureus strains belonging to multilocus sequence type 59 in Taiwan. Antimicrob Agents Chemother 52: 837–45.
27. Harmsen D, Claus H, Witte W, Rothganger J, Claus H, et al. (2003) Typing of methicillin-resistant Staphylococcus aureus in a university hospital setting by using novel software for spa repeat determination and database management. J Clin Microbiol 41: 5442–5448.
28. Enright MC, Day NP, Davies CE, Peacock SJ, Spratt BG (2000) Multilocus sequence typing for characterization of methicillin-resistant and methicillin-susceptible clones of Staphylococcus aureus. J Clin Microbiol 38: 1008–1015.
29. Klevens RM, Morrison MA, Nadle J, Petit S, Gershman K, et al. (2007) Invasive methicillin-resistant Staphylococcus aureus infections in the United States. JAMA 298: 1763–1771.
30. Davis SL, Rybak MJ, Amjad M, Kaatz GW, McKinnon PS (2006) Characteristics of patients with healthcare-associated infection due to SCCmec type IV methicillin-resistant Staphylococcus aureus. Infect Control Hosp Epidemiol 27: 1025–1031.
31. Fowler VG, Jr., Nelson CL, McIntyre LM, Kreiswirth BN, Monk A, et al. (2007) Potential associations between hematogenous complications and bacterial genotype in Staphylococcus aureus infection. J Infect Dis 196: 738–747.
32. Edgeworth J, Yadegarfar G, Pathak S, Batra R, Cockfield JD, et al. (2007) An outbreak in an intensive care unit of a strain of methicillin-resistant Staphylococcus aureus sequence type 239 associated with an increased rate of vascular access device-related bacteremia. Clin Infect Dis 44: 493–501.
33. Seybold U, Blumberg HM (2007) Reading the tea leaves or deciphering DNA microarrays: are certain methicillin-resistant Staphylococcus aureus clones adapted to cause specific infections? Clin Infect Dis 44: 502–505.
34. Zetola N, Francis JS, Nuermberger EL, Bishai WR (2005) Community-acquired methicillin-resistant Staphylococcus aureus: an emerging threat. Lancet Infect Dis 5: 275–286.
35. Okuma K, Iwakawa K, Turnidge JD, Grubb WB, Bell JM, et al. (2002) Dissemination of new methicillin-resistant Staphylococcus aureus clones in the community. J Clin Microbiol 40: 4289–94.
36. Laurent F, Lelievre H, Cornu M, Vandenesch F, Carret G, et al. (2001) Fitness and competitive growth advantage of new gentamicin-susceptible MRSA clones spreading in French hospitals. J Antimicrob Chemother 47: 277–283.
37. Ma XX, Ito T, Tiensasitorn C, Jamklang M, Chongtrakool P, et al. (2002) Novel type of staphylococcal cassette chromosome mec identified in community-acquired methicillin-resistant Staphylococcus aureus strains. Antimicrob Agents Chemother 46: 1147–1152.
38. Diep BA, Otto M (2008) The role of virulence determinants in community-associated MRSA pathogenesis. Trends Microbiol 16: 361–369.

6

Pediatric Vancomycin Use in 421 Hospitals in the United States, 2008

Tamar Lasky[1]*, Jay Greenspan[2], Frank R. Ernst[3], Liliana Gonzalez[4]

1 MIE Resources, Kingston, Rhode Island, United States of America, **2** Thomas Jefferson University, Nemours Children's Clinics, Wilmington, Delaware, United States of America, **3** Clinical and Outcomes Research, Premier Research Services, Premier Healthcare Alliance, Charlotte, North Carolina, United States of America, **4** Computer Science and Statistics, University of Rhode Island, Kingston, Rhode Island, United States of America

Abstract

Background: Recommendations to prevent the spread of vancomycin resistance have been in place since 1995 and include guidelines for inpatient pediatric use of vancomycin. The emergence of large databases allows us to describe variation in pediatric vancomycin across hospitals. We analyzed a database with hospitalizations for children under 18 at 421 hospitals in 2008.

Methodology/Principal Findings: The Premier hospital 2008 database, consisting of records for 877,201 pediatric hospitalizations in 421 hospitals, was analyzed. Stratified analyses and logistic mixed effects models were used to calculate the probability of vancomycin use while considering random effects of hospital variation, hospital fixed effects and patient effects, and the hierarchical structure of the data. Most hospitals (221) had fewer than 10 hospitalizations with vancomycin use in the study period, and 47 hospitals reported no vancomycin use in 17,271 pediatric hospitalizations. At the other end of the continuum, 21 hospitals (5.6% of hospitals) each had over 200 hospitalizations with vancomycin use, and together, accounted for more than 50% of the pediatric hospitalizations with vancomycin use. The mixed effects modeling showed hospital variation in the probability of vancomycin use that was statistically significant after controlling for teaching status, urban or rural location, size, region of the country, patient ethnic group, payor status, and APR-mortality and severity codes.

Conclusions/Significance: The number and percentage of pediatric hospitalizations with vancomycin use varied greatly across hospitals and was not explained by hospital or patient characteristics in our logistic models. Public health efforts to reduce vancomycin use should be intensified at hospitals with highest use.

Editor: Adam J. Ratner, Columbia University, United States of America

Funding: Funded by AHRQ grant R03 HS017998 "Measuring Pediatric Inpatient Use" to Tamar Lasky, Principal Investigator, http://www.ahrq.gov. The funders had no role in study design, data collection and analysis, decision to publish, or preparation of the manuscript.

Competing Interests: The authors have the following interests. Frank Ernst is employed by Premier Research Services, the company that produced the database used in the analysis. Tamar Lasky is President and owner of MIE Resources. There are no further patents, products in development or marketed products to declare.

* E-mail: tlasky@mie-epi.com

Introduction

Vancomycin is indicated for the treatment of serious or severe infections caused by susceptible strains of methicillin-resistant (beta-lactam-resistant) staphylococci. It is indicated for patients who cannot receive or who have failed to respond to other drugs, including the penicillins or cephalosporins, and for infections caused by vancomycin-susceptible organisms that are resistant to other antimicrobial drugs. Because of concerns about the development of drug-resistant bacteria, vancomycin should be used only to treat or prevent infections that are proven or strongly suspected to be caused by susceptible bacteria. Recommendations to prevent the spread of vancomycin resistance have been in place since 1995 and include guidelines for inpatient pediatric use of vancomycin [1,2,3,4,5,6,7].

In 1999 Shah and colleagues described vancomycin use in one hospital's pediatric neurosurgery unit and noted vancomycin was used primarily for prophylaxis and was inconsistent with the Hospital Infection Control Practices Advisory Committee recommendations [8]. Hopkins and colleagues evaluated use in one hospital's pediatric hematology-oncology unit, and concluded that 100% of the use was not consistent with CDC recommendations [9]. Keyserling and colleagues (2003) studied 22 hospitals belonging to the Pediatric Prevention Network (PPN) [10]. They described series of 25 patients receiving vancomycin at each hospital, and surveyed the physicians who prescribed the vancomycin. They did not categorize adherence to guidelines, but noted general patterns of use such as the low percentage (7%) with laboratory-confirmed β-lactam-resistant organisms isolated at the time vancomycin was prescribed, or the association of vancomycin use with presence of indwelling vascular catheters. Bolon and colleagues evaluated vancomycin use in children older than 1 year at a pediatric tertiary care medical center in 2000 and 2001 [11]. They developed algorithms to evaluate whether use was appropriate, and concluded that 35% of the initial courses were inappropriate. Patel and colleagues studied the medical records of 200 neonates born after Septermber 2005 at 4 tertiary care (NICUs) and concluded that 32% of the days of vancomycin use were inappropriate and non-adherent to the Centers for Disease Control and Prevention 12 Step Campaign to Prevent Antimicrobial Resistance [3,12]. They noted non-adherence to steps 4 (Target the pathogen) and 8 (Treat infection, not contamination or colonization). Other studies have described use, but have not assessed guideline adherence [13,14]. The emergence of large multi-hospital databases in the past decade offers new opportunities to study patterns of vancomycin use across hospitals. In this study, we analyzed a large database and describe variation in pediatric vancomycin use in all children under 18 hospitalized at 421 hospitals in 2008.

Methods

We analyzed vancomycin use occurring in pediatric hospitalizations in 2008 using the Premier hospital database, a large US hospital-based, service-level, all-payer database, containing information from primarily non-profit, non-governmental, community and teaching hospitals and health systems [15]. Detailed service level information was available for each hospital day and included medication information and central supplies. Patient information collected included, but was not limited to, patient demographics (age, gender, race/ethnicity), principal and secondary diagnoses, principal and secondary procedures, payor, length of stay, cost of care, drug utilization, department cost and charge detail, day-of-stay data, and physician specialty. In addition to the service-level data recorded in most standard hospital discharge files, the database provided a daily log of all billed items, including procedures, medications, laboratory tests and diagnostic and therapeutic services, at the individual patient level. Hospitals were self-selected, choosing to provide their own data to Premier as part of agreements by which they received access to analytic tools developed and offered by Premier. In the study year, 2008 423 hospitals participated (99.1% with pediatric hospitalizations). Data were entered into a hospital's core information system, fed into their decision support system (DSS), then sent to Premier on a monthly or quarterly basis via a secure FTP site. Upon receiving data from participating hospitals, Premier undertook an extensive seven phase data validation and correction process that included more than 95 quality assurance checks. Deidentified data were extracted and used for statistical analysis. The study proposal was approved by the University of Rhode Island Institutional Review Board and informed consent requirements were waived, as permitted under 45 CFR 46.116(c) or (d).

We calculated the number of unique hospitalizations with any use of vancomycin and estimated the prevalence of vancomycin use (number of hospitalizations with documentation of any vancomycin use per 100 hospitalizations). We also estimated the percentages vancomycin use in children over and under 1 year of age, and the percentages of hospitalizations with use longer than 3 days duration. Patient characteristics were: age in years, gender, race (White, African-American, other), and type of insurance (private, government or none). Hospital characteristics were size (small, medium, large), teaching or non-teaching, urban or rural, and region of the country (Northeast, Midwest, South and West, as defined by the US Census).

Logistic mixed effects modeling with two levels of hierarchy (hospital and patient) were used to calculate the probability of vancomycin use while considering the random effects of hospital variation, as well as hospital fixed effects and patient effects. In our models we included the 3 M^{TM} All Patient Refined Diagnosis Related Groups (APR DRGs) severity and mortality (as 4 level, ordered categories), and International Classification of Diseases – 9th Revision – Clinical Modification (ICD-9-CM) Group Codes. The 3 M^{TM} APR DRGs expand the basic DRG structure and address patient differences relating to severity of illness and risk of mortality [16]. Severity of illness was defined as the extent of physiologic decompensation or organ system loss of function. Risk of mortality was defined as the likelihood of dying. The SAS procedure, GLIMMIX was run using the events/trial syntax to maintain the hierarchical structure of the data [17,18,19]. Models were run in subsets of hospitalizations, for children under 1 year of age, and further separated by ICD-9 Group Codes. Plots of odds ratios were produced using SAS Graphics [20]. All statistical analyses were conducted using SAS 9.2 [21].

Results

The dataset contained records for 877,201 hospitalizations of children under 18 at time of admission with 50,879 (5.8%) being repeat admissions. The study population was 50.9% male and 49.1% female, 48.5% white, 16.1% African-American, 12.2% Hispanic, 3.6% Asian/Pacific Islander, 18.7% other and less than 1% American Indian. The average length of stay was 3.7 days (median 2 days, interquartile range 2–3 days). Private insurance paid for 46.2% of the hospital stays, government paid for 45.9% and self-pay, no charge or other sources accounted for 7.9% of the hospital stays. Most of the hospitalizations took place in urban areas (89.2%) compared to rural areas (10.8%).

We validated the Premier sample of hospitalizations by comparing characteristics of the sample to the HCUP KID sample of pediatric hospitalizations for 2006 and details of the validation are available in a previous publication (Lasky et al., 2011). The Premier sample included a greater proportion of infants born in the hospital, from Southern hospitals, from non-teaching hospitals, and from large size hospitals compared to the HCUP KID sample. The two samples were similar with regards to proportions male, routine discharge status, APR-DRGs severity and proportions urban. We did not compare the proportions of different racial and ethnic groups in Premier to the KID because of well documented limitations in racial and ethnic data within the KID, high rates of missing data resulting from state differences in collection and reporting of race and ethnicity. Vancomycin was administered in 19,775 hospitalizations, or 2.3% of 877,201 pediatric hospitalizations in the database in 2008. In 98% of cases, vancomycin was administered parenterally or "other" (this includes ophthalmic solutions, intraocular/intravitreal injections, catheter flushes, inhalation formulations, rectal formulations and topical gels compounded by pharmacy) and in less than 2% of cases, vancomycin was administered orally. Half (10,033 or 50.7%) of the courses of vancomycin were less than 3 days duration. Males had higher prevalence of use than did females (2.5%, 95% CI 2.5–2.6 compared to 2.0%, 95% CI 2.0–2.0), African-Americans had higher use than did whites or other groups (3.1%, 95% CI 3.0–3.2, 2.3%, 95% CI 2.3–2.4 and 1.8%, 95% CI 1.8–1.9 respectively), and children in the age groups 2–4 and 5–11 had higher prevalence compared to children under 2, or children age 12–17 (6.8%, 95% CI 6.5–7.1, 6.6%, 95% CI 6.4–6.8, 1.5%, 95% CI 1.5–1.5, and 4.3%, 95% 4.2–4.4). The greatest number of hospitalizations with vancomycin use occurred to children under 2 (10,282 or 52% of hospitalizations), however the highest prevalence of use occurred in children age 2–4, and 5–11 (Figure 1). Children age 2–4 were 4.5 times more likely, children 5–11 were 4.4 times more likely, and children 12–17 were 2.9 times more likely to receive vancomycin compared to children under 2. In hospitalizations of children under one year with vancomycin use, the four most frequent ICD-9 group diagnoses were: "Liveborn infants according to type of birth" (ICD-9-CM V30–39) (51.83%),

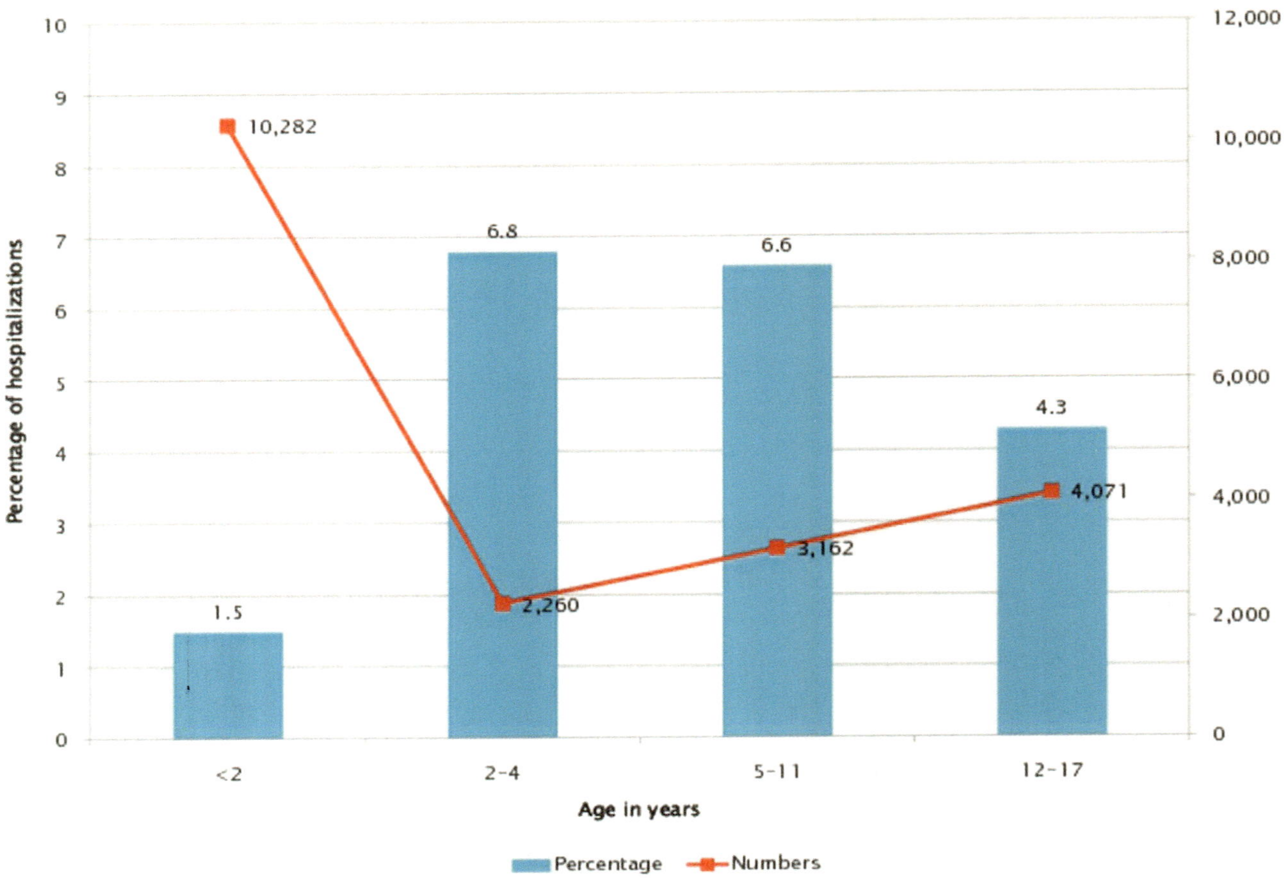

Figure 1. Vancomycin use by age group.

"Other conditions originating in the perinatal period" (ICD-9-CM 760–779) (14.29%), "Infections of skin and subcutaneous tissue" (ICD-9-CM 680–709) (6.07%), and "Congenital anomalies" (5.91%) (ICD-9-CM 740–759). In children age 1 or over, the four most frequent diagnoses were: "Infections of skin and subcutaneous tissue" (23.32%), "Pneumonia and influenza", (9.41%) (ICD-9-CM 480–488), "Complications of surgical and medical care, not elsewhere classifiable" (7.58%) (ICD-9-CM 996–999), and "Other bacterial diseases" (4.41%) (030–041).

Vancomycin was administered to children at 374 hospitals in the Premier hospital database; another 47 hospitals with 17,271 pediatric hospitalizations (13,233 under age 2) reported no vancomycin use during 2008. The number of hospitalizations with vancomycin use ranged from 0 to 1225 at individual hospitals, and percentage of hospitalizations with vancomycin use ranged from 0.0% to 33.3%. Twenty one hospitals (5.6%) had more than 200 hospitalizations with vancomycin use, accounting for 9,979 (50%) of the pediatric hospitalizations with vancomycin use. Because of the skewness in distribution of vancomycin use, we stratified hospitals by number of hospitalizations with vancomycin use. Low volume was defined as 0 to 10, medium volume as 11–100, and high volume as over 100. Most hospitals were

Table 1. The estimates and 95% Confidence Bounds of the variance of the random hospital intercepts on the logit scale in four models for individual diagnostic groups in children under 1.

ICD-group included in model	Estimate of Random Intercept	95% Confidence Bounds
Liveborn infants according to type of birth ICD-9-CM V30–39	1.5	1.2–1.9
Infections of skin and subcutaneous tissue ICD-9-CM 680–709	1.5	1.1–2.2
Other conditions originating in perinatal period ICD-9-CM 760–779	0.4	0.3–0.7
Congenital anomalies ICD-9-CM 740–759	0.3	0.2–0.9

categorized as low volume (221 hospitals), 155 hospitals were categorized as medium volume, and 45 hospitals categorized as high volume. Within high volume hospitals, percentage of hospitalizations with vancomycin use ranged from 1.3–12.9 (mean percentage was 4.6, 95% CI = 3.9–5.4). Within medium volume hospitals, percentage of hospitalizations with vancomycin use ranged from 0.3 to 9.5 (mean percentage was 1.7, 95% CI = 1.5–1.9). The hospitals with high volume of vancomycin use were predominantly large (73.3%), teaching (68.9%), and urban (97.8%) compared to the hospitals with low volume of vancomycin use, which were 45.7% large, 19.91% teaching, and 74.21% urban, and 95% Confidence Intervals of estimates generally did not overlap. In 2008, 47 hospitals, or 11.16% of the hospitals in the database, reported no vancomycin use in the entire year.

The logistic mixed effects modeling showed hospital variation in vancomycin use. The estimated variance of the random effects hospital intercepts for models run for children under 1, and for the four most frequent ICD-9 Code Groups are summarized in Table 1. The intercept estimates and the 95% Confidence Bounds for each model do not include zero, indicating hospital variation that is statistically significant after controlling for the other variables in the model. The lower limits of the 95 percent confidence intervals are above zero, indicating statistically significant variability in the use of vancomycin depending on the hospital in which a patient was treated.

The Odds Ratios for hospital and patient fixed effects for two of the models are plotted in Figures 2 and 3. Variables associated with vancomycin use were different in each of the age and ICD groups. For example, in children under 1 year with ICD-9 group "Liveborn infants according to type of birth" increased APR-DRG severity of illness was associated with over 6 times the use of vancomycin, but in children under 1 year with ICD-9 group "Infections of skin and subcutaneous tissue" use of vancomycin was almost 2 times as frequent in children with increased APR-DRG severity (although the 95%CI slightly overlapped 1). Both models showed an association between increased APR-DRG severity of illness and vancomycin use, but the magnitude of the effect differed greatly in the two patient groups. Another example is the effect of rural vs. urban status of the hospital. Rural or urban status of the hospital was statistically significant in predicting vancomycin use in children under 1 year with ICD-9 group "Liveborn infants according to type of birth" and with ICD-9 group "Infections of skin and subcutaneous tissue", but the direction of the effect was different in each group of patients. For children under 1 year with ICD-9 group "Liveborn infants according to type of birth" rural hospitals had lower vancomycin use than did urban hospitals, but for children under 1 year with ICD-9 group "Infections of skin and subcutaneous tissue" rural hospitals had higher vancomycin use than did urban hospitals. Another example can be seen with patient's insurance coverage. In

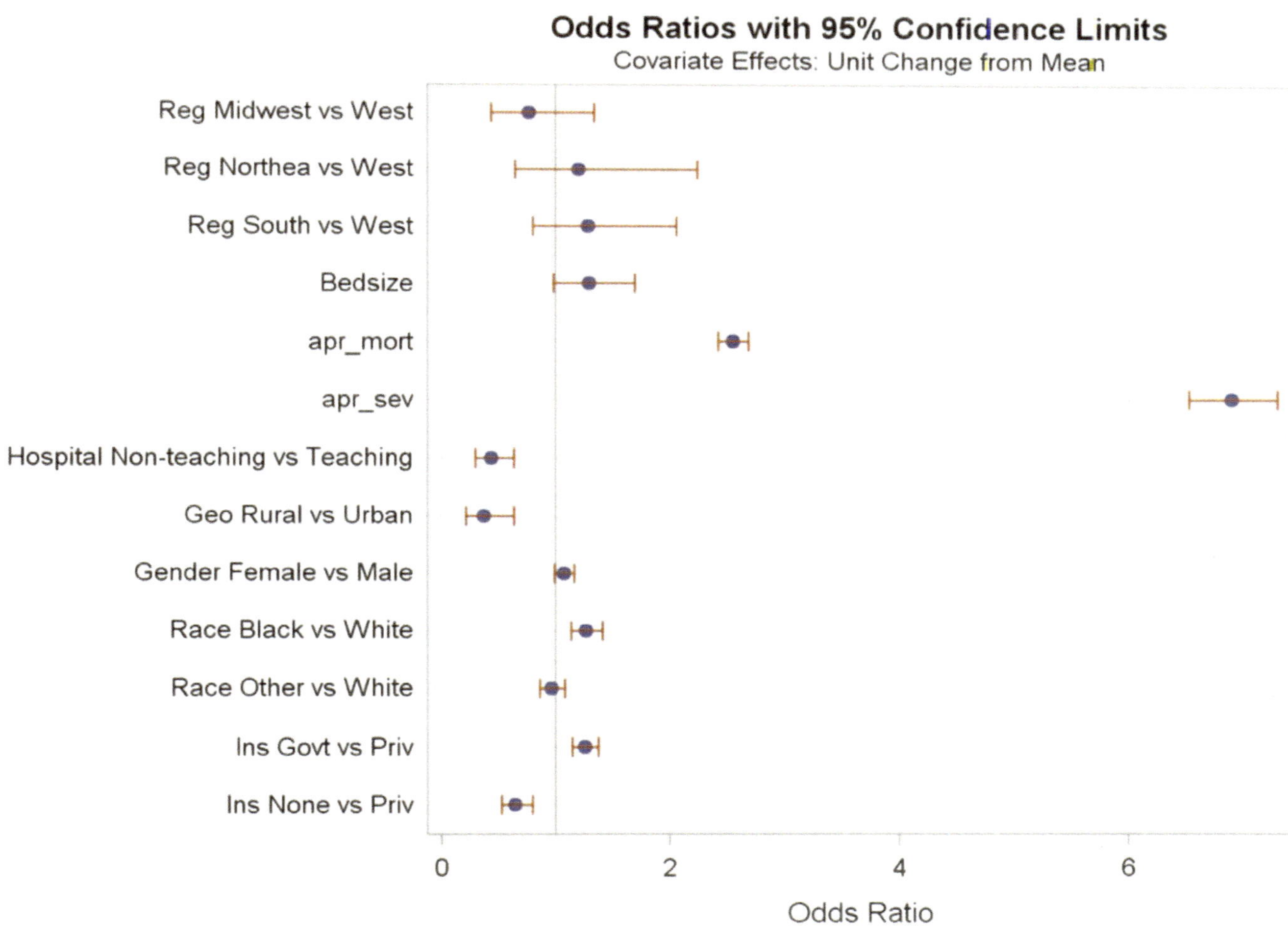

Figure 2. Odds Ratios for models in patients under 1 year of age ICD-9-CM group "Liveborn infants according to type of birth".

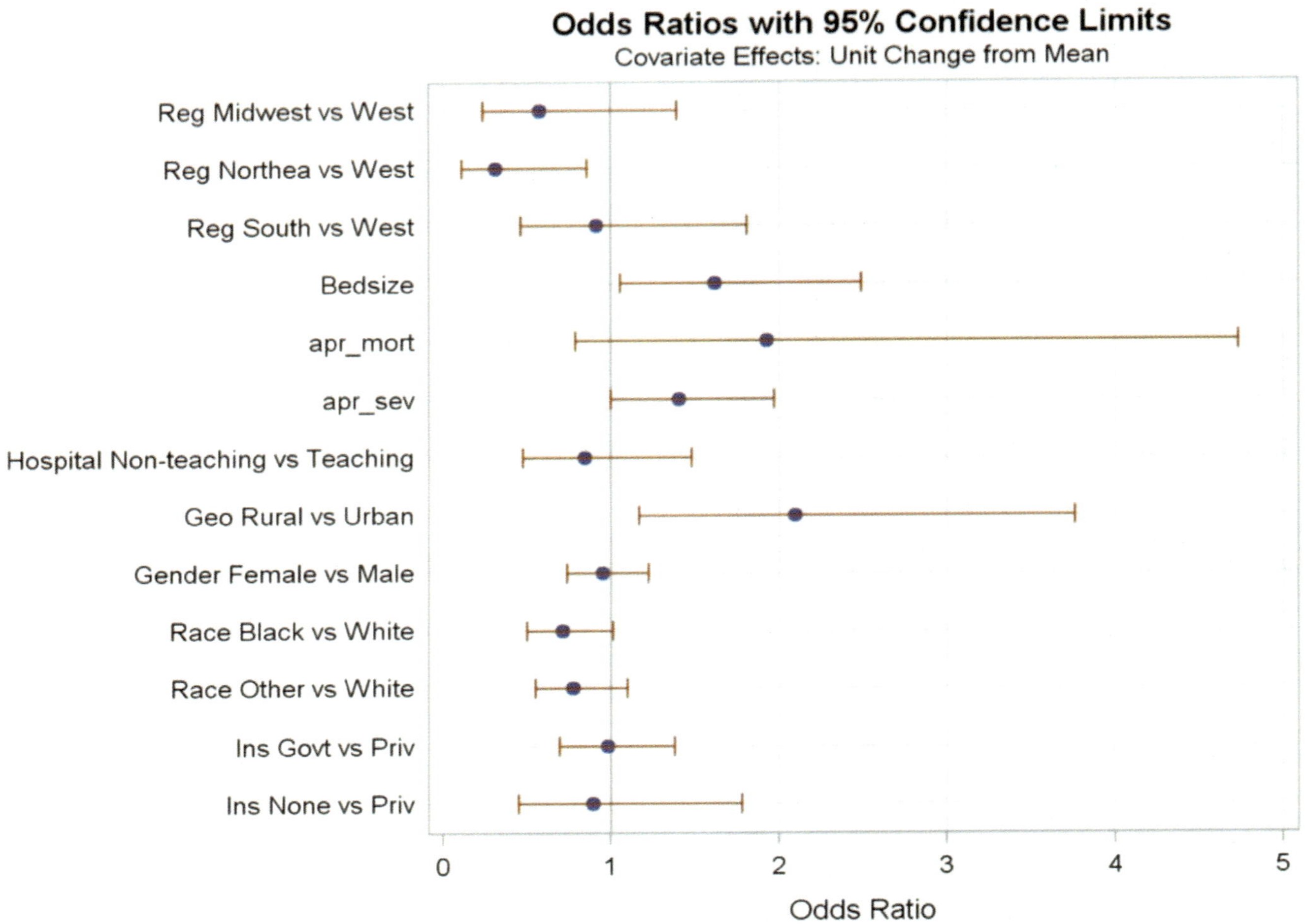

Figure 3. Odds Ratios for models in patients under 1 year of age ICD-9-CM group "Infections of skin and subcutaneous tissue".

children under 1 year with ICD-9 group "Liveborn infants according to type of birth" those with government insurance had slightly higher vancomycin use than did those with private insurance, and those with no insurance had less vancomycin use than those with private insurance. In children under 1 year with ICD-9 group "Infections of skin and subcutaneous tissue" insurance coverage was not associated with vancomycin use.

Discussion

Most hospitals (221) had fewer than 10 hospitalizations with vancomycin use in the study period, and 47 hospitals reported no vancomycin use in 17,271 pediatric hospitalizations. At the other end of the continuum, 21 hospitals (5.6% of hospitals) each had over 200 hospitalizations with vancomycin use, and together, accounted for more than 50% of the pediatric hospitalizations with vancomycin use. Percentage of hospitalizations with vancomycin use ranged up to 33.3% when hospitals with few pediatric hospitalizations were kept in the sample, and for this reason, percentage, by itself, may not be a useful indicator in small hospitals. In hospitals with more than 100 hospitalizations with vancomycin use, the percentage with vancomycin use ranged from 1.26 to 12.90, a 10 fold range in the probability of vancomycin use. Without knowing how percentage correlates with inappropriate use, one might begin by evaluating vancomycin use in hospitals with greater than 100 hospitalizations with vancomycin use and greater than 4 or 5% of hospitalizations having vancomycin. The two measures, absolute number of hospitalizations and percentage of hospitalizations with vancomycin use, can be used to identify and target hospitals for evaluation and potential interventions.

The limitations of the study include those inherent in secondary analysis of large databases. In this database, the ICD-9 code referred to the entire hospitalization rather than the indication for medication use, and we were unable to analyze the relationship between Methicillen-resistant Staphylococcus aureus (MRSA) occurrence and vancomycin use. The Premier database codes for MRSA changed during 2008 and future analyses will be able to describe MRSA variation. Although we could not analyze the data from our study year, 2008, a preliminary analysis of 2011 data showed MRSA codes in only 9.6% of hospitalizations with vancomycin use. Future analyses whether this is explained by undercoding MRSA, inappropriate use of vancomycin, or some other difference.

The definition of vancomycin use as any use during the hospital stay is both a weakness and a strength. It does not permit analysis of dose or duration which will be of interest in future studies, but it does permit estimates of percentages of hospitalized children exposed to vancomycin use. This is of interest when planning clinical studies, comparative effectiveness research, policy and labeling priorities, and other issues. The percentage (or prevalence) may provide a different perspective than that developed as a result of using numerator data only. For example, Keyserling and colleagues (2003) tabulated vancomycin courses and identified the largest number as occurring in neonatology services, and then suggested that neonatal intensive care units (NICUs) improve their vancomycin use [10]. We also found the highest number of uses in children under 2 years of age, but the lowest probability of use in children under 2 years of age (1.5%) compared to other age groups (4.3–6.8%). This may reflect the large number of healthy newborns in databases and programs to measure use of vancomycin in neonates will need to define a denominator, in addition to measuring the numerator, as is currently done.

The stratified analysis and the logistic modeling consistently document variation in vancomycin use by individual hospital, after considering independent effects of hospital and patient characteristics. The mixed models allowed us to estimate variation in the use of vancomycin by hospital in children with the same ICD-9 group codes. The intercepts measure the differences between hospitals, controlling for other effects in the model such as hospital and patient characteristics [18]. For every ICD-9 Group modeled, hospital-to-hospital variation and 95% Confidence Bounds of the intercept excluded zero, after controlling for hospital and patient effects.

Until recently, few studies have compared antibiotic use across large numbers of hospitals or geography, however the establishment of the National Healthcare Safety Network by the Centers for Disease Control and Prevention will allow regular comparisons across hospitals [22]. Geographic variation in use of antibiotics has also recently been documented in the United States [23].

The analyses presented here are also a step forward in studying pediatric hospital variation; previous researchers have used hierarchical models to consider hospital variation in adults, for example by studying maternity length of stay or mortality in patients undergoing coronary artery bypass surgery (CABG) [18,24]. Hospital variation in care of adults has been studied for several decades, much of it made possible by large Medicare claims databases [25]. Only recently have aggregated data for pediatric hospitalizations been available. Bowman and colleagues (2005) recently demonstrated variation in management of pediatric splenic injuries and Weiss et al (2009) have demonstrated variation in use of corticosteroids, opioids and nonsteroidal anti-inflammatory drug, diagnostic imaging, and renal biopsy in children with Henoch Schönlein purpura [26,27]. The public health implications of these data are that efforts to control vancomycin use may be channeledo hospitals with high numbers and prevalence of vancomycin use. While it seems intuitive that high prevalence will lead to high volume, and vice versa, some high volume hospitals maintain a prevalence below 3 per cent, while others range above 7 percent, almost to 13 percent. Presently, the message to reduce vancomycin use is broadcast to the entire healthcare community [2,28]. General principles of judicious antibiotic use are applicable to all hospitals and providers for all antibiotics, and these data may be used to channel intensive stewardship activities and intervention research data to hospitals with the highest volume and prevalence of vancomycin use.

While the Premier hospital database contains information about presence or absence of laboratory testing, it does not include information about test results. Future research relating vancomycin use to laboratory test results may need to budget for and obtain access to hospital charts or to laboratory-based infection surveillance data. We restricted the current analysis to one year, 2008; access to other years of data would permit assessment of trends over the last several years. Finally, further study may prepare the way for comparative effectiveness research, by identifying and comparing children with similar conditions treated with and without vancomycin, and relating the treatment patterns to outcomes.

Our key findings include the skewness of the distribution of vancomycin use throughout hospitals, the importance of denominator data in assessing vancomycin use, and hospital variation in vancomycin use, not explained by hospital or patient characteristics including: bed size, teaching status, region of the country, rural or urban geography, and patient sex, race, APR-DRG risk of mortality and APR-DRG severity of illness.

Acknowledgments

We would like to thank Cecilia Di Pentima, MD, MPH, FAAP, for her comments and careful reading of the manuscript. At the time when she reviewed the manuscript, she was Associate Professor, Department of Pediatrics, Infectious Disease Division, Alfred I. duPont Hospital for Children, Jefferson Medical College, Thomas Jefferson University.

Author Contributions

Conceived and designed the experiments: TL JG FE LG. Performed the experiments: TL JG FE LG. Analyzed the data: TL LG. Wrote the paper: TL JG FE LG.

References

1. Goldmann DA, Weinstein RA, Wenzel RP, Tablan OC, Duma RJ, et al. (1996) Strategies to Prevent and Control the Emergence and Spread of Antimicrobial-Resistant Microorganisms in Hospitals. A challenge to hospital leadership. Jama 275: 234–240.
2. Di Pentima M, Chan S (2010) Impact of Antimicrobial Stewardship Program on Vancomycin Use in a Pediatric Teaching Hospital. Pediatr Infect Dis J.
3. Centers for Disease Control and Prevention (2002) 12-Step Program to Prevent Antimicrobial Resistance in Health Care Settings. Department of Health and Human Services.
4. Centers for Disease Control and Prevention (1995) Recommendations for preventing the spread of vancomycin resistance: recommendations of the Hospital Infection Control Practices Advisory Committee (HICPAC). Morbidity and Mortality Weekly Reports 44: 1–12.
5. Shlaes DM, Gerding DN, John JF, Jr., Craig WA, Bornstein DL, et al. (1997) Society for Healthcare Epidemiology of America and Infectious Diseases Society of America Joint Committee on the Prevention of Antimicrobial Resistance: guidelines for the prevention of antimicrobial resistance in hospitals. Infect Control Hosp Epidemiol 18: 275–291.
6. American Academy of Pediatrics Committee on Infectious Diseases (1997) Therapy for children with invasive pneumococcal infections. Pediatrics 99: 289–299.
7. Rybak MJ, Lomaestro BM, Rotschafer JC, Moellering RC, Jr., Craig WA, et al. (2009) Therapeutic monitoring of vancomycin in adults summary of consensus recommendations from the American Society of Health-System Pharmacists, the Infectious Diseases Society of America, and the Society of Infectious Diseases Pharmacists. Pharmacotherapy 29: 1275–1279.
8. Shah SS, Sinkowitz-Cochran RL, Keyserling HL, Jarvis WR (1999) Vancomycin use in pediatric neurosurgery patients. Am J Infect Control 27: 482–487.
9. Hopkins HA, Sinkowitz-Cochran RL, Rudin BA, Keyserling HL, Jarvis WR (2000) Vancomycin use in pediatric hematology-oncology patients. Infect Control Hosp Epidemiol 21: 48–50.
10. Keyserling HL, Sinkowitz-Cochran RL, Harris JM, 2nd, Levine GL, Siegel JD, et al. (2003) Vancomycin use in hospitalized pediatric patients. Pediatrics 112: e104–111.
11. Bolon MK, Arnold AD, Feldman HA, Rehkopf DH, Strong EF, et al. (2005) Evaluating vancomycin use at a pediatric hospital: new approaches and insights. Infect Control Hosp Epidemiol 26: 47–55.
12. Patel SJ, Oshodi A, Prasad P, Delamora P, Larson E, et al. (2009) Antibiotic use in neonatal intensive care units and adherence with Centers for Disease Control and Prevention 12 Step Campaign to Prevent Antimicrobial Resistance. Pediatr Infect Dis J 28: 1047–1051.
13. Grohskopf LA, Huskins WC, Sinkowitz-Cochran RL, Levine GL, Goldmann DA, et al. (2005) Use of antimicrobial agents in United States neonatal and pediatric intensive care patients. Pediatr Infect Dis J 24: 766–773.

14. Pakyz AL, Gurgle HE, Ibrahim OM, Oinonen MJ, Polk RE (2009) Trends in antibacterial use in hospitalized pediatric patients in United States academic health centers. Infect Control Hosp Epidemiol 30: 600–603.
15. (2008) Premier Perspective Database. Charlotte, North Carolina: Premier Research Services, Premier, Inc.
16. Hughes J (2008) Development of the 3 M TM All Patient Refined Diagnosis Related Groups (APR DRGs). Mortality Measurement Meeting. Cambridge, Massachusetts: Department of Health and Human Services.
17. Schabenberger O (2005) Introducing the GLIMMIX Procedure for General Linear Mixed Models. Cary, North Carolina: SAS Institute Inc.
18. Dai J, Li Z, Rocke D (2006) Hierarchical Logistic Regression Modeling with SAS GLIMMIX. Proceedings of the Thirty-first Annual SAS Users Group International Conference. Cary, North Carolina: SAS Institute Inc.
19. Li J, Alterman T, Deddens JA (2006) Analysis of Large Hierarchical Data with Multilevel Logistic Modeling Using PROC GLIMMIX. SAS Conference Proceedings: Western Users of SAS Software 2006. Irvine, California.
20. SAS Institute Inc. (2009) SAS/GRAPH 9.2: StatisticalGraphics Procedures Guide. Cary: SAS Institute Inc.
21. SAS Institute Inc. (2009) Base SAS 9.2 Procedures Guide: Statistical Procedures, Second Edition. Cary: SAS Institute Inc.
22. Kuehn BM (2011) Antibiotic Use Tracking. Jama 306: 2661.
23. Titus A (2011) National Antibiotic Use at a Glance: How Does Your State Compare? Extending the Cure. Washington, DC: Center for Disease Dynamics, Economics & Policy.
24. Leung K-M, Elashoff RM, Rees KS, Hasan MM, Legorreta AP (1998) Hospital- and Patient-Related Characteristics Determining Maternity Length of Stay: A Hierarchical Linear Model Approach. American Journal of Public Health 88: 377–381.
25. Wennberg JE, Fisher ES, Stukel TA, Sharp SM (2004) Use of Medicare claims data to monitor provider-specific performance among patients with severe chronic illness. Health Aff (Millwood) Suppl Web Exclusives: VAR5–18.
26. Bowman SM, Zimmerman FJ, Christakis DA, Sharar SR, Martin DP (2005) Hospital characteristics associated with the management of pediatric splenic injuries. JAMA 294: 2611–2617.
27. Weiss PF, Klink AJ, Hexem K, Burnham JM, Leonard MB, et al. (2009) Variation in inpatient therapy and diagnostic evaluation of children with Henoch Schonlein purpura. J Pediatr 155: 812–818 e811.
28. Hersh AL, Beekmann SE, Polgreen PM, Zaoutis TE, Newland JG (2009) Antimicrobial stewardship programs in pediatrics. Infect Control Hosp Epidemiol 30: 1211–1217.

Panton-Valentine Leukocidin Is Not the Primary Determinant of Outcome for *Staphylococcus aureus* Skin Infections: Evaluation from the CANVAS Studies

Amy Tong[1], Steven Y. C. Tong[1,4], Yurong Zhang[1], Supaporn Lamlertthon[1,3], Batu K. Sharma-Kuinkel[1], Thomas Rude[1], Sun Hee Ahn[1], Felicia Ruffin[1], Lily Llorens[5], Ganesh Tamarana[5], Donald Biek[5], Ian Critchley[5], Vance G. Fowler Jr.[1,2]*

1 Division of Infectious Diseases, Department of Medicine, Duke University Medical Center, Durham, North Carolina, United States of America, **2** Duke Clinical Research Institute, Durham, North Carolina, United States of America, **3** Naresuan University, Phitsanulok, Phitsanulok Province, Thailand, **4** Menzies School of Health Research, Darwin, Northern Territory, Australia, **5** Cerexa, Inc., Oakland, California, United States of America

Abstract

The impact of Panton-Valentine leukocidin (PVL) on the severity of complicated skin and skin structure infections (cSSSI) caused by *Staphylococcus aureus* is controversial. We evaluated potential associations between clinical outcome and PVL presence in both methicillin-resistant *S. aureus* (MRSA) and methicillin-susceptible *S. aureus* (MSSA) isolates from patients enrolled in two large, multinational phase three clinical trials assessing ceftaroline fosamil for the treatment of cSSSI (the CANVAS 1 and 2 programs). Isolates from all microbiologically evaluable patients with monomicrobial MRSA or MSSA infections (n = 473) were genotyped by PCR for *pvl* and underwent pulsed-field gel electrophoresis (PFGE). Genes encoding *pvl* were present in 266/473 (56.2%) isolates. Infections caused by *pvl*-positive *S. aureus* were associated with younger patient age, North American acquisition, and presence of major abscesses ($P<0.001$ for each). Cure rates of patients infected with *pvl*-positive and *pvl*-negative *S. aureus* were similar overall (93.6% versus 92.8%; $P = 0.72$), and within MRSA-infected (94.5% vs. 93.1%; $P = 0.67$) and MSSA-infected patients (92.2% vs. 92.7%; $P = 1.00$). This finding persisted after adjustment for multiple patient characteristics. Outcomes were also similar when USA300 PVL+ and non-USA300 PVL+ infections were compared. The results of this contemporary, international study suggest that *pvl* presence was not the primary determinant of outcome in patients with cSSSI due to either MRSA or MSSA.

Editor: Herminia de Lencastre, Rockefeller University, United States of America

Funding: V.G.F. was supported in part by K24-AI093969 (http://grants.nih.gov/). S.Y.C.T. was supported by an Australian National Health and Medical Research Council Postdoctoral Training Fellowship (508829) (http://www.nhmrc.gov.au/grants), an Australian-American Fulbright Scholarship and a Royal Australasian College of Physicians Bayer Australia Medical Research Fellowship. This work was supported by Cerexa, Inc., Oakland, CA, (http://www.cerexa.com/) wholly owned subsidiary of Forest Laboratories, Inc. (New York, NY). The CANVAS clinical program was funded by Forest Laboratories, Inc., New York, NY. Forest Laboratories, Inc., was involved in the design, collection, analysis, and decision to present these results. Forest Laboratories, Inc., had no involvement in the interpretation of the data. Scientific Therapeutics Information, Inc., provided editorial coordination, which was funded by Forest Research Institute, Inc. Laboratory isolates were obtained from Network on Antimicrobial Resistance in Staphylococcus aureus (NARSA).

Competing Interests: L.L., G.T., D.B., and I.C. are employees of Cerexa, Inc. V.G.F. has received grants or research support from Astellas Pharma, Inc., Cubist Pharmaceuticals, Merck & Co., Inc., Theravance, Inc., MedImmune, Cerexa, Inc., Pfizer, and the United States National Institutes of Health. He is a consultant for Astellas Pharma, Inc., Biosynexus, Novartis, Cubist Pharmaceuticals, Inimex, Merck & Co., Inc., Galderma, Johnson & Johnson, Medicines Company, Novartis and is on the speaker's bureau and advisory committee for Cubist Pharmaceuticals. He has received honoraria from Achaogen, Arpida, Astellas Pharma, Inc., Cubist Pharmaceuticals, Durata, Inhibitex, Leo Pharma, Merck & Co., Inc., Pfizer, Targanta, Theravance, Inc., and Ortho-McNeil. Scientific Therapeutics Information, Inc., provided editorial coordination (which was funded by Forest Research Institute, Inc.). A.T., S.Y.C.T., Y.Z., S.L., B.K.S., T.R., and F.R. have no competing interests to declare.

* E-mail: fowle003@mc.duke.edu

Introduction

Staphylococcus aureus is the leading cause of complicated skin and skin structure infections (cSSSI) in the United States [1–4]. A number of studies have reported a high prevalence of Panton-Valentine leukocidin (PVL), a pore-forming, bi-component toxin that causes neutrophil lysis [5], among bacterial isolates causing cSSSI [6]. While the association between cSSSI and presence of *pvl* is particularly strong with community-acquired methicillin-resistant *S. aureus* (MRSA) [7], it has also been described among methicillin-susceptible *S. aureus* (MSSA) isolates causing cSSSI [3,8].

The role of PVL in determining the outcome and severity of *S. aureus* cSSSI remains one of the most controversial topics in the field of staphylococcal research [9]. The presence of *pvl* in *S. aureus* strains has been associated with severe infections in some [10–15] but not all [9,16,17] previous studies. For example, our group has reported that *pvl* presence was paradoxically associated with a better clinical outcome than cSSSI infections caused by *pvl*-negative MRSA [17,18]. For this reason, the role of *pvl* in cSSSI is unresolved.

The goal of the current study was to evaluate the impact of *pvl* presence on the outcome of patients with cSSSI caused by both MRSA and MSSA. To accomplish this goal, we used clinically well-characterized *S. aureus* isolates collected from patients with cSSSI who were enrolled in two phase 3 multinational clinical trials. The objectives of the current study were: 1) to confirm our previous observations that *pvl* is not the primary determinant of clinical outcome in patients with cSSSI due to MRSA, and 2) to test whether this same finding is also encountered in MSSA-infected patients. In addition, we aimed to evaluate whether outcomes of infections caused by USA300 PVL+ isolates differed from those caused by non-USA300 PVL+ isolates.

Methods

Patients and settings

CANVAS 1 (NCT00424190) and CANVAS 2 (NCT00423657; Ceftaroline versus Vancomycin in Skin and Skin-Structure Infection) were two methodologically identical, randomized, double-blind, multinational phase 3 clinical trials that compared the efficacy and safety of intravenous ceftaroline fosamil monotherapy with intravenous vancomycin plus aztreonam combination therapy for the treatment of adults with cSSSI caused by gram-positive and gram-negative organisms. The study designs of the CANVAS trials have been published in detail [19–21].

A total of 1378 patients from 111 participating centers in 12 countries were enrolled from February 2007 through December 2007 [19,20]. Men and non-pregnant women aged ≥18 years and diagnosed with cSSSI severe enough to require initial hospitalization or treatment in an emergency department and ≥5 days of intravenous antimicrobial therapy and that involved either (1) deep soft tissue or required deep surgical intervention, or (2) cellulitis or abscess of a lower extremity in patients with diabetes mellitus (DM) or well-documented peripheral vascular disease (PVD), were eligible for the study. Purulent or seropurulent drainage and/or collection or the presence of at least three of the following signs or symptoms was also required for participation: erythema, fluctuance, heat and/or localized warmth, pain and/or tenderness to palpation, fever (temperature >38°C) or hypothermia, white blood cell (WBC) count of $>10{,}000$ / mm^3, or >10% immature neutrophils irrespective of WBC count.

Patients were randomized to receive either ceftaroline fosamil (600 mg every 12 h) followed by normal saline placebo or vancomycin followed by aztreonam (1 g each every 12 h) for 5–14 days. Bacterial isolates were obtained from all patients at baseline by needle aspiration or a surgical procedure. Test-of-cure evaluation was performed 8 to 15 days after administration of the last dose of the study drug. The clinical response at the test of cure was classified as cure, failure, or indeterminate [21]. Clinical cure was defined as total resolution of all signs and symptoms of the baseline infection or improvement such that no further antimicrobial therapy was necessary. The microbiologically evaluable (ME) population was defined as clinically evaluable patients with ≥1 bacterial pathogen isolated from blood or the cSSSI site at baseline, excluding patients whose baseline cultures revealed monomicrobial *Pseudomonas aeruginosa* or anaerobic infection. In the present investigation, the analysis population was defined as microbiologically evaluable patients with cSSSI due to monomicrobial *S. aureus* and a clinical response at test of cure evaluation. The investigation was approved by the Duke University Medical Center Institutional Review Board.

Pulsed Field Gel Electrophoresis

Pulsed-field gel electrophoresis (PFGE) with the restriction enzyme *SmaI* was performed as previously described [22]. The PFGE profiles were analyzed using BioNumerics software (Applied Maths, Kortrijk, Belgium). A similarity coefficient of 80% was used to define pulsed-field type clusters. Dice coefficients (pairwise similarity) were calculated for each pair of isolates, and a dendrogram was constructed using an optimization value of 0.50% and a position tolerance ranging from 1.25% to 1.35% (the end of the fingerprint). PFGE profiles were interpreted according to a published typing schema [22].

PCR assays for genotyping

S. aureus genomic DNA was extracted using an ultraclean microbial DNA kit (MO BIO Laboratories, Inc., Carlsbad, CA) in accordance with the manufacturer's instructions. PCR assays were used to screen the *S. aureus* genome for the putative bacterial virulence toxin *pvl* for all *S. aureus* isolates using previously described methods [17,18].

Statistical methods

Cure rate by *pvl* status was stratified by markers of severity, including abscess versus non-abscess infection type, presence of fever, white blood cells ($>10{,}000$/ mm^3), infection size (baseline infection area of >100 cm^2), presence of diabetes, patient age, and study medication. Infection size was calculated as the product of the length and width of the primary infection site at its longest and widest axes, respectively. Continuous variables were compared between groups by using the two-sample t test. Categorical variables were analyzed using Fisher's exact test, its 2-by-K extension, or the Cochran-Mantel-Haenszel test, as appropriate, for stratified analyses. Our *a priori* hypothesis, that the presence of *pvl* in MRSA cSSSI is not associated with a worse clinical outcome, was tested using Fisher's exact test. All reported P values are two sided. P values of <0.05 were deemed statistically significant. Since subjects were not randomized on the basis of *pvl* status, all P values calculated should be considered descriptive and not inferential. Results were obtained using SAS software, version 9.1.3 (SAS Institute Inc, Cary, NC, USA).

Results

Study population and baseline characteristics

A total of 473 patients from the CANVAS studies with cSSSI due to monomicrobial *S. aureus* (280 MSSA, 59.2%; 193 MRSA, 40.8%) and for whom clinical outcome were available, were included in the current study. Among these 473 study patients, 253 (53.5%) received ceftaroline fosamil and 220 (46.5%) received vancomycin plus aztreonam. Patients were predominantly white, male, and North American, with an average age of 45 years. The majority of infections were either major abscesses (202 [42.7%]) or deep/extensive cellulitis (144 [30.4%]) (Table 1).

Patient characteristics according to *pvl* presence and methicillin-susceptibility

Overall, *pvl* was detected in 266/473 (56.2%) of the *S. aureus* isolates (Table 1; MRSA 164/193 [85.0%], MSSA 102/280 [36.4%]). In both the MRSA-infected and MSSA-infected cohorts, presence of *pvl* was associated with younger age, and major abscess ($P<0.001$). Patients with *pvl*-positive MRSA were significantly more likely to be from North America, and less likely to have been hospitalized or have PVD (all $P<0.001$) than patients with *pvl*-negative MRSA infections. Patients with *pvl*-positive MSSA were less likely to have other comorbid conditions, including DM ($P<0.001$) or PVD ($P=0.03$) than patients with *pvl*-negative MSSA infections.

Table 1. Baseline characteristics of 473 patients with *S. aureus* complicated skin and skin structure infections (cSSSI) stratified by methicillin-resistance and *pvl* gene status of the infecting pathogen.

Parameter	*Value for indicated patient group; n(%) except where noted* MRSA (n = 193) *pvl*-negative (n = 29)	*pvl*-positive (n = 164)	P-Value*	MSSA (n = 280) *pvl*-negative (n = 178)	*pvl*-positive (n = 102)	P-Value*
Demographic characteristics						
Mean age(yr) ± SD	53.1±17.2	40.6±14.0	<0.0001**	51.2±15.1	40.2±16.0	<0.0001**
Male	15 (51.7%)	96 (58.5%)	0.5440	119 (66.9%)	55 (53.9%)	0.0403
White race	27 (93.1%)	94 (57.3%)	0.0053	148 (83.1%)	87 (85.3%)	0.2357
Source of infection			<0.0001î			<0.0001î
Infected Wound	1 (3.4%)	19 (11.6%)		30 (16.9%)	6 (5.9%)	
Major Abscess	4 (13.8%)	95 (57.9%)		46 (25.8%)	57 (55.9%)	
Infected Ulcer	11 (37.9%)	0 (0.0%)		11 (6.2%)	2 (2.0%)	
Infected Burn	10 (34.5%)	2 (1.2%)		6 (3.4%)	0 (0.0%)	
Infected Bite	0 (0.0%)	9 (5.5%)		1 (0.6%)	3 (2.9%)	
Deep/Extensive Cellulitis	2 (6.9%)	36 (22.0%)		72 (40.4%)	34 (33.3%)	
Lower Extremity SSSI in Diabetic Subject	1 (3.4%)	3 (1.8%)		7 (3.9%)	0	
Geographical location			<0.0001§			0.0046§
Eastern Europe	20 (69.0%)	4 (2.4%)		94 (52.8%)	67 (65.7%)	
Latin America	2 (6.9%)	3 (1.8%)		18 (10.1%)	1 (1.0%)	
Western Europe	2 (6.9%)	0 (0.0%)		24 (13.5%)	8 (7.8%)	
US	5 (17.2%)	157 (95.7%)		42 (23.6%)	26 (25.5%)	
Prior antibiotic use			<0.0001±			0.2323±
No prior therapy	22 (75.9%)	52 (31.7%)		121 (68.0%)	59 (57.8%)	
≤24 hours of treatment	6 (20.7%)	84 (51.2%)		45 (25.3%)	34 (33.3%)	
>24 hours of treatment	1 (3.4%)	28 (17.1%)		12 (6.7%)	9 (8.8%)	
MRSA risk factors						
Hospitalization	27 (93.1%)	73 (44.5%)	<0.0001	156 (87.6%)	85 (83.3%)	0.3704
Antibiotic use in 4 weeks prior	16 (55.2%)	111 (67.7%)	0.2071	62 (34.8%)	38 (37.3%)	0.6990
Diabetes Mellitus	4 (13.8%)	20 (12.2%)	0.7642	43 (24.2%)	7 (6.9%)	0.0003
Peripheral Vascular Disease	9 (31.0%)	2 (1.2%)	<0.0001	24 (13.5%)	5 (4.9%)	0.0250
Infection characteristics						
Fever (temp of >38°C)[1]	19 (65.5%)	14 (8.6%)	<0.0001	69 (38.8%)	43 (42.2%)	0.6131
White Blood Cells >10,000 /mm^3 **, 1	9 (34.6%)	72 (46.2%)	0.2954	49 (30.4%)	34 (41.5%)	0.1152
Baseline infection area of >100 cm^2 **	22 (75.9%)	101 (61.6%)	0.2079	121 (68.0%)	60 (58.8%)	0.1529
Duration of antibiotic treatment (days median) ***	8.0	9.5	0.1836	7.0	7.0	0.0054
Study medication			0.5401			1.0000
Ceftaroline	19 (65.5%)	94 (57.3%)		89 (50.0%)	51 (50.0%)	
Vancomycin plus Aztreonam	10 (34.5%)	70 (42.7%)		89 (50.0%)	51 (50.0%)	

* = P-Value from generalized 2-sided Fishers Exact Test. Calculated using 7×2 table ( ), 4×2 table (§) and 3×2 table (±).
** = P-Value from 2-sided T-test.
*** = P-value from Wilcoxon Rank Sum test.
1 = Subjects with missing data were not included in these summaries.

Association of *pvl* gene status and patient clinical outcome

Overall, cure rates among patients with cSSSI due to *pvl*-positive and *pvl*-negative *S. aureus* did not differ significantly (*pvl*-positive *S. aureus* 93.6% [249/266] vs. *pvl*-negative *S. aureus* 92.8% [192/207]; $P = 0.72$). Cure rates remained similar when stratified by methicillin-resistance (Table 2). Similar findings also persisted in both the MRSA and MSSA populations after stratification by infection type (abscess versus non-abscess), presence of fever, leukocytosis, infection size (baseline infection area of >100 cm^2), patient age, or DM (Table 2).

Table 2. Clinical outcome of cure for 473 patients with methicillin-resistant and methicillin-susceptible *S. aureus* complicated skin and skin structure infections by *pvl* gene status, stratified by infection severity, diabetes, patient age, and study medication.

	No. of cured patients/total no. of patients (%) with indicated status					
	MRSA (n = 193)			MSSA (n = 280)		
Covariate	pvl-negative (n = 29)	pvl-positive (n = 164)	P-Value*	pvl-negative (n = 178)	pvl-positive (n = 102)	P-Value*
Overall	27/29 (93.1%)	155/164 (94.5%)	0.6722	165/178 (92.7%)	94/102 (92.2%)	1.0000
Type of infection						
Abscess	3/4 (75.0%)	90/95 (94.7%)	0.2244	42/46 (91.3%)	53/57 (93.0%)	1.0000
Non-abscess	24/25 (96.0%)	65/69 (94.2%)	1.0000	123/132 (93.2%)	41/45 (91.1%)	0.7412
Baseline fever (temp >38°C)	19/19 (100.0%)	13/14 (92.9%)	0.4242	65/69 (94.2%)	40/43 (93.0%)	1.0000
White blood cells >10,000 / mm^3	7/9 (77.8%)	68/72 (94.4%)	0.1306	45/49 (91.8%)	30/34 (88.2%)	0.7107
Baseline infection area of >100 cm^2	21/22 (95.5%)	95/101 (94.1%)	1.0000	113/121 (93.4%)	59/60 (98.3%)	0.2753
Diabetes	3/4 (75.0%)	18/20 (90.0%)	0.4368	39/43 (90.7%)	7/7 (100.0%)	1.0000
Patient age (<65 y)	18/19(94.7%)	150/159(94.3%)	1.0000	136/145 (93.8%)	84/92 (91.3%)	0.6065
Study medication						
Ceftaroline	17/19 (89.5%)	91/94 (96.8%)	0.1962	82/89 (92.1%)	46/51 (90.2%)	0.7578
Vancomycin plus Aztreonam	10/10 (100.0%)	64/70 (91.4%)	1.0000	83/89 (93.3%)	48/51 (94.1%)	1.0000

* = P-Value from generalized 2-sided Fishers Exact Test.
Missing categories are not in the analyses.

PFGE profiles

A total of 470 isolates successfully underwent PFGE genotyping (three isolates failed *smaI* digestion). Of these 470 isolates, 231 (49.1%) were typeable by the USA typing schema. Among the typeable isolates, 171 (74.0%) were USA300. Other strain types identified included USA100 (2 isolates; 0.9%), USA200 (19 isolates; 8.2%); USA400 (6 isolates; 2.6%); USA600 (29 isolates; 12.6%); USA700 (1 isolate; 0.4%); and USA800 (3 isolates; 1.3%).

A comparison of infections caused by USA300 PVL+ with non-USA300 PVL+ isolates (Table 3) demonstrated that USA300 PVL+ infections were associated with non-Caucasian ethnicity, North America, prior antibiotic use, MRSA, and the absence of hospitalization as a risk factor (all $P<0.001$). Neither the presence of a deep abscess, the receipt of surgical intervention nor the antibiotic regimen received differed between the two groups. Outcomes from USA300 PVL+ and non-USA300 PVL+ infections were similar overall ($P=0.80$) and when stratified across multiple sub-groups including methicillin-susceptibility (Table 4).

Discussion

The significance of PVL in the outcome of staphylococcal infections remains unresolved. The present study used a large, contemporary, multinational collection of MRSA and MSSA isolates to evaluate the impact of *pvl* presence on clinical outcome of patients with cSSSI. Despite adjustment for a number of clinically relevant variables, *pvl* presence was not associated with a higher risk of failure. This finding has several implications.

This analysis of the isolates collected in the CANVAS 1 and 2 studies add to an increasing body of evidence [17,18,23] that the simple presence of *pvl* is not the primary outcome determinant in all *S. aureus* infections. This finding persisted after adjusting for patient comorbidities, infection type, infection severity, and patient age. The results of this study are consistent with two previous reports by our group evaluating potential associations between *pvl* and cSSSI caused by MRSA [17,18]. However, the current investigation extends our understanding of the role of *pvl* in staphylococcal pathogenesis by considering its relevance in MSSA infections. While *pvl* is currently considered primarily in the setting of MRSA infections [1–4], its presence in MSSA is also well established [3,6,8,24–26]. Collectively, these results underscore the recent conclusions of Otto [9] that factors other than the mere presence of *pvl* are the primary determinants of clinical outcome in patients with *S. aureus* cSSSI.

However, the infections process is a continuum from onset to resolution and while outcomes did not differ, the presence of *pvl* was associated with important clinical characteristics in patients with *S. aureus* cSSSI. Patients with *pvl*-positive cSSSI were younger, more likely to have major abscess, more likely to be North American and less likely to have health care contact, findings that have been previously noted [17,26]. In contrast, patients with *pvl*-negative strains tended to be older and have comorbidities such as diabetes or peripheral vascular disease. These differences persisted in both the MRSA and MSSA subgroups, and may reflect in part the epidemiologic settings in which the infections were acquired. Healthcare-associated *S. aureus* infections are less likely to contain *pvl* [2] and are also more likely to cause cSSSI in older patients with more comorbid conditions. By contrast, presence of *pvl* is often associated with community-acquired infection. Thus, the presence of *pvl* is associated with a different spectrum of disease in a distinct subgroup of patients and also influences the treatment received in that *pvl*+ cSSSI more frequently required surgical management. However, the need for surgical intervention is a clinical decision and prior knowledge of *pvl* status is unlikely to be of assistance at the time this decision is made.

Following the provision of appropriate management, the current investigation underscores the fact that *pvl* is not the principle determinant of clinical outcome in patients with either MRSA or MSSA cSSSI. Factors other than *pvl* should be

Table 3. Baseline characteristics of 266 patients with *pvl* positive *S. aureus* complicated skin and skin structure infections (cSSSI) stratified by pulsed-field gel electrophoresis type.

Parameter	*Value for indicated patient group; n(%) except where noted* *USA300 (n = 162)*	*Non-USA300 (n = 104)*	*P-Value**
Demographic characteristics			
Mean age(yr) ± SD	40.1 (13.9)	41.1 (16.1)	0.6012
Male	90 (55.6)	61 (58.7)	0 7037
White race	94 (58.0)	87 (83.7)	<0.0001
Source of infection			0.0283
Infected Wound	16 (9.9)	9 (8.7)	
Major Abscess	99 (61.1)	53 (51.0)	
Infected Ulcer	0 (0)	2 (1.9)	
Infected Burn	0 (0)	2 (1.9)	
Infected Bite	9 (5.6)	3 (2.9)	
Deep/Extensive Cellulitis	35 (21.6)	35 (33.7)	
Lower Extremity SSSI in Diabetic Subject	3 (1.9)	0 (0)	
Geographical location			<0.0001§
Eastern Europe	1 (0.6)	70 (67.3)	
Latin America	0 (0)	4 (3.8)	
Western Europe	0 (0)	8 (104)	
US	161 (99.4)	22 (21.2)	
Prior antibiotic use			<0.0001±
No prior therapy	49 (30.2)	62 (59.6)	
≤24 hours of treatment	84 (51.9)	34 (32.7)	
>24 hours of treatment	29 (17.9)	8 (7.7)	
MRSA risk factors			
Hospitalization	69 (42.6)	89 (85.6)	<0.0001
Antibiotic use in 4 weeks prior	108 (66.7)	41 (39.4)	<0.0001
Diabetes Mellitus	18 (11.1)	9 (8.7)	0.6779
Peripheral Vascular Disease	2 (1.2)	5 (4.8)	0.1144
Infection characteristics			
Fever (temp of >38°C)	13 (8.0)	44 (42.3)	<0.0001
White Blood Cells >10,000 / mm^3 **	76 (46.9)	30 (28.8)	0.1006
MRSA	141 (87)	23 (22.1)	<0.0001
Surgical intervention	115 (71.0)	64 (61.5)	0.7919
Study medication			0.5294
Ceftaroline	91 (56.2)	54 (51.9)	
Vancomycin plus Aztreonam	71 (43.8)	50 (48.1)	

* = P-Value from generalized 2-sided Fishers Exact Test. Calculated using 7×2 table (^), 4×2 table (§) and 3×2 table (±).
** = P-Value from 2-sided T-test.

considered for future therapeutic and diagnostic strategies in combating *S. aureus* cSSSI. For example, other characteristics including alpha hemolysin [27], a new bicomponent leukotoxin [28], the antagonistic effects of antibody to control proliferation of PVL-producing *S. aureus* [29], and host species specificity of the neutrophil lysis properties of PVL [30], may also be associated with the clinical outcome of *S. aureus* cSSSI. It is also possible that the genes coding for PVL may simply be markers of particular bacterial clones and are not themselves directly involved in the pathogenesis of more severe infection.

Due to the predominance of USA300 in North America as previously described and also in this study, most reports regarding PVL from this region focus on this strain of *S. aureus*. The multinational nature of the CANVAS studies allowed us to compare infections caused by USA300 PVL+ with non-USA300 PVL+ isolates. Despite some differences in epidemiology regarding the likelihood of community-acquisition, deep abscesses were the main clinical manifestation of both groups and, importantly, the need for surgery and outcomes were equivalent. This suggests that findings relating to the clinical manifestations and outcomes of cSSSI due to USA300 are likely to be generalizable to other PVL+

Table 4. Clinical outcome of cure for 266 patients with *pvl* positive *S. aureus* complicated skin and skin structure infections by pulsed-field gel type, stratified by infection severity, diabetes, patient age, methicillin-susceptibility and study medication.

Covariate	No. of cured patients/total no. of patients (%) with indicated status		
	USA300 *(n = 162)*	**Non-USA300** *(n = 104)*	*P-Value**
Overall	151/162 (93.2)	98/104 (94.2)	0.8030
Type of infection			
Abscess	96/101 (95.0)	49/53 (92.5)	0.4954
Infection wound	13/16 (81.3)	8/9 (88.9)	1.0000
Other non-abscess	42/45 (93.3)	41/42 (97.6)	0.6171
Baseline fever (temp >38°C)	12/13 (92.3)	41/44(93.2)	1.0000
White blood cells >10,000 /mm^3	70/76 (92.1)	28/30 (93.3)	1.0000
Baseline infection area of>100 cm^2	92/98 (93.9)	62/63 (98.4)	0.2478
Diabetes	16/18 (88.9)	9/9 (100.0)	0.5385
Patient age (<65 y)	147/158 (93.0)	87/93 (93.5)	1.0000
Surgical intervention**	109/115 (94.8)	60/64 (93.8)	0.7466
MRSA	132/141 (93.6)	23/23 (100.0)	0.3623
Study medication			
Ceftaroline	87/91 (95.6)	50/54 (92.6)	0.4707
Vancomycin plus Aztreonam	64/71 (90.1)	48/50 (96.0)	0.3039

* = P-Value from generalized 2-sided Fishers Exact Test.
**Receipt of a surgical procedure ≤48 hours post enrolment.
Missing categories are not in the analyses.

infections. However, the epidemic spread of USA300 in North America compared to PVL+ clones elsewhere in the world remains unexplained and our data indicate that factors other than PVL may play a more important role in the success of USA300.

The *S. aureus* isolates collections used in this study are large, contemporary, multinational, cSSSI specific, and clinically characterized to the level of rigor of a U.S. Food and Drug Administration (FDA) registrational trial. Limitations include the fact that we did not evaluate quantitative *pvl* expression or the presence of *pvl* polymorphisms, as these properties may influence the function of gene products [31,32], although *pvl* polymorphisms have not been found to be of clinical importance [26]. By design, this investigation focused only upon infections in which the causative pathogen was available for culture. We were also unable to consider potential relationships between vancomycin trough levels and outcome.

In summary, this study has demonstrated that presence of *pvl* in *S. aureus* strains is not associated with a worse outcome in patients with cSSSI. This finding persisted regardless of methicillin-resistance status. These findings indicate that factors other than the presence of *pvl* are the primary determinants of clinical outcome in *S. aureus* cSSSI. Future efforts are necessary for a more complete understanding of the role of *pvl* in the pathogenesis of serious infections due to *S. aureus*.

Acknowledgments

Charlotte L. Nelson served in the lead data management role for this project.

Author Contributions

Conceived and designed the experiments: AT DB VGF. Performed the experiments: AT SYCT YZ SL BKS TR SA. Analyzed the data: SYCT GT DB. Contributed reagents/materials/analysis tools: FR. Wrote the paper: AT SYCT DB VGF. Critical review of the manuscript: LL IC.

References

1. Daum RS (2007) Skin and Soft-Tissue Infections Caused by Methicillin-Resistant *Staphylococcus aureus*. N Engl J Med 357: 380–390.
2. Naimi TS, LeDell KH, Como-Sabetti K, Borchardt SM, Boxrud DJ, et al. (2003) Comparison of community- and health care-associated methicillin-resistant *Staphylococcus aureus* infection. JAMA 290: 2976–2984.
3. Moran GJ, Krishnadasan A, Gorwitz RJ, Fosheim GE, McDougal LK, et al. (2006) Methicillin-resistant *S. aureus* infections among patients in the emergency department. N Engl J Med 355: 666–674.
4. Stryjewski ME, Chambers HF (2008) Skin and soft-tissue infections caused by community-acquired methicillin-resistant *Staphylococcus aureus*. Clin Infect Dis 46 Suppl 5: S368–377.
5. Genestier AL, Michallet MC, Prevost G, Bellot G, Chalabreysse L, et al. (2005) *Staphylococcus aureus* Panton-Valentine leukocidin directly targets mitochondria and induces Bax-independent apoptosis of human neutrophils. J Clin Invest 115: 3117–3127.
6. Lina G, Piemont Y, Godail-Gamot F, Bes M, Peter MO, et al. (1999) Involvement of Panton-Valentine leukocidin-producing *Staphylococcus aureus* in primary skin infections and pneumonia. Clin Infect Dis 29: 1128–1132.
7. King MD, Humphrey BJ, Wang YF, Kourbatova EV, Ray SM, et al. (2006) Emergence of community-acquired methicillin-resistant *Staphylococcus aureus* USA 300 clone as the predominant cause of skin and soft-tissue infections. Ann Intern Med 144: 309–317.
8. Tinelli M, Monaco M, Vimercati M, Ceraminiello A, Pantosti A (2009) Methicillin-susceptible *Staphylococcus aureus* in skin and soft tissue infections, Northern Italy. Emerg Infect Dis 15: 250–257.
9. Otto M (2011) A MRSA-terious enemy among us: end of the PVL controversy? Nat Med 17: 169–170.
10. Labandeira-Rey M, Couzon F, Boisset S, Brown EL, Bes M, et al. (2007) *Staphylococcus aureus* Panton-Valentine leukocidin causes necrotizing pneumonia. Science 315: 1130–1133.
11. Diep BA, Chan L, Tattevin P, Kajikawa O, Martin TR, et al. (2010) Polymorphonuclear leukocytes mediate *Staphylococcus aureus* Panton-Valentine

leukocidin-induced lung inflammation and injury. Proc Natl Acad Sci U S A 107: 5587–5592.
12. Gillet Y, Issartel B, Vanhems P, Fournet JC, Lina G, et al. (2002) Association between *Staphylococcus aureus* strains carrying gene for Panton-Valentine leukocidin and highly lethal necrotising pneumonia in young immunocompetent patients. Lancet 359: 753–759.
13. Bocchini CE, Hulten KG, Mason EO Jr., Gonzalez BE, Hammerman WA, et al. (2006) Panton-Valentine leukocidin genes are associated with enhanced inflammatory response and local disease in acute hematogenous *Staphylococcus aureus* osteomyelitis in children. Pediatrics 117: 433–440.
14. Cremieux AC, Dumitrescu O, Lina G, Vallee C, Cote JF, et al. (2009) Panton-valentine leukocidin enhances the severity of community-associated methicillin-resistant *Staphylococcus aureus* rabbit osteomyelitis. PLoS ONE 4: e7204.
15. Miller LG, Perdreau-Remington F, Rieg G, Mehdi S, Perlroth J, et al. (2005) Necrotizing fasciitis caused by community-associated methicillin-resistant *Staphylococcus aureus* in Los Angeles. N Engl J Med 352: 1445–1453.
16. Li M, Cheung GY, Hu J, Wang D, Joo HS, et al. (2010) Comparative analysis of virulence and toxin expression of global community-associated methicillin-resistant *Staphylococcus aureus* strains. J Infect Dis 202: 1866–1876.
17. Bae IG, Tonthat GT, Stryjewski ME, Rude TH, Reilly LF, et al. (2009) Presence of genes encoding the Panton-Valentine leukocidin exotoxin is not the primary determinant of outcome in patients with complicated skin and skin structure infections due to methicillin-resistant *Staphylococcus aureus*: results of a multinational trial. J Clin Microbiol 47: 3952–3957.
18. Campbell SJ, Deshmukh HS, Nelson CL, Bae IG, Stryjewski ME, et al. (2008) Genotypic characteristics of *Staphylococcus aureus* isolates from a multinational trial of complicated skin and skin structure infections. J Clin Microbiol 46: 678–684.
19. Corey GR, Wilcox MH, Talbot GH, Thye D, Friedland D, et al. (2010) CANVAS 1: the first Phase III, randomized, double-blind study evaluating ceftaroline fosamil for the treatment of patients with complicated skin and skin structure infections. J Antimicrob Chemother 65 Suppl 4: iv41–51.
20. Wilcox MH, Corey GR, Talbot GH, Thye D, Friedland D, et al. (2010) CANVAS 2: the second Phase III, randomized, double-blind study evaluating ceftaroline fosamil for the treatment of patients with complicated skin and skin structure infections. J Antimicrob Chemother 65 Suppl 4: iv53–iv65.
21. Corey GR, Wilcox M, Talbot GH, Friedland HD, Baculik T, et al. (2010) Integrated analysis of CANVAS 1 and 2: phase 3, multicenter, randomized, double-blind studies to evaluate the safety and efficacy of ceftaroline versus vancomycin plus aztreonam in complicated skin and skin-structure infection. Clin Infect Dis 51: 641–650.
22. McDougal LK, Steward CD, Killgore GE, Chaitram JM, McAllister SK, et al. (2003) Pulsed-field gel electrophoresis typing of oxacillin-resistant *Staphylococcus aureus* isolates from the United States: establishing a national database. J Clin Microbiol 41: 5113–5120.
23. Bubeck Wardenburg J, Palazzolo-Ballance AM, Otto M, Schneewind O, DeLeo FR (2008) Panton-Valentine leukocidin is not a virulence determinant in murine models of community-associated methicillin-resistant *Staphylococcus aureus* disease. J Infect Dis 198: 1166–1170.
24. Fontanilla JM, Kirkland KB, Talbot EA, Powell KE, Schwartzman JD, et al. (2010) Outbreak of skin infections in college football team members due to an unusual strain of community-acquired methicillin-susceptible *Staphylococcus aureus*. J Clin Microbiol 48: 609–611.
25. Perez-Roth E, Alcoba-Florez J, Lopez-Aguilar C, Gutierrez-Gonzalez I, Rivero-Perez B, et al. (2010) Familial furunculosis associated with community-acquired leukocidin-positive methicillin-susceptible *Staphylococcus aureus* ST152. J Clin Microbiol 48: 329–332.
26. Tong SY, Lilliebridge RA, Bishop EJ, Cheng AC, Holt DC, et al. (2010) Clinical correlates of Panton-Valentine leukocidin (PVL), PVL isoforms, and clonal complex in the *Staphylococcus aureus* population of Northern Australia. J Infect Dis 202: 760–769.
27. Kennedy AD, Bubeck Wardenburg J, Gardner DJ, Long D, Whitney AR, et al. (2010) Targeting of alpha-hemolysin by active or passive immunization decreases severity of USA300 skin infection in a mouse model. J Infect Dis 202: 1050–1058.
28. Ventura CL, Malachowa N, Hammer CH, Nardone GA, Robinson MA, et al. (2010) Identification of a novel *Staphylococcus aureus* two-component leukotoxin using cell surface proteomics. PLoS ONE 5: e11634.
29. Yoong P, Pier GB (2010) Antibody-mediated enhancement of community-acquired methicillin-resistant *Staphylococcus aureus* infection. Proc Natl Acad Sci U S A 107: 2241–2246.
30. Loffler B, Hussain M, Grundmeier M, Bruck M, Holzinger D, et al. (2010) *Staphylococcus aureus* Panton-Valentine leukocidin is a very potent cytotoxic factor for human neutrophils. PLoS Pathog 6: e1000715.
31. Kennedy AD, Otto M, Braughton KR, Whitney AR, Chen L, et al. (2008) Epidemic community-associated methicillin-resistant *Staphylococcus aureus*: Recent clonal expansion and diversification. Proc Natl Acad Sci U S A 105: 1327–1332.
32. Xu Y, Rivas JM, Brown EL, Liang X, Hook M (2004) Virulence potential of the staphylococcal adhesin CNA in experimental arthritis is determined by its affinity for collagen. J Infect Dis 189: 2323–2333.

8

Panton-Valentine Leukocidin Does Play a Role in the Early Stage of *Staphylococcus aureus* Skin Infections: A Rabbit Model

Urszula Lipinska[1]*, Katleen Hermans[1], Lieve Meulemans[1], Oana Dumitrescu[3,4,5], Cedric Badiou[3,4], Luc Duchateau[2], Freddy Haesebrouck[1], Jerome Etienne[3,4,5], Gerard Lina[3,4,5]

1 Department of Pathology, Bacteriology and Avian Diseases, Faculty of Veterinary Medicine, Ghent University, Merelbeke, Belgium, **2** Department of Physiology and Biometry, Faculty of Veterinary Medicine, Ghent University, Merelbeke, Belgium, **3** Centre National de Référence des Staphylocoques, Université Lyon 1, Lyon, France, **4** INSERM U851, IFR128, Lyon, France, **5** Hospices Civils de Lyon, Lyon, France

Abstract

Despite epidemiological data linking necrotizing skin infections with the production of Panton-Valentine leukocidin (PVL), the contribution of this toxin to the virulence of *S. aureus* has been highly discussed as a result of inconclusive results of in vivo studies. However, the majority of these results originate from experiments using mice, an animal species which neutrophils - the major target cells for PVL - are highly insensitive to the action of this leukocidin. In contrast, the rabbit neutrophils have been shown to be as sensitive to PVL action as human cells, making the rabbit a better experimental animal to explore the PVL role. In this study we examined whether PVL contributes to *S. aureus* pathogenicity by means of a rabbit skin infection model. The rabbits were injected intradermally with 10^8 cfu of either a PVL positive community-associated methicillin-resistant *S. aureus* isolate, its isogenic PVL knockout or a PVL complemented knockout strain, and the development of skin lesions was observed. While all strains induced skin infection, the wild type strain produced larger lesions and a higher degree of skin necrosis compared to the PVL knockout strain in the first week after the infection. The PVL expression in the rabbits was indirectly confirmed by a raise in the serum titer of anti-LukS-PV antibodies observed only in the rabbits infected with PVL positive strains. These results indicate that the rabbit model is more suitable for studying the role of PVL in staphylococcal diseases than other animal models. Further, they support the epidemiological link between PVL producing *S. aureus* strains and necrotizing skin infections.

Editor: Binh An Diep, University of California San Francisco, United States of America

Funding: This research was funded by the Special Research Fund of Ghent University (01J.055.06), the grant European Community (EC 222718), Pfizer, bioMerieux and Novartis. The funders had no role in study design, data collection and analysis, decision to publish, or preparation of the manuscript.

Competing Interests: Gerard Lina received grants from Pfizer and Novartis to examine the impact of their molecule on PVL production, and from bioMerieux to develop rapid test for PVL detection. There is no relationship between these projects and the manuscript.

* E-mail: urszula.lipinska@ugent.be

Introduction

Staphylococcus aureus is a potent human pathogen causing various medical conditions, from minor skin infections (i.a. pimples, impetigo, abscesses) to life-threatening diseases (i.a. bacteraemia, endocarditis and sepsis) [1]. The capacity of *S. aureus* to evoke such a wide range of clinical manifestations may be attributed to the production of numerous exoproteins. One of them, Panton-Valentine leukocidin (PVL), is a two-component (LukS-PV and LukF-PV), pore-forming toxin with affinity for neutrophils and macrophages - cells responsible for the first line defence against invading bacteria [2–5]. Epidemiologically, PVL-producing strains have been linked with necrotizing 'skin and soft tissues infections' (SSTI) already in the 1990s [6–10]. More recently, the emergence of community-associated methicillin-resistant *S. aureus* (CA-MRSA) strains containing PVL determinants and their association with a rapid growing number of skin infections [11], severe necrotising pneumonia [12] and necrotizing fasciitis [13] raised an interest in the importance of PVL in staphylococcal infections.

One of the first *in vivo* studies evaluating the role of PVL in staphylococcal skin infections showed that intradermal injection of PVL provokes widespread and infiltrated erythema followed by skin necrosis in rabbits [6]. In contrast, subsequent *in vivo* experiments using murine models failed to uniformly prove the PVL contribution to the development of staphylococcal skin infections [14–17]. The reason for this inconsistency has been linked to a species-specific susceptibility of the host cells to PVL [18,19]. Since neutrophils isolated from mice have been reported to be relatively insensitive to the leukotoxic effect of PVL in contrast to human and rabbit cells [2,18], the latter has been postulated to be a better model for studying the role of PVL [18,19].

Therefore, we employed a rabbit skin infection model in order to evaluate the contribution of PVL to the pathogenicity of the *S. aureus* USA300 strain, a predominant cause of community-associated staphylococcal infections in Northern America [20], using isogenic PVL positive and negative strains.

Materials and Methods

Bacterial strains and culture

To provide optimal conditions for the production of PVL, all strains used in this study were cultivated in CCY medium [3]. LAC is a USA300 pulsotype community-associated methicillin resistant *S. aureus* (CA-MRSA) isolate, LACΔ*pvl* is its isogenic PVL knockout strain constructed as described elsewhere [14]. LUG1515 was obtained by trans-complementation of PVL in the LACΔ*pvl* strain using a pLUG534 plasmid [21]. To support plasmid maintenance, all growth media for the LUG1515 strain were supplemented with chloramphenicol (10 µg/ml).

To prepare the bacterial inoculum, a single colony was propagated in 5 ml of casein hydrolysate and yeast extract medium (CCY) medium with constant shaking at 200 revolutions per minute (rpm) at 37°C. The overnight culture was diluted 1:200 in CCY, incubated till the mid-exponential growth phase ($OD_{600} = 0.8$) and harvested by centrifugation. The pelleted bacteria were washed once, resuspended in sterile phosphate buffered saline (PBS) to a concentration of about 2×10^9 colony-forming units (cfu) per ml and immediately used for inoculation. The exact number of bacteria used was determined by plating out serial dilutions of the inocula.

Experimental animals

Thirty-three twelve-week-old albino hybrid rabbits of either sex, weighing 2.5–3 kg, were purchased from ILVO (Melle, Belgium). These animals do not carry rabbit-associated high virulence *S. aureus* strains evoking i.a. skin lesions, as was confirmed by the absence of such strains in swab samples taken from nine different body sites from all animals [22,23]. The rabbits were divided randomly into three groups of eleven animals, which were kept in separate HEPA-filtered rooms with negative pressure and light-dark cycles of 12 h per 12 h. The rabbits were housed individually with water and feed provided *ad libitum*.

Experimental design

From each animal 4 ml of blood was collected from the marginal ear vein before the onset of the experiment. On the day of the infection, the hair on the right flank of each rabbit was shaved with electric clippers (Wella Contura Hair Clipper, Wella) and the skin was disinfected thoroughly with 70% ethanol (Chem-Lab NV, Zedelgem, Belgium). After evaporation of the ethanol, 50 µl of PBS containing 10^8 cfu of either the knockout strain LACΔ*pvl*, the PVL producing strain LAC or the complemented strain LUG1515 were injected intradermally in the right flank of the rabbits of the respective groups.

During the following 14 days the behavior of the animals and their rectal temperature were examined daily, and the appearance of the lesions was noted. Width and length of the lesions and the necrotic areas were measured, and their surface was calculated as described earlier [15], using the formula $A = \pi(l \times w)/2$, where A is a surface, l is a length and w is a width of the lesion. At day 4 after inoculation (p.i.) three randomly selected animals per group were euthanized. Skin biopsies from the inoculation site were taken aseptically and preserved until further analysis. From the remaining animals, blood samples were collected at day 21 p.i., preceding euthanasia and collection of skin biopsies.

The experimental protocol was approved by the ethical committee of the Faculties of Veterinary Medicine and Bioscience Engineering, Ghent University (permit number 2009_121). The animal studies were performed following the EU legislation being the Council Directive 86/609 EEC covering the protection of animals used for experimental and other scientific purposes. Housing and care of the rabbits was in conformity with the adapted Appendix A of the European Convention ETS 123 of the council of Europe, as approved by the multilateral consultation in 2007.

Histological analysis

Following fixation in 10% buffered formalin, the skin samples were dehydrated with increasing concentrations of ethanol, cleared with Histosolve (Thermo Shandon, Pittsburgh, PA) and embedded in paraffin. Four microns sections were used to perform hematoxylin-eosin staining. All samples were examined by light microscopy in the absence of any information about their origin.

Hematoxylin-eosin stained sections were evaluated according to the following parameters: degree of dermal necrosis, degree of dermal inflammation and inflammatory cell type, degree of fibrosis and epidermal changes present.

Detection of anti-PVL antibodies

Blood samples collected during the experiment were incubated for 30 min at room temperature in glass tubes with inert gel barrier and activated disc (Venoject VT109SAS, Terumo). Next, the sera were separated by centrifugation at 1500 rpm for 10 min and stored at −20°C until use.

Antibodies against PVL (before *S. aureus* challenge and at sacrifice) were measured in rabbit sera using an ELISA protocol adapted from Croze et al. [24], with a peroxidase-conjugated swine anti-rabbit polyvalent IgG diluted $1{:}10^3$ (DAKO). Serial dilutions of anti-LukS-PV polyclonal rabbit serum (bioMérieux) were used for calibration. The results were expressed in arbitrary units per liter (AU/L), with one arbitrary unit corresponding to the amount of anti-LukS-PV antibodies present in a $1{:}10^7$ dilution of the polyclonal rabbit reference serum.

Statistical analysis

The comparison between strains with respect to diameter of the necrotic area, diameter and surface of the lesion was based on the linear mixed model with strain, time and their interaction as categorical fixed effects and rabbit as random effect. A global significance level of 5% was used. For multiple comparisons (the comparison of the 3 strains at each of the 14 times separately), Bonferroni's adjustment technique was used leading to a comparisonwise significance level of $0.5\%/(5 \times 14) = 0.096\%$.

Antibody levels were compared pairwise between strains at 0 and 21 days after infection using a t-test.

Results

Clinical observations

The rectal temperature registered for all rabbits during the experiment was within the normal range [25], with an exception of the first day after the infection. On that day, two animals in group LACΔ*pvl* and one animal in group LUG1515 developed fever (above 40.6°C).

Despite the developing lesions and the raised temperature on day 1 p.i., all animals remained alert, showed normal grooming behavior and appetite throughout the entire experiment.

Macroscopic description of the lesion development

All 33 rabbits developed an inflammatory reaction at the site of injection of the bacteria within the first 24 h, which within the following days evolved into fully grown lesions. The lesions appeared as a central necrotic area surrounded by a region of inflamed skin. The areas of necrosis became encrusted in all animals by day 5 p.i. (photos in fig. 1 show the appearance of the

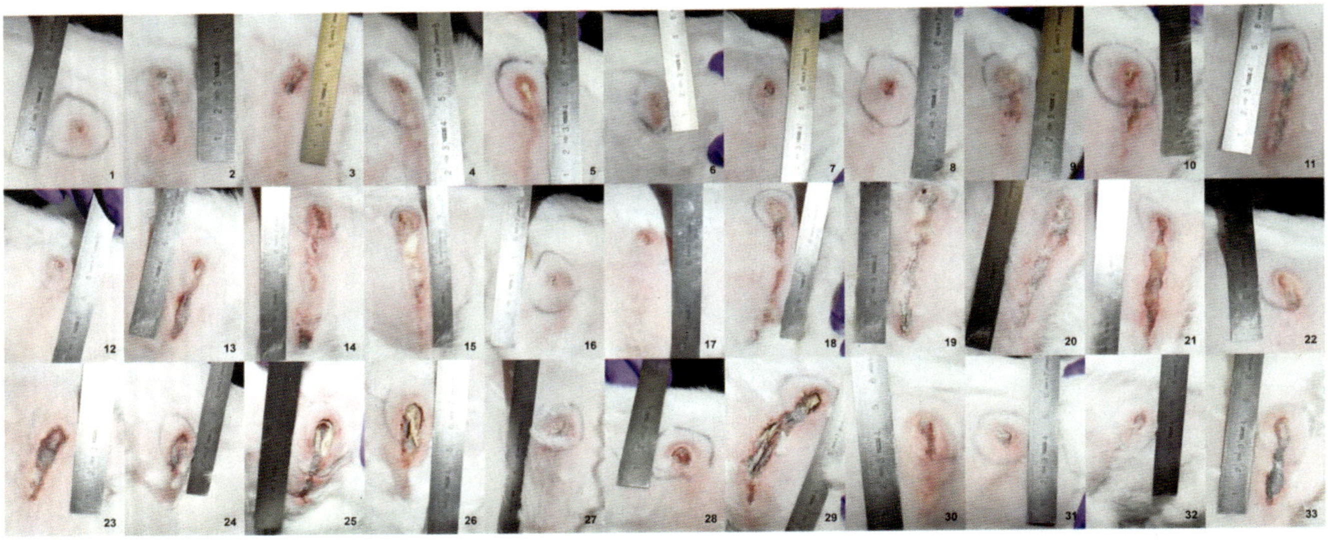

Figure 1. The appearance of lesions on day 4 after infection. The appearance of the lesions on day 4 p.i. in rabbits infected with LACΔ*pvl* (1–11), LAC (12–22) and LUG1515 (23–33). The unit of length of used measuring rod is centimetre.

lesions on day 4). The crusts in the LUG1515 group were situated deeper in the surrounding inflamed skin (fig. 1C), which was not the case in the remaining two groups. Periodic loss of the crusts in all groups revealed purulent material, whereafter a new crust was formed within the following 24 h. Before the end of the observation period (day 14 p.i.) the purulent material within the lesions was replaced by fibrotic scarring tissue.

A graphic overview of the mean surface of the lesions and necrotic areas in different groups during 14 days after infection is presented in figure 2.

The maximal mean diameter of the lesions was observed for all three infection groups on day 3 p.i. and reached 41 (range 7–75), 80 (range 38–115) and 58 mm (range 25–90) in group LACΔ*pvl*, LAC and LUG1515, respectively. On the last day of the observation the mean diameter of the lesions had decreased to 22 mm (range 10–38) in group LACΔ*pvl*, 35 mm (range 15–55) in group LAC and 30 mm (range 16–63) in group LUG1515. The mean diameter of the lesions in group LACΔ*pvl* was significantly smaller than in group LAC from day 3 till 6 p.i. ($P<0.00096$). As the surface of the lesions is a function of their diameter, a similar tendency was observed for the mean surface of the lesions, where a significant difference was observed between group LACΔ*pvl* and LAC from day 3 till 5 p.i. The difference between the surface of the lesions of group LACΔ*pvl* and LUG1515 was significant only on day 3 p.i.

The maximal mean diameter of the necrotic area was observed in group LACΔ*pvl* on day 6 p.i., in group LAC on day 2 and in group LUG1515 on day 5, reaching a diameter of 20 (range 7–47), 47 (range 6–92) and 30 mm (range 9–69), respectively. On the last day of the observation the mean diameter of the dermonecrosis had decreased to 12 mm in group LACΔ*pvl*, 23 in group LAC and 17 in group LUG1515. The mean diameter of the necrotic area in group LACΔ*pvl* was significantly smaller than in group LAC on day 2 p.i. ($P<0.00096$). For days 3–7 p.i. the results were similar, but the difference was not significant. The surface of the dermonecrosis showed a similar tendency with significant difference between LACΔ*pvl* and LAC on day 2 and 3 p.i., and similar but not significant results for days 4–6 p.i.

In the course of the experiment one animal in group LACΔ*pvl*, three in group LAC and two in group LUG1515 developed a secondary lesion on their abdomen. This was possibly a result of gravity-enhanced transport of the bacteria through the lymphatic system. Those lesions were not included in the statistical analysis as there was no physical connection of those lesions with the lesion at the original inoculation site.

Histological examination

The histopathological changes observed in skin samples collected from animals euthanized at day 4 p.i. are presented in table 1, and photos of the representative histological sections are shown in figure 3.

For rabbits euthanized at the end of the experiment (day 21 p.i.), the following histological findings were noted in the skin. In all samples from the LACΔ*pvl* and LAC inoculated groups there was a marked epidermal hyperplasia and the dermis showed moderate to marked fibrosis with mild perivascular infiltrations of mainly monocytes and lymphocytes. Similar findings were noted in the LUG1515 group, except for one biopsy where there was only a mild dermal fibrosis. In three biopsies from each group some PMNs were present as well. In four LAC, two LUG1515 and one LACΔ*pvl* inoculated skin samples, macrophages were noted. In one biopsy from the LUG1515 group, an old organised intravascular thrombus was present.

Detection of anti-PVL antibodies in the sera

The distribution of the titers of the anti-PVL antibodies detected in the sera collected from the rabbits from LACΔ*pvl*, LAC and LUG1515 group before challenge and at euthanasia are presented in figure 4.

There was no statistical difference between the groups in the titer of anti-PVL antibodies in the sera collected before challenge. While in group LACΔ*pvl* there was no statistical difference in the level of antibody before infection and at day 21 p.i., in group LAC and LUG1515 the mean antibody titers were significantly higher in the samples collected at the end of the experiment (8.4 and 19.6 times, respectively).

A

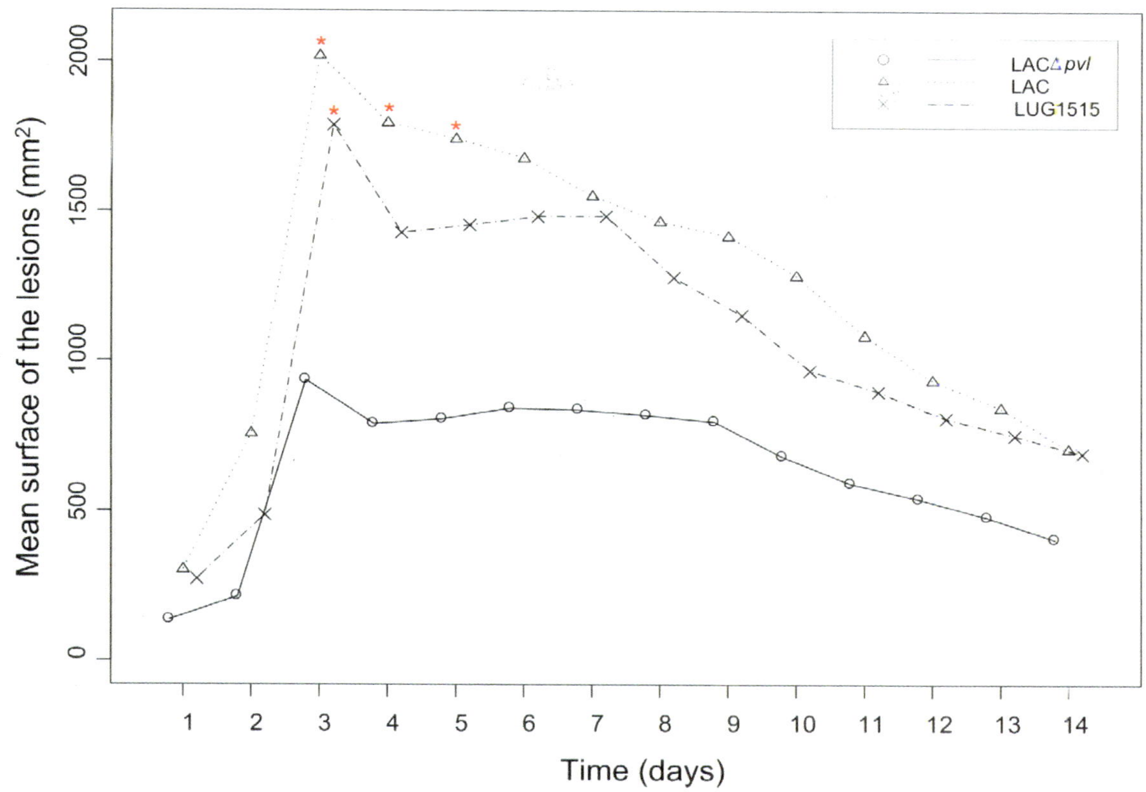
Mean surface of the lesions (mm²)
Time (days)
LACΔpvl
LAC
LUG1515

B

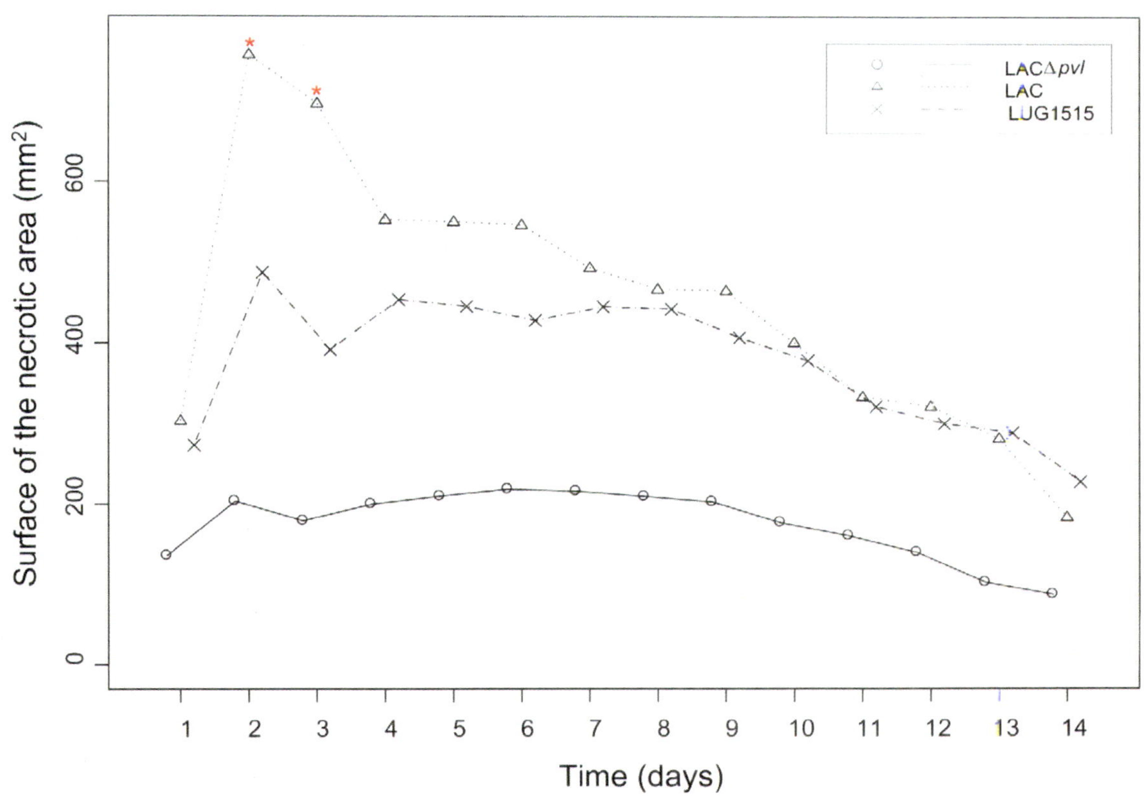
Surface of the necrotic area (mm²)
Time (days)
LACΔpvl
LAC
LUG1515

Figure 2. The size of the lesions and skin necrosis over the time. Mean surface of the lesions (a) and necrotic areas (b) evoked by intradermal injection of LAC (Δ), LACΔ*pvl* (o) and LUG1515 (x) in the rabbits. Asterisk (*) represents a statistically significant result in comparison to LACΔ*pvl* group.

Discussion

Involvement of PVL in the virulence of *S. aureus* has been a controversial topic for many scientists searching for factors responsible for the high pathogenicity of community associated *S. aureus* strains. Inasmuch as murine models have been delivering inconclusive results on the PVL contribution to the staphylococcal skin infections, we examined the role of this toxin using a rabbit - an animal species whose neutrophils are as sensitive to the action of PVL as those of humans [18]. We found that the CA-MRSA USA300 isolate expressing PVL produced lesions with significantly bigger surface than the isogenic PVL knockout strain in the first week after inoculation. Those data suggest that PVL has an impact on the early development of *S. aureus* skin infections in rabbits. In line with our results are the conclusions drawn from other studies investigating the role of PVL in rabbit models. Diep et al. depicted a modest, but measurable role of PVL in the pathogenesis during the early stages of bacteremic seeding in the kidney [26], and Cremieux et al. demonstrated PVL contribution to the local extension of osteomyelitis during the early phase of bone infection [27]. With regard to skin infections, our results are the first showing the capability of PVL producing strain to produce bigger lesions in rabbits, in comparison to their isogenic PVL knockout.

Recently, Li et al. published a study showing that rabbits infected with another USA300-type isolate produced lesions with a surface corresponding to that observed in our study in animals infected with LAC [28]. However, in the same study a PVL negative USA500 isolate evoked comparable lesions, which prompted the authors to the conclusion that PVL does not contribute to the development of skin lesions. The variation between the conclusions of the above mentioned and our study could be attributed to the study set up. While strains used in our study varied only upon PVL expression, those used by Li et al. may differ in respect to other determinants as well. Moreover, the latter failed to detect any PVL mRNA by qRT-PCR in the abscesses of PVL positive strains in their experimental model.

As the PVL determinants have been linked with necrotizing infections, the development of skin necrosis was evaluated during our study. The animals in all experimental groups initially developed necrotic lesions in the place of injection of bacteria. Interestingly, the majority of animals inoculated with the PVL knockout strain developed skin necrosis restricted to the surrounding of the inoculation spot. In contrast, the animals injected with PVL producing strains (LAC and LUG1515) developed necrotic lesions largely exceeding the inoculation area, suggesting that PVL activity accounts for development of severe

Table 1. Histopathological changes in rabbit skin produced by PVL-positive or -negative *S. aureus* strains.

Rabbit belonging to group	Necrosis		Inflammation			Remarks
	location	level	location	level	cell type	
LACΔ*pvl*	dermis	++	dermis	++	PMN ++, MF +/−, LF +/−	
	muscle	−	muscle	+	PMN +/−, MF +	
LACΔ*pvl*	dermis	+++	dermis	+++	PMN +++, MF +/−, LF +/−	
	muscle	−	muscle	+	PMN +/−, MF +	
LACΔ*pvl*	dermis	+++	dermis	+++	PMN +++, MF +, LF +	
	muscle	−	muscle	+/−	PMN +/−, MF +	
LAC	dermis	++++	dermis	++++	PMN ++++, MF +, LF +/−	bacteria observed
	muscle	+++	muscle	+++	PMN ++, MF +	
LAC	dermis	+++++	dermis	++	PMN ++, MF +	bacteria observed
	muscle	+++	muscle	+++	PMN +++	
LAC	dermis	+++++	dermis	++++	PMN +++, MF +/−, LF +/−	
	muscle	+	muscle	++	PMN +/−, MF +	
LUG1515	dermis	++++	dermis	++++	PMN +++, MF +, LF +	bacteria observed
	muscle	+++	muscle	++	PMN ++	
LUG1515	dermis	++	dermis	+++	PMN +++, MF +/−, LF +	bacteria observed
	muscle	+	muscle	+	PMN +/−, MF +	
LUG1515	dermis	+++	dermis	++++	PMN +++, MF +, LF +	
	muscle	++	muscle	+	PMN +	

From animals euthanized at day 4 p.i. lesions samples were used to prepare histological slides and the histopathological changes observed are summarized in the table. The grading system used was as follows: for necrosis (−) absent, (+) mild, (++) mild to moderate, (+++) moderate, (++++) pronounced, (+++++) severe; for inflammation (+/−) several inflammatory cells present, (+) mild, (++) moderate, (+++) pronounced and (++++) severe inflammation; presence of specific cell populations (+/−) few cells present, (+) several, (++) some, (+++) many cells present, (++++) big population of cells observed. Abbreviations: PMN = Polymorphonuclear cells; MF = macrophages; LF = lymphocytes.

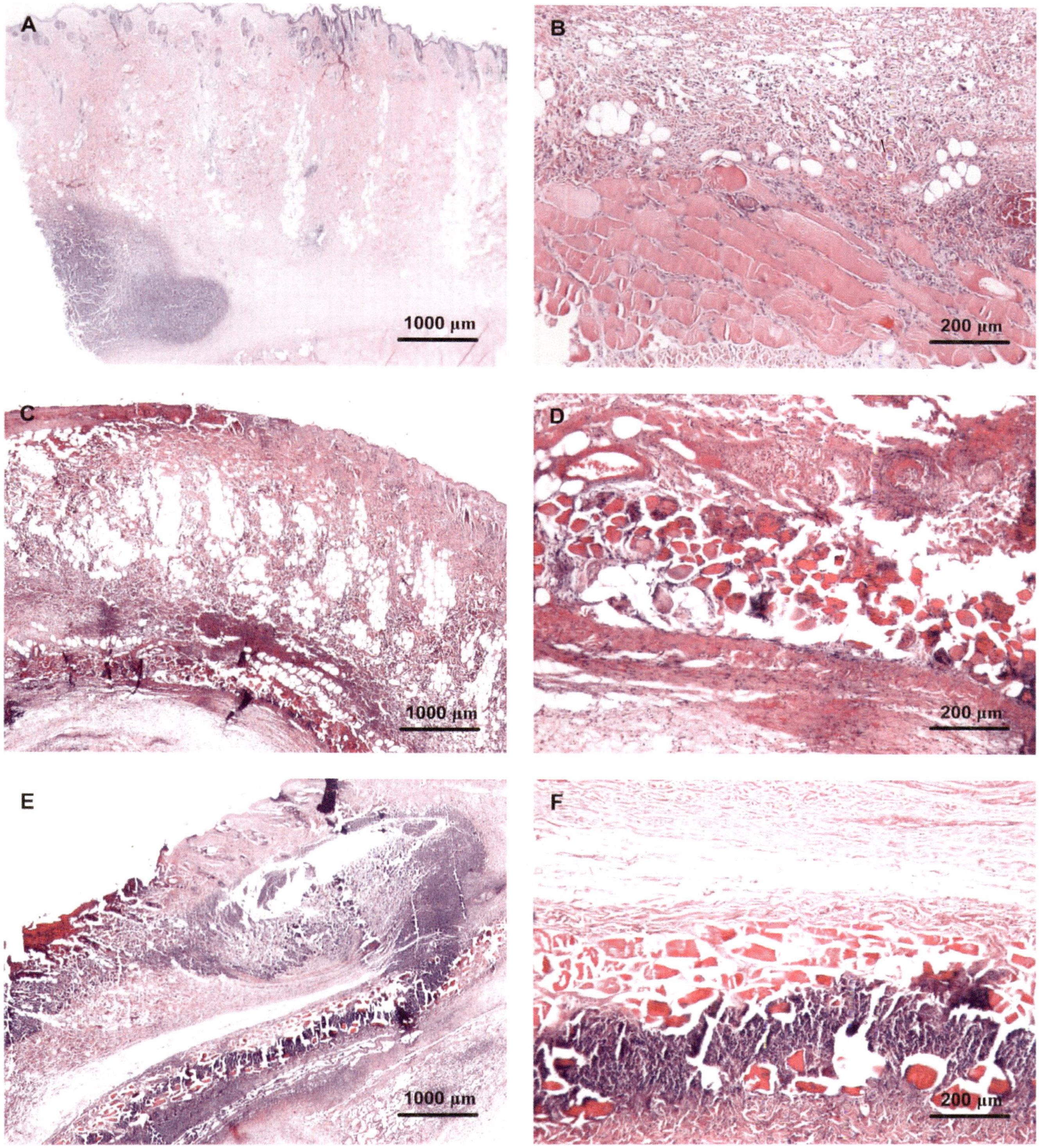

Figure 3. Microscopic appearance of skin lesions on day 4 after infection. The sections of the skin lesions collected from rabbits euthanized at day 4 p.i. were stained with hematoxylin and eosin, and observed under light microscope. A, C and E present the sections from the skin of rabbits infected with LACΔ*pvl*, LAC and LUG1515, respectively. B, D and F show the appearance of the skin muscle layer in animals inoculated with the strains mentioned above.

necrotizing lesions. Obtained results are consistent with those of Cribier et al. [6] who observed development of skin necrosis in rabbits injected with purified PVL and observations from a rabbit model of necrotizing pneumonia where a PVL-producing strain caused more lung necrosis than its PVL knockout [19]. Moreover, the histological analysis of skin biopsies collected at day 4 p.i. from

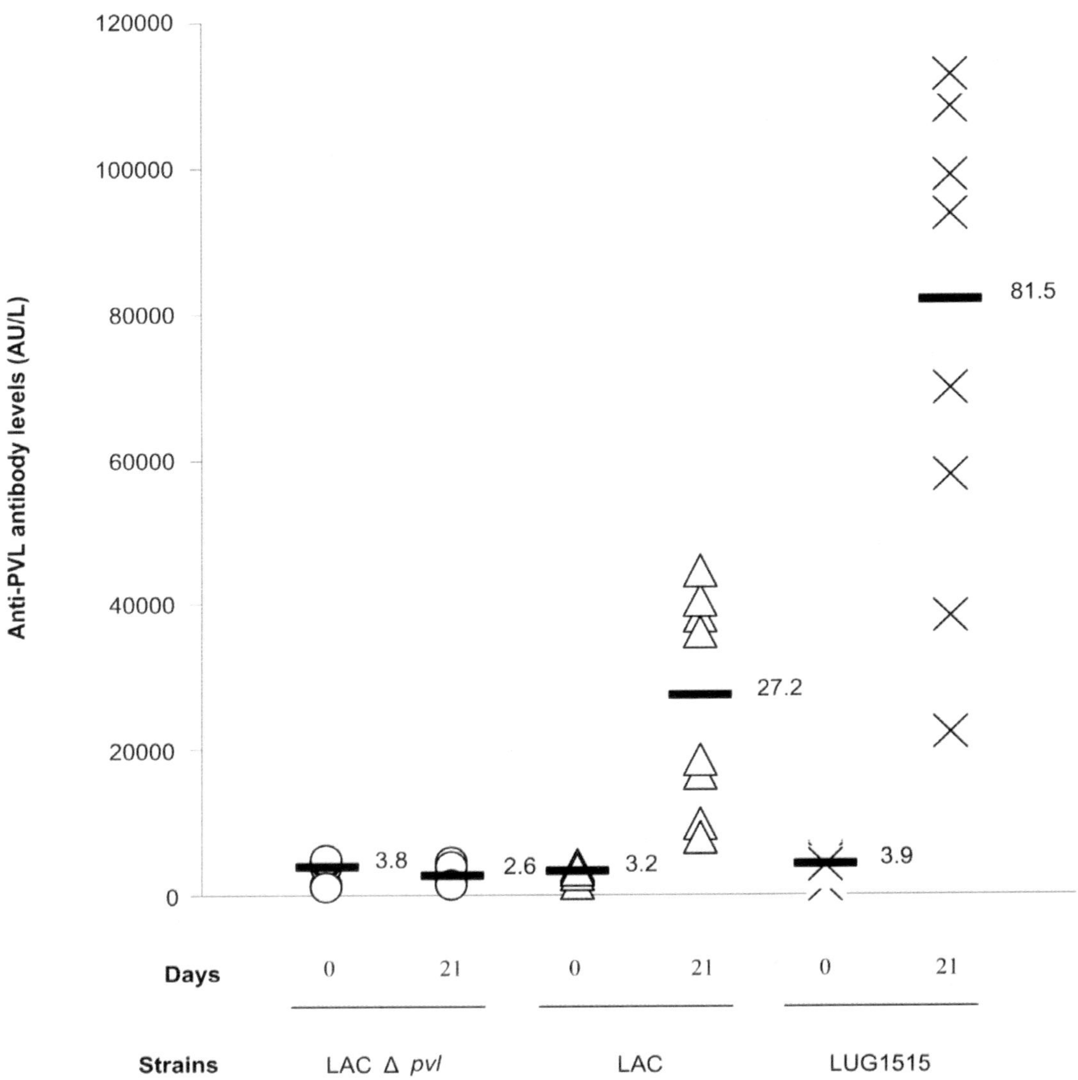

Figure 4. Production of anti-PVL antibodies. Distribution of anti-PVL antibody levels in the sera collected before challenge and at day 21 p.i. from rabbits infected with LACΔ*pvl*, LAC and LUG1515. Bars show the mean value.

the inoculation spot revealed slightly more pronounced damage and inflammatory response in animals infected with PVL positive *S. aureus* strains. The fact that some necrosis and inflammation was observed in the group infected with the PVL knockout strain indicates that other staphylococcal factors (i.e. phenol-soluble modulin, α-toxin) may contribute to the lesion development [28,29]. In conclusion, the presented results endorse the epidemiological link between PVL-producing strains and necrotizing skin infections [6–8,10].

Interestingly, while only minor histopathological differences have been noted for the dermis, necrosis of the skin muscle layer was observed for animals infected with PVL positive strains, in contrast to the PVL knockout where normal muscle was observed. Similarly, Tseng at al. observed damage of the muscle underlying inoculation spot in mice infected with high doses of PVL producing *S. aureus* [16]. Those data indicate that PVL may contribute to the damage of both the dermis and the skin muscle layer during skin infection.

To confirm the fact that differences between the wild type CA-MRSA strain and its PVL knockout could be accounted to PVL action, our study included a PVL knockout strain expressing PVL from a plasmid (LUG1515). Although the lesions produced by that strain differed macroscopically (smaller, but deeper - see fig. 1 and fig. 2a) from those evoked by the wild type strain, both strains produced bigger lesions in the early phase of infection than the PVL negative strain. Despite the fact that the PVL genes were accompanied by the original promoter and translator, the difference in the structure of the lesions produced by the wild type and the complemented strain could be result of a difference in the amount of PVL produced.

In order to confirm the *in vivo* expression of PVL, blood samples collected from the rabbits were analysed for the presence of antibodies directed against PVL. The anti-PVL antibody level in the rabbits infected with the PVL positive strains increased significantly in the course of the infection, while no shift in the titer of the antibody was observed for the rabbits infected with the PVL knockout strain. This raise in the titer of anti-PVL antibody is an indirect proof for production of this toxin during the infection. In line with our results are the observations from human patients where the anti-PVL antibody titers were demonstrated to be higher in patients with PVL positive *S. aureus* infection and to rise 4.6 times in the course of a skin infection [24].

Our results indicate that the rabbit is a better model than the mouse to study the contribution of PVL in the pathogenesis of skin infections by *S. aureus*. It is important that attention is paid to use animals free of high virulence rabbit *S. aureus* strains [30]. Those can be isolated from different body sites in carrier rabbits and can lead to the development of massive skin infection when introduced into the skin lesion. Through the collection of skin swabs from rabbits prior to the experiment, followed by bacteriological examination and molecular analysis of detected staphylococci, high virulence rabbit *S. aureus* strains can be identified [23] and their interference in the studies of human isolates can be avoided.

Although it could be remarked that the evaluation of the lesions was not performed blinded during this experiment, the significant difference in the size of the lesions evoked by wild type strain and its PVL knockout, in combination with the histological observations, indicate that PVL contributes to the severity of skin infections evoked by the CA-MRSA USA300 strain. As USA300 type isolates are epidemic in the USA and are responsible for a growing number of infections worldwide, further studies concerning community-associated staphylococcal infections should not neglect the impact of PVL.

Acknowledgments

We would like to acknowledge Dr. Frank DeLeo for providing us with *S. aureus* strains LAC and LACΔ*pvl*.

Author Contributions

Conceived and designed the experiments: UL GL KH. Performed the experiments: UL OD CB LM. Analyzed the data: UL KH GL JE FH LD. Contributed reagents/materials/analysis tools: UL OD CB. Wrote the paper: UL.

References

1. Lowy FD (1998) Medical progress - *Staphylococcus aureus* infections. New England Journal of Medicine 339: 520–532.
2. Gladstone GP, Van Heyningen WE (1957) Staphylococcal leucocidins. British Journal of Experimental Pathology 38: 123–137.
3. Woodin AM (1959) Fractionation of a leucocidin from *Staphylococcus aureus*. Biochemical Journal 73: 225–237.
4. Szmigielski S, Sobiczewska E, Prévost G, Monteil H, Colin DA, et al. (1998) Effect of purified staphylococcal leukocidal toxins on isolated blood polymorphonuclear leukocytes and peritoneal macrophages *in vitro*. Zentralblatt Fur Bakteriologie-International Journal of Medical Microbiology Virology Parasitology and Infectious Diseases 288: 383–394.
5. Hongo I, Baba T, Oishi K, Morimoto Y, Ito T, et al. (2009) Phenol-soluble modulin alpha 3 enhances the human neutrophil lysis mediated by Panton-Valentine leukocidin. Journal of Infectious Diseases 200: 715–723.
6. Cribier B, Prévost G, Couppie P, Finckbarbancon V, Grosshans E, et al. (1992) *Staphylococcus aureus* leukocidin - a new virulence factor in cutaneous infections - an epidemiologic and experimental study. Dermatology 185: 175–180.
7. Couppie P, Cribier B, Prévost G, Grosshans E, Piemont Y (1994) Leukocidin from *Staphylococcus aureus* and cutaneous infections - an epidemiologic study. Archives of Dermatology 130: 1208–1209.
8. Prévost G, Supersac G, Colin DA, Couppie P, Sire S, et al. (1994) The new family of leucotoxins from *Staphylococcus aureus* - structural and biological properties. In: Freer J, Aitken R, Alouf JE, Boulnois G, Falmagne P, et al. (1994) Bacterial Protein Toxins - Sixth European Workshop. Stuttgart 70: Gustav Fischer Verlag. pp 284–293.
9. Prévost G, Couppie P, Prévost P, Gayet S, Petiau P, et al. (1995) Epidemiologic data on *Staphylococcus aureus* strains producing synergohymenotropic toxins. Journal of Medical Microbiology 42: 237–245.
10. Lina G, Piemont Y, Godail-Gamot F, Bes M, Peter MO, et al. (1999) Involvement of Panton-Valentine leukocidin-producing *Staphylococcus aureus* in primary skin infections and pneumonia. Clinical Infectious Diseases 29: 1128–1132.
11. Diep BA, Sensabaugh GF, Somboona NS, Carleton HA, Perdreau-Remington F (2004) Widespread skin and soft-tissue infections due to two methicillin-resistant Staphylococcus aureus strains harboring the genes for Panton-Valentine leucocidin. Journal of Clinical Microbiology 42: 2080–2084.
12. Gillet Y, Issartel B, Vanhems P, Fournet JC, Lina G, et al. (2002) Association between *Staphylococcus aureus* strains carrying gene for Panton-Valentine leukocidin and highly lethal necrotising pneumonia in young immunocompetent patients. Lancet 359: 753–759.
13. Miller LG, Perdreau-Remington F, Rieg G, Mehdi S, Perlroth J, et al. (2005) Necrotizing fasciitis caused by community-associated methicillin-resistant *Staphylococcus aureus* in Los Angeles. New England Journal of Medicine 352: 1445–1453.
14. Voyich JM, Otto M, Mathema B, Braughton KR, Whitney AR, et al. (2006) Is Panton-Valentine leukocidin the major virulence determinant in community-associated methicillin-resistant *Staphylococcus aureus* disease? Journal of Infectious Diseases 194: 1761–1770.
15. Wardenburg JB, Palazzolo-Ballance AM, Otto M, Schneewind O, DeLeo FR (2008) Panton-Valentine leukocidin is not a virulence determinant in murine models of community-associated methicillin-resistant *Staphylococcus aureus* disease. Journal of Infectious Diseases 198: 1166–1170.
16. Tseng CW, Kyme P, Low J, Rocha MA, Alsabeh R, et al. (2009) *Staphylococcus aureus* Panton-Valentine leukocidin contributes to inflammation and muscle tissue injury. Plos One 4(7): e6387.
17. Brown EL, Dumitrescu O, Thomas D, Badiou C, Koers EM, et al. (2009) The Panton-Valentine leukocidin vaccine protects mice against lung and skin infections caused by *Staphylococcus aureus* USA300. Clinical Microbiology and Infection 15: 156–164.
18. Löffler B, Hussain M, Grundmeier M, Bruck M, Holzinger D, et al. (2010) *Staphylococcus aureus* Panton-Valentine leukocidin is a very potent cytotoxic factor for human neutrophils. Plos Pathogens 6(1): e1000715.
19. Diep BA, Chan L, Tattevin P, Kajikawa O, Martin TR, et al. (2010) Polymorphonuclear leukocytes mediate Staphylococcus aureus Panton-Valentine leukocidin-induced lung inflammation and injury. Proceedings of the National Academy of Sciences of the United States of America 107: 5587–5592.
20. Tenover FC, Goering RV (2009) Methicillin-resistant Staphylococcus aureus strain USA300: origin and epidemiology. Journal of Antimicrobial Chemotherapy 64: 441–446.
21. des Horts TB, Dumitrescu O, Badiou C, Thomas D, Benito Y, et al. (2010) A histidine-to-arginine substitution in Panton-Valentine leukocidin from USA300 community-acquired methicillin-resistant *Staphylococcus aureus* does not impair its leukotoxicity. Infection and Immunity 78: 260–264.
22. Hermans K, De Herdt P, Devriese LA, Hendrickx W, Godard C, et al. (1999) Colonization of rabbits with *Staphylococcus aureus* in flocks with and without chronic staphylococcosis. Veterinary Microbiology 67: 37–46.
23. Vancraeynest D, Haesebrouck F, Hermans K (2007) Multiplex PCR assay for the detection of high virulence rabbit *Staphylococcus aureus* strains. Veterinary Microbiology 121: 368–372.
24. Croze M, Dauwalder O, Dumitrescu O, Badiou C, Gillet Y, et al. (2009) Serum antibodies against Panton-Valentine leukocidin in a normal population and during *Staphylococcus aureus* infection. Clinical Microbiology and Infection 15: 144–148.
25. Harcourt-Brown F (2002) The rabbit consultation and clinical techniques. In: Textbook of rabbit medicine. London, . pp 52–93.
26. Diep BA, Palazzolo-Ballance AM, Tattevin P, Basuino L, Braughton KR, et al. (2008) Contribution of Panton-Valentine leukocidin in community-associated methicillin-resistant *Staphylococcus aureus* pathogenesis. Plos One 3(9): e3198.
27. Cremieux AC, Dumitrescu O, Lina G, Vallee C, Cote JF, et al. (2009) Panton-Valentine leukocidin enhances the severity of community-associated methicillin-resistant *Staphylococcus aureus* rabbit osteomyelitis. Plos One 4(9): e7204.
28. Li M, Cheung GY, Hu J, Wang D, Joo H, et al. (2010) Comparative analysis of virulence and toxin expression of global community-associated methicillin-resistant *Staphylococcus aureus* strains. Journal of Infectious Diseases 202: 1866–1876.
29. Wang R, Braughton KR, Kretschmer D, Bach THL, Queck SY, et al. (2007) Identification of novel cytolytic peptides as key virulence determinants for community-associated MRSA. Nature Medicine 13: 1510–1514.
30. Hermans K, Devriese LA, Haesebrouck F (2003) Rabbit staphylococcosis: difficult solution for serious problems. Veterinary Microbiology 91: 57–64.

9

Some Are More Equal - A Comparative Study on Swab Uptake and Release of Bacterial Suspensions

Philipp Warnke*, Liesa Warning, Andreas Podbielski

Institute of Medical Microbiology, Virology, and Hygiene, Rostock University Hospital, Rostock, Germany

Abstract

Objectives: Swabs are widely used to collect samples for microbiological analyses from various clinical settings. They vary by material, size, and structure of the tip. This study investigates the uptake and release capacities for liquid and bacteria.

Methods: Five swabs were analyzed for their uptake and release capacities of *Staphylococcus aureus* and *Staphylococcus epidermidis* suspensions. Two approaches were investigated providing volume-restricted and unrestricted amounts of bacterial suspensions to mimic various clinical situations. Volume and bacterial uptake and release were measured in milligrams and by counting colony forming units (CFU), respectively.

Results: Volume uptake and release in the unrestricted setting varied highly significant between 239.6 mg and 88.7 mg ($p<0.001$) and between 65.2 mg and 2.2 mg ($p<0.001$), respectively. In the volume-restricted setting the complete volume was absorbed by all swabs, volume release could only be detected for flocked swabs (2.7 mg; $p<0.001$). Highest amount of CFU release was detected for the MWE Dryswab in the unrestricted setting for both *S. aureus* and *S. epidermidis* with 1544 CFU and 553 CFU, respectively, lowest release for the Sarstedt neutral swab with 32 CFU and 17 CFU, respectively ($p<0.001$). In the volume-restricted setting MWE Σ-Swab released the highest bacterial amount with 135 CFU *S. aureus* and 55 CFU *S. epidermidis*, respectively, the lowest amount was released by Mast Mastaswab with 2 CFU *S. aureus* and 1 CFU *S. epidermidis*, respectively ($p<0.001$). Within the range of the utilized bacterial concentrations, uptake/release ratios were identical for the particular swab types and independent of the bacterial species.

Conclusions: The influence of the swab type on subsequent diagnostic results is often underestimated. Uptake and release of the investigated bacteria vary significantly between different swab types and sampling conditions. For best diagnostic outcome swabs should be chosen according to the examined situation and the swab performance profile.

Editor: Jan Kluytmans, Amphia Ziekenhuis, Netherlands

Funding: The authors have no support or funding to report.

Competing Interests: The authors have declared that no competing interests exist.

* Email: philipp.warnke@med.uni-rostock.de

Introduction

Microbiological diagnostics are divided in three steps, i.e. (i) pre-analysis, (ii) analysis, and (iii) post-analysis. Optimum performance of the later steps is based on the performance of the previous ones. While steps (ii) and (iii) are exclusively in the hands of the laboratory, step (i) is typically performed at the patient and therefore, is at best partly under quality control of the laboratory. Thus, if the preanalytical step is performed with suboptimal quality, even the highest standards of laboratory quality management cannot compensate the initial flaws.

Swabs are frequently used to collect specimen for cultural as well as molecular microbiological analysis. Different swabs and transport systems have been evaluated for some in vitro and in vivo performance data in the past [1,2,3,4,5,6,7,8]. Yet, in medical facilities often only one swab type is used to cover all needs for microbiological analysis, for example in screening tests for a bacterial carrier status, for the diagnosis of skin or mucosa infections, or to obtain specimens during operations. These situations completely differ in their general presence and amounts of body fluids. The upper limit for volume uptake of the swab is determined by its size and material. Common swab materials are for example rayon, Dacron, cotton, or nylon fibers or alternatively, cellular foam. The modes by which this material is applied to the swab shaft differs. While tips with wound fibers were used for decades, a novel swab type was recently introduced. On such swabs with so-called flocked tips the fibers are arranged in a perpendicular fashion with respect to its shaft, resulting in enhanced uptake and facilitated release of cellular specimens [9,10,11,12].

Obviously, different tip materials have different physical and chemical characteristics which in turn individually influence the process of specimen collection. Additionally, swab handling techniques could significantly affect the recovery rates for microorganisms [13]. Thus, the seemingly simple process of sample collection by swab techniques is influenced by a complex array of parameters which, depending on additive or subtractive effects, could largely change the sensitivity of microbiological assays.

Aim of this study was to characterize swab type-dependent uptake and release rates for fluids and bacteria as important parameters of the preanalytical process in microbiological diagnostics. To address this issue, five commonly used swab types were tested in settings providing unrestricted and restricted volumes of bacterial, i.e. *S. aureus* and *S. epidermidis*, suspensions to mimic various clinical situations. Handling of the swabs followed a strict standardized protocol. Parameters analyzed were volume uptake and release as measured by weight in milligrams as well as uptake and release of different bacterial species as measured by CFU counting.

Materials and Methods

Swabs

The following swabs were tested:

1. MWE medical wire, Corsham Wiltshire England, Tubed Sterile Dryswab, rayon, ref. MW102;
2. MWE medical wire, Corsham Wiltshire England, Sigma Dry Swab Tubed, Σ-Swab, cellular foam, ref. MW941;
3. Mast Group Ltd., Reinfeld, Germany, MASTASWAB MD 555, via Copan, Brescia, Italy, ref. 800155;
4. Copan, Brescia, Italy, FLOQSwabs, nylon fiber, cat. no. 502CS01;
5. Sarstedt, Nuembrecht, Germany, neutral swab, rayon, via Copan, Brescia, Italy, cat.no. 80.1301.

Bacterial culture techniques

Staphylococcus aureus strain ATCC 25923 and *Staphylococcus epidermidis* strain DSMZ 1798 were separately propagated at 37°C in Caso broth (Roth, Karlsruhe, Germany) as overnight standing cultures in ambient air. Early stationary phase cells were harvested, washed in phosphate-buffered saline (PBS; NaCl (137 mmol/l), KCl (2.7 mmol/l), $Na_2HPO_4 \times 2\ H_2O$ (10 mmol/l), KH_2PO_4 (2.0 mmol/l)) at pH 7.4 and resuspended in PBS+ 10% glycerol. Aliquots were stored at −80°C for up to 3 months. After 3 d conservation in the freezer, the viable cell count of 3 tubes was determined according to standard techniques. Bacterial suspensions were prepared for each test series at the day of usage, with a mixed suspension of *S. aureus* ATCC 25923 and *S. epidermidis* DSMZ 1798 bacterial strains at amounts of 2.6×10^4 and 1×10^4 colony-forming units (CFU)/ml, respectively.

Experimental setting

Volume uptake and release. 5 ml Falcon round-bottom tubes (Becton Dickinson, Heidelberg, Germany) were filled with 1000 µl or 10 µl bacteria suspended in PBS, respectively. To analyze volume uptake, swabs were placed into bacterial suspension for 15 seconds and then removed. After establishing the direct 1:1 correlation of bacterial suspension volumes and masses by ten repeated measurements with a 0.1% error range (not shown), tube weight was quantified on a scale (Sartorius Excellence, Sartorius, Göttingen, Germany) prior to introduction and after removal of the swabs. To analyze volume release, inoculated swabs were placed into empty sterile round-bottom tubes, agitated at maximum speed on a lab mixer (Vortex Mixer, neoLab, Heidelberg, Germany) for 10 sec while exerting gentle pressure to the tube wall (swab shaft started to bend) and afterwards removed. Released volumes as measured by masses were then calculated by comparing tube weights before and after the procedure.

Bacterial uptake and release. In the unrestricted volume (1000 µl) setting, CFU were counted from the initial suspensions, the remaining volume and the released volume by plating 100 µl aliquots from ten-fold serial dilutions using PBS as the diluent on Columbia agar supplemented with 5% sheep blood (Becton Dickinson).

In the restricted volume (10 µl) setting, CFU were counted from the initial suspensions. As most of the swabs did not release any liquid, CFU were determined by streaking swabs in a standardized fashion onto Columbia agar supplemented with 5% sheep blood in 5 streaks with a length of 5 cm while constantly rotating the swab shaft in an angle of 45° to the plate and exerting gentle pressure (swab shaft was slightly bended).

For the elution of Copan FLOQSwabs according to manufacturer's instructions, the swabs were rotated (10 turns) in eSwab liquid Amies preservation medium, Copan, Brescia, Italy, ref. 490CE.A. CFU were then counted by ten-fold serial dilution steps and plating of 200 µl aliquots onto Columbia agar supplemented with 5% sheep blood.

Iteration of experiments. All experiments were performed in triplicate (technical replicates) and repeated on three independent time points (biological replicates).

Detection of bacteria

CFU of each bacterial strain were analyzed for every swab used in the experiments. Therefore, bacteria were cultured on Columbia agar supplemented with 5% sheep blood at 37°C under ambient atmosphere for 48 h. CFU were then counted by macroscopic inspection. *Staphylococcus aureus* was distinguished from *Staphylococcus epidermidis* by hemolysis (β-hemolysis vs. no hemolysis) and colony color (golden yellow vs. white), if necessary by agglutination assay (Slidex Staph Plus, bioMérieux, Marcy l'Etoile, France). Additionally, purity controls were performed by analyzing ten arbitrarily chosen colonies of five randomly selected plates with MALDI-TOF mass spectrometry (AXIMA Assurance, Shimadzu).

Statistical analysis

Data were analyzed using nonparametric Mann-Whitney U test. All p values resulted from two-tailed statistical test. p-values of <0.05, <0.01, and <0.001 were considered to be marginally significant, significant, and highly significant, respectively.

Regarding reproducibility of the technical and biological replicates, we tested by using Kruskal-Wallis-Test for each parameter and received no significant results (significance, if $p < 0.01$ because of Bonferroni correction for 5 tests, that means $p < 0.05/5$).

Ethics statement

The study was performed without using human or animal subjects and/or tissues.

For swabbing experiments of healthy humans (table S11) all volunteers provided written informed consent. This study was approved by the ethics committee of Rostock University Hospital (A 2014-0096).

Results

To mimic different clinical situations, settings were chosen providing an unrestricted (1000 µl) and a restricted (10 µl) supply of bacterial suspensions. Since bacterial suspension volumes correlated to respective masses, volume uptake and release was measured in milligrams. Further, uptake and release of bacteria (for both settings) was analyzed by CFU counting.

Volume-unrestricted setting (1000 µl)

Volume uptake. Mean volume uptake by the different swab-types as measured by masses varied highly significant between 239.6 mg and 88.7 mg ($p<0.001$). Mean volume uptake by each swab-type was measured as followed: MWE Dryswab 239.6 mg; MWE Σ-Swab 131.3 mg; Mast Mastaswab 89.4 mg; Copan FLOQSwabs 89.7 mg; Sarstedt neutral swab 88.7 mg (figure 1, table S1 and table S9).

The highest amount was absorbed by the MWE Dryswab. The difference was highly significant compared to all other swabs ($p<0.001$).

The second highest amount was absorbed by the MWE Σ-Swab. Compared to Mast Mastaswab, Copan FLOQSwabs, and Sarstedt neutral swab the difference was highly significant ($p<0.001$). No significant difference in volume uptake could be observed between Mast Mastaswab, Copan FLOQSwabs, and Sarstedt neutral swab ($p>0.05$) (table S1).

Volume release. Mean volume release by the different swab-types varied highly significant between 65.2 mg and 2.2 mg ($p<0.001$). Mean volume release by each swab-type was measured as followed: MWE Dryswab 65.2 mg; MWE Σ-Swab 51.2 mg; Mast Mastaswab 3.1 mg; Copan FLOQSwabs 20.1 mg; Sarstedt neutral swab 2.2 mg (figure 1, table S1 and table S9).

The highest amount was released by the MWE Dryswab. The difference was highly significant compared to Mast Mastaswab and Sarstedt neutral swab ($p<0.001$), and significant compared to Copan FLOQSwabs ($p<0.01$). No significant difference in volume release could be observed compared to MWE Σ-Swab ($p>0.05$).

The second highest amount was released by the MWE Σ-Swab. Compared to Mast Mastaswab and Sarstedt neutral swab the difference was highly significant ($p<0.001$), and significant compared to Copan FLOQSwabs ($p<0.01$). Mast Mastaswab released highly significant less volume compared to Copan FLOQSwabs ($p<0.001$), and a similar amount compared to Sarstedt neutral swab ($p>0.05$). Differences between Copan FLOQSwabs and Sarstedt neutral swab were also highly significant ($p<0.001$) (table S1).

Release of bacteria in absolute numbers. In this assay, each swab was immersed in a suspension containing $2.6\pm0.8\times10^4$ CFU *S. aureus* and $1.0\pm0.2\times10^4$ CFU *S. epidermidis* per ml. Mean release of bacteria by the different swab-types varied highly significant between 1544 to 32 CFU for *S. aureus* ($p<0.001$), and 553 to 17 CFU for *S. epidermidis*, respectively (figure 2, table S2 and table S9).

The following mean quantitative release for each swab-type was measured for *S. aureus*: MWE Dryswab 1544 CFU; MWE Σ-Swab 916 CFU; Mast Mastaswab 59 CFU; Copan FLOQSwabs 242 CFU; Sarstedt neutral swab 32 CFU (figure 2, table S9), and for *S. epidermidis*: MWE Dryswab 553 CFU; MWE Σ-Swab 463 CFU; Mast Mastaswab 25 CFU; Copan FLOQSwabs 138 CFU; Sarstedt neutral swab 17 CFU (figure 2, table S9). The highest bacterial numbers were released by the MWE Dryswab for both *S. aureus* and *S. epidermidis*. The differences were highly significant compared to Mast Mastaswab and Sarstedt neutral swab for both bacterial species ($p<0.001$), highly significant compared to Copan FLOQSwabs for *S. aureus* ($p<0.001$) and significant for *S. epidermidis* ($p<0.01$). Compared to MWE Σ-Swab the difference was only marginal significant for *S. aureus* ($p<0.05$) and not significant for *S. epidermidis* ($p>0.05$) (table S2).

The second highest bacterial amounts were released by the MWE Σ-Swab. Compared to Mast Mastaswab, Copan FLOQSwabs, and Sarstedt neutral swab the differences were highly significant for both bacterial species ($p<0.001$). Mast Mastaswab released significantly less bacteria compared to Copan FLOQSwabs ($p<0.01$), and a similar amount compared to Sarstedt neutral swab ($p>0.05$). Differences between Copan FLOQSwabs and Sarstedt neutral swab were also highly significant for *S. aureus* and *S. epidermidis*, respectively ($p<0.001$) (table S2).

Relative release of bacteria compared to uptake. Mean release of bacteria compared to initial mean uptake varied swabtype-dependent between 27.2% and 0.7% for *S. aureus* and 30.8% and 1.6% for *S. epidermidis*, respectively (figure 3). Since statistical analysis was performed on absolute CFU counts (figure 2, table S2), it was not repeated on the relative ratios.

With respect to the two staphylococcal species, the relative uptake/release ratios did not show significant differences, thereby confirming nonselective interaction of the tip material with the bacteria. Since *S. aureus* and *S. epidermidis* cells were used in a ratio

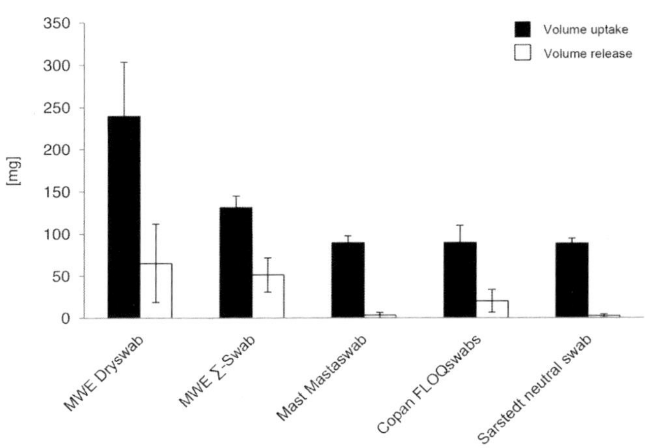

Figure 1. Volume uptake and release (volume-unrestricted setting). Volumes were determined by measuring weight [mg] of round-bottom tubes before and after uptake or deposition of fluids by 5 different swab types. Results from statistical analysis are shown in table S1.

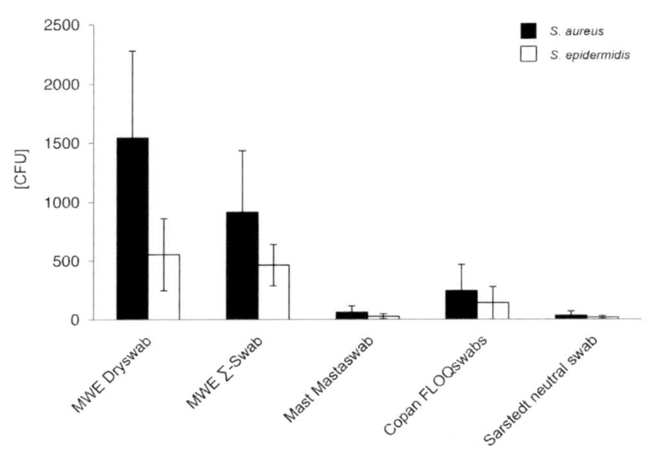

Figure 2. Release of bacteria in absolute numbers (volume-unrestricted setting). Viable counts of bacterial suspension after release by 5 different swab types were determined by serial dilutions and plate counting as described in the methods section. CFU = colony forming units. Results from statistical analysis are shown in table S2.

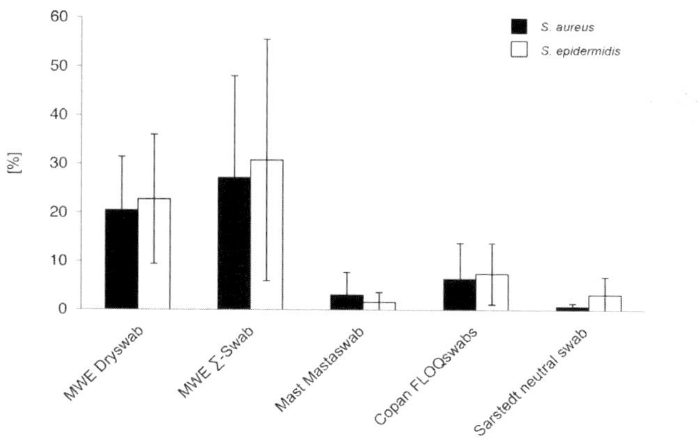

Figure 3. Relative bacterial release compared to initial uptake (volume-unrestricted setting). Ratios were determined by comparison of viable counts of absorbed and released bacteria. Results from statistical analysis are shown in table S3.

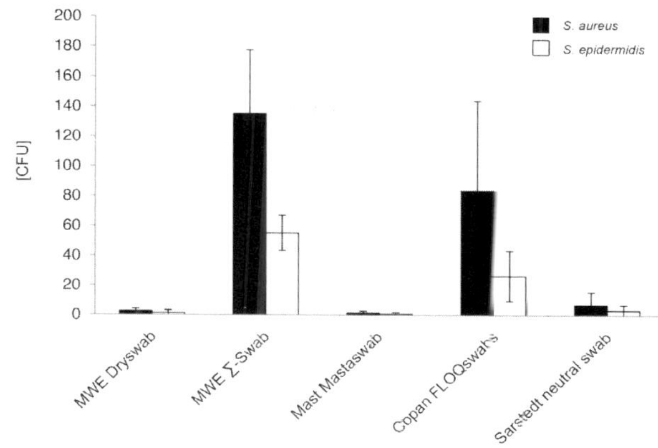

Figure 5. Release of bacteria in absolute numbers (volume-restricted setting). Viable counts of bacterial suspension after release by 5 different swab types were determined by serial dilutions and plate counting as described in the methods section. CFU = colony forming units. Results from statistical analysis are shown in table S5.

of approximately 2.5: 1, within this range, the tip material did not display a dose-dependency for bacterial uptake or release ($p>0.05$) (table S3).

Volume-restricted setting (10 µl)

Volume uptake. All swabs completely absorbed the offered volume, thus no difference between the swabs could be observed (figure 4, table S4 and table S10).

Volume release. No volume was released by the swabs except for Copan FLOQSwabs, which released a mean mass of 2.7 mg. This was highly significant compared to the other swabs ($p<0.001$) (figure 4, table S4 and table S10).

Release of bacteria in absolute numbers. Since the complete offered volumes of bacterial suspensions were soaked up by the swaps, quantitation of absorbed bacteria was not performed, assuming that the major portion entered the tip material. Even when no volume could be extracted from most swab types, bacteria were expected to be released under typical diagnostic conditions. After directly streaking the swabs onto

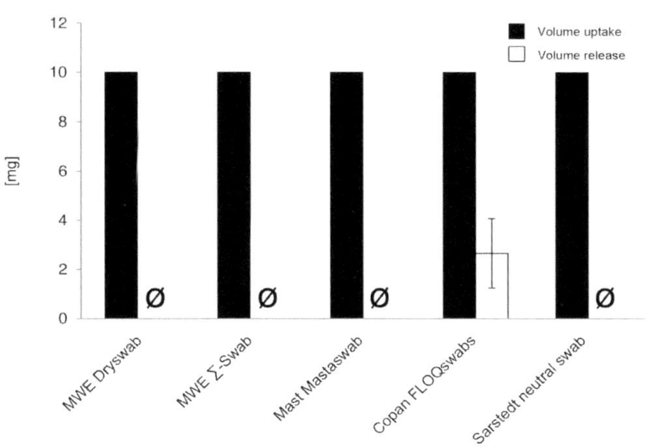

Figure 4. Volume uptake and release (volume-restricted setting). Volumes were determined by measuring weight [mg] of round-bottom tubes before and after uptake or deposition of fluids by 5 different swab types. Results from statistical analysis are shown in table S4.

Columbia agar by a standardized technique, determined mean release of bacterial counts by the different swab-types ranged with highly significant differences for *S. aureus* and *S. epidermidis* from 135 to 2 CFU, and from 55 to 1 CFU, respectively ($p<0.001$) (figure 5, table S5 and table S10).

Mean counts for released *S. aureus* and *S. epidermidis* cells by each swab-type were: MWE Dryswab 3 CFU; MWE Σ-Swab 135 CFU; Mast Mastaswab 2 CFU; Copan FLOQSwabs 84 CFU; Sarstedt neutral swab 7 CFU and MWE Dryswab 1 CFU; MWE Σ-Swab 55 CFU; Mast Mastaswab 1 CFU; Copan FLOQSwabs 26 CFU; Sarstedt neutral swab 3 CFU, respectively (figure 5, table S10).

The highest bacterial numbers were released by the MWE Σ-Swab for both *S. aureus* and *S. epidermidis*. The differences were highly significant compared to MWE Dryswab, Mast Mastaswab, and Sarstedt neutral swab for both bacterial species ($p<0.001$), significant compared to Copan FLOQSwabs for *S. epidermidis* ($p<0.01$) and not significant for *S. aureus* ($p>0.05$) (table S5).

The second highest bacterial amounts were released by the Copan FLOQSwabs. Compared to MWE Dryswab, Mast Mastaswab, and Sarstedt neutral swab the bacterial release was significantly higher for both species ($p<0.01$), compared to the *S. aureus* release of Mast Mastaswab even highly significant ($p<0.001$). Between MWE Dryswab, Mast Mastaswab, and Sarstedt neutral swab no significant difference in the release of the two bacterial species could be observed ($p>0.05$) (table S5).

Relative release of bacteria compared to uptake. Mean release of bacteria compared to postulated initial uptake varied swabtype-dependent between 53.9% and 0.6% for *S. aureus* and 58.5% and 0.9% for *S. epidermidis*, respectively (figure 6). Again, statistical analysis was not performed here because already introduced for the corresponding absolute CFU numbers (figure 5, table S5).

Also again, relative release rates were species-independent for each swab-type. Considering a quantitative ratio of approximately 2.5: 1 between absorbed *S. aureus* and *S. epidermidis* cells, within this range a dose-dependent release could also be excluded ($p>0.05$) (table S6).

Release of bacteria into Amies preservation medium. Release of bacterial numbers by rotating the swabs into Amies preservation medium was analyzed for Copan FLOQSwabs (figure 7, table S10) and compared to the released numbers using the same swab-type without medium. Mean release

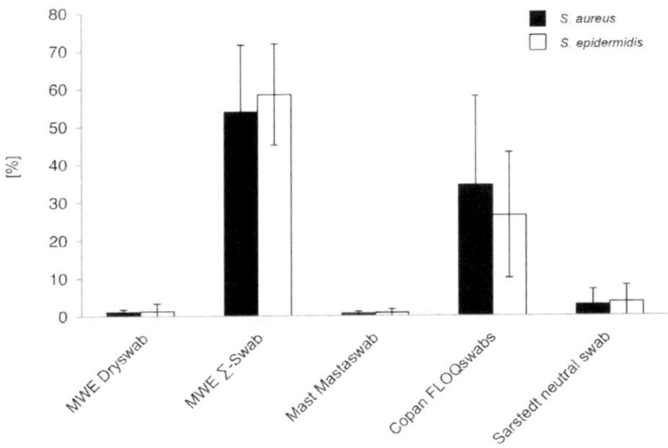

Figure 6. Relative bacterial release compared to initial uptake (volume-restricted setting). Ratios were determined by comparison of viable counts of absorbed and released bacteria. Results from statistical analysis are shown in table S6.

of 197 CFU *S. aureus* and 77 CFU *S. epidermidis* cells was significant higher, compared to 84 CFU and 26 CFU without medium, respectively ($p<0.01$) (table S7). Similar to the results obtained

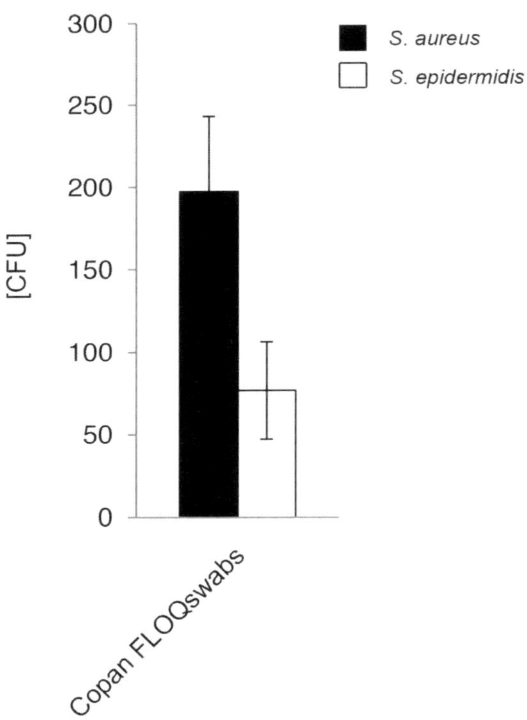

Figure 7. Bacterial release into Amies medium (volume-restricted setting). Viable counts of bacterial suspension after release by flocked swabs were determined by serial dilutions and plate counting as described in the methods section. CFU = colony forming units. Results from statistical analysis are shown in table S7.

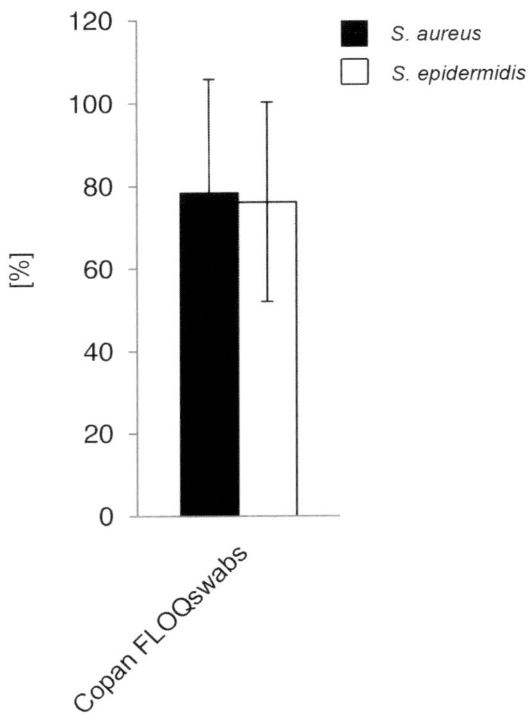

Figure 8. Relative bacterial release into Amies medium compared to initial uptake (volume-restricted setting). Ratios were determined by comparison of viable counts of absorbed and released bacteria. Results from statistical analysis are shown in table S8.

without using Amies medium, release rates were species- and dose-independent ($p>0.05$) (figure 8, table S8).

Discussion

In contrast to massive recent changes in microbiological analysis and postanalysis due to the introduction of exciting novel techniques with high impact on test duration, sensitivity and specificity, the initial step of sample collection has undergone few if any principal changes. However, sample collection quality is crucial for the quality of the subsequent analytical steps and therefore, any improvements of this first step will benefit the whole diagnostic process. Although often leading to inferior diagnostic quality, sample collection utilizing swabs is the preferred technique for most clinicians because of its performance ease and swiftness. Thus, if the general approach for sample collection cannot be changed, it appears prudent to optimize swabs and swabbing techniques [13] especially with respect to test sensitivity. As a prerequisite for optimization, test sensitivities of presently available swabs should be quantified under conditions close to natural circumstances.

Swabs based on a new production technique, so called flocked swabs, have recently been introduced on a commercial basis. Several publications have shown the high performance rates of these swabs with respect to specimen uptake and release by in vitro and in vivo approaches [10,14,15,16,17,18]. In the present study we intended to determine the test sensitivity of routinely used swabs produced by established procedures (i.e. fibers wound onto the swab tip), swabs with a foam tip and the flocked swabs by using two different protocols mimicking sample collection from comparatively dry surfaces such as skin and other epithelia (see table S11) and from wet surfaces such as operation wounds or operative sites [19,20], conditions which so far have not been addressed in a single study.

In this study we separately monitored volume as well as bacterial uptake and release, since each parameter could differ between swabs due to unspecific interaction of fluids or microorganisms with the swab material. For test organisms, we chose *Staphylococcus aureus* as the most frequent causative agent of purulent infections on the skin or mucosa as well as in organ tissues and therefore diagnostic techniques should include detection of this species [21,22,23]. In addition, this species transiently or persistently colonizes especially the anterior nares of 20 to 30% of the human population and therefore is the target for the majority of screening assays for human carrier detection, especially in the nosocomial setting with respect to the MRSA-subset of *S. aureus* strains [21,24,25,26,27,28,29,30,31]. Since *S. aureus* is often associated with the resident microflora of skin and mucosa, we also included *S. epidermidis* [32,33,34,35,36,37,38] as the major representative species into our test format to monitor potential interactions affecting test sensitivity. The inoculum concentrations were between 10^3–10^5 CFU as recommended for swab evaluation testing by the Clinical and Laboratory Standards Institute for aerobic and facultative anaerobic bacteria [39]. To put emphasis on the clinical relevance of *S. aureus*, this strain was used in a ratio of 2.5: 1 compared to *S. epidermidis*, i.e. 2.6×10^4 CFU/ml *S. aureus* and 1×10^4 CFU/ml *S. epidermidis*, respectively, were offered in each test to the swabs.

Utilizing the unrestricted volume test format, absorbed and released volumes significantly differed between the tested swab types. The relative rates of absorbed and released bacterial numbers correlated quite well for each swab type, indicating that swab materials could behave differently towards fluid volumes and bacteria, and these differences comprise both the absorption and release steps. The differences between the swab types could add up to two orders of magnitude. Under these conditions, MWE Dryswab absorbed and released the highest amount of bacteria, while Mast Mastaswab and Sarstedt neutral swab carried the lowest amounts. This indicated, that in a clinical setting with ample fluid supply, swabs with the highest liquid uptake rates such as MWE Dryswab and MWE Σ-Swab would perform best with respect to highest diagnostic yield.

These conclusions cannot be applied to clinical settings with restricted volume amounts. In such a setting, only the Copan FLOQSwabs released some fluid. When testing bacterial release upon contact to an agar surface, only MWE Σ-Swabs and Copan FLOQSwabs released mentionable bacterial numbers. Thus, under such conditions and in the presence of only low bacterial counts, usage of MWE Dryswab, Mast mastaswab and Sarstedt neutral swab could lead to false negative results. Under routine diagnostic conditions, most microbiological specimens are processed by semiquantitative methods [40]. For instance, in a recent study, nasal colonization was categorized as low, 1+, 2+, 3+, and 4+. Then low colonization was described in 31% of patients [41], a situation when the above mentioned disclaimer for the latter three swab types would apply.

The performance of Copan FLOQSwabs under volume-restricted conditions was further improved by applying the tip into Amies medium directly after the absorption of bacterial suspensions as also described when employing other bacterial species [42]. With this specific protocol, this swab type led to the best results – similar to the results of an in vivo study on swabs for nasal MRSA screening [43]. However, this protocol requires usage of the complete set of swab and transport tubes offered by the manufacturer. If the tubes are not available or the laboratory procedures are not set to deal with liquid specimens, MWE Σ-Swabs offer a similarly efficient alternative. The present experimental settings did not stress the swab surface during absorption of bacterial suspensions. Contact to rough surfaces obviously affects the tip structures to a varying degree (more so for wound fibers than for flocked ones), which in turn would additionally effect bacterial recovery rates in a swab type-dependent manner [44]. That phenomenon would additionally favor usage of flocked swabs for examination of (relatively) dry surfaces. However, the advantage of flocked swaps for test sensitivity is limited to such surfaces and does not extend to situations of ample surface supply.

Importantly, for all tested swab types bacterial release was staphylococcal species and, within the tested range, dose independent. Thus, frequent *S. epidermidis* presence in skin, mucosa and wound material should not affect detection of the most important pathogen *S. aureus*.

There are limitations to this study. Here we focused on bacterial species important in MRSA screening examinations. Yet, for some of tested swab types the results apparently apply to other bacterial species [42], although that study used bacterial suspensions in volumes between the extreme boundaries of the present study. Also, bacterial release was analyzed shortly after inoculation of the tips to simulate optimum transport conditions, thereby omitting potential interactions between tip material and drying bacteria during variable transport periods [45]. Suboptimum transport conditions lead to reduced survival rates of bacteria and consecutively to a decline in analytical sensitivity [2,46,47]. This would especially affect swab types with low numbers of collected bacteria. However, examination of these circumstances would dramatically increase the complexity of results because of the different transport vials and media used in the clinical setting.

Conclusion

This study emphasizes the role of preanalytical parameters on the corresponding diagnostic results. Commonly used swabs vary significantly with respect to uptake and release of liquid and bacteria. Definitely, the clinical setting influences the results obtained by swabbing specimens and should be considered when choosing a swab-type. Obviously, one swab type does not fit all needs and careful selection of swab types for the specific clinical setting plus thorough education of clinical staff for choice of the appropriate swab type as well as its proper usage appears to be necessary for optimal diagnostic results in clinical microbiology.

Supporting Information

Table S1 Volume uptake and release (volume-unrestricted setting). All p values result from nonparametric, two-tailed Wilcoxon-Mann-Whitney U-test.

Table S2 Release of bacteria in absolute numbers (volume-unrestricted setting). All p values result from nonparametric, two-tailed Wilcoxon-Mann-Whitney U-test. CFU = colony forming units.

Table S3 Relative bacterial release compared to initial uptake (volume-unrestricted setting). All p values result from nonparametric, two-tailed Wilcoxon-Mann-Whitney U-test.

Table S4 Volume uptake and release (volume-restricted setting). All p values result from nonparametric, two-tailed Wilcoxon-Mann-Whitney U-test.

Table S5 Release of bacteria in absolute numbers (volume-restricted setting). All p values result from nonparametric, two-tailed Wilcoxon-Mann-Whitney U-test. CFU = colony forming units.

Table S6 Relative bacterial release compared to initial uptake (volume-restricted setting). All p values result from nonparametric, two-tailed Wilcoxon-Mann-Whitney U-test.

Table S7 Bacterial release into Amies medium compared to direct plating (volume-restricted setting). All p values result from nonparametric, two-tailed Wilcoxon-Mann-Whitney U-test. CFU = colony forming units.

Table S8 Relative bacterial release into Amies medium compared to initial uptake (volume-restricted setting). All p values result from nonparametric, two-tailed Wilcoxon-Mann-Whitney U-test.

Table S9 Mean values of volume and bacterial uptake and release (volume-unrestricted setting). CFU = colony forming units.

Table S10 Mean values of volume and bacterial uptake and release (volume-restricted setting). CFU = colony forming units. n.d. = not detected.

Table S11 Amounts of specimen uptaken by pharynx-, nose-, and skin-swabs. 3 healthy volunteers were swabbed at different anatomical locations as indicated. Specimen uptake was measured in milligrams [mg]. SD = standard deviation.

Acknowledgments

We would like to thank George Orwell for the inspiring idea.

Author Contributions

Conceived and designed the experiments: PW LW AP. Performed the experiments: PW LW AP. Analyzed the data: PW LW AP. Contributed reagents/materials/analysis tools: PW LW AP. Contributed to the writing of the manuscript: PW AP.

References

1. Osterblad M, Jarvinen H, Lonnqvist K, Huikko S, Laippala P, et al. (2003) Evaluation of a new cellulose sponge-tipped swab for microbiological sampling: a laboratory and clinical investigation. J Clin Microbiol 41: 1894–1900.
2. Barber S, Lawson PJ, Grove DI (1998) Evaluation of bacteriological transport swabs. Pathology 30: 179–182.
3. Brook I (1987) Comparison of two transport systems for recovery of aerobic and anaerobic bacteria from abscesses. J Clin Microbiol 25: 2020–2022.
4. Citron DM, Warren YA, Hudspeth MK, Goldstein EJ (2000) Survival of aerobic and anaerobic bacteria in purulent clinical specimens maintained in the Copan Venturi Transystem and Becton Dickinson Port-a-Cul transport systems. J Clin Microbiol 38: 892–894.
5. Farhat SE, Thibault M, Devlin R (2001) Efficacy of a swab transport system in maintaining viability of Neisseria gonorrhoeae and Streptococcus pneumoniae. J Clin Microbiol 39: 2958–2960.
6. Hindiyeh M, Acevedo V, Carroll KC (2001) Comparison of three transport systems (Starplex StarSwab II, the new Copan Vi-Pak Amies Agar Gel collection and transport swabs, and BBL Port-A-Cul) for maintenance of anaerobic and fastidious aerobic organisms. J Clin Microbiol 39: 377–380.
7. Olsen CC, Schwebke JR, Benjamin WH Jr, Beverly A, Waites KB (1999) Comparison of direct inoculation and Copan transport systems for isolation of Neisseria gonorrhoeae from endocervical specimens. J Clin Microbiol 37: 3583–3585.
8. Roelofsen E, van Leeuwen M, Meijer-Severs GJ, Wilkinson MH, Degener JE (1999) Evaluation of the effects of storage in two different swab fabrics and under three different transport conditions on recovery of aerobic and anaerobic bacteria. J Clin Microbiol 37: 3041–3043.
9. Abu-Diab A, Azzeh M, Ghneim R, Zoughbi M, Turkuman S, et al. (2008) Comparison between pernasal flocked swabs and nasopharyngeal aspirates for detection of common respiratory viruses in samples from children. J Clin Microbiol 46: 2414–2417.
10. Chernesky M, Castriciano S, Jang D, Smieja M (2006) Use of flocked swabs and a universal transport medium to enhance molecular detection of Chlamydia trachomatis and Neisseria gonorrhoeae. J Clin Microbiol 44: 1084–1086.
11. Dalmaso G, Bini M, Paroni R, Ferrari M (2008) Qualification of high-recovery, flocked swabs as compared to traditional rayon swabs for microbiological environmental monitoring of surfaces. PDA J Pharm Sci Technol 62: 191–199.
12. Krech T, Castriciano S, Jang D, Smieja M, Enders G, et al. (2009) Detection of high risk HPV and Chlamydia trachomatis in vaginal and cervical samples collected with flocked nylon and wrapped rayon dual swabs transported in dry tubes. J Virol Methods 162: 291–293.
13. Warnke P, Harnack T, Ottl P, Kundt G, Podbielski A (2014) Nasal Screening for Staphylococcus aureus - Daily Routine with Improvement Potentials. PLoS One 9: e89667.
14. Daley P, Castriciano S, Chernesky M, Smieja M (2006) Comparison of flocked and rayon swabs for collection of respiratory epithelial cells from uninfected volunteers and symptomatic patients. J Clin Microbiol 44: 2265–2267.
15. Tan TY, Ng LS, Sim DM, Cheng Y, Min MO (2014) Evaluation of bacterial recovery and viability from three different swab transport systems. Pathology 46: 230–233.
16. Wiley DJ, Hsu H, Bolan R, Voskanian A, Elashoff D, et al. (2013) Comparison of 2 anal cytology protocols to predict high-grade anal intraepithelial neoplasia. J Low Genit Tract Dis 17: 414–424.
17. Hernes SS, Quarsten H, Hagen E, Lyngroth AL, Pripp AH, et al. (2011) Swabbing for respiratory viral infections in older patients: a comparison of rayon and nylon flocked swabs. Eur J Clin Microbiol Infect Dis 30: 159–165.
18. Hedin G, Rynback J, Lore B (2010) New technique to take samples from environmental surfaces using flocked nylon swabs. J Hosp Infect 75: 314–317.
19. Stahl DL, Groeben H, Kroepfl D, Gautam S, Eikermann M (2012) Development and validation of a novel tool to estimate peri-operative blood loss. Anaesthesia 67: 479–486.
20. Tjeenk RM, Vrancken Peeters MP, van den Ende E, Kastelein GW, Breslau PJ (2005) Wound drainage versus non-drainage for proximal femor fractures. A prospective randomised study. Injury 36: 100–104.
21. Wertheim HF, Melles DC, Vos MC, van Leeuwen W, van Belkum A, et al. (2005) The role of nasal carriage in Staphylococcus aureus infections. Lancet Infect Dis 5: 751–762.
22. Kluytmans JA, Wertheim HF (2005) Nasal carriage of Staphylococcus aureus and prevention of nosocomial infections. Infection 33: 3–8.
23. Peacock SJ, de Silva I, Lowy FD (2001) What determines nasal carriage of Staphylococcus aureus? Trends Microbiol 9: 605–610.
24. Eriksen NH, Espersen F, Rosdahl VT, Jensen K (1995) Carriage of Staphylococcus aureus among 104 healthy persons during a 19-month period. Epidemiol Infect 115: 51–60.
25. Wertheim HF, Vos MC, Boelens HA, Voss A, Vandenbroucke-Grauls CM, et al. (2004) Low prevalence of methicillin-resistant Staphylococcus aureus (MRSA) at hospital admission in the Netherlands: the value of search and destroy and restrictive antibiotic use. J Hosp Infect 56: 321–325.
26. Davis KA, Stewart JJ, Crouch HK, Florez CE, Hospenthal DR (2004) Methicillin-resistant Staphylococcus aureus (MRSA) nares colonization at hospital admission and its effect on subsequent MRSA infection. Clin Infect Dis 39: 776–782.
27. Huang SS, Platt R (2003) Risk of methicillin-resistant Staphylococcus aureus infection after previous infection or colonization. Clin Infect Dis 36: 281–285.
28. Gupta K, Strymish J, Abi-Haidar Y, Williams SA, Itani KM (2011) Preoperative nasal methicillin-resistant Staphylococcus aureus status, surgical prophylaxis, and risk-adjusted postoperative outcomes in veterans. Infect Control Hosp Epidemiol 32: 791–796.
29. Safdar N, Bradley EA (2008) The risk of infection after nasal colonization with Staphylococcus aureus. Am J Med 121: 310–315.
30. Klein E, Smith DL, Laxminarayan R (2007) Hospitalizations and deaths caused by methicillin-resistant Staphylococcus aureus, United States, 1999–2005. Emerg Infect Dis 13: 1840–1846.
31. Klevens RM, Morrison MA, Nadle J, Petit S, Gershman K, et al. (2007) Invasive methicillin-resistant Staphylococcus aureus infections in the United States. JAMA 298: 1763–1771.
32. Uehara Y, Nakama H, Agematsu K, Uchida M, Kawakami Y, et al. (2000) Bacterial interference among nasal inhabitants: eradication of Staphylococcus aureus from nasal cavities by artificial implantation of Corynebacterium sp. J Hosp Infect 44: 127–133.

33. Grice EA, Segre JA (2011) The skin microbiome. Nat Rev Microbiol 9: 244–253.
34. Chiller K, Selkin BA, Murakawa GJ (2001) Skin microflora and bacterial infections of the skin. J Investig Dermatol Symp Proc 6: 170–174.
35. Fredricks DN (2001) Microbial ecology of human skin in health and disease. J Investig Dermatol Symp Proc 6: 167–169.
36. Roth RR, James WD (1988) Microbial ecology of the skin. Annu Rev Microbiol 42: 441–464.
37. Roth RR, James WD (1989) Microbiology of the skin: resident flora, ecology, infection. J Am Acad Dermatol 20: 367–390.
38. Cogen AL, Nizet V, Gallo RL (2008) Skin microbiota: a source of disease or defence? Br J Dermatol 158: 442–455.
39. NCCLS (2003) Quality Control of Microbiological Transport Systems; Approved Standard. NCCLS document M40-A. NCCLS, Wayne, Pennsylvania.
40. York MK (2010) Processing, isolation, detection, and interpretation of aerobic bacteriology cultures. In: Garcia LS, Clinical microbiology procedures handbook, ed., vol. 1. American Society for Microbiology, Washington, D.C. 3319–3324.
41. Datta R, Shah A, Huang SS, Cui E, Nguyen V, et al. (2014) High nasal burden of methicillin-resistant Staphylococcus aureus increases risk of invasive disease. J Clin Microbiol 52: 312–314.
42. Van Horn KG, Audette CD, Tucker KA, Sebeck D (2008) Comparison of 3 swab transport systems for direct release and recovery of aerobic and anaerobic bacteria. Diagn Microbiol Infect Dis 62: 471–473.
43. Smismans A, Verhaegen J, Schuermans A, Frans J (2009) Evaluation of the Copan ESwab transport system for the detection of methicillin-resistant Staphylococcus aureus: a laboratory and clinical study. Diagn Microbiol Infect Dis 65: 108–111.
44. Probst A, Facius R, Wirth R, Moissl-Eichinger C (2010) Validation of a nylon-flocked-swab protocol for efficient recovery of bacterial spores from smooth and rough surfaces. Appl Environ Microbiol 76: 5148–5158.
45. Morosini MI, Loza E, Gutierrez O, Almaraz F, Baquero F, et al. (2006) Evaluation of 4 swab transport systems for the recovery of ATCC and clinical strains with characterized resistance mechanisms. Diagn Microbiol Infect Dis 56: 19–24.
46. Drake C, Barenfanger J, Lawhorn J, Verhulst S (2005) Comparison of Easy-Flow Copan liquid Stuart's and Starplex swab transport systems for recovery of fastidious aerobic bacteria. J Clin Microbiol 43: 1301–1303.
47. Perry JL (1997) Assesment of swab transport systems for aerobic and anaerobic organism recovery. J Clin Microbiol 35: 1269–127 .

10

Fermentation of *Propionibacterium acnes,* a Commensal Bacterium in the Human Skin Microbiome, as Skin Probiotics against Methicillin-Resistant *Staphylococcus aureus*

Muya Shu[1]❡, Yanhan Wang[1]❡, Jinghua Yu[2], Sherwin Kuo[1], Alvin Coda[1], Yong Jiang[3], Richard L. Gallo[1], Chun-Ming Huang[1,4]*

1 Division of Dermatology, Department of Medicine, University of California San Diego, La Jolla, California, United States of America, **2** Sanford-Burnham Institute for Medical Research, La Jolla, California, United States of America, **3** Surface Bioadvances Inc., San Diego, California, United States of America, **4** Moores Cancer Center, University of California San Diego, La Jolla, California, United States of America

Abstract

Bacterial interference creates an ecological competition between commensal and pathogenic bacteria. Through fermentation of milk with gut-friendly bacteria, yogurt is an excellent aid to balance the bacteriological ecosystem in the human intestine. Here, we demonstrate that fermentation of glycerol with Propionibacterium acnes (P. acnes), a skin commensal bacterium, can function as a skin probiotic for in vitro and in vivo growth suppression of USA300, the most prevalent community-acquired methicillin-resistant Staphylococcus aureus (CA-MRSA). We also promote the notion that inappropriate use of antibiotics may eliminate the skin commensals, making it more difficult to fight pathogen infection. This study warrants further investigation to better understand the role of fermentation of skin commensals in infectious disease and the importance of the human skin microbiome in skin health.

Editor: Riccardo Manganelli, University of Padova, Medical School, Italy

Funding: This work was supported by NIH Grants (STTR and 1R21AI088147). The funders had no role in study design, data collection and analysis, decision to publish, or preparation of the manuscript.

Competing Interests: The authors would like to declare the affiliation(s) to Surface Bioadvances Inc. The manuscript did not have the affiliations to Surface Bioadvances Inc. in terms of employment, consultancy, patents, products in development or marketed products.

* E-mail: chunming@ucsd.edu

❡ These authors contributed equally to this work.

Introduction

Bacterial interference, or bacteriotherapy, in which commensal bacteria are used to prevent colonization of the host by pathogens, has been shown to be a promising modality for prevention and treatment of infections [1,2]. Yogurts containing live probiotic strains, the best examples of bacterial interference, have been used for centuries to maintain the digestive microbial ecosystem. Bacterial interference via fermentation commonly takes place in natural ecosystems as well. For instance, microorganisms both on and inside fruits metabolize sugars to produce fermentation products including short-chain fatty acids (SCFAs) during ripening. These fermentation products have been found to inhibit activity of bacterial competitors within ripe fruit [3]. Although not identical microenvironments, reports show that SCFAs produced by fermentation of microorganisms have been detected in pus from deep-seated abscesses, anaerobic microenvironments in the context of human bacterial infection [4].

Each individual carries approximately ten times more bacterial cells than human cells [5]. The skin is the human body's largest organ, colonized by a diverse milieu of microorganisms (skin microbiome), most of which are commensals as they are harmless and even beneficial to their host. Propionibacterium acnes (*P. acnes*) is a predominant bacterium in skin microbiome [5,6]. Everyone hosts *P. acnes* [5,6] which accounts for approximately half of the total skin microbiome, with an estimated density of 10^2 to 10^{5-6} cm^2 [7–9]. *Staphylococcus aureus* (S. aureus) is a Gram-positive bacterium and one of the major causes of both hospital- and community-acquired infections worldwide. This bacterium is responsible for a broad range of infections such as skin wound and disseminated systemic infections leading to organ failure and death [10]. It is estimated that *S. aureus* accounts for 12 million outpatient visits and 292,000 hospitalizations of which 126,000 are due to methicillin-resistant *S. aureus* (MRSA) annually in the United States (US) alone [11]. The Center for Disease Control Prevention (CDC) estimates that more than 90,000 people die from hospital-acquired bacterial infections in US each year [12]. Community-acquired MRSA (CA-MRSA) is reported as the most common cause of purulent skin and soft tissue infections in the US [13]. These infections are particularly difficult to treat because the bacterium has become resistant to many commonly used antibiotics.

Previous studies indicated that *P. acnes* was found in the human skin wounds [14]. *P. acnes* and *S. aureus* were co-isolated from both shoulder sepsis [15] and prosthetic hip infections [15,16] in adult patients. Although *P. acnes* predominates on the skin surface and is exposed to atmospheric oxygen, we hypothesize that *P. acnes* enters the dermis when a deep wound is created by pathogen infection. The anaerobic microenvironment in deep-seated abscesses may trigger P. acnes to undergo fermentation using carbon sources (such as glycerol and glucose) naturally produced in skin. Human hosts exploit P. acnes fermentation in deep-seated abscesses to prevent the entry of S. aureus into the bloodstream and reduce the risk of systemic S. aureus infections.

Propionibacterium acnes was so-named for its ability to ferment carbohydrates to propionic acid, a SCFA known to have antimicrobial activity [17,18]. Our results demonstrated that P. acnes can fermentatively metabolize glycerol, an endogenous skin metabolite, in mouse skin. The fermentation products of *P. acnes* significantly suppress the *in vitro* and *in vivo* growth of USA300, a CA-MRSA. These results show that fermentation of *P. acnes* in the human skin microbiome may play a role in human innate immunity against *S. aureus*. The use of *P. acnes* fermentation for bacterial interference therapy leverages evolutionary medicine by lowering selective pressure for antibiotic resistance and developing therapeutics with negligible side effect profiles.

Results

P. acnes Fermentation Counteracts USA300

To examine if *P. acnes* fermentation affects the growth of USA300, *P. acnes* or Micrococcus luteus (M. luteus), a Gram-positive, non-fermenting skin commensal bacterium, was grown on agar plates in the presence or absence of glycerol, a naturally occurring metabolite found in human skin [19], for three days before growing USA300 in the overlaid agar. As shown in Figure 1A, only *P. acnes* grown with glycerol showed visible inhibitory effects against USA300. No inhibitory effect was observed when *P. acnes* was grown in the absence of glycerol (Figure 1C). M. luteus grown with or without glycerol did not display inhibitory effects against the growth of USA300 (Figure 1B and D). These findings suggest that glycerol fermentation is required for inhibitory effect of *P. acnes* against USA300.

To test the probiotic effect of *P. acnes* fermentation products, *P. acnes* was incubated in rich medium under anaerobic conditions in the presence of glycerol as the carbon source. Rich medium plus glycerol and rich medium plus *P. acnes* were used as controls. To monitor the fermentation process, cultures were tested with phenol red, a fermentation indicator, to assess SCFA production as a result of glycerol fermentation. Only media in the culture of *P. acnes* with glycerol turned yellow (more acidic) ten days following incubation (Figure 2A), demonstrating *P. acnes* fermentation. This was further validated quantitatively by pH values in rich medium containing glycerol, *P. acnes* and glycerol plus *P. acnes* of 6.6, 6.5, and 5.6 respectively, following 17 days of incubation. To assess the anti-CA-MRSA activity of *P. acnes* fermentation products, USA300 [1×10^5 colony-forming unit (CFU)/ml] was then incubated with each group and their respective serial two-fold dilutions (1/2 to 1/16) overnight. Initial fermented media and its ½ dilution markedly suppressed the growth of USA300 (Figure 2B).

Ferments of *P. acnes* Reduce the Intracellular pH of USA300

SCFAs are the principal end products of bacterial fermentation [20]. The antimicrobial effects of SCFAs result mainly from the un-dissociated form of SCFAs [21,22]. Non-dissociated SCFAs passively diffuse through the cell wall of bacteria. Once internalized into the neutral pH of the cell cytoplasm, they can dissociate into anions and protons. Elevation of both anions and protons is a potentially lethal factor to bacteria that must maintain a near neutral pH cytoplasm to sustain functional macromolecules. Export of excess protons requires consumption of cellular adenosine triphosphate (ATP) and may result in depletion of cellular energy [21]. To determine the action mechanism of fermentation products of *P. acnes* against CA-MRSA, we loaded USA300 with an internally conjugated fluorescent pH probe, carboxyfluorescein succinimidyl ester (cFSE). Compared to control media, fermented media of *P. acnes* significantly lowered the intracellular pH of USA300 (Figure 2C). consistent with previous findings that a lowered intracellular pH of bacteria is a lethal mechanism of SCFA [22].

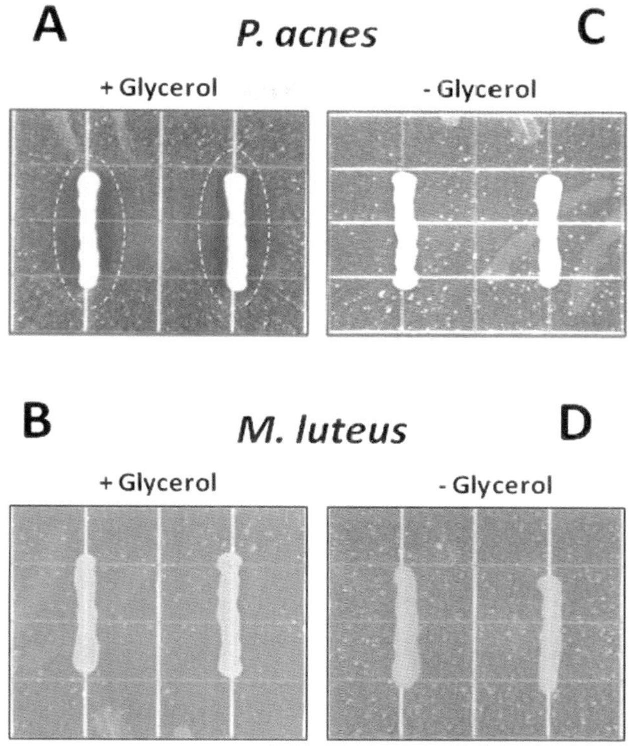

Figure 1. *P. acnes* interferes with the growth of USA300 in the presence of glycerol. An overlay assay reveals zones (circles) of inhibition of USA300 growth when *P. acnes* (ATCC6919, 10^5 CFU) (A), not *M. luteus* (B), was grown with USA300 in the presence of glycerol in agar plates under anaerobic conditions at 30°C. No inhibition zones were developed when *P. acnes* (C) or *M. luteus* (D) was grown with USA300 in the absence of glycerol.

Identification of SCFAs in Fermentation Products of *P. acnes* by Nuclear Magnetic Resonance (NMR) Analysis

To identify the SCFAs in bacterial fermentation, *P. acnes* (ATCC6919) was incubated in rich media under anaerobic conditions in the presence of $^{13}C_3$-glycerol (20 g/l) for 17 days. The ^{13}C-labeled metabolites in the fermentation products of *P. acnes* were identified by NMR analysis. In addition to un-metabolized ^{13}C-glycerol (62.3 and 72.5 ppm), three SCFAs (acetic acid, lactic acid, and propionic acid) were detected in the fermentation productions of *P. acnes*. In a one-dimensional (1-D) ^{13}C NMR spectrum using an NMR spectrometer (400 MHz

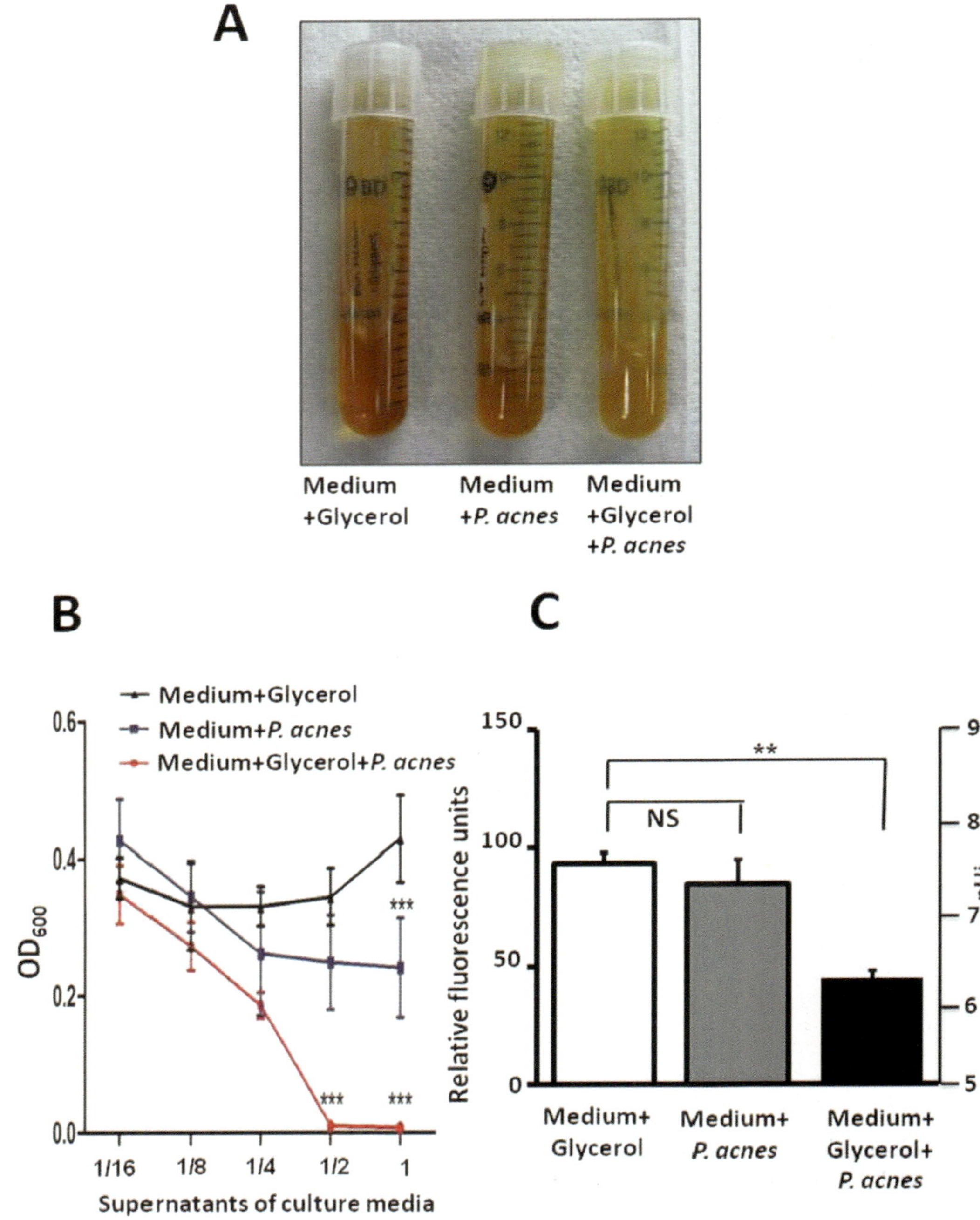

Figure 2. Probiotic effects of *P. acnes* fermentation against USA300 accompanied by a decrease in intracellular pH. (A) P. acnes (10^5 CFU/ml), was incubated in rich medium in the absence (■) and presence (●) of glycerol under anaerobic conditions for ten days. Rich medium plus glycerol without P. acnes (▲) was included as a control. (B) After a 17-day incubation, fermented or control media were then collected, diluted (1/2 to 1/16) and added to cultures of USA300 (10^5 CFU/ml) overnight. The inhibitory growth of USA300 was defined as a decline in OD_{600}. (C) The cFSE-loaded USA300 (3×10^4 CFU) was treated with 100 μl fermented (Medium+glycerol+P. acnes; solid bar) or control [(Medium+glycerol (open bar) and Medium+P. acnes (grey bar)] media. The change in the relative fluorescence units corresponding to intracellular pH of USA300 was measured 5 min after treatment. $^{**}P<0.01$; $^{***}P<0.001$ (two-tailed t-tests). Data are the mean ± standard deviation (SD) of three individual experiments. NS: Non-significant.

JEOL JNM-ECS) (Figure S1A), two signals at 21.2 and 69.5 ppm corresponded to ^{13}C-labeled lactic acid. Two ^{13}C-labeled propionic acids appeared at 8.9 and 31.0 ppm. Acetic acid was detected at 24.3 ppm. The signals of acetic acid (1.90 ppm), lactic acid (1.33 and 4.09 ppm), and propionic acid (1.15 and 2.38) in a 1-D ^{1}H NMR spectrum were displayed in Figure S1B. Three major SCFAs including propionic acid in the fermentation products of *P. acnes* were shown in a two-dimensional (2-D) ^{1}H-^{13}C HSQC NMR spectrum (Figure S1C). Propionibacterium including *P. acnes* produces propionic acid as the end product of its anaerobic fermentation [23]. Thus, the results above demonstrate that *P. acnes* fermentatively metabolizes $^{13}C_3$-glycerol into SCFAs.

Fermentation Products of *P. acnes* Suppress USA300-infected Lesions and Bacterial Colonization

Although *S. aureus* can cause a life-threatening and systemic infection (bacteremia), skin and soft tissue are the most common sites of *S. aureus* infection and comprise more than 75% of MRSA disease [24]. Eradication of infected *S. aureus* in skin will prevent the bacteria entering the bloodstream. To mimic the natural route of CA-MRSA infection, a 5 mm wound was made on the dorsal skin of Institute of Cancer Research (ICR) mice and USA300 bacteria were topically applied onto the wound. To test the potency of *P. acnes* fermentation products against CA-MRSA *in vivo*, we inoculated USA300 (2×10^6 CFU) to skin wounds 10 min after topical application of *P. acnes* ferments or controls. Application of fermented media, but not controls, considerably decreased the sizes of USA300-infected skin lesions (Figure 3A and B). To determine the intensity of bacterial colonization, wounds were homogenized to estimate the CFU. The USA300 counts in wounds applied with culture supernatants of medium plus glycerol, medium plus *P. acnes* or medium plus glycerol and *P. acnes* were $4.8\pm0.9\times10^6$, $4.9\pm2.6\times10^6$ and $9.4\pm4.5\times10^5$ CFU/g, respectively. These result show that application of fermented media of *P. acnes* decreased 80% of USA300 colonization in the lesions as compared to application of control media (Figure 3C).

To examine if propionic acid exerts antimicrobial activity against CA-MRSA, we determined the minimal bactericidal concentration (MBC) value of propionic acid for USA300. Bacteria were incubated with propionic acid at various concentrations in their media overnight at 37°C. After incubation, the bacteria were diluted with PBS and spotted on an agar plate to count CFU. We found that propionic acid effectively suppressed the growth of USA300 (Figure 3D) at a concentration greater than 25 mM and completely killed all of bacteria at a concentration greater than 100 mM. To assess the antimicrobial activity of propionic acid *in vivo*, USA300 (2×10^6 CFU) was inoculated to the wounded areas of ICR mice 10 min following topical application of either propionic acid (100 mM), PBS (pH 7.1) or acidic PBS (pH 3.5, corresponding to pH for 100 mM propionic acid). Application of propionic acid significantly reduced the size of USA300-infected skin lesions as compared to application of both PBS solutions (Figure 3E). On Day 1, the sizes of USA300-infected skin lesions in PBS (pH 7.1)-, acidic PBS (pH 3.5)-, or propionic acid-treated wounds were 4.6 ± 0.6, 4.0 ± 0.8, and 3.2 ± 0.8 mm^2, respectively. A significant decrease in the size of USA300-infected skin lesion was detected two days following application of PBS (pH 3.5). Histological observation [hematoxylin and eosin (H&E) staining] revealed that the propionic acid-treated wounds had an attenuated inflammatory response and improved integrity of epidermis and hair follicle compared to PBS-treated wounds (Figure S2). This suggests that propionic acid reduced USA300-induced damage of the epidermal layers and inflammation. To determine the bacterial colonization, USA300-infected skin lesions treated with propionic acid and controls were homogenized to estimate CFU. The bacterial numbers in lesions were: $1.9\pm1.0\times10^9$ (PBS, pH 7.1), $1.7\pm1.5\times10^9$ (PBS, pH 3.5) and $1.4\pm1.4\times10^7$ (propionic acid) CFU/g (Figure 3F), suggesting that propionic acid significantly decreased the growth of USA300 in the skin lesions.

Fermentation of *P. acnes* Occurs in Mouse Skin

To date, no evidence demonstrates that bacteria can employ the fermentative process to produce SCFAs *in vivo*. To determine if *P. acnes* is able to ferment carbon sources *in vivo*, ear of ICR mice was intradermally injected with $^{13}C_3$-glycerol (0.2 mg) immediately before injection of P. acnes (ATCC6919; 10^7 CFU in 10 µl PBS). As a control, the same amount of $^{13}C_3$-glycerol and PBS was injected to the other ear. One, two and three days after injection, ears were excised, homogenized, and then centrifuged. Supernatants of ear homogenates in 10% deuterium oxide (D_2O) were subjected to 1-D ^{13}C NMR analysis. In addition to $^{13}C_3$-glycerol (62.3 and 72.5 ppm), two strong signals of ^{13}C-labeled metabolites were detected at 17.1 and 58.4 ppm (Figure 4B) in the mice injected with $^{13}C_3$-glycerol plus *P. acnes* for three days. These two signals were undetectable in the mice injected with $^{13}C_3$-glycerol plus *P. acnes* for one or two day(s) (data not shown). No ^{13}C-labeled metabolites, except $^{13}C_3$-glycerol, were detected in the mice injected with $^{13}C_3$-glycerol plus PBS (Figure 4A). These two signals at 17.1 and 58.4 ppm correspond to the chemical groups (-CH_3 and -CH_2OH) of ethanol. In 1-D ^1H NMR analysis, two detected signals at 1.15 and 3.64 ppm validate the production of ethanol (data not shown). To identify the SCFAs in the fermentation products, supernatants of ear homogenates in D_2O were subjected to 2-D ^{13}C and ^1H NMR analysis. In addition to ethanol, four SCFAs (butyric acid, 3-hydroxy-butyric acid, lactic acid, and propionic acid) were detected in the ear injected with $^{13}C_3$-glycerol plus *P. acnes* (Figure 4C). The results demonstrate that *P. acnes* is able to undergo fermentation *in vivo*.

P. acnes Fermentation in Skin Wounds Diminishes the Colonization of USA300

Although we demonstrated that *P. acnes* grown with glycerol developed inhibition zones against USA300 in an overlay assay *in vitro* (Figure 1), it is unclear if *P. acnes* fermentation in skin wounds can prevent or mitigate a subsequent infection of CA-MRSA. A wound made on the dorsal skin of ICR mice was topically applied with *P. acnes* (10^7 CFU in 5 µl PBS) or P. acnes and glycerol (0.2 mg) for three days. USA300 (10^7 CFU in 5 µl PBS) was subsequently administered onto the same wounds for additional three days. Compared to application of *P. acnes* alone, application of P. acnes and glycerol showed improved healing of the USA300-infected skin lesions (Figure 5A). In addition, application of P. acnes and glycerol onto the wounds prior to administration of USA300 reduced more than 50% of USA300 colonization in comparison with application of P. acnes alone (Figure 5C). To investigate the effects of glycerol on the USA300 colonization, PBS (5 µl) or glycerol (0.2 mg) was topically applied to skin wounds for three days followed by a 3-day USA300 infection. Compared to PBS, glycerol did not significantly alter the size of USA300-infected lesions (Figure 5B) and USA300 colonization (Figure 5D). These findings indicate that the suppression of USA300 may be due to glycerol fermentation of *P. acnes* creating an unfavorable environment for USA300, rather than glycerol weakening the defense system of USA300.

Discussion

Mounting evidence demonstrates that human commensal bacteria may be part of human immunity by exhibiting bacterial interference against pathogens [25]. For example, Staphylococcus epidermidis (*S. epidermidis*), a human commensal bacterium commonly found in the skin, can activate Toll-like receptor 2 (TLR2) signaling and induce antimicrobial peptide expression, thus enabling the skin to mount an enhanced response to pathogens including *S. aureus* [26]. *S. epidermidis* in the nasal cavity can secrete serine protease Esp to inhibit biofilm formation and nasal colonization by *S. aureus* [27]. Here we introduce a novel

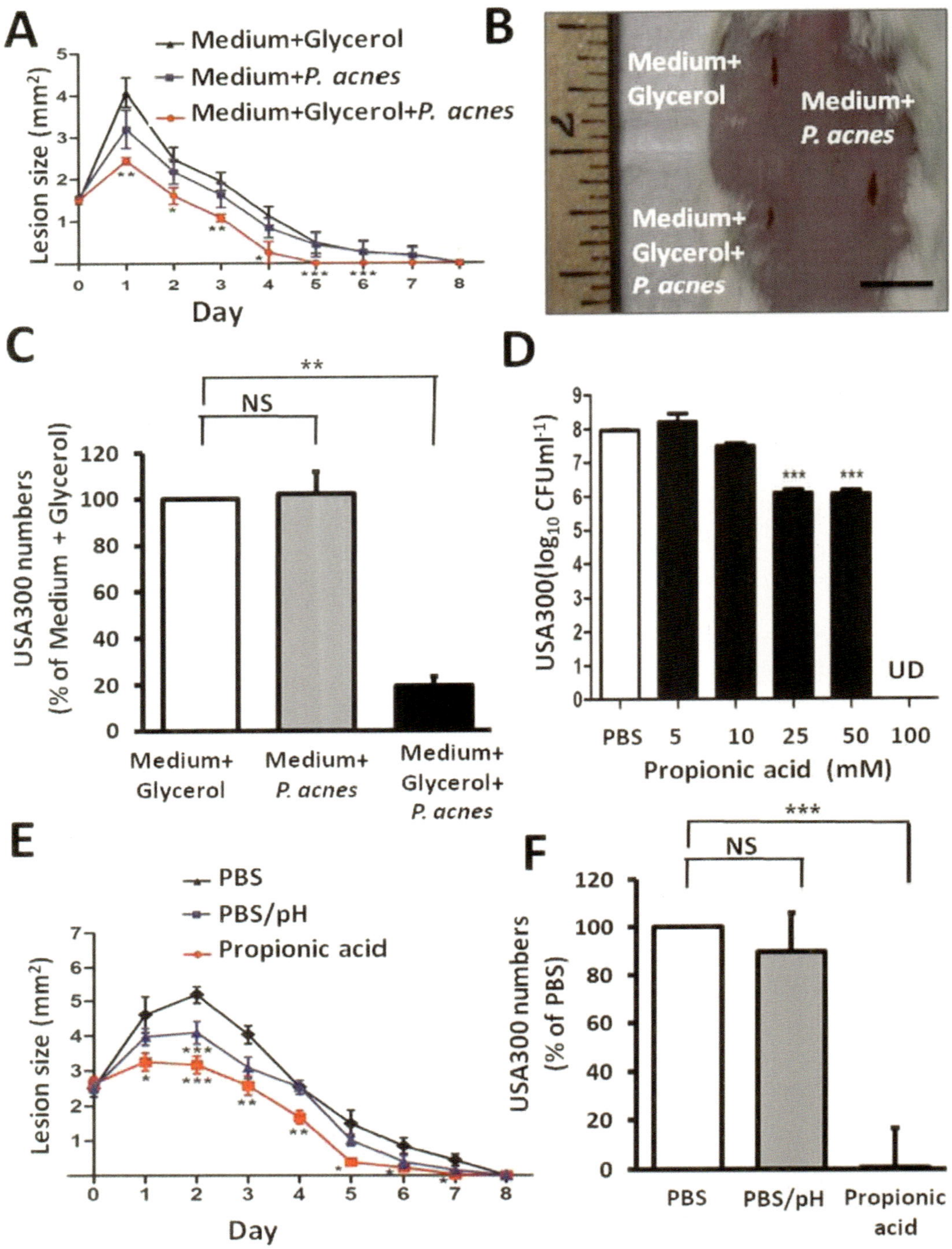

Figure 3. Fermented media of *P. acnes* and propionic acid suppress the infection of USA300 in mouse skin. (A) USA300 bacteria (2×10^6 CFU) were applied onto the wounded areas 10 min after application of culture supernatants of *P. acnes* in the absence and presence of glycerol or a control (medium plus glycerol). The lesion size was recorded daily for 8 days. (B) Skin lesions pictured on day 1 after bacterial application were illustrated. Bar = 1 cm. (C) Three days after bacterial application, the USA300 numbers in the skin were enumerated and presented as % of control. (D) For MBC assays, USA300 (10^6 CFU/ml) was incubated with propionic acid (5–100 mM in PBS) in media on a 96-well microplate overnight. Bacteria incubated with PBS alone served as a control. After incubation, USA300 was diluted 1:10–1:10^6 with PBS, and 5 μl of the dilutions were spotted on an agar plate for CFU counts. $^{**}P<0.01$; $^{***}P<0.001$ (two-tailed t-tests). Data are the mean ± SD of three individual experiments. UD, undetectable. (E) USA300 bacteria (2×10^6 CFU) were applied onto the wounded areas 10 min after application of propionic acid (5 μl; 100 mM) or PBS (5 μl). The lesion size was measured daily for 8 days. $^{*}P<0.05$; $^{**}P<0.01$; $^{***}P<0.001$ (A, E). (F) Three days after bacterial application, the USA300 numbers in the skin were counted and presented as % of PBS control. $^{**}P<0.01$; $^{***}P<0.001$ (C, F). *P*-values were evaluated using two-tailed *t*-tests. Data are the mean ± SD of lesions from three separate experiments performed with five mice per group. NS: Non-significant.

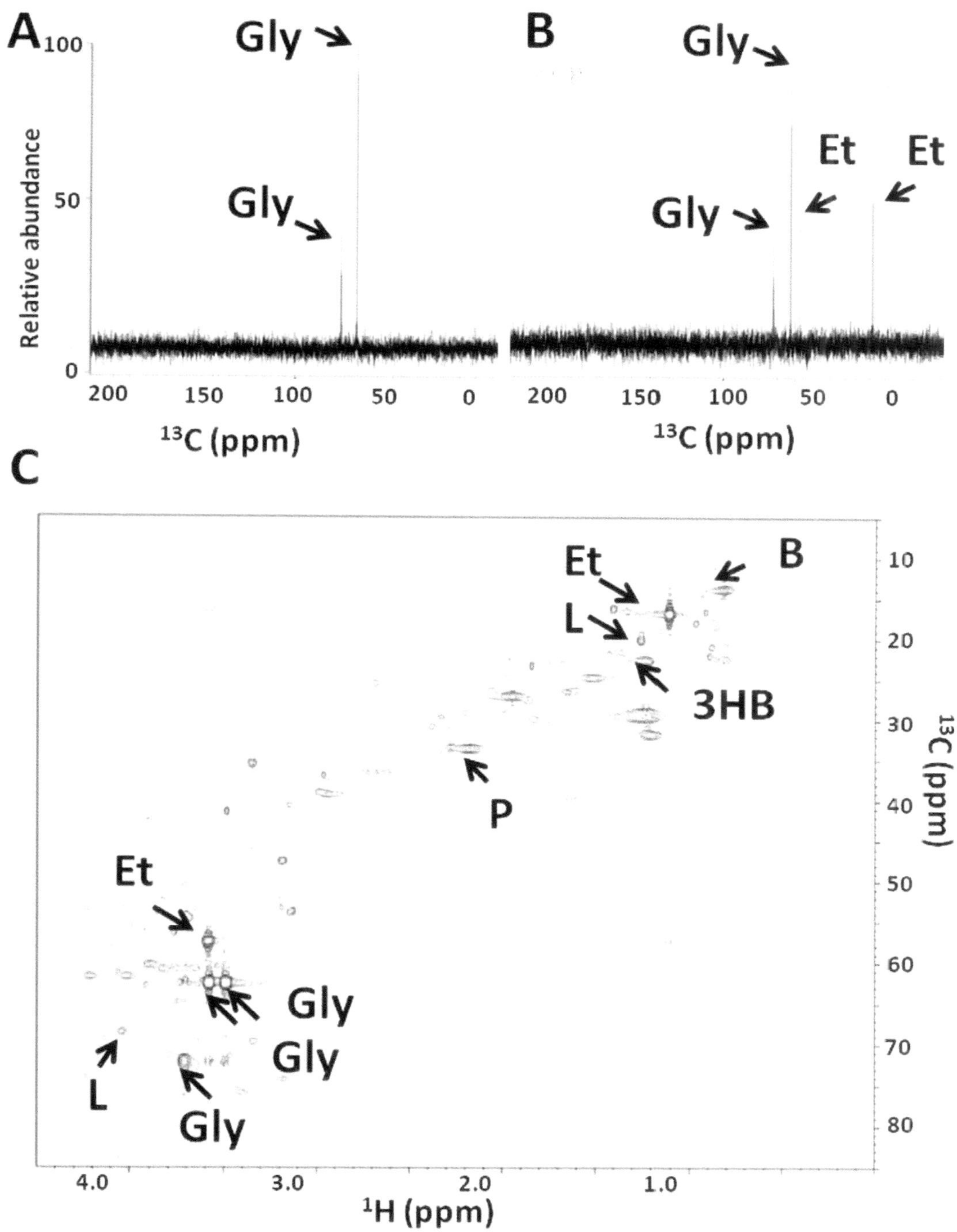

Figure 4. NMR validation of fermentation of *P. acnes* in mouse skin. (B) The ear of ICR mice was intradermally injected with $^{13}C_3$-glycerol (0.2 mg) and P. acnes (ATCC6919; 10^7 CFU in 10 μl PBS) for 3 days. (A) The other ear of the same mouse received $^{13}C_3$-glycerol (0.2 mg) and PBS (10 μl) as a control. Supernatants of ear homogenates were mixed with 10% D_2O and analyzed by a NMR (400 MHz JEOL JNM-ECS) spectrometer. Data from 1,024 scans were accumulated. The NMR signals (17.1 and 58.4 ppm) of ^{13}C-ethanol (Et) metabolized from $^{13}C_3$-glycerol (Gly) were detected exclusively in the mice injected with $^{13}C_3$-glycerol and *P. acnes*. The un-metabolized $^{13}C_3$-glycerol appears between 60 and 80 ppm in the ^{13}C-NMR spectrum. (C) A 2-D ^{1}H-^{13}C HSQC NMR spectrum (600 MHz) was displayed. In addition to glycerol (Gly), ethanol (Et), four SCFAs [butyric acid (B), 3-hydroxy-butyric acid (3HB), lactic acid (L), and propionic acid (P)] were detected in the ear injected with glycerol and *P. acnes*.

mechanism by which the skin commensal *P. acnes* makes use of fermentative processes to hinder the colonization of CA-MRSA in the skin wounds. In mouse skin, *P. acnes* can ferment glycerol to various SCFAs including propionic acid (Figure 4). Previous studies indicated that SCFAs in skin play a crucial role in influencing the predominant residence of bacteria on normal human skin [18]. It is known that *P. acnes* and *S. epidermidis* have higher tolerances to propionic acid than other pathogens [28]. In

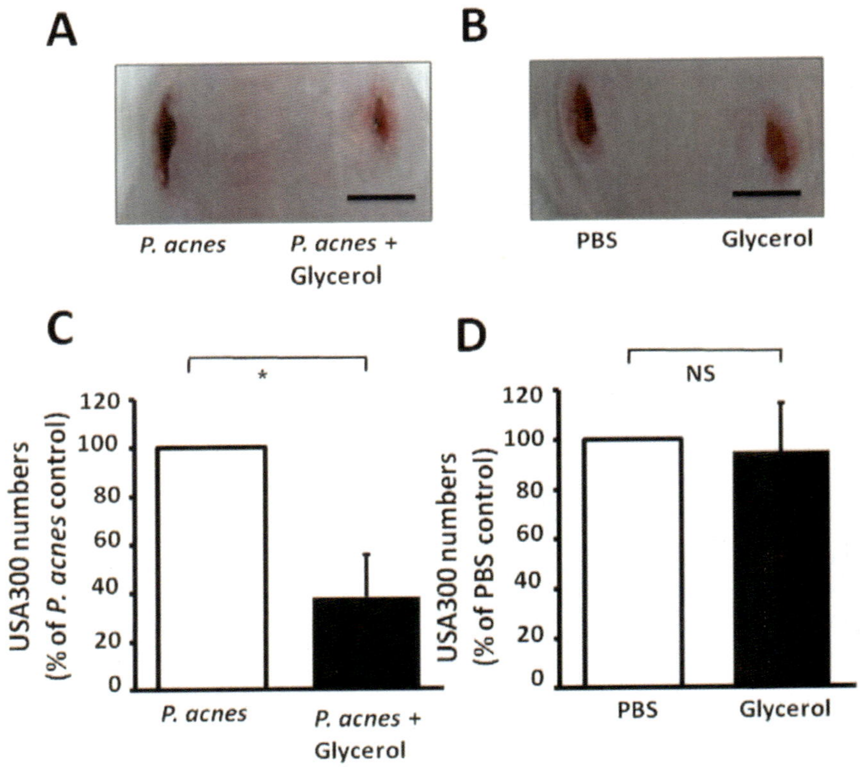

Figure 5. Glycerol fermentation of *P. acnes* in skin wounds diminishes the colonization of USA300. *P. acnes* (10^7 CFU in 5 µl PBS), P. acnes and glycerol (0.2 mg), PBS (5 µl) alone or glycerol alone were applied onto the skin wounds for 3 days before administration of USA300 (10^7 CFU in 5 µl PBS) onto the wounded areas. (A, B) Skin lesions pictured 3 days after USA300 application were illustrated. Bar = 0.5 cm. (C) The USA300 numbers in the skin wounds were enumerated 3 days after USA300 application and presented as % of those in skin applied with *P. acnes* (C) or PBS (D). *$P<0.05$. *P*-values were evaluated using two-tailed *t*-tests. Data are the mean ± SD of lesions from five mice per group. NS: Non-significant.

fact, as shown in Figure 3D, propionic acid (25 mM) exerted excellent antimicrobial activity against USA300, but did not affect the growth of *P. acnes* (data not shown). Thus, *P. acnes* fermentation may have a low risk of disrupting the balance of skin microbiome. It has been documented that propionic acid inhibited the various strains (e.g. ATCC29247 [29] and CMCC(B)26003 [30]) of *S. aureus* besides USA300, suggesting the broad spectrum anti-*S. aureus* activity of propionic acid.

The identified ^{13}C-labeled SCFAs in Figure 4 were not directly derived from $^{13}C_3$-glycerol metabolism by mouse skin cells since no ^{13}C-labeled SCFAs were detected in the mice injected with $^{13}C_3$-glycerol plus PBS. Furthermore, the presence of ^{13}C-labeled propionic acid in the mice injected with $^{13}C_3$-glycerol plus *P. acnes* validated that the identified ^{13}C-labeled SCFAs resulted from the *P. acnes* fermentation. However, the SCFA profile of $^{13}C_3$-glycerol fermentation by *P. acnes in vivo* (Figure 4) was not exactly the same as that *in vitro* (Figure S1). Although propionic acid was measureable in the products of both *in vivo* and *in vitro* glycerol fermentation, ethanol, butyric acid and 3-hydroxy-butyric acid were only detected when $^{13}C_3$-glycerol plus *P. acnes* were injected into mice. *P. acnes* HL027PA2 (NCBI Taxon ID 765112) expressed butyryl-CoA dehydrogenase, an enzyme involved in the production of butyric acid during a fermentation process of anaerobic bacteria. A *P. acnes* strain from health cow rumen fluid had the capability to ferment carbohydrates to butyric acid [31]. Some *P. acnes* strains were able to produce butyric acid when they were incubated in culture media containing glucose and tributyrin, a triglyceride which can be converted to butyric acid by *P. acnes* lipase [32]. *P. acnes* (KPA171202) expressed alcohol dehydrogenase [33], a key enzyme for production of ethanol. Despite the presence of ethanol and butyric acid in mouse skin injected with $^{13}C_3$-glycerol plus *P. acnes* in this study, the metabolites of glycerol fermentation of *P. acnes in vivo* were not well characterized in the literature. We cannot rule out the possibility that host (e.g. pH in skin) affects the *in vivo* fermentation properties of *P. acnes* [34].

SCFAs can regulate several leukocyte functions including production of cytokines [(tumor necrosis factor (TNF)-α, interleukins (IL)-2, IL-6 and IL-10]. The ability of leukocytes to migrate to the foci of inflammation and destroy microbial pathogens can be affected by SCFAs [28]. In addition, SCFA and butyric acid, in particular, significantly reduce expression of *S. aureus*-induced IL-2 and interferon (IFN)-γ [35]. SCFAs have been demonstrated as ligands for free fatty acid receptor 1 (Ffar1) [also called G-protein-coupled receptor 40 (GPR40)] [36]. Previous studies indicated that GW9508 (GlaxoSmithKline), an arylalkyl derivative of the propionic acid, activated the Ffar1 receptor, suppressed chemokine induction in keratinocytes and attenuated cutaneous immune inflammation [37]. Thus, the use of Ffar1 knockout [Ffar1(−/−) mice may be able to determine if Ffar1 is essential for anti-inflammatory action of SCFAs. As shown in Figures 1 and 5, the inhibitory effect of *P. acnes* on the growth of USA300 was detectable exclusively through glycerol fermentation. Glycerol itself did not influence the growth of *P. acnes* (Figure S3) and USA300 (data not shown). It was reported that glycerol can be produced endogenously by the breakdown of triglycerides by sebaceous gland-associated lipase in human skin [38]. Bacteria also produce glycerol during fermentation of glucose to ethanol [39]. Aquaporin-3 functions as a glycerol transporter in mammalian skin [40]. It is known that glycerol helps maintain healthy skin integrity [19]. Aquaporin 3-deficient mice exhibit skin defects, including impairment of water holding capacity, barrier recovery, and wound healing [40]. Thus, glycerol naturally produced in skin maybe acts as a bi-functional molecule that serves as a humectant to promote a healthy skin barrier and a fermentation inducer to trigger the probiotic activity of skin commensals. Although propionic acid exerted antimicrobial activity against USA300 *in vitro* (Figure 3D) and *in vivo* (Figure 3F), we cannot exclude the possibility that a mixture of SCFAs and/or other secretory proteins [41] or metabolites in glycerol fermentation products of *P. acnes* also contributed to the anti-USA300 effects of fermented media (Figure 2B and Figure 3C). Propionic acid in lesser amounts may be produced by *P. acnes* in the TBS culture media in the absence of glycerol since TSB contains dextrose (2.5 g/l), a D-glucose monohydrate, as a carbon source for bacterial growth. The presence of propionic acid and/or other secretory proteins or metabolites may explain a slight suppression of UCA300 growth *in vitro* by undiluted and glycerol-free media of *P. acnes* (Figure 2C).

It has been reported that bacteria possess metabolic capabilities to respond to low external pH [42]. This adaptation permits the induction of genes involved in an acid-tolerance response and synthesis of a series of acid shock proteins that are protective for extreme acidic conditions [42]. Mutants defective in AtrB lack an acid tolerance response to propionic acid, indicating that AtrB protein is necessary for the full induction of acid resistance by exposure to propionic acid [43]. Inactivation of PhoP significantly increased bacterial resistance to propionic acid [43]. Recently, *S. aureus* gene profile expression was investigated in a condition of acidification [44]. Results revealed that the expression of several genes was affected by a variation in pH from 7.5 to 5.5. Among these genes, one can find genes involved in maintaining the intracellular pH, such as the urease operon (ure) and genes encoding intracellular chaperones (clpB). Thus, although our results demonstrate that fermented media of *P. acnes* decrease the intracellular pH of *S. aureus* (Figure 2C), the effects of long-term use of skin probiotics containing SCFAs as antimicrobials induces an acid tolerance/resistance response are unknown. Although SCFAs are normal human metabolites and theoretically less toxic, SCFAs at high doses may create an extremely acid solution, which causes skin irritation and/or corrosion [45].

Future work will include developing anti-*S. aureus* skin probiotics containing live *P. acnes*, glycerol and/or SCFAs. Even though skin immune cells may block the entrance of *P. acnes* into bloodstream, it is worth examining if live *P. acnes* in the anti-*S. aureus* skin probiotics can enter bloodstream when skin probiotics are applied onto the skin wounds for consecutive days. The application of bacterial-free fermented media or a fermentation inducer (e.g. glycerol) that did not affect the growth of *P. acnes* (Figure S3) may be a safer approach. A recent study using a multilocus sequence typing scheme (MLST) for *P. acnes* has suggested that pathogenic versus truly commensal lineages of *P. acnes* may exist [33,46]. *P. acnes* type IA_1 strains including ATCC6919 in this study were found predominantly both in healthy skin and acne vulgaris [33]. Several strains of *P. acnes* were only ever isolated from healthy skin, particularly CC72 (type II) and CC77 (type III) strains, although whether they truly represent commensal lineages still remains to be firmly established. Besides *P. acnes*, other *Propionibacterium* species including *P. granulosum* and *P. avidum* found in human skin have the capability of utilizing carbohydrates for anaerobic fermentation [47,48]. Therefore, as far as safety is concerned, the use of skin commensal strains of *P. acnes* or other *Propionibacterium* species as anti-*S. aureus* skin probiotics will be included in future development.

In human healthy skin, an immune response is not generally mounted against commensal *P. acnes*. Mice can display a robust inflammatory response to *P. acnes* [49] since *P. acnes* bacteria do not reside naturally in the mouse skin. Although a mouse wound model recapitulated human *S. aureus* infection (Figure 5) and the effects of *P. acnes*-induced inflammatory responses on skin lesions were subtracted from controls, injection of *S. aureus* with glycerol into an *ex vivo* human skin explant [50] that harbors commensal *P. acnes* will be part of future studies. To support our hypothesis that deep-seated abscesses create an anaerobic microenvironment, thus facilitating P. acnes fermentation to interfere with S. aureus, future work will also include collecting various skin biopsies from patients with S. aureus infection. Impetigo, a superficial infection of the skin that bacteria have a chance to expose to oxygen, while cellulitis is a deep-seated infection that invaded bacteria live in an anaerobic microenvironment around the deeper layers (connective tissue) of skin [51]. The abundance of bacteria (*P. acnes* and *S. aureus*) and SCFAs including propionic acid in the skin infections of impetigo and cellulitis should be compared. The significance in this study includes 1) validating the effectiveness of *P. acnes* fermentation as anti-*S. aureus* skin probiotics; and 2) providing a novel approach to treat *S. aureus* infections, thereby benefiting the large community of patients with *S. aureus*/MRSA infections [11]. Microbial fermentation has been widely employed in the development of various products including yogurt, wine, and vinegar. The concept of fermentation of skin commensals against pathogens not only creates potentially a new skin industry but also generates a new area of investigation into the biological function of skin microbiome for promoting human health.

Materials and Methods

Ethics Statement

This study was carried out in strict accordance with the recommendations in the Guide for the Care and Use of Laboratory Animals of the National Institutes of Health (NIH). Experiments of using mice were performed at University of California, San Diego (UCSD). The UCSD ethics committee specifically approved this study under an approved Institutional Animal Care and Use Committee (IACUC) protocol (no. S10058).

Culture of Microorganisms

USA300 or *M. luteus* (ATCC9341) was cultured on 3% tryptic soy broth (TSB) (Sigma, St. Louis, MO, USA) agar overnight at 37°C. *P. acnes* (ATCC6919) was cultured on Reinforced Clostridium Medium (RCM, Oxford, Hampshire, England) under anaerobic conditions using Gas-Pak (BD, Sparks, MD, USA) at 37°C. All microorganisms from a single colony were cultured in their media. Overnight cultures were diluted 1:100 and cultured to an absorbance at 600 nm [optical density $(OD)_{600}$] = 1.0. Microorganisms were harvested by centrifugation at 5,000 g for 10 min, washed with PBS, and suspended in PBS.

Anti-USA300 Overlay Assay

The *P. acnes* (10^5 CFU) or *M. luteus* was inoculated in two parallel 2-cm streaks on 1.5% agar (Oxoid. Ltd., London, UK) plates containing rich medium [10 g/l yeast extract (Biokar Diagnostics, Beauvais, France), 5 g/l TSB, 2.5 g/l K_2HPO_4 and 1.5 g/l KH_2PO_4] in the absence and presence of 20 g/l glycerol under anaerobic conditions using Gas-Pak (BD, Sparks, MD, USA) at 30°C for three days. Soft agar (1%) was cooled to 45°C before USA300 bacteria were added to obtain a concentration of

(10^4 CFU/ml). The soft agar (10 ml) was then poured onto the plates to overlay the rich medium agar. After incubation at 30°C for 40 h under anaerobic conditions, the plates were examined visually.

Probiotic Effects of *P. acnes* Fermentation Against USA300

P. acnes (10^5 CFU/ml) was incubated in rich medium (10 ml) in the absence and presence of 20 g/l glycerol under anaerobic conditions using Gas-Pak (BD, Sparks, MD, USA) at 30°C. Rich medium plus 20 g/l glycerol without *P. acnes* was included as a control. The 0.001% (w/v) phenol red (Sigma, St. Louis, MO, USA) in rich medium with 20 g/l glycerol served as an indicator, converting from red-orange to yellow when fermentation occurs. To assess the probiotic activity of fermentation products, *P. acnes* was incubated in phenol red-free rich medium with/without glycerol for seventeen days. After fermentation, *P. acnes* was discarded by centrifugation at 5,000 g for 30 min. Media were then passed through 0.2-μm-pore-size filters. After filtration, the initial medium or its dilution (1/2 to 1/16) was added to USA300 (10^5 CFU/ml in TSB) on a 96-well microplate overnight. The plates were mixed well and then OD_{600} was measured by a microplate reader to estimate bacterial growth.

Measurement of Intracellular pH

Measurement of intracellular pH of USA300 using a cFSE florescence probe (Life Technologies, Grand Island, NY, USA) was previously described [52]. Briefly, USA300 bacteria were loaded with cFSE (5 μM) for 30 min at 37°C in 50 mM HEPES and 5 mM ethylenediaminetetraacetic acid (EDTA). To eliminate unbound probe, bacteria were incubated with glucose (10 mM) for an additional 30 min, washed twice in 50 mM PBS with 10 mM $MgCl_2$, pH 7.0, and then re-suspended in 1 mM PBS. The cFSE-loaded bacteria (3×10^4 CFU) were dispensed in on a 96-well microplate containing 100 μl/per well of rich medium plus 20 g/l glycerol, or culture supernatants of *P. acnes* in rich medium in the absence and presence of 20 g/l glycerol. Fluorescence intensities were measured immediately and every min for 5 min using an excitation wavelength of 490 nm and emission wavelength of 520 nm. A drop in relative fluorescence indicates the decrease in intracellular pH. Fluorescence of the bacteria-free filtrate (background fluorescence) was measured after the 5-min assay. In this case, treated suspensions were centrifuged at 5,000 g for 5 min. The fluorescence of the bacteria-free supernatant was measured and deducted from values for the treated suspensions. Calibration curves were obtained by incubation of un-treated, cFSE-loaded bacteria in buffers of various pHs. The buffer containing glycine (50 mM), citric acid (50 mM), $Na_2HPO_4.2H_2O$ (50 mM), and KCl (50 mM) was adjusted to various pH values ranging from 4 to 10. Equilibration of the intracellular and extracellular pH was conducted by addition of 1 μM valinomycin and nigericin (Sigma, St. Louis, MO, USA).

In vivo Effects of Fermented Media and Propionic Acid on Skin Infection of USA300

ICR mice (2–3 month-old females; Harlan Labs, Placentia, CA, USA) were anesthetized by isoflurane. A 5 mm wound was made on the dorsal skin following shaving with electrical clippers. Following skin wounding, we applied 5 μl of media of *P. acnes* (10^5 CFU/ml in 10 ml) incubated with/without glycerol or media plus glycerol (control) for 17 days to the wounded areas. To determine if propionic acid can prevent or mitigate the infection of CA-MRSA, 5 μl of 100 mM propionic acid was applied to the wounded areas. Application of PBS (pH 3.5, corresponding to pH for 100 mM propionic acid) or PBS (pH 7.1) to the wounded areas served as controls. The wounds were left uncovered throughout the experimental period. To simulate bacterial infection, USA300 (2×10^6 CFU in 5 μl PBS) was applied to the wounds 10 min after application of media, propionic acid or PBS controls. To measure the extent of wound closure, a transparent parafilm was placed over the wounded skin and the area was marked by outlining the area of the wound. The lesion size (mm^2) was measured daily for 8 days then calculated with ImageJ software (NIH, Bethesda, MD, USA). Five mice per group per experiments were used. We used a Student's *t*-test to determine the significance of the differences between groups. Data represent the mean ± SD from three independent experiments. All experiments using mice were conducted in a biosafety level 2 (BSL-2) facility and in accordance with institutional guidelines for animal experiments. To determine the bacterial counts in infected skin, the infected skin was excised 72 h following bacterial application. The excised skin was weighted and homogenized in 200 μl of sterile PBS with a tissue grinder. Bacterial CFUs in the skin were enumerated by plating serial dilutions ($1:10^1$–$1:10^6$) of the homogenate on a TSB agar plate. The plate was incubated for 24 h at 37°C to count colonies. The bacterial numbers (CFUs) per gram of excised skin were calculated and presented as % of control.

MBC Assays

To determine the MBC of propionic acid, bacteria (10^6 CFU/ml) were incubated with propionic acid at various concentrations (5–100 mM in PBS) in media on a 96-well microplate (100 μl per well) overnight. The control received only PBS. After incubation, bacteria were diluted $1:10$–$1:10^6$ with PBS. MBC was finally examined at a 99.9% killing level and determined by spotting the dilution (5 μl) on an agar plate supplemented with media for the counting of CFUs.

Validation of *P. acnes* Glycerol Fermentation *in vivo* by NMR Analysis

The ear of ICR mice was intradermally injected with $^{13}C_3$-glycerol (0.2 mg) and P. acnes (ATCC6919; 10^7 CFU in 10 μl PBS) for one, two or three days. The other ear of the same mouse received $^{13}C_3$-glycerol (0.2 mg) and PBS (10 μl) as a control. Supernatants (500 μl) of ear homogenates were mixed with 10% D_2O for NMR analysis. The 1-D NMR spectra were measured on a JEOL-ECS NMR spectrometer (JEOL USA, Inc., Peabody, MA, USA) operating at resonance frequency of 400 MHz with a repetition delay of 3 sec for ^{13}C NMR. The 2-D ^1H-^{13}C heteronuclear single quantum correlation (HSQC) NMR spectra were acquired on a Bruker Avance 600 MHz NMR spectrometer (Bruker Daltonics Inc., Fremont, CA, USA) with a triple resonance inverse (TCI) cryo-probe and recorded as 2048×256 complex points with 32 scans and 1 sec repetition time. Newly appearing signals belong to the intermediates or final products resulting from $^{13}C_3$-glycerol fermentation by P. acnes [53].

Interference of *P. acnes* Fermentation with the Colonization of USA300 *in vivo*

A 5 mm wound made on the dorsal skin of ICR mice were described above. *P. acnes* (10^7 CFU in 5 μl PBS), P. acnes and glycerol (0.2 mg), PBS (5 μl) alone or glycerol alone were applied onto the skin wounds for 3 days. USA300 (10^7 CFU in 5 μl PBS) was administered onto the same wounds. The wounds were excised, weighted and homogenized 3 days after USA300 administration. Bacterial CFUs in the wounds were enumerated by plating serial dilutions ($1{:}10^1$–$1{:}10^6$) of the homogenate on a TSB agar plate. The plate was incubated for 24 h at 37°C to count colonies of USA300. After 24 h incubation, only USA300 colonies were formed. It normally takes more than 3 days for *P. acnes*, a relatively slow-growing bacterium, to form visible colonies on TSB agar plates.

Statistical Analysis

To determine significances between groups, comparisons were made using the two-tailed *t*-test. For all statistical tests, the *P*-values of <0.05 (*), <0.01 (**), and <0.001 (***) were accepted for statistical significance.

Supporting Information

Figure S1 Validation of *P. acnes* glycerol fermentation via identification of SCFAs in the fermented media by NMR analysis. Fermented media of *P. acnes* were centrifuged and passed through a 0.2 µm filter. Supernatants were then mixed with 10% D_2O and analyzed by NMR spectrometers. Representative 1-D ^{13}C- (A) and 1H- (B) NMR spectra (400 MHz JEOL JNM-ECS) that reveal the principal SCFAs in the fermented media seventeen days after addition of $^{13}C_3$-glycerol. (C) A 2-D ^{1}H-^{13}C HSQC NMR spectrum (600 MHz) was displayed. In addition to glycerol (Gly), three SCFAs [acetic acid (Ac), lactic acid (L), and propionic acid (P)] were detected in the fermentation products of *P. acnes*.

Figure S2 Suppression of USA300-infected lesions by propionic acid. A 5-mm long excision wound will be created on the back of ICR mice. To assess if propionic acid alleviates the lesions caused by USA300 infection, USA300 bacteria (2×10^6 CFU) were applied onto the wounded areas 10 min after application of propionic acid (5 µl; 100 mM) or PBS (5 µl). (A) Skin lesions were pictured on day 1 after bacterial application. (B) Inflammation (arrows) surrounding the skin lesions (▼) was observed in the H&E-stained frozen sections [low (upper panels) and high (lower panels) powers] of skins applied with USA300 and controls. The scale bars of low power and high power were 40 µm, respectively.

Figure S3 Comparison of growth curves of *P. acnes* in the absence of presence of glycerol. *P. acnes* was incubated in rich medium in the absence (□) and presence (■) of glycerol on a 96-well microplate under anaerobic conditions at 30°C. The OD_{600} was read at the indicated time points. Data are the mean ± SD of three separate experiments. Glycerol did not change significantly in the growth of *P. acnes*.

Methods and Materials S1 Confirmation of *P. acnes* fermentation by NMR analysis.

Acknowledgments

We thank Dr. Y.T. Liu for providing comments on this manuscript and A. Dai for reading and editing this manuscript.

Author Contributions

Conceived and designed the experiments: CHM. Performed the experiments: MS YW CMH JY SK. Analyzed the data: AC YJ CMH. Contributed reagents/materials/analysis tools: RLG CMH. Wrote the paper: CMH.

References

1. Ji G, Beavis R, Novick RP (1997) Bacterial interference caused by autoinducing peptide variants. Science 276: 2027–2030.
2. Falagas ME, Rafailidis PI, Makris GC (2008) Bacterial interference for the prevention and treatment of infections. Int J Antimicrob Agents 31: 518–522.
3. Ingram LO, Buttke TM (1984) Effects of alcohols on micro-organisms. Adv Microb Physiol 25: 253–300.
4. Demaerel P, Van Hecke P, Van Oostende S, Baert AL, Jacken J, et al. (1994) Bacterial metabolism shown by magnetic resonance spectroscopy. Lancet 344: 1234–1235.
5. Grice EA, Segre JA (2011) The skin microbiome. Nat Rev Microbiol 9: 244–253.
6. Ahn CY, Ko CY, Wagar EA, Wong RS, Shaw WW (1996) Microbial evaluation: 139 implants removed from symptomatic patients. Plast Reconstr Surg 98: 1225–1229.
7. Evans CA (1975) Persistent individual differences in the bacterial flora of the skin of the forehead: numbers of propionibacteria. J Invest Dermatol 64: 42–46.
8. Evans CA, Crook JR, Strom MS (1984) The bacterial flora of the forehead and back of Alaskan native villagers in summer and in winter. J Invest Dermatol 82: 294–297.
9. Ramstad S, Futsaether CM, Johnsson A (1997) Porphyrin sensitization and intracellular calcium changes in the prokaryote Propionibacterium acnes. J Photochem Photobiol B 40: 141–148.
10. Malani PN, Rana MM, Banerjee M, Bradley SF (2008) Staphylococcus aureus bloodstream infections: the association between age and mortality and functional status. J Am Geriatr Soc 56: 1485–1489.
11. Goetghebeur M, Landry PA, Han D, Vicente C (2007) Methicillin-resistant Staphylococcus aureus: A public health issue with economic consequences. Can J Infect Dis Med Microbiol 18: 27–34.
12. Gilbert M, MacDonald J, Gregson D, Siushansian J, Zhang K, et al. (2006) Outbreak in Alberta of community-acquired (USA300) methicillin-resistant Staphylococcus aureus in people with a history of drug use, homelessness or incarceration. CMAJ 175: 149–154.
13. Kaplan SL, Hulten KG, Gonzalez BE, Hammerman WA, Lamberth L, et al. (2005) Three-year surveillance of community-acquired Staphylococcus aureus infections in children. Clin Infect Dis 40: 1785–1791.
14. Saleh K, Sonesson A, Persson B, Riesbeck K, Schmidtchen A (2011) A descriptive study of bacterial load of full-thickness surgical wounds in dermatologic surgery. Dermatol Surg 37: 1014–1022.
15. Bashir A, Mujahid TY, Jehan N (2007) Antibiotic resistance profile: isolation and characterization of clinical isolates of staphylococci from patients with community-acquired skin infections. Pak J Pharm Sci 20: 299–304.
16. Ramage G, Tunney MM, Patrick S, Gorman SP, Nixon JR (2003) Formation of Propionibacterium acnes biofilms on orthopaedic biomaterials and their susceptibility to antimicrobials. Biomaterials 24: 3221–3227.
17. Higaki S, Nakamura M, Morohashi M, Yamagishi T (2004) Propionibacterium acnes biotypes and susceptibility to minocycline and Keigai-rengyo-to. Int J Dermatol 43: 103–107.
18. Ushijima T, Takahashi M, Ozaki Y (1984) Acetic, propionic, and oleic acid as the possible factors influencing the predominant residence of some species of Propionibacterium and coagulase-negative Staphylococcus on normal human skin. Can J Microbiol 30: 647–652.
19. Fluhr JW, Darlenski R, Surber C (2008) Glycerol and the skin: holistic approach to its origin and functions. Br J Dermatol 159: 23–34.
20. Millet S, Van Oeckel MJ, Aluwe M, Delezie E, De Brabander DL (2010) Prediction of in vivo short-chain fatty acid production in hindgut fermenting mammals: problems and pitfalls. Crit Rev Food Sci Nutr 50: 605–619.
21. Ostling CE, Lindgren SE (1993) Inhibition of enterobacteria and Listeria growth by lactic, acetic and formic acids. J Appl Bacteriol 75: 18–24.
22. Ricke SC (2003) Perspectives on the use of organic acids and short chain fatty acids as antimicrobials. Poult Sci 82: 632–639.
23. Dishisha T, Alvarez MT, Hatti-Kaul R (2012) Batch- and continuous propionic acid production from glycerol using free and immobilized cells of Propionibacterium acidipropionici. Bioresour Technol 118: 553–562.
24. Cohen AL, Shuler C, McAllister S, Fosheim GE, Brown MG, et al. (2007) Methamphetamine use and methicillin-resistant Staphylococcus aureus skin infections. Emerg Infect Dis 13: 1707–1713.
25. Gallo RL, Nakatsuji T (2011) Microbial symbiosis with the innate immune defense system of the skin. J Invest Dermatol 131: 1974–1980.
26. Lai Y, Cogen AL, Radek KA, Park HJ, Macleod DT, et al. (2010) Activation of TLR2 by a small molecule produced by Staphylococcus epidermidis increases antimicrobial defense against bacterial skin infections. J Invest Dermatol 130: 2211–2221.
27. Iwase T, Uehara Y, Shinji H, Tajima A, Seo H, et al. (2010) Staphylococcus epidermidis Esp inhibits Staphylococcus aureus biofilm formation and nasal colonization. Nature 465: 346–349.

28. Vinolo MA, Rodrigues HG, Nachbar RT, Curi R (2011) Regulation of inflammation by short chain fatty acids. Nutrients 3: 858–876.
29. Raftari M, Jalilian FA, Abdulamir AS, Son R, Sekawi Z, et al. (2009) Effect of organic acids on Escherichia coli O157:H7 and Staphylococcus aureus contaminated meat. Open Microbiol J 3: 121–127.
30. Zhang H, Shen Y, Weng P, Zhao G, Feng F, et al. Antimicrobial activity of a food-grade fully dilutable microemulsion against Escherichia coli and Staphylococcus aureus. Int J Food Microbiol 135: 211–215.
31. Wu L, Zhao M, Xia C, Ni H, Zhang H (2009) Isolation, identification and rumen fermentation characteristics of Propionibacterium acnes. Wei Sheng Wu Xue Bao 49: 168–173.
32. Higaki S, Hasegawa Y, Morohashi M, Sakamoto K, Yamagishi T (1990) The influence of coptidis rhizoma to lipase activity of Propionibacterium acnes. Nihon Hifuka Gakkai Zasshi 100: 883–886.
33. Lomholt HB, Kilian M (2010) Population genetic analysis of Propionibacterium acnes identifies a subpopulation and epidemic clones associated with acne. PLoS One 5: e12277.
34. Louis P, Scott KP, Duncan SH, Flint HJ (2007) Understanding the effects of diet on bacterial metabolism in the large intestine. J Appl Microbiol 102: 1197–1208.
35. Park JS, Lee EJ, Lee JC, Kim WK, Kim HS (2007) Anti-inflammatory effects of short chain fatty acids in IFN-gamma-stimulated RAW 264.7 murine macrophage cells: involvement of NF-kappaB and ERK signaling pathways. Int Immunopharmacol 7: 70–77.
36. Hara T, Hirasawa A, Ichimura A, Kimura I, Tsujimoto G (2011) Free fatty acid receptors FFAR1 and GPR120 as novel therapeutic targets for metabolic disorders. J Pharm Sci 100: 3594–3601.
37. Fujita T, Matsuoka T, Honda T, Kabashima K, Hirata T, et al. (2011) A GPR40 agonist GW9508 suppresses CCL5, CCL17, and CXCL10 induction in keratinocytes and attenuates cutaneous immune inflammation. J Invest Dermatol 131: 1660–1667.
38. Smith KR, Thiboutot DM (2008) Thematic review series: skin lipids. Sebaceous gland lipids: friend or foe? J Lipid Res 49: 271–281.
39. Wang ZX, Zhuge J, Fang H, Prior BA (2001) Glycerol production by microbial fermentation: a review. Biotechnol Adv 19: 201–223.
40. Zheng X, Bollinger Bollag W (2003) Aquaporin 3 colocates with phospholipase d2 in caveolin-rich membrane microdomains and is downregulated upon keratinocyte differentiation. J Invest Dermatol 121: 1487–1495.
41. Kabongo Muamba ML. (1982) Exoenzymes of Propionibacterium acnes. Can J Microbiol 28: 758–761.
42. Slonczewski (1992) pH-regulated genes in enteric bacteria. Am Soc Microbial News 58: 140–144.
43. Kwon YM, Ricke SC (1998) Induction of acid resistance of Salmonella typhimurium by exposure to short-chain fatty acids. Appl Environ Microbiol 64: 3458–3463.
44. Weinrick B, Dunman PM, McAleese F, Murphy E, Projan SJ, et al. (2004) Effect of mild acid on gene expression in Staphylococcus aureus. J Bacteriol 186: 8407–8423.
45. Kidd DA, Johnson M, Clements J (2007) Development of an in vitro corrosion/irritation prediction assay using the EpiDerm skin model. Toxicol In Vitro 21: 1292–1297.
46. McDowell A, Barnard E, Nagy I, Gao A, Tomida S, et al. (2012) An expanded multilocus sequence typing scheme for propionibacterium acnes: investigation of 'pathogenic', 'commensal' and antibiotic resistant strains. PLoS One 7: e41480.
47. Cummins CS (1976) Identification of Propionibacterium acnes and related organisms by precipitin tests with trichloroacetic acid extracts. J Clin Microbiol 2: 104–110.
48. Cummins CS, Johnson JL (1974) Corynebacterium parvum: a synonym for Propionibacterium acnes? J Gen Microbiol 80: 433–442.
49. Kitagawa H, Yamanaka K, Kakeda M, Inada H, Imai Y, et al. (2011) Propionibacterium acnes vaccination induces regulatory T cells and Th1 immune responses and improves mouse atopic dermatitis. Exp Dermatol 20: 157–158.
50. Curry JL, Qin JZ, Robinson J, Nickoloff BJ (2003) Reactivity of resident immunocytes in normal and prepsoriatic skin using an ex vivo skin-explant model system. Arch Pathol Lab Med 127: 289–296.
51. Odell CA (2010) Community-associated methicillin-resistant Staphylococcus aureus (CA-MRSA) skin infections. Curr Opin Pediatr 22: 273–277.
52. Chitarra LG, Breeuwer P, Van Den Bulk RW, Abee T (2000) Rapid fluorescence assessment of intracellular pH as a viability indicator of Clavibacter michiganensis subsp. michiganensis. J Appl Microbiol 88: 809–816.
53. Lind H, Broberg A, Jacobsson K, Jonsson H, Schnurer J (2010) Glycerol enhances the antifungal activity of dairy propionibacteria. Int J Microbiol 2010: 430873.

11

Staphylococcal Panton-Valentine Leucocidin as a Major Virulence Factor Associated to Furuncles

Lamine Baba-Moussa[1]*, Haziz Sina[1], Jean-Michel Scheftel[2], Brigitte Moreau[3], Dominique Sainte-Marie[4], Simeon O. Kotchoni[5], Gilles Prévost[2], Pierre Couppié[4]

1 Département de Biochimie et de Biologie Cellulaire, Université d'Abomey-Calavi, Cotonou, Benin, **2** Institut de Bactériologie, Unité EA-4438 Physiopathologie et Médecine, Strasbourg, France, **3** Service de Biologie Polyvalente, Centre Hospitalier de Cayenne, Cayenne, Guyane Française, **4** Service de Dermatologie, Centre Hospitalier de Cayenne et Institut Guyanais de Dermatologie Tropicale, Cayenne, Guyane Française, **5** Department of Biology, Rutgers University, Camden, New Jersey, United States of America

Abstract

Panton-Valentine Leucocidin (PVL), one of the β-barrel pore-forming staphylococcal leucotoxins, is known to be associated to furuncles and some severe community pneumonia. However, it is still uncertain how many other virulence factors are also associated to furuncles and what the risk factors of furuncles are in immuno-compromised status of patients, especially the HIV (+) patients. In this paper, we use antigen immunoprecipitation and multiplex PCR approach to determine the presence of 19 toxins, 8 adhesion factors and the PFGE profiles associated to furuncles in three independent patient study groups of *S. aureus* (SA) isolates collected from the Cayenne General Hospital (French Guiana). The patient groups were made of: 16 isolates from HIV (−) patients, 9 from HIV (+) patients suffering from furuncles, and 30 control isolates from patients with diverse secondary infected dermatitis. Our data reveals that the majority (96%) of *SA* strains isolated from HIV patient-derived furuncles significantly produced PVL ($p<10^{-7}$), whereas only 10% of *SA* strains produced this toxin in secondary infected dermatosis. A high prevalence of LukE-LukD-producing isolates (56 to 78%) was recorded in patient groups. Genes encoding clumping factor B, collagen- and laminin-binding proteins (*clfB, cna, lbp*, respectively) were markedly frequent (30 to 55%), without being associated to a specific group. Pulse field gel electrophoresis evidenced 24 overall pulsotypes, whereas the 25 PVL-producing isolates were distributed into 15 non clonal fingerprints. These pulsotypes were not specific PVL-producing isolates. PVL appears to be the major virulence factor associated to furuncles in Europe and in South America regardless of the immune status of the HIV patients.

Editor: Paulo Lee Ho, Instituto Butantan, Brazil

Funding: These authors have no support or funding to report.

Competing Interests: The authors have declared that no competing interests exist.

* E-mail: laminesaid@yahoo.fr

Introduction

Staphylococcus aureus (*SA*) are known to produce a large series of toxins [1,2] and adhesion factors [3,4] considered as virulence-associated factors. Among the virulence factors associated to clinical syndromes, only few were initially considered in most of original studies [5,6,7]. For example, the Panton Valentine leucocidin (PVL)-producing *SA* strains were successively associated to furuncles and carbuncles [5,6,8,9] and/or to community pneumonia with lung abscesses [10,11,12].

PVL was initially identified because of the acute cytotoxicity of some culture supernatants of *SA* isolates from furuncles and staphylococcal necrotizing follicular infections of the skin [13,14]. PVL is a skin-necrotizing toxin when intradermally injected into rabbits [15]. This bipartite toxin is an active pore-forming toxin against human polymorphonuclear cells, monocytes and macrophages [16]. However, the two protein components of PVL, LukS-PV and LukF-PV, may recombine with other related leucotoxins components, to generate new leucotoxins with specific cell spectra [17]. The newly formed toxins such as PVL and gamma-hemolysins (HlgA-HlgB or HlgC-HlgB sometimes called LukS-LukF) may be expressed at different levels [18] with highly variable binding constants to cells [19]. Sequence and three-dimensional structures of LukS-PV and LukF-PV have been determined [20,21], and the interaction of LukS-PV with a membrane receptor was strongly suggested [19].

The origin and recurrence of furuncles as primary infections, and their severity in some patients remain unclear. This has been related to the nasal carriage of the bacterium [14], but this may suggest a role of innate immunity. Immunosuppressed HIV (+) patients develops frequently SA skin infections such as folliculitis and sometimes furuncle [22]. There is still no evidence of virulence factors in *SA* isolated from staphylococcal infections in HIV (+) patients. In addition, the possibility that immunodeficiency status of the patient may modify susceptibility to *SA* virulence has never been proved.

In this work we analyzed the toxin profile and adhesion factors of *SA* isolated from HIV positive and negative patients at the Cayenne General Hospital, the principal hospital in French Guiana, in South America, where HIV prevalence in adults was 1,6%. *SA* was isolated from independent furuncle and furuncle free patients. A comparative study of different *SA* toxins and adhesion factors was performed in order to establish the eventual association of virulence factors other than PVL, especially in HIV positive and negative patients with respect to secondary skin infections.

Materials and Methods

Ethics Statement

Samples collected from patients at French Guiana hospital center were anonymously sent to the University of Abomey-Calavi, Benin (West Africa) for microbial screening, while PFGE analysis were performed at Strasbourg University, Strasbourg, France. The authors had no access to the patient medical data, with the exception of anonymous clinical sample data such as ages, HIV status, skin infections. This work is mainly focused on the bacterium SA virulence factors and not on the patients, and was therefore exempted from ethical approval.

Collected samples and clinical data

We collected *SA* isolates from 55 patients in Cayenne General Hospital (French Guiana). These patients were classified in three groups according to infectious origin: 30 patients with staphylococcal secondary skin infections (eczema: 13, wound: 7, prurigo: 6 and diverse dermatosis: 4), 16 HIV (−) patients with furuncles and 9 HIV (+) patients with furuncles. The HIV (+) status was discovered for 2 patients with furuncles by ELISA and Western blot, consecutively confirmed by dermatology consultation test (where HIV test was systematically proposed when a furuncle was diagnosed) and 7 patients were previously diagnosed as HIV (+) and they were regularly followed at hospital. The median of the CD4+ lymphocytes in HIV (+) patients was 225 U/mm3 (42–896). Four patients had CD4+ lymphocytes $<200/mm^3$ and one $<100/mm^3$. Among the HIV (+) patients, only one suffered of cerebellar toxoplasmosis.

The other patients were consecutively seen at dermatological consultation. In this study, only patients presenting lesions like furuncles or secondary skin infections of a pre-existing non infectious dermatosis due to *SA* were included. The demographic and clinical characteristics of patients were recorded before the bacteriological sampling on the lesion. The mean age of all 55 patients was 25.4 year old (1–69). It was 18.3 (1–55), 28.8 (2–56), 44.6 (20–69), respectively, for the patients with secondary infections, HIV (−) patients and HIV (+) patients. The sex ratio was 1.3.

Susceptibility to antibiotics

Antibiograms for the isolates were obtained by the disk diffusion method (Bio-Rad-Diagnostic Pasteur, Marnes la Coquette, France). Isolates were inoculated and antibiotics were tested according to the 2010 Antiobiogram Committee of the French Society of Microbiology and the NCCLS recommendations [23]: Oxacillin (Oxa), Penicillin G (PeG), Vancomycin (Va), Teicoplanin (Tec), Kanamycin (Kan), Tobramycin (Tob), Chloramphenicol (Chl), Rifampicin (Rif), Fusidic acid (Fus), Gentamicin (Gm), Trimetroprim Sulfamethozolin (Sxt), Ofloxacin (OXF), Pristinamycin (Pt), Linezolide (Lzd) and Erythromicin (Ery) have been tested. Evaluation of methicillin resistance was performed by plating the strains on buffered Mueller-Hinton agar with 2% (wt/vol) NaCl at 37°C for 24 h.

Phenotypic detection of toxins

Enterotoxins A, B, C, and D and TSST-1. *SA* cultures were carried out overnight in 3 mL of Brain-Heart (Difco) medium under shaking, and toxins were detected using the semi-quantitative reversed passive latex agglutination detection kits SET-RPLA™ and TST-RPLA™ (Oxoid, Basingstoke, England). These tests were reported to be sensitive and specific, although large amounts of enterotoxin E may be detected as low levels of enterotoxin A [24].

Bicomponent leucotoxins and epidermolysins. The different leucotoxins (PVL, LukE-LukD, LukM-LukF-PV, and the gamma-hemolysin proteins HlgA, HlgB, and HlgC), epidermolysins A and B were evidenced from culture supernatants after 18 h of growth in YCP medium [19] by radial gel immunodiffusion in 0.6% (wt/vol) agarose in 10 mM Hepes, 150 mM NaCl, pH 7.5 with component-specific rabbit polyclonal and affinity-purified antibodies [14]. For a better determination, gels were dried, stained in Coomassie blue, and destained in 10% (vol/vol) acetic acid.

Genotype detection of toxins and adhesion factors

Presence of genes encoding entorotoxins SEE, SEG, SEH, SEK, SEL, SET, epidermolysin D (*etd*), Edin factors (*edinA*, *edinB*, *edinC*) and of genes encoding eight adhesion factors: Collagen Binding Protein (*Cna*), Fibronectin Binding Proteins A and B (*fnbA and fnbB*), Bone Sialoprotein Binding Protein (*bbp*), Clumping Factor B (*clfb*), Fibrinogen Binding Protein (*fib*), Elastin Binding Protein (*ebp*) and Laminin Binding Protein (*lbp*) was detected by Multiplex PCR (Table 1). Additionally, genes encoding PVL were also detected with oligonucleotides previously used for expression studies [18]. Total DNA was purified using QIAamp® DNA Mini Kit (Qiagen, GmbH, Germany) with a Gene Amp® PCR System 9700 (Perkin-Elmer, Norwalk, USA) and amplified in a total volume of 50 µl containing 25 pmoles of each primer, 50 ng of total DNA, 1.5 mM $MgCl_2$, 200 µM of dNTP mixture, 1× PCR reaction Buffer and 5 units of FastTaq™ DNA polymerase (Roche Applied Science, GmbH, Germany). The thermal cycling conditions included an initial denaturation step (2 min at 92°C) followed by 35 cycles of amplification comprising three steps: 2 min denaturation for 92°C, 1 min annealing at 50°C, 2 min extension at 72°C. The reaction was terminated with 3 min extension at 72°C. PCR products were analysed by electrophoresis through 1.4% (wt/vol) agarose gel (Euromedex, Mundolsheim, France).

Pulse Field Gel Electrophoresis (PFGE)

SA strains at mid-exponential growth in 25 ml of TY (1.6% [w/v] BioTrypcase, 1% [w/v] yeast extract, 0.5% [w/v] NaCl,) were embedded in agarose plugs as described previously [25]. After lysis of plugs by proteinase K (Sigma) for 18 h at 56°C, plugs were washed and stored at 4°C in 10 mM Tris-HCl, 1 mM EDTA (pH 8.0). Plugs (agarose plugs, 2.5 by 5.0 by 1 mm) were equilibrated in 300 µL of restriction enzyme buffer for 30 min at 4°C. DNA macro-restriction was then accomplished in 60 µL with 10 U of *Sma* I (New England Biolabs, Beverly, Mass.) for 4 h at room temperature. Electrophoresis was performed at 12°C with a Beckman Geneline™ Transverse Alternating Field Electrophoresis (TAFE) system at 150 mA in 0.5× TAFE system buffer (TAFE buffer is 0.2 M Tris, 10 mM free acid EDTA, and 87 mM CH_3COOH [pH 8.2]) in a 1% (w/v) agarose gel. Electrophoresis of *Sma*I-fragmented DNA was carried out with 2-s pulses for 1 h, followed by 14-s pulses for 1 h, 12-s pulses for 1.5 h, 10-s pulses for 2.5 h, 8-s pulses for 6 h, and 6-s pulses for 6 h. Bacteriophage lambda PFG Marker (New England Biolabs) was used as a molecular marker. The gels were stained with ethidium bromide and photographed under UV trans-illumination. Pulsotypes were compared and classified in a dendrogram using the Dice coefficient and the unweighted pair group method with arithmetic mean clustering provided by Molecular Analyst™ (version 1.5) and Fingerprinting™ (version 1.12) softwares (Bio-Rad, Ivry sur Seine, France). Isolates that differed by no more than three fragments were considered to be subtypes of a given clonal type.

Table 1. Primers used for PCR detection of genes encoding virulence factors.

Oligonucleotides sequences	size pb/ PCR set	accession n°
edinA 1: 5'-TCATAGAAGTATCTAATACTTCTTTAGCA-3'	604/2	M63917
edinA 2 : 5'-TCCAACACGGTATTCTGTGCCTCTAGGTA-3'		
edinb 1: 5'-ACAGACTTAGTTGAAGCTACT-AAATG-3'	522/5	AB057421
edinb 2: 5'-TGTCCCTGTAGGCAAAAGAAC-TTCTTG-3'		
edinC 1: 5'-AGGTCTTCCAGCTAATGCAGC-TCCTT-3'	543/6	NC 003265
edinC 2: 5'-ACAGTTCAAAAGACAAAGAA-GCTATT-3'		
etd 1: 5'-AATACATATGAAGAATCTGAAATTTTA3'	800/4	AB057421
etd 2: 5'-AAGTTATTCCATAATGATTAGAATGA-3'		
lukE-lukD 1: 5'-AATACTAATATTGAAAATATTGGTGATGG-3'	1882/8	Y13225
lukE-lukD 2: 5'-CTTAAATTTCGGGTTTAACTCCTCTATTTC-3'		
see 1: 5'-CTTACCGCCAAAGCTGTCG-3'	159/3	M21319
see 2: 5'-GTCCACTTGTAAATGGTAGCGAGAA-3'		
seg 1: 5'-AATTATGTGAATGCTCAACCCGAT-3'	408/3	AF064773
seg 2: 5'-CTTTAGTGAGCCAGTGTCTTGCTTTG-3'		
seh 1: 5'-CATCTACCCAAACATTAGCACC-3'	222/5	U11702
seh 2: 5-TAGAAATCAAGGTGATAGTGGCAA-3'		
sek 1: 5'-TGATACTCCTATAGCTAATCAACTACA-3'	300/3	U93688
sek 2: 5-ACATCAATCTCTTGAGCGGTAACA-3'		
sel 1: 5'-ACCAGAATCACACCGCTTAGAATAC-3'	422/2	AF217235
sel 2: 5'-TGGAATACTACACTCCCCTTATCAAAAG-3'		
set1-1: 5'-GAAGGTCTACAAGGCCAAAATGTCT-3'	363/6	BX571856
set1-2: 5'-TCAACACATCGCCCATGCGCTCGA-3'		
bbp 1: 5'-CGGCTAGTGATAATAAAGAAGTAGTG-3'	550/1	BA000018
bbp 2: 5'-CTTGTTGGAGCTGTAGCAACTGGTTT-3'		
clfB 1: 5'-ATTAGTGCAAACACAAACAGTGCG-3'	305/4	AJ224764
clfB 2: 5'-AGTTCCTTGCGCATTGGAAATCGT-3'		
cna 1: 5'-CGGGAGATATGCTACCAGAAGATA-3'	278/1	BX571857
cna 2: 5'-ATAGCCTTGTGGAATTGTTACATCA-3'		
ebp 1: 5'-AGACCAATCAGAATTAGAACATCA-3'	378/4	U48826
ebp2: 5'-TCAGAAACTGTTGAATGCTCAGTGT-3'		
fib 1: 5'-AGCGGCAATAGGTATTACTACAACT3'	220/2	X72013
fib 2: 5'-CGAATGTACCATCGTTAAATTCAT-3'		
fnbA 1: 5'-TTAACTTGGGATAATGGTTTAGTTT-3'	273/7	AJ629521
fnbA 2: 5'-GCTGATGAATCCGTTTCTTCTATTG-3'		
fnbB 1: 5'-TGGAAGAAACTAAAGCGACAGGTAC-3'	317/1	AJ629502
fnbB 2: 5'-TTCTTTAAACGTATATCTAACTTTTC-3'		
lbp 1: 5'-TGGTGTATATGACTACAGTAAGTT-3'	410/5	AF065394
lbp 2: 5'-CGTTTGTAGCAACAGCAATATCAGC-3'		

Other virulence factors have been detected by multiplex PCR onto purified total DNA (Qiagen). Presence of genes encoding enterotoxins E, G, H, K, L, T, epidermolysin D (Etd), genes encoding Edin A and EDIN B and the genes encoding seven adhsesion factors (Cna, FnbA, FnbB Bbp, Clfb, Fib, Ebp and Lbp) was checked in 8 set in function of base size.

Statistical analysis

For comparison tests of positive isolates of each patient group, we used the Student T test, and the Fischer's test for lower number series (SPSS Ltd software, version 10.1). P<0.05 was considered statistically significant.

Results

Susceptibility to antibiotics

In this study, no isolate was resistant to oxacillin or gentamicin. However, production of β-lactamase was observed for all isolates of the three groups with the exception of one isolate of the control group. In addition, the isolates were generally sensitive to all tested antimicrobials with the exception of few SA that were resistant to fusidic acid, *i.e.* 9 of the 10 fusidic acid resistant isolates were from the control group, or to erythromycin, *i.e.* 9 of the 11 erythromycin resistant isolates were also issued from the control group.

Comparative analysis of toxins production

The presence of the staphylococcal toxins in the different groups is detailed in the Table 2. A great majority (96%) of the *SA* strains isolated from furuncles regardless of status of the HIV patient produced PVL, while only 10% of the isolates originated from secondary infected dermatosis produced this toxin (Table 2). This difference between furuncles and non-furuncles populations was significant ($p<10^{-7}$). All the strains isolated from furuncles of HIV (−) patients produced PVL, while it is produced by 89% of the isolates obtained from furuncles of HIV (+) patients. Only PVL-producing isolates were also detected for the presence of corresponding genes, conversely to the LukE/LukD leucotoxin. In fact, the *lukE/lukD* locus was detected in most *SA* isolates (92%), but the effective production of the corresponding LukE/LukD leucotoxin was observed only for 64% of isolates obtained from furuncles and for 76% of those from secondary infected dermatosis (Table 2). Therefore, no noticeable difference between groups could be drawn in this study. This result illustrates heterogeneity between *SA* isolates from our sample collection in regards to the occurrence of LukE/LukD production [24,26,27]. Epidermolysin A (ETA) is produced by 16% of isolates from secondary infected dermatosis. The presence of enterotoxins A and G yielded 23% and 16% in the group of secondary infections respectively, while only 4% and 16% in the cumulated groups of furuncles, respectively. Finally, no more than 40% (12/30) of the secondary dermatitis- and no more than 36% (9/25) of the furuncle-originated isolates produced one at least of the most encountered superantigens.

Comparative analysis of the presence of adhesion factors

The distribution of 8 genes encoding adhesion factors were examined (Table 3). Gene encoding *FnBA* was carried out in all tested isolates. In the groups of the strains isolated from furuncles and the secondary infected dermatitis, no isolate carries genes encoding *Fib*, *Cna*, *FnBb*, *Bbp*. The presence of *ClfB* seemed to be linked to the presence of *Lbp*, since all the strains carrying *clfB* also carried *lbp*. Ebp is produced by 48% of the isolates from furuncles, while it is produced by 30% in the case of non-infected dermatitis. Concerning the two HIV (+) and HIV (−) patient groups, the genes encoding the adhesion factors ClfB, Lbp, and EBP are present respectively at 6/16, 6/16 and 7/16 for HIV (−) group and 4/9, 4/9 and 5/9 for HIV (+) group.

Pulsed Field Gel Electrophoresis (PFGE)

Pulsed field gel electrophoresis defined 24 *SmaI*-pulsotypes differing by more than two DNA fragments for the 55 different isolates, which

Table 2. Production of toxins and identification of genes encoding toxins in *Staphylococcus aureus*.

Toxins and genes encoding toxins	Infected dermatosis (n = 30)	Furuncles (n = 25)		
		All	HIV (−) (n = 16)	HIV (+) (n = 9)
SEA	7 (23.3%)	1 (4.0%)	1 (6.3%)	0
SEB	3 (10.0%)	5 (20.0%)	2 (12.5%)	3 (33.3%)
SEC	4 (13.3%)	4 (16.0%)	1 (6.3%)	3 (33.3%)
SED	2 (6.7%)	1 (4.0%)	1 (6.3%)	0
TSST1	1 (3.3%)	0	0	0
ETA	5 (16.7%)	0	0	0
ETB	0	1 (4.0%)	1 (6.3%)	0
PVL	3 (10.0%)	24 (96.0%)	16 (100.0%)	8 (88.9%)
LukE/LukD	23 (76.7%)	16 (64.0%)	9 (56.3%)	7 (77.8%)
lukE-lukD	29 (96%)	22 (88%)	13 (81.5%)	9 (100%)
etd	0	0	0	0
see	0	0	0	0
seg	5 (16.7%)	7 (28.0%)	2 (12.5%)	5 (55.6%)
seh	0	0	0	0
sek	0	0	0	0
sel	0	0	0	0
set	0	0	0	0
edinB	0	0	0	0
edinC	0	0	0	0
edinA	0	0	0	0

The majority of *SA* strains isolated from HIV patient-derived furuncles significantly produced PVL ($p<0.05$), whereas only 10% of *SA* strains produced this toxin in secondary infected dermatosis. A high prevalence of LukE-LukD-producing isolates (56 to 78%) was recorded in patient groups.

therefore, exclude clonal relationships between isolates (Figure 1). Among the different pulsotypes, which account for a diverse collection of SA genotypes in French Guiana, some were identified in both furuncles and secondary pyodermites isolates. Therefore, PVL-producing isolates cannot be referred to as a specific category of pulsotype. According to the isolates, 9 to 14 defined DNA fragments of lengths comprised between 20 kb and 600 kb after *Sma*I restriction. Six of these pulsotypes were displayed by isolates belonging to different groups including secondary dermatitis. The most represented pulsotypes n° 1, 8, 13 are composed of 7, 6, and 6 isolates respectively. The diversity of the pulsotypes accounts for an endemic polymorphic SA isolates in French Guiana and reinforces the PVL as a main causative agent of furuncles.

Discussion

This study reinforces PVL as probably the major staphylococcal virulence factor in furuncles as it is produced by almost all *SA*

Table 3. Presence of genes encoding adhesion factors of *Staphylococcus aureus*.

Gene encoding adhesion factors	Infected dermatosis (n = 30)	Furuncles (n = 25)		
		All	HIV (−) (n = 16)	HIV (+) (n = 9)
bbp	0	0	0	0
cna	0	0	0	0
clfb	16 (53.3%)	10 (40%)	6 (37.5%)	4 (44.4%)
ebp	9 (30%)	12 48%)	7 (43.8%)	5 (55.6%)
fib	0	0	0	0
fnbA	30 (100%)	25 (100%)	16 (100%)	9 (100%)
fnbB	0	0	0	0
lbp	16 (53.3%)	10 (40%)	6 (37.5%)	4 (44.4%)

Genes encoding clumping factor B, collagen- and laminin-binding proteins (*clfB*, *cna*, *lbp*, respectively) were markedly frequent (30 to 55%), without being associated with a specific group.

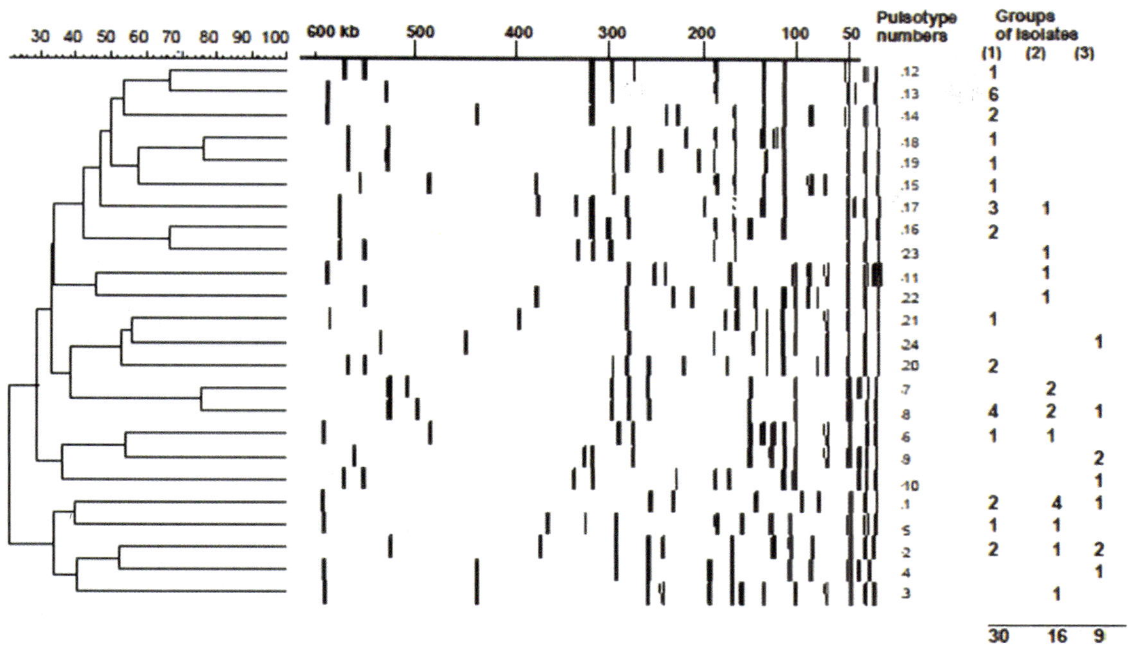

Figure 1. Pulsed field gel electrophoresis (PFGE) dependent dendogram of isolated *Staphylococcus aureus*. Pulsed field gel electrophoresis (PFGE) proves no specific clonal relationship between PVL-producing isolates issued from furuncles or secondary dermatosis. The similarity of the different pulsotypes was established by using Molecular Analyst™ software. Twenty four pulsotypes corresponded to the 55 isolates and their distribution is given according to the groups of isolates issued from secondary infected dermatosis (1), furuncles from HIV (−)(2) or HIV (+)(3) patients.

isolates, i.e. 96% from furuncles and (10%) ($p<10^{-7}$) from control group constituted of *SA* isolates from non furunculous skin infections. These results are comparable with those previously obtained in Europe [28,29,30]. In Strasbourg (France), 85.7% of *SA* strains isolated from a series of 35 furuncles produced this toxin, while it was produced by less than 2% of strains issued from healthy patients or patients with other staphylococci affections [8,14]. In former studies, PVL production from routine isolates represented 3 to 12% of isolates according to collections [14,31]. Other authors established the association with furuncles at 93% within a series of 30 furuncles [11]. Together with other research group, we have previously noticed that isolates obtained simultaneously from different furuncles, or from different episodes or in a same fratry were comparable. However, they are less comparable if they are isolated from individuals, except when they were obtained from outbreaks [6,32,33]. All together, the absence of clonal relationships between these American isolates confirms the significance of the association of PVL with furuncles.

A furuncle is characterized by necrosis of body hair follicles and adjacent tissues. In rabbit skin, PVL induces necrosis after intradermal injection [14,15]. The *SA* PVL-producing strains were also associated to severe primitive staphylococci pneumonia with high mortality rate, and with multiple consecutive lung abscesses to metastastic diffusion from furuncles [10]. However, it could not be excluded from any of these studies that another virulence factor may be also associated with PVL. We almost excluded the role of superantigens and other major toxins, while no specific adhesion factor can be suspected. In fact, despite the presence of such a factor, adhesion of *SA* provides a benefit to the bacterial colonisation, but a specific adhesion remains questionable.

Our study did not found a significant difference ($p=0.36$) between the PVL produced by *SA* strains responsible for the furuncles regardless of the status of HIV patient considered: HIV (+) (89%), HIV (−) (100%). Among HIV (+) patients, the chronic nasal carriage of *S. aureus* is more frequent [34]. The frequency of *SA* infections increased with the decreasing of immunity. Severe *SA* infections are generally described among the patients with CD4+ lymphocytes less than 100 cells/mm^3 [22,35]. In the case of a chronic nasal carriage, the risk for *SA* infection rose to 20% per year among patients with CD4+ <100 cell/mm3 [35]. The frequency of *SA* skin infections increased with the immunodeficiency. At an advanced stage of the disease, 20% of the patients may be concerned by a *SA* skin infection [22]. The furuncles or carbuncles are within the first reported *SA* skin infections among the HIV (+) patients [35,36]. Like in HIV (−) patients, in HIV (+) patients the principal bacterial factor associated with furuncle is PVL-producing *SA* infecting a follicle body hair. This data argued for the association of PVL-production with some necrotic lesions like furuncles and carbuncles.

For HIV (+) patients and others, furuncle is a sign of the presence of a virulent *SA*-strain, which produces PVL. In the context of advanced immunodeficiency, this infection must be particularly cured as well as the bacterial carriage, because of the risk of consecutive septicaemia due to this kind of strain. Recently, the emergence of Methicillin Resistant *SA* (*MRSA*) isolates producing Panton-Valentine Leucocidin (PVL) have been observed [37,38,39], thus highlighting additional seriousness of potential complication.

In our study, the *SA* strains isolates involved in furuncles did not harbour any specific resistance to antibiotics. The high frequency of LukE/LukD-producing isolates observed in the groups of strains (55 to 85%), may be due to an endemic situation, which should be further confirmed. A markedly high frequency of some adhesion factors *Clf*, *Lbp* and *Ebp* does not seem to be associated to any particular group of isolates.

In conclusion, and like in Europe, we demonstrate here a strong association between SA-producing PVL isolates in South America and necrotic skin lesions such as furuncles. This association is similar in HIV (+) and in HIV (−) patients. It remains unclear whether such skin lesions might be considered as risk markers in exposed patient's populations. Absence of clonal relationships between SA strains isolated from furuncles is an important argument for a causal relationship between capacity of PVL production by the SA and the development of furuncles.

Acknowledgments

The authors acknowledge the skillful technical assistance of D. Keller.

Author Contributions

Conceived and designed the experiments: LBM GP PC. Performed the experiments: LBM GP BM DSM PC HS. Analyzed the data: LBM JMS SOK GP PC. Contributed reagents/materials/analysis tools: GP PC. Wrote the paper: LBM PC GP SOK.

References

1. Prévost G (2005) Toxins in *Staphylococcus aureus* pathogenesis. In: Proft T, ed. Microbial toxins: molecular and cellular biology. Norfolk: Horizon Bioscience Press. pp 243–83.
2. Baba-Moussa L, Anani L, Scheftel JM, Couturier M, Riegel P, et al. (2008) Virulence factors produced by strains of *Staphylococcus aureus* isolated from urinary tract infections. J Hosp Infect 68: 32–38.
3. Foster JT, Höök M (1998) Surface protein adhesions of *S. aureus*. Trends Microbiol 6: 484–488.
4. Baba-Moussa L, Ahissou H, Azokpota P, Assogba B, Atindéhou M, et al. (2010) Toxins and adhesion factors associated with *Staphylococcus aureus* strains isolated from diarrheal patients in Benin. Afr J Biotechnol 9: 604–611.
5. Yamasaki O, Kaneko J, Morizane S, Akiyama H, Arata J, et al. (2005) The association between *Staphylococcus aureus* strains carrying Panton-Valentine leukocidin genes and the development of deep-seated follicular infection. Clin Infect Dis 40: 381–395.
6. Baggett HC, Hennessy TW, Rudolph K, Bruden D, Reasonover A, et al. (2004) Community-onset methicillin-resistant *Staphylococcus aureus* associated with antibiotic use and the cytotoxin Panton-Valentine leukocidin during a furunculosis outbreak in rural Alaska. J Infect Dis 189: 1565–1573.
7. Seiberling KA, Conley DB, Tripathi A, Grammer LC, Shuh L, et al. (2005) Superantigens and chronic rhinosinusitis: detection of staphylococcal exotoxins in nasal polyps. Laryngoscope 115: 1580–1585.
8. Couppié P, Cribier B, Prévost G (1994) Leucocidin from *Staphylococcus aureus* and skin infections: an epidemiological study. Arch Dermatol 130: 1208–1209.
9. Carré N, Herbreteau N, Askeur N, Dabas JP, Sillam F, et al. (2011) Outbreak of skin infections due to *Staphylococcus aureus* carrying Panton-Valentine leukocidin genes in pupils and their relatives. Med Mal Infect 10: 1016–1017.
10. Defres S, Marwick C, Nathwani D (2009) MRSA as a cause of lung infection including airway infection, community-acquired pneumonia and hospital-acquired pneumonia. Eur Respir J 34: 1470–1476.
11. Lina G, Piémont Y, Godail-Gamot F, Bes M, Peter MO, et al. (1999) Involvement of Panton-Valentine leukocidin-producing *Staphylococcus aureus* in primary skin infections and pneumonia. Clin Infect Dis 29: 1128–1132.
12. Gillet Y, Issartel B, Vanhems P, Fournet JC, Lina G, et al. (2002) Association between *Staphylococcus aureus* strains carrying gene for Panton-Valentine leukocidin and highly lethal necrotising pneumonia in young immunocompetent patients. Lancet 359: 753–759.
13. Panton PN, Valentine FCO (1932) Staphylococcal toxin. Lancet 222: 506–508.
14. Prévost G, Couppié P, Prévost P, Gayet S, Petiau P, et al. (1995) Epidemiological data on *Staphylococcus aureus* strains producing synergohymenotropic toxins. J Med Microbiol 42: 237–245.
15. Ward PD, Turner WH (1980) Identification of staphylococcal Panton–Valentine leukocidin as a potent dermonecrotic toxin. Infect Immun 28: 393–397.
16. Prévost G, Cribier B, Couppié P, Petiau P, Supersac G, et al. (1995) Panton-Valentine leucocidin and gamma-haemolysin from *Staphylococcus aureus* ATCC 49775 are encoded by distinct genetic loci and have different biological activities. Infect Immun 63: 4121–4129.
17. Gravet A, Colin DA, Keller D, Girardot R, Monteil H, et al. (1998) Characterization of a novel structural member, LukE-LukD, of the bi-component leucotoxins family. FEBS Lett 436: 202–208.
18. Bronner S, Stoessel P, Gravet A, Monteil H, Prévost G (2000) Variable expressions of *Staphylococcus aureus* bicomponent leucotoxins semiquantified by competitive reverse transcription-PCR. Appl Environ Microbiol 66: 3931–3938.
19. Gauduchon V, Werner S, Prévost G, Monteil H, Colin DA (2001) Flow cytometric determination of Panton-Valentine leucocidin S component binding. Infect Immun 69: 2390–2395.
20. Pédelacq JD, Maveyraud L, Prévost G, Baba-Moussa L, Gonzalez A, et al. (1999) The structure of a *Staphylococcus aureus* leucocidin component (LukF-PV) reveals the fold of the water-soluble species of a family of transmembrane pore-forming toxins. Structure 7: 277–287.
21. Guillet V, Roblin P, Werner S, Coraiola M, Menestrina G, et al. (2004) Crystal Structure of Leucotoxin S Component: New Insight into the Staphylococcal Beta-Barrel Pore-Forming Toxins. J Biol Chem 279: 41028–41037.
22. Smith KJ, Wagner KF, Yeager J, Skelton HG, Ledsky R (1994) *Staphylococcus aureus* carriage and HIV-1 disease: association with increased mucoskin infections as well as deep soft-tissue infections and sepsis. Arch Dermatol 130: 521–522.
23. National Committee for Clinical Laboratory Standards. (2010) Performance standards for antimicrobials susceptibility testing. NCCLS, Wayne, Pa. Supplement; M100-S12.
24. Gravet A, Rondeau M, Harf-Monteil C, Grunenberger F, Monteil H, et al. (1999) Predominant *Staphylococcus aureus* isolated from antibiotic-associated diarrhea is clinically relevant and produces enterotoxin A and the bicomponent toxin LukE-LukD. J Clin Microbiol 37: 4012–4019.
25. Prévost G, Pottecher B, Dahlet M, Bientz M, Mantz JM (1991) Pulsed field gel electrophoresis as a new epidemiological tool for monitoring methicillin-resistant Staphylococcus aureus in an intensive care unit. J Hosp Infect 17: 255–269.
26. Gravet A, Couppié P, Meunier O, Clyti E, Moreau B, et al. (2001) *Staphylococcus aureus* isolated from impetigo produces both epidermolysins A or B and LukE+LukD in 78% of 131 retrospective and prospective cases. J Clin Microbiol 39: 4349–4356.
27. von Eiff C, Friedrich AW, Peters G, Becker K (2004) Prevalence of genes encoding for members of the staphylococcal leukotoxin family among clinical isolates of *Staphylococcus aureus*. Diagn Microbiol Infect Dis 49: 157–162.
28. Naas T, Fortineau N, Spicq C, Robert J, Jarlier V, et al. (2005) Three-year survey of community-acquired methicillin-resistant *Staphylococcus aureus* producing Panton-Valentine leukocidin in a French university hospital. J Hosp Infect 61: 321–329.
29. Holmes A, Ganner M, McGuane S, Pitt TL, Cookson BD, et al. (2005) *Staphylococcus aureus* isolates carrying Panton-Valentine leucocidin genes in England and Wales: frequency, characterization, and association with clinical disease. J Clin Microbiol 43: 2384–2390.
30. Del Giudice P, Bes M, Hubiche T, Blanc V, Roudière L, et al. (2011) Panton-Valentine leukocidin-positive *Staphylococcus aureus* strains are associated with follicular skin infections. Dermatology 222: 167–170.
31. Baba-Moussa L, Sanni A, Dagnra AY, Anagonou S, Prince-David M, et al. (1999) Approche épidémiologique de l'antibiorésistance et de la production de leucotoxines par les souches de *Staphylococcus aureus* isolées en Afrique de l'Ouest. Med Mal Infect 29: 689–696.
32. Diep BA, Sensabaugh GF, Somboona NS, Carleton HA, Perdreau-Remington F (2004) Widespread skin and soft-tissue infections due to two methicillin-resistant *Staphylococcus aureus* strains harboring the genes for Panton-Valentine leucocidin. J Clin Microbiol 42: 2080–2084.
33. Linde H, Wagenlehner F, Strommenger B, Drubel I, Tanzer J, et al. (2005) Healthcare-associated outbreaks and community-acquired infections due to MRSA carrying the Panton-Valentine leucocidin gene in southeastern Germany. Eur J Clin Microbiol Infect Dis 24: 419–422.
34. Raviglione MC, Mariuz P, Pablos-Mendez A, Battan R, Ottuso P, et al. (1990) High *Staphylococcus aureus* nasal carriage rate in patients with acquired immunodeficiency syndrome or AIDS-related complex. Am J Infect Control 18: 64–69.
35. Nguyen MH, Kauffman CA, Goodman RP, Squier C, Arbeit RD, et al. (1999) Nasal carriage of and infection with *Staphylococcus aureus* in HIV-infected patients. Ann Intern Med 130: 221–225.
36. Pitche P, Tchangai-Walla K, Napo-Koura G, Mijiyawa M, Agbere A, et al. (1995) Prevalence of skin manifestations in AIDS patients in the Lomé-Tokoin University Hospital (Togo). Santé 5: 349–352.
37. Vandenesch F, Naimi T, Enright M, Lina G, Nimmo GR, et al. (2003) Community acquired methicillin-resistant *Staphylococcus aureus* carrying Panton-Valentine leukocidin genes: worldwide emergence. Emerg Infect Dis 9: 978–984.
38. Liassine N, Auckenthaler R, Descombes MC, Bes M, Vandenesch F, et al. (2004) Community-acquired methicillin-resistant *Staphylococcus aureus* isolated in Switzerland contains the Panton-Valentine leukocidin or exfoliative toxin genes. J Clin Microbiol 42: 825–828.
39. Mithoe D, Rijnders MI, Roede BM, Stobberingh E, Möller AV (2011) Prevalence of community-associated meticillin-resistant *Staphylococcus aureus* and Panton-Valentine leucocidin-positive *S. aureus* in general practice patients with skin and soft tissue infections in the northern and southern regions of The Netherlands. Eur J Clin Microbiol Infect Dis;doi: 10.1007/s10096-011-1316-9O.

12

The Zwitterionic Cell Wall Teichoic Acid of *Staphylococcus aureus* Provokes Skin Abscesses in Mice by a Novel CD4+ T-Cell-Dependent Mechanism

Christopher Weidenmaier, Rachel M. McLoughlin, Jean C. Lee*

Channing Laboratory, Department of Medicine, Brigham and Women's Hospital and Harvard Medical School, Boston, Massachusetts, United States of America

Abstract

Zwitterionic polysaccharide (ZPS) components of the bacterial cell envelope have been shown to exert a major histocompatibility complex (MHC) II-dependent activation of CD4+ T cells, which in turn can modulate the outcome and progression of infections in animal models. We investigated the impact of zwitterionic cell wall teichoic acid (WTA) produced by *Staphylococcus aureus* on the development of skin abscesses in a mouse model. We also compared the relative biological activities of WTA and capsular polysaccharide (CP), important *S. aureus* pathogenicity factors, in abscess formation. Expression of both WTA and CP markedly affected the ability of *S. aureus* to induce skin abscess formation in mice. Purified wild-type zwitterionic WTA was more active in inducing abscess formation than negatively charged mutant WTA or purified CP8. To assess the ability of purified native WTA to stimulate T cell proliferation in vitro, we co-cultivated WTA with human T-cells and antigen presenting cells in the presence and absence of various inhibitors of MHC-II presentation. Wild-type WTA induced T cell proliferation to a significantly greater extent than negatively charged WTA. T cell activation was dependent on the presentation of WTA on MHC II, since inhibitors of MHC II-dependent presentation and antibodies to MHC II significantly reduced T cell proliferation. T cells activated in vitro with wild-type WTA, but not negatively charged WTA, induced abscess formation when injected subcutaneously into wild-type mice. CD4−/− mice similarly injected with WTA failed to develop abscesses. Our results demonstrate that the zwitterionic WTA of *S. aureus* induces CD4+ T-cell proliferation in an MHCII-dependent manner, which in turn modulates abscess formation in a mouse skin infection model. An understanding of this novel T cell-dependent host response to staphylococcal abscess formation may lead to the development of new strategies to combat *S. aureus* skin and soft tissue infections.

Editor: Michael Otto, National Institutes of Health, United States of America

Funding: CW was supported by a fellowship from the Deutsche Forschungsgesellschaft (http://www.dfg.de/en/index.jsp). The funders had no role in study design, data collection and analysis, decision to publish, or preparation of the manuscript.

Competing Interests: The authors have declared that no competing interests exist.

* E-mail: jclee@rics.bwh.harvard.edu

Introduction

Wall teichoic acid (WTA) of *Staphylococcus aureus* is a zwitterionic cell wall glycopolymer composed of ~40 ribitol phosphate repeating units modified with *N*-acetylglucosamine and D-alanine [1,2]. The negatively charged phosphate groups in the ribitol repeating unit and the ester-linked D-alanine residues contribute to the zwitterionic charge of WTA (Fig. 1). The presence of WTA-like molecules in most Gram-positive bacteria prompted scientists to focus on the role of WTA in cell wall function [3,4] and turnover [5]. More recently, defined mutants of *S. aureus* that lack WTA or have altered WTA structures have facilitated experiments to elucidate in greater detail the role of WTA in staphylococcal pathogenesis [6–10]. WTA has been implicated in the adhesion of *S. aureus* to human epithelial and endothelial cells [9–11], and expression of WTA has been shown to be essential for *S. aureus* nasal colonization of cotton rats [9,11]. A *S. aureus* mutant lacking WTA showed attenuated virulence in a rabbit model of endocarditis [10]. Moreover, purified WTA was able to induce intraabdominal abscesses when rats were inoculated by the intraperitoneal route [12]. *S. aureus* mutants in the *dlt* operon, which mediates D-alanylation of WTA, exhibit a negatively charged cell surface and are more sensitive to cationic antimicrobial peptides than the parental strain [13,14].

WTA is expressed constitutively [1], whereas *S. aureus* capsular polysaccharides (CPs) are expressed in a tightly regulated manner [15,16]. Most clinical isolates of *S. aureus* express either capsule type 5 (CP5) or 8 (CP8). However, 20–25% of clinical isolates produce no capsule due to a variety of mutations within the conserved capsule biosynthesis operon [17,18].

WTA exhibits a zwitterionic charge, and advances in the field of glyco-immunology have led to the finding that zwitterionic polysaccharides (ZPS) exert a direct activity on the adaptive immune system, thereby modulating the development of bacterial infections [19]. ZPS, such as complex CPs produced by specific bacterial pathogens, directly elicit immune responses by activating various T cells subtypes in the absence of protein carriers [20,21]. ZPS activated T cells modulate the outcome of infection or colonization by different bacterial species [19,22]. CP5 and CP8 produced by *S. aureus* enhance staphylococcal virulence [23–25], and purified zwitterionic CP8 induces intraabdominal abscesses in rats in a CD4 T cell dependent manner [12]. In a wound infection

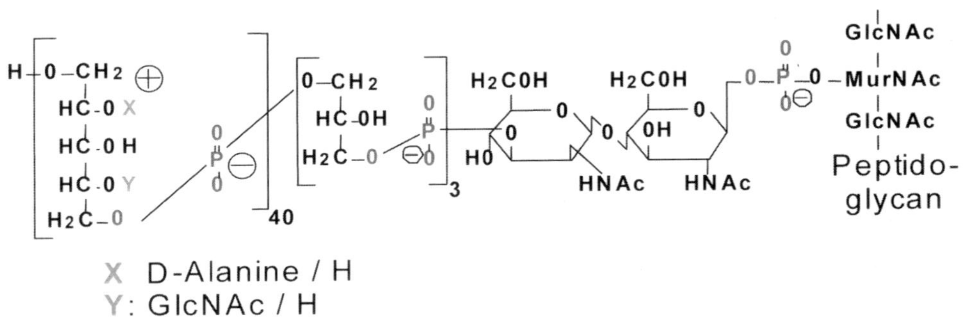

Figure 1. *Staphylococcus aureus* WTA is a zwitterionic cell wall polymer composed of ~40 ribitol phosphate repeating units modified with *N*-acetylglucosamine and D-alanine. The negatively charged phosphodiester bonds and the positively charged D-alanine residues are responsible for the zwitterionic nature of the polymer.

model, McLoughlin et al. demonstrated that the presence of CD4 T cells modulated CXC chemokine production at the *S. aureus* infection site in an IFN-γ dependent manner, which led to a massive recruitment of neutrophils, and this effect was mediated by CP8 [26]. These findings suggest that staphylococcal ZPS are important factors for T cell dependent immune stimulation, which strongly influences the outcome of infections.

Skin and soft tissue infections are the most common types of *S. aureus* infections and occur in the hospital as well as in the community, affecting hosts without predisposing risk factors [27,28]. Since bacterial ZPS are associated with abscess formation [12,29], we explored the contribution of zwitterionic WTA and CPs in a mouse skin infection model. We demonstrate here that WTA activates T cells in a MHC II dependent manner, and that T cells activated in vitro by WTA induce skin abscesses in mice. These novel findings link staphylococcal skin infections to recent discoveries of glyco-immunology and may lead to novel approaches to combat skin infections by *S. aureus*.

Results

WTA and Capsule Impact Abscess Formation When Live Bacteria Are Injected Subcutaneously into the Flanks of Mice

We used a mouse model to study the ability of various *S. aureus* strains to induce skin infections that closely resemble staphylococcal skin infections in humans. *S. aureus* cells mixed with cytodex beads were injected subcutaneously into the flanks of mice. The cytodex beads allow for formation of a localized abscess even at low inocula or with low concentrations of purified WTA.

To assess the relative roles played by *S. aureus* WTA and CPs in skin infections, we transduced the *tagO* mutation into the CP5+ strain Newman and its isogenic acapsular *cap5O* mutant. The resulting *tagO* deletion mutants lacked WTA in their cell wall as evidenced by the low phosphorus content of cell wall fractions, but their doubling times were similar to that of the parental strains under in vitro conditions (Fig. S1). The Newman *tagO* mutant was complemented by introducing a wild-type copy of *tagO* on plasmid prB*tagO*. In addition, we used previously described mutants of the acapsular SA113 strain that either lack WTA (*tagO*) [9] or the D-alanine esters (*dltA*) [13] in the repeating WTA subunits. The *dltA* mutation was transduced into Newman, and the phenotype of the resulting mutant was consistent with the absence of positive charges in the teichoic acids (Fig. S1).

S. aureus wild-type strains SA113 and Newman at inocula ranging from 10^6 to 10^4 cfu were potent inducers of subcutaneous abscesses in mice (Fig. 2). The *tagO* mutants of both bacterial strains were significantly attenuated in their ability to induce abscesses, whereas the *dltA* mutants showed an intermediate phenotype at the lower inocula (Figs. 2A and 2B and Supplemental Fig. 2). Consistent with previous data with a CP8+ strain [22], the acapsular Newman *cap5O* mutant was also attenuated for subcutaneous abscess formation (Fig. 2C). When the bacteria were grown on Columbia salt agar to enhance capsule expression (Fig. 2C), strain Newman provoked a higher bacterial burden per abscess than when it was grown on tryptic soy agar (Fig. 2B). The Newman *tagO* and *cap5O* mutants were both significantly attenuated for abscess induction when compared to the parental strain. A double mutant of Newman that expresses neither capsule nor WTA was more attenuated for abscess formation than the single mutants (Fig. 2C), but the differences did not reach statistical significance. These data suggest that both WTA and CP promote *S. aureus* skin abscess formation when live bacteria are used as the inocula.

Purified WTA Induces Skin Abscesses More Efficiently than Purified CP8

To further assess its biological activity, we purified WTA from the acapsular strains SA113 wild-type (zwitterionic WTA) and SA113 *dltA* (anionic WTA). WTA purity was assessed by ^{1}H NMR, phosphate content, the absence of nucleic acids (<0.1%), protein (<0.1%), and endotoxin (<1 EU/mg). Sterile abscesses were induced by injection of sterile cytodex beads mixed with purified wt WTA at doses ranging from 200 to 0.02 μg. After 48 h, abscesses were excised and quantified by their weight. Purified wt WTA was a potent inducer of abscess formation at doses as low as 0.02 μg (Fig. 3A). WTA purified from the *dltA* mutant or beads alone showed minimal activity under these conditions (Fig. 3A). Administration of *dltA* WTA resulted in the recruitment of fewer neutrophils in the abscessed tissue than wt WTA (Fig. S2). We quantified the host response by measuring neutrophil accumulation at the infection site with the myeloperoxidase (MPO) assay (Fig. 3B) [30]. MPO is present in the azurophilic granules of neutrophils and is routinely used to assess the tissue inflammatory responses [31] and abscess formation. MPO activity in abscesses provoked by 20 μg wt WTA after 48 h was significantly ($P<0.0001$) higher than that induced by 20 μg *dltA* WTA. Despite its potent activity in the induction of intraabdominal abscesses [12], purified CP8 exhibited only minimal potency in the s.c. abscess model, even at a 50 μg dose.

Purified WTA Fails to Induce Neutrophil Chemotaxis or Proinflammatory Cytokines

To investigate whether purified WTA exhibited direct chemotactic activity, we assayed chemotaxis of human neutrophils in response to

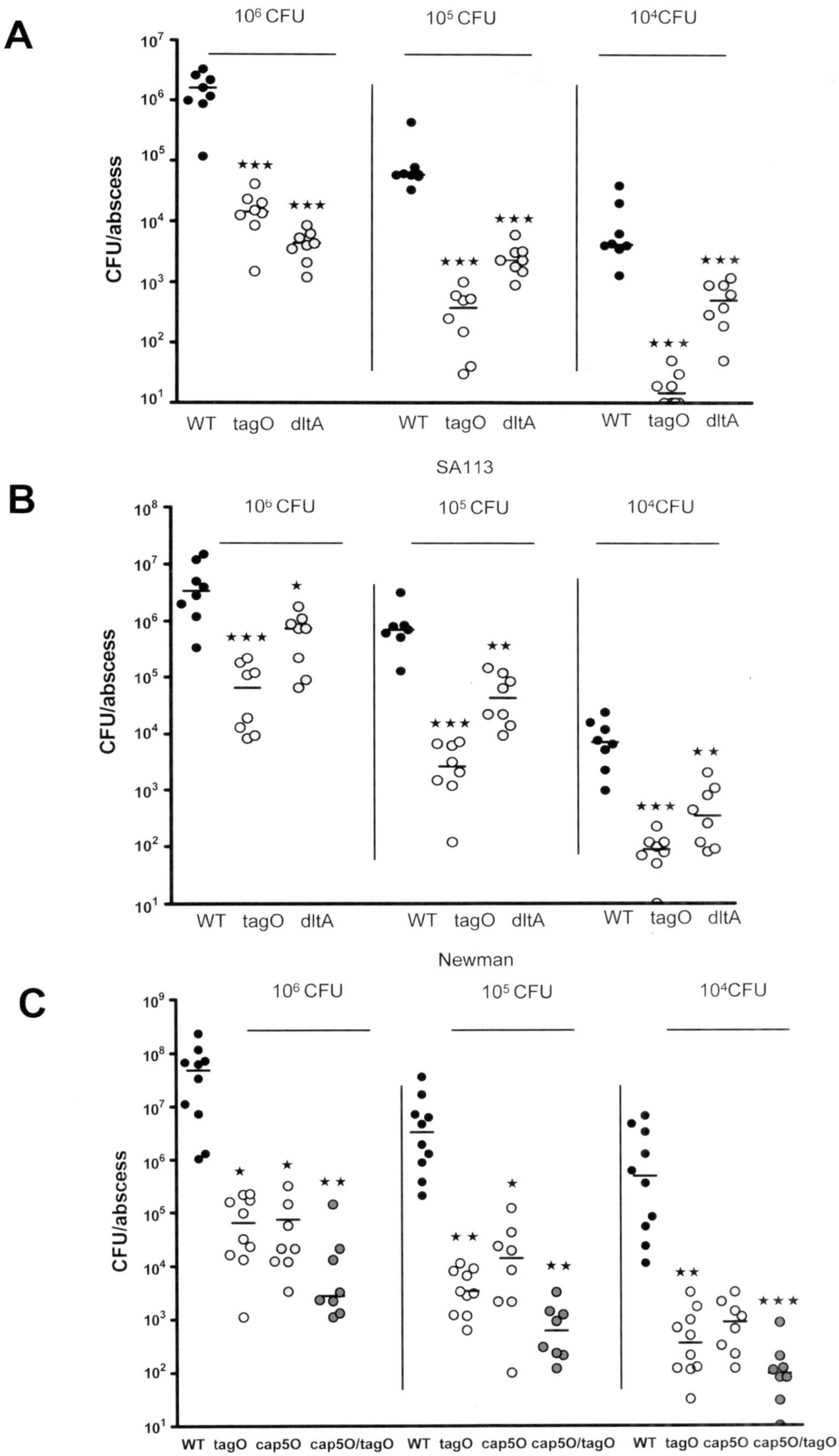
A
10⁶ CFU
10⁵ CFU
10⁴CFU
CFU/abscess
WT tagO dltA
WT tagO dltA
WT tagO dltA
SA113
B
10⁶ CFU
10⁵ CFU
10⁴CFU
CFU/abscess
WT tagO dltA
WT tagO dltA
WT tagO dltA
Newman
C
10⁶ CFU
10⁵ CFU
10⁴CFU
CFU/abscess
WT tagO cap5O cap5O/tagO
WT tagO cap5O cap5O/tagO
WT tagO cap5O cap5O/tagO

Figure 2. Strains with no WTA or structurally altered WTA are deficient in induction of s.c. abscesses. 10^6 to 10^4 CFU *S. aureus* was injected s.c into the flanks of mice. After 48 h, the mice were euthanized, and each abscess was excised, homogenized, and cultured quantitatively. Horizontal bars represent group median values, n = 8. A) The Sa113*dltA* mutant (negatively charged teichoic acids) and the *tag*O mutant (no WTA) were attenuated compared to the wt (all *p*-values are 0.0002). B) Newman *tagO* ($p = 0.0002$ at 10^6; $p = 0.0003$ at 10^5, $p = 0.0002$ at 10^4) and the *dltA* mutant ($p = 0.0047$ at 10^6; $p = 0.0006$ at 10^5, $p = 0.007$ at 10^4) were significantly less virulent in the abscess model compared to the wt, n = 8. All *p*-values were determined by Mann-Whitney analysis. C) Newman wt, *tagO*, isogenic acapsular mutant *cap5O* and the *cap5O/tagO* double mutant were grown on CSA plates to enhance CP production. The Newman *tagO* ($p<0.05$ at 10^6; $p<0.01$ at 10^5, $p<0.01$ at 10^4) and *cap5O* ($p<0.01$ at 10^6; $p<0.05$ at 10^5, $p>0.05$ at 10^4) mutants and the double mutant ($p<0.001$ at 10^6; $p<0.001$ at 10^5, $p<0.001$ at 10^4) were significantly inhibited in abscess formation compared to the wt. The mutants showed no significant difference when compared to each other. P-values for Figure 2C were determined by Kruskal-Wallis one-way ANOVA with Dunn's multiple comparison test. ★$p<0.05$; ★★$p<0.01$, ★★★$p<0.001$.

WTA in a transwell assay. WTA purified from *S. aureus* SA113 or the SA113 *dltA* mutant failed to induce significant chemotaxis compared to the authentic chemoattractant fMLP (Fig. 4A).

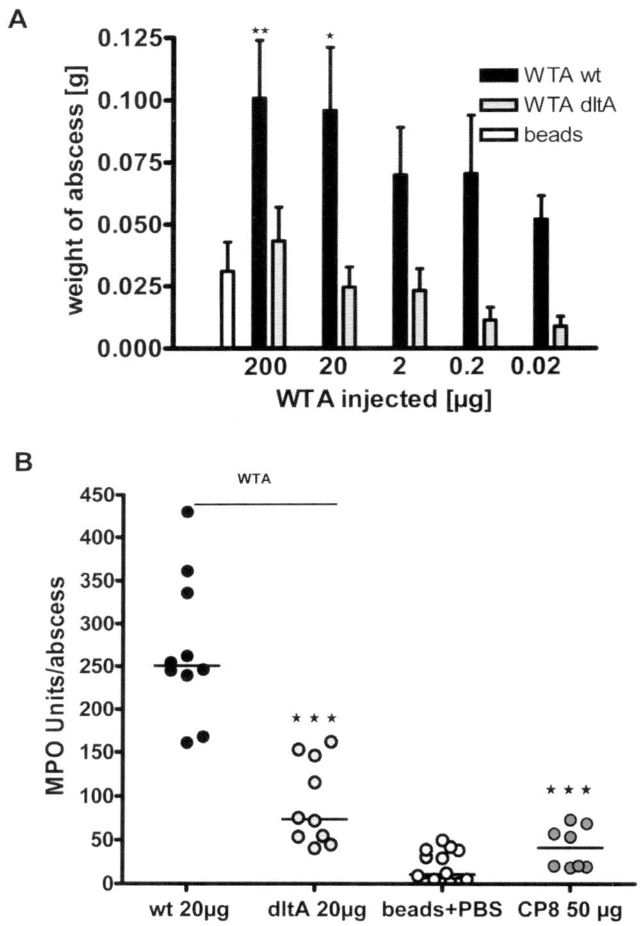

Figure 3. Purified WTA is a potent abscess inducer. WTA was purified from wt SA113 or the *dltA* mutant, mixed with cytodex beads, and injected s.c. into mouse flanks. A) The weights of the abscesses were determined after 48 h and expressed as mean ± SEM, n = 8. The zwitterionic WTA purified from SA113 induced well-defined abscesses, whereas the negatively charged *dltA* WTA was only a weak abscess inducer (wt WTA compared to beads $p = 0.0062$ at 200 µg; $p = 0.0381$ at 20 µg. *dltA* WTA compared to beads yielded p values >0.05 at all doses. All *p*-values were determined by two-tailed Student t-tests). B) 20 µg WTA purified from wild-type SA113 or the *dltA* mutant was mixed with cytodex beads and injected into the flanks of mice. After 48 h, the abscesses were excised, homogenized, and MPO activity was determined to assess the intensity of the host response. Wt WTA induced strong MPO activity, indicative of neutrophil recruitment, whereas *dltA* WTA and CP8 were considerably less active (*p*-values <0.0001 by Mann-Whitney analyses). ★$p<0.05$; ★★$p<0.01$, ★★★$p<0.001$.

Activation of pro-inflammatory responses via pattern recognition receptors like Toll-like receptors (TLRs) could also lead to pronounced inflammation and modulate abscess formation. Therefore, we tested whether purified WTA stimulates pro-inflammatory cytokines in macrophages or in HEK293 cells transfected with TLR-2. These experiments not only interrogated WTA proinflammatory activity but also enabled us to exclude functional contaminants in our purified WTA preparation. We measured production of TNF-α by human monocytes (THP-1 cells) or mouse macrophages (RAW 264.7 cells) after stimulation with WTA or with the TLR agonists LPS, MALP-2, or Pam3Cys as positive controls. We stimulated HEK293 cells transfected with TLR-2 with WTA, MALP-2, or Pam3Cys, and assayed for IL-8 production in the culture supernatants. Purified WTA at concentrations as high as 100 µg/ml showed no proinflammatory activity in THP-1 or RAW 264.7 cells (Fig. 4B) or in TLR-2 expressing HEK293 cells (Fig. 4C). This is consistent with previous reports that demonstrated the inability of WTA to directly activate host cells in a manner typical of classical pathogen associated molecular pattern molecules [32].

WTA activates proliferation of human T cells in a MHC II dependent manner

The induction of intraperitoneal abscesses by other zwitterionic polysaccharides is based on their ability to directly activate T-cells, which in turn modulate cellular responses at the infection site [14,28]. Therefore, we cultured nylon wool-purified human T-cells or column-purified CD4+ T cells with irradiated antigen-presenting cells (APCs) and wt or *dltA* WTA. *S. aureus* enterotoxin A (SEA) and polygalacturonic acid (GalU) were used as positive and negative controls, respectively. Wt WTA elicited a potent dose-dependent proliferative response in human T cells on day 6 (Fig. 5A). The T-cell response to wt WTA was significantly higher than that exhibited by CP8, *dltA* WTA, or beads alone (Fig. 5A). The negatively charged polygalacturonic acid failed to induce T-cell proliferation, and the *S. aureus* superantigen SEA induced a significantly higher T-cell response than proliferation induced by either of the WTA antigens (Fig. 5D).

To determine whether T-cell proliferation induced by purified WTA was mediated by MHC class I or II molecules, we performed assays in the presence of blocking antibodies (Abs) and isotype control Abs. Wt WTA induced T-cell proliferation was dependent on the MHC class II molecule HLA-DR since T cell proliferation was reduced significantly in the presence of blocking Abs to HLA-DR (Fig. 5B), but not with Abs to HLA-DP, HLA-DQ, or HLA-A, -B, or –C (data not shown). The residual activity of the *dltA* WTA was not inhibited by any of the Abs. In assays utilizing the human Burkitt lymphoma cell line (Raji) and its MHC class II transcriptional mutant cell line (RJ2.2.5), WTA stimulated T-cell proliferation only when the MHC-II–expressing Raji cells, but not the RJ2.2.5 cells, were incubated with T-cells and WTA (Fig. 5C). Inhibitors of the intracellular antigen-processing pathways that are required for MHC II-dependent antigen

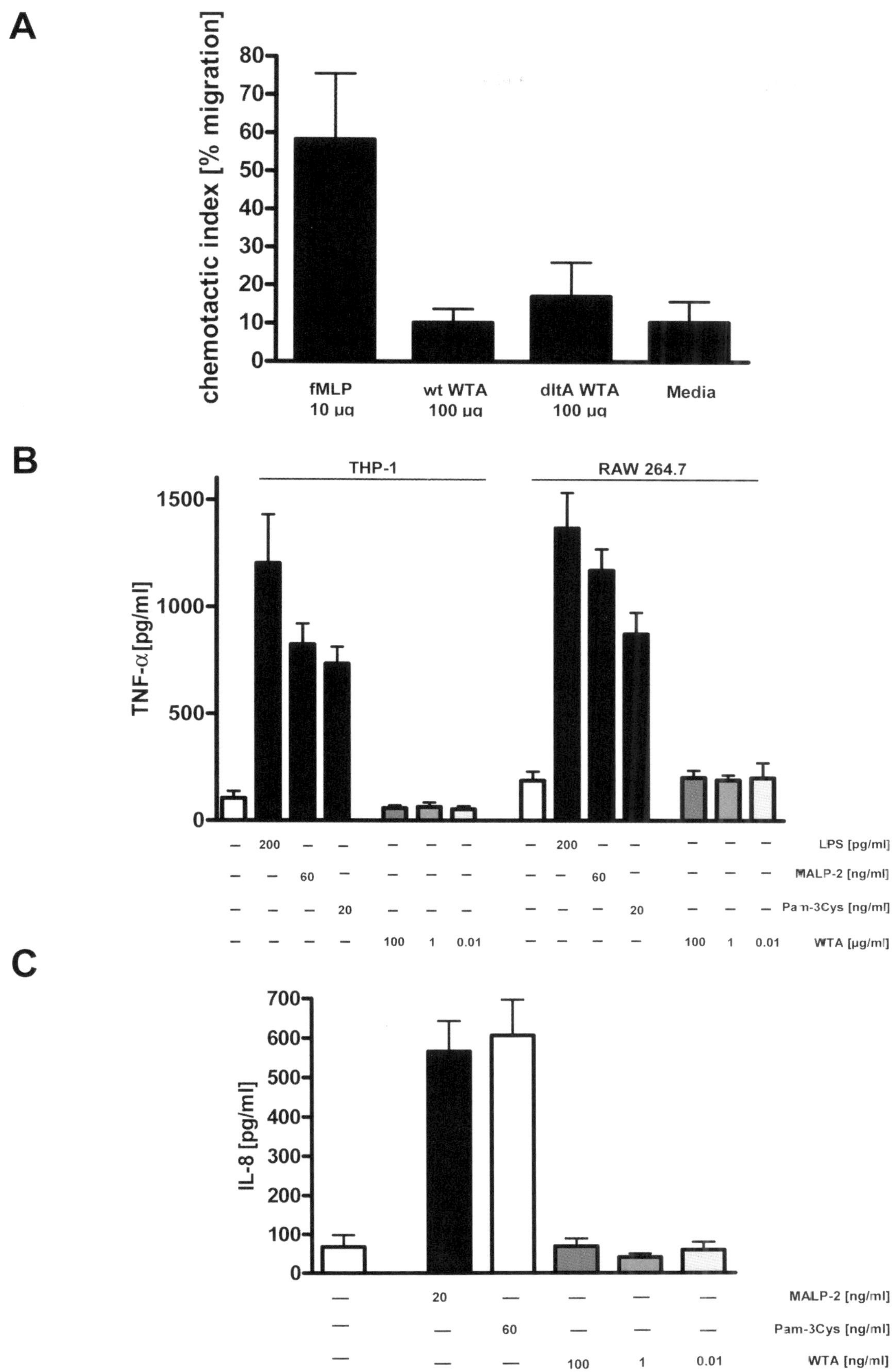
A
chemotactic index [% migration]
0
10
20
30
40
50
60
70
80
fMLP 10 µg
wt WTA 100 µg
dltA WTA 100 µg
Media
B
THP-1
RAW 264.7
TNF-α [pg/ml]
0
500
1000
1500
LPS [pg/ml]
MALP-2 [ng/ml]
WTA [µg/ml]
200
60
20
100
1
0.01
C
IL-8 [pg/ml]
0
100
200
300
400
500
600
700
MALP-2 [ng/ml]
Pam-3Cys [ng/ml]
WTA [ng/ml]
20
60
100
1
0.01

Figure 4. WTA fails to directly induce chemotactic migration or cytokine induction. A) The chemotactic activity of WTA was assessed in a transwell assay. Shown are means (n = 3) and SD of the chemotactic index (% of cells that migrated from the upper compartment towards the stimulus in the lower compartment). The positive control fMLP induced strong chemotactic migration whereas wt and *dltA* WTA failed to affect neutrophil migration ($p>0.05$ for WTA vs. media by Mann-Whitney analyses). B) Production of TNF-α in the human monocyte cell line THP-1 and the mouse macrophage cell line RAW 264.7 after stimulation for 8 h. LPS, Pam3Cys and MALP-2 stimulated a potent response whereas wt WTA at 100, 1 or 0.01 μg/ml failed to induce cytokine production (WTA vs. media >0.05 by two-tailed Student t-test). Shown are means and SD, n = 3. C) Production of IL-8 in TLR-2 transfected HEK293 cells after stimulation for 10 h. Pam3Cys, MALP-2 stimulated a potent response whereas wt WTA failed to induce cytokine production at concentrations of 100,1 or 0.01 μg/ml. Shown are means and SD, n = 3 (WTA vs. media $p>0.05$ by two-tailed Student t-test).

presentation were used at concentrations that had no effect on the stimulatory activity of the *S. aureus* superantigen SEA (Fig. 5D). The inhibitors Bafilomycin A (BafA), Brefeldin A (BrefA), Colchicine, and Cytochalasin D (CytoCalD) reduced the T-cell proliferation induced by wt WTA and *dltA* WTA, providing evidence that, unlike superantigens, WTA requires intracellular processing for efficient MHC II presentation to T cells.

WTA Stimulated Mouse T Cells Modulate Abscess Formation in the S.C Abscess Model

The role of T-cell activation in the modulation of WTA-induced abscess formation was assessed by T-cell transfer experiments. *S. aureus* wt WTA stimulated a potent proliferative response in mouse T cells after 6 days, whereas *dltA* WTA was less active (Fig. 6A). In T cell transfer assays, purified mouse CD4+ T cells were cultured in vitro for 6 days with WTA and irradiated APCs. The stimulated T cells were then purified, assayed for purity by FACS analysis, mixed with cytodex beads, and injected s.c. into mouse flanks. Abscess formation was quantified by MPO activity in the abscessed tissue after 48 h. In dose-dependency experiments, we found that 3×10^5 activated T cells were sufficient to induce an abscess after 48 h (data not shown). T cells stimulated with wt WTA induced abscess formation in mice, whereas T cells stimulated with *dltA* WTA, naive T-cells, or APCs incubated with WTA in the absence of T cells were significantly less potent (Fig. 6B).

To lend further evidence to the premise that T cells are crucial for *S. aureus* abscess formation, we used CD4 T cell deficient mice. As predicted, WTA provoked abscesses in C57Bl/6 mice, but not in CD4-deficient C57Bl/6 tm1mac mice (Fig. 6C). These in vivo data clearly demonstrate the link between WTA dependent T cell activation and the modulation of abscess formation by activated CD4 T cells.

Discussion

Ribitol-phosphate WTA is a conserved cell wall-associated ZPS produced by *S. aureus*. CP produced by the majority of staphylococcal strains may mask WTA on the bacterial surface. However, neither CP5 nor CP8 is expressed by 20–25% of clinical isolates [17,18]. Even in encapsulated strains, WTA is most likely surface exposed during the logarithmic growth phase when little CP is produced [16,17,33]. WTA is present both in the logarithmic and stationary phases of bacterial growth, and it appears to be expressed constitutively by the bacterial cell. Structural genes encoding enzymes of WTA biosynthesis machinery can be upregulated under certain in vivo conditions, such as the early phases of nasal colonization, as demonstrated in the cotton rat model [34].

We were interested in the role of WTA in the development of skin infections caused by *S. aureus*, since these are among the most frequent staphylococcal infections. Moreover, WTA was shown to induce abscesses in a rat model of intraabdominal abscess formation [12]. Our data demonstrate that *S. aureus* WTA plays a critical role in the development of staphylococcal skin lesions. Mutants that lack WTA (*tagO*) or have an altered WTA structure (*dltA*) are significantly impaired in the mouse s.c. abscess model. The attenuated phenotype of the *dltA* mutant may be partially attributed to its susceptibility to killing by neutrophils and cationic microbial peptides [9,13], which are highly abundant in skin infections [35]. The absence of *S. aureus* WTA or the presence of an altered WTA structure influences the molecular events that modulate abscess formation since purified wt WTA induced abscesses more efficiently than *dltA* WTA. T cells have previously been shown to play a role in animal models of *S. aureus* intraperitoneal and subcutaneous abscess formation [12,22] and in a staphylococcal surgical wound infection model [22]. In this study we identify a novel role for zwitterionic WTA, together with CP, in the induction of subcutaneous abscess formation through a mechanism dependant upon T-cell activation. We demonstrated that purified WTA stimulated CD4+ T-cell proliferation in vitro, and that this was dependent upon the zwitterionic charge of WTA. WTA was unable to induce T cell proliferation when APCs lacking MHC II were used in co–culture, and the stimulatory activity of wt WTA, but not the residual activity of the *dltA* WTA, was diminished by HLA-DR blocking Abs. In contrast, inhibitors of intracellular processing pathways blocked the activity of wt WTA and the residual activity of *dltA* WTA. This argues for a charge-dependency of WTA presentation but not intracellular processing, which is consistent with reports characterizing other bacterial ZPS polymers [36]. Thus, WTA qualifies as a bacterial ZPS that is processed and presented by APCs via the MHCII pathway [19]. Having defined a mechanism by which WTA can activate T-cells, we then established that the T cell stimulatory activity of WTA could modulate skin abscess formation. CD4 T cells activated by purified wt WTA were sufficient to provoke abscesses when injected s.c. into the flanks of healthy mice. Moreover, CD4−/− mice injected with WTA failed to develop abscesses. Taken together, we present a novel function of WTA as a ZPS that can modulate CD4 T cell-dependent development of skin abscesses in mice.

S. aureus mutants defective in CP production were attenuated in the s.c. abscess model of infection, but purified CP8 was less active than WTA in T-cell proliferation assays and in the skin abscess model. Both CP8 and WTA showed similar potency in the rat intraperitoneal abscess model [12], suggesting that the underlying molecular mechanisms leading to abscess formation differ between the skin and peritoneal cavity. USA300 strains that are responsible for most SSTIs in the U.S. are negative for CP production [37], and thus WTA may be a critical factor that promotes USA300 abscess formation in humans.

The molecular effector mechanisms that are downstream of WTA-induced T cell activation and lead to abscess formation have yet to be resolved. CD4+ T cells have been shown to influence neutrophil recruitment into *S. aureus*–infected wound tissues via production of IFN-γ [26]. High local IFN-γ production leads to upregulation of CXC chemokines, thereby resulting in a pronounced neutrophil influx into the infected host tissues [26]. Here we provide evidence that *S. aureus* WTA and CP are both crucial for SSTIs provoked by *S. aureus*, and that WTA induces

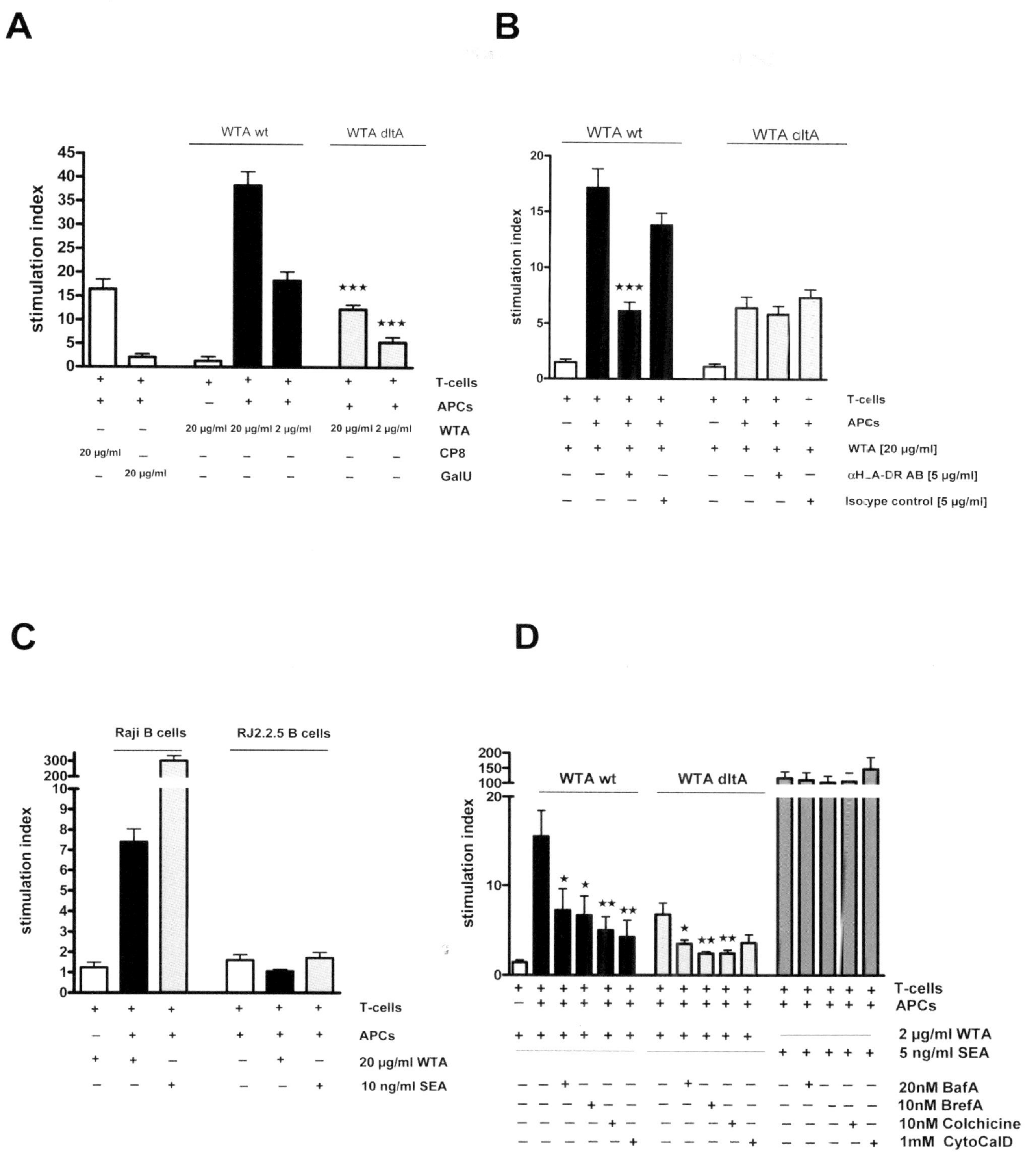

Figure 5. WTA stimulates in vitro T-cell activation by a MHC-II dependent mechanism. T cells and APCs were incubated with different concentrations of WTA purified from SA113 wt or the *dltA* mutant. The stimulation index was calculated by normalizing on wells with APCs and T-cells but no stimulating antigen. A) wt WTA stimulated T-cell proliferation in a dose-dependent manner, whereas *dltA* WTA and CP8 were considerably less active ($p<0.0001$ for wt WTA vs. *dltA* WTA at 20 and 2 µg, $p=0.0003$ for wt WTA vs. CP8). The negatively charged GalU showed no activity. SEA was considerably more active than WTA (panel D). Values represent means ± SEM, n = 6. B) T-cell proliferation assays with WTA from wt and *dltA* were performed in the presence of blocking Abs to the MHC class II molecules and the appropriate isotype control. An antibody to HLA-DR (5 µg/ml) inhibited T-cell proliferation induced by zwitterionic wt WTA ($p<0.0001$) but not negatively charged *dltA* WTA. Shown are means ± SEM. n = 5. C). WTA induced T-cell proliferation only with Raji cells as APCs but not when APCs were from the MHC II negative cell line RJ2.5.5. Shown are means and SEM, n = 4. D) T cells were incubated with different inhibitors of the MHC II antigen processing pathway. The inhibitors bafilomycin A (BafA), brefeldin A (BrefA), colchicine, and cytochalasin D (CytoCalD) decreased T-cell proliferation induced by wt WTA (wt WTA with BafA: $p=0.0399$; wt WTA with BrefA: $p=0.0230$; wt WTA with Colchicine: $p=0.0042$; wt WTA with CytoCalD; $p=0.0036$) and *dltA* WTA (*dlt* WTA with BafA: $p=0.0220$; *dlt* WTA with

BrefA: $p = 0.0026$; *dlt* WTA with Colchicine: $p = 0.0032$; *dlt* WTA with CytoCalD: $p = 0.0527$). Shown are means ± SEM, n = 4. All *p*-values were determined by the two-tailed Student t-test. ★$p < 0.05$; ★★$p < 0.01$, ★★★$p < 0.001$.

skin abscesses through MHC II–dependent activation of CD4+ T cells. A recent study by Cho et al. demonstrated the importance of γδ T cells in controlling neutrophil recruitment and influencing the outcome of intradermal *S. aureus* infections in mice [38]. The discrepancies between the results of Cho et al. and our own results may reflect subtle differences between the two infection models, as well as characteristics of the *S. aureus* strains utilized by the different labs. The immune mechanisms modulating the onset of infection likely differ depending on the site of infection, the specific virulence factors produced by the microbe, and the repertoire of effector cells responding to the bacterial insult.

Multiple virulence determinants likely affect *S. aureus* induction of SSTIs [39], and the host response to infection is currently under investigation by several laboratories. WTA is present in all *S. aureus* strains, and synergistic interactions among leukocidins, CPs, α-toxin [40], phenol-soluble modulins [41] and WTA may increase the frequency or severity of staphylococcal SSTIs. The ribitol phosphate WTA produced by *S. aureus* differs from the glycerol phosphate WTA polymer synthesized by *Staphylococcus epidermidis*, the most common staphylococcal species found on human skin [42,43]. Whether the biological properties of the two polymers differ is a question that has not yet been addressed.

Our results demonstrate a novel function for the zwitterionic WTA polymer of *S. aureus*. We link the novel finding that WTA can stimulate CD4+ T cells to the development of staphylococcal SSTIs in an *in vivo* infection model. We offer new insights into the pathology of SSTIs caused by *S. aureus* and propose a novel host mechanism involved in staphylococcal skin infections.

Methods

Ethics Statement

Human blood was collected from healthy volunteers giving written informed consent for venipuncture, as approved by the Institutional Review Board of The Brigham and Women's Hospital (Human Subject Assurance Number 00000484). Animal experiments were performed in accordance with the guidelines of the Harvard Medical School Standing Committee on Animals (Animal Welfare Assurance Number A3431-01) under approved protocol 86-02131. The Harvard Medical School animal management program is accredited by the American Association for Accreditation of Laboratory Animal Care and meets National Institutes of Health standards as set forth in "Guide for the Care and Use of Laboratory Animals" (DHSS Publication No. (NIH) 85-23 Revised 1985). The institution also accepts as mandatory the Public Heath Service "Policy on Humane Care and Use of Laboratory Animals by Awardee Institutions" and NIH "Principles for the Utilization and Care of Vertebrate Animals Used in Testing, Research and Training."

Bacterial Strains and Growth Conditions

S. aureus SA113 (ATCC 35556) is a previously described laboratory strain [44]. The WTA-deficient Sa113 *tagO* mutant was generated by replacing the *tagO* gene with an erythromycin resistance cassette [9]. The Δ*dltA* mutant of *S. aureus* SA113 was generated by replacing the *dltA* gene with a spectinomycin resistance cassette [13], and this mutation was transduced into strain Newman with phage 80α. The phenotype of the *dltA* mutant was assessed by its ability to bind more positively charged cytochrome C (Sigma) than the wildtype strain, as described previously [45]. *S. aureus* Newman and the isogenic Newman *cap5O* mutant were described previously [46]. The *tagO::tet* mutation from RN4220 *tagO::tet geh::tagO* (kindly provided by Drs. Timothy Meredith and Suzanne Walker, Harvard Medical School) was introduced into strain Newman by transduction with phage 80α. The strain Newman *tagO* mutation was verified by PCR, and the absence of WTA was confirmed by measuring the phosphorus content of cell wall fractions prepared from the isogenic wild-type and mutant strains [9]. For genetic complementation studies, the mutants were complemented with a plasmid containing a wild-type copy of the *tagO* gene (pRB*tagO*) [9]. Bacterial strains were grown in tryptic soy broth (BBL) or B-Medium BM [9] unless otherwise noted.

WTA Isolation and Purification

Staphylococcal WTA was isolated and analyzed as described [9]. The phosphorus content in WTA samples was determined by colorimetric assays [9,13]. WTA was then dialyzed against 20 mM Bis/Tris buffer and run on a Q-Sepharose column with a NaCl gradient (0–1 M) followed by a Sephacryl S-300 size exclusion column. All buffers and water were pyrogen-free. The instruments and devices used in the WTA purification process were deproteinated by treatment with sulfuric acid and depyrogenated by heat inactivation for 4 h at 240°C or by treatment with a 1–2 M sodium hydroxide buffer. WTA was analyzed for protein by the Biorad method and by UV absorbance at 280 nm; for nucleic acid by UV absorbance at 260 nm and by agarose gel electrophoresis; and for endotoxin by the Limulus amebocyte lysate test (Charles River Laboratories, Charleston, SC). ^{1}H-nuclear magnetic resonance spectroscopy (NMR) was performed for structural evaluation.

Mouse Model of Subcutaneous Abscess Formation

Male Swiss Webster ND4 mice (4–6 weeks old) were purchased from Charles River or Harlan, and C57Bl/6 and C57Bl/6 tm1mac CD4−/− mice were purchased from The Jackson Laboratory. 10^4 to 10^6 CFU *S. aureus* or purified WTA was mixed with sterile dextran beads (Cytodex 1, Sigma), and the mixture (0.2 ml) was injected s.c. into the shaved flanks of mice as described previously [47]. The abscesses were either weighed or homogenized in TSB for quantitative culture. Alternatively, the myeloperoxidase (MPO) activity in abscess homogenates was measured with a colorimetric assay [48]. For histological analysis, excised tissue was fixed in formalin, embedded in paraffin, and stained with hematoxylin and eosin for microscopic examination.

T-Cell Activation, Neutrophil Chemotaxis, and Cytokine Production Assays

Mononuclear cells were purified by density gradient centrifugation in Polymorphoprep (Axis-Shield) from blood drawn from various healthy human donors. Total T cells were purified from the mononuclear cell fraction with nylon wool columns (Polysciences, Inc.), and CD4 T cells were purified with CD4 enrichment columns (R&D Systems). Purity was assessed by FACS with CD3 and CD4 antibody staining. T cells (1×10^5) were cultured with 1×10^5 irradiated antigen-presenting cells and *S. aureus* WTA. Dose-dependency experiments were performed using WTA at concentrations of 20 and 2 µg/ml using SEA (5 ng/ml) and polygalacturonic acid (20 µg/ml) as positive and negative controls,

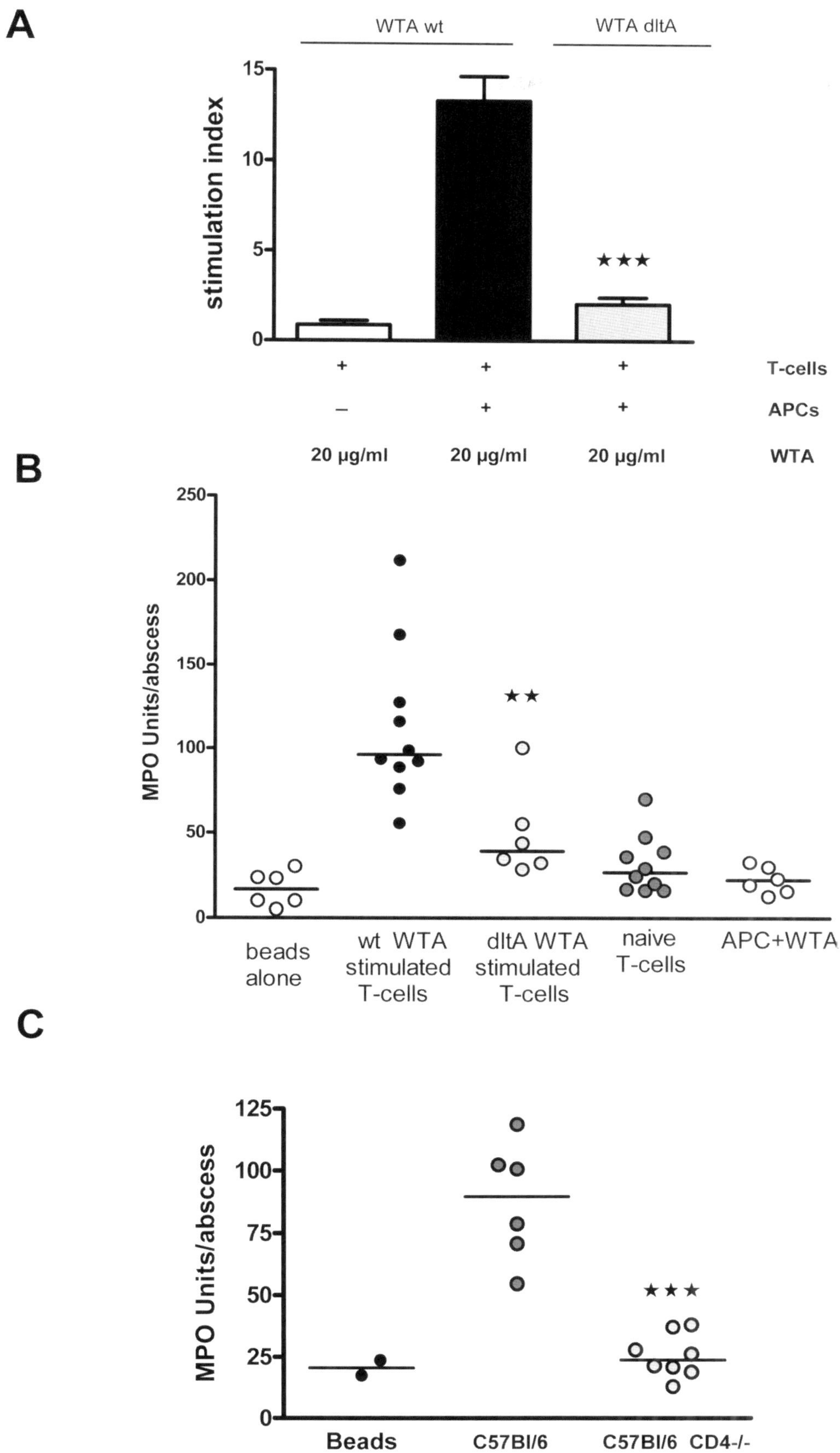
A
WTA wt
WTA dltA
stimulation index
15
10
5
0
★★★
+ + + T-cells
– + + APCs
20 µg/ml 20 µg/ml 20 µg/ml WTA
B
MPO Units/abscess
250
200
150
100
50
0
★★
beads alone
wt WTA stimulated T-cells
dltA WTA stimulated T-cells
naive T-cells
APC+WTA
C
MPO Units/abscess
125
100
75
50
25
0
★★★
Beads
C57Bl/6
C57Bl/6 CD4-/-

Figure 6. WTA-stimulated mouse T cells modulate abscess formation. A) T cells and APCs were incubated with 20 μg WTA purified from SA113 wt or the *dltA* mutant. The stimulation index was calculated by normalizing on wells with APCs and T-cells but no stimulating antigen. wt WTA stimulated T-cell proliferation more efficiently than *dltA* WTA ($p<0.0001$ for wt WTA vs. *dltA* WTA at 20 μg). Values represent means ± SEM, n = 3. B) Mouse T cells were incubated with APCs in the presence of WTA purified from wild-type SA113 or the *dltA* mutant. Additional T cells were incubated with APCs and no stimulus. After 6 days CD4+ T cells were purified, and 3×10^5 cells were mixed with cytodex beads and injected s.c. into mice. The abscesses were excised after 48 h, and MPO activity was measured in the abscess homogenate. T cells stimulated with wt WTA showed a significantly greater ability to provoke abscess formation than T cells stimulated with *dltA* WTA ($P=0.0075$ by Mann Whitney analysis). Shown are the values for individual mouse samples, and horizontal bars represent the medians. C) 20 μg of purified WTA or PBS was mixed with cytodex beads and injected into the flanks of C57BL/6 mice or isogenic mice with no functional CD4+ T cells. Shown are the values for individual mouse abscesses, and horizontal bars represent the medians. Abscess MPO activity was higher in WT vs. CD4 −/− mice ($P=0.0007$) by Mann Whitney analysis. ★$p<0.05$; ★★$p<0.01$, ★★★$p<0.001$.

respectively. Cellular proliferation was measured after 6 days by a ^{3}H-thymidine incorporation method [21]. In some experiments splenic mouse T cells were purified over nylon wool columns and stimulated with WTA as described above. In addition, T-cell proliferation assays were performed in the presence of blocking Abs to the MHC class I molecules HLA-A, HLA-B, and HLA-C, the MHC class II molecules HLA-DR, HLA-DP, and HLA-DQ, and their respective isotype controls. The human Burkitt lymphoma cell line (Raji) expressing MHC class II and MHC class I molecules and its MHC class II transcriptional mutant cell line (RJ2.2.5) were used as APCs in certain experiments [21]. WTA was incubated with T cells purified from human blood and either MHCII+/+ Raji B-cells or MHCII−/− RJ 2.5.5 cells for 6 days, and cellular proliferation was measured as described above. WTA was tested for chemotactic activity on human neutrophils as previously described [49].

For cytokine detection assays HEK293 cells were cultured in Iscove's Modified Dulbecco's Medium (Invitrogen) with 10% fetal calf serum. THP-1 human monocytes were cultured in RPMI 1640 medium supplemented with 2 mM L-glutamine and 10% fetal calf serum. RAW 264.7 mouse macrophages were cultured in Dulbecco's modified Eagle's medium (GIBCO) with 10% fetal calf serum.

After stimulation with purified WTA, LPS, MALP-2 or Pam3Cys for 8 h (TNF alpha) or 10 h (IL-8), supernatants were harvested and stored at −20°C until assayed by ELISA (R&D Biosystems) according to the manufacturer's instructions. All assays were performed with triplicate or quadruplicate replicas.

Adoptive Transfer Assays

The role of T-cell activation by WTA in the modulation of abscess formation was determined by transferring T cells stimulated with WTA into mice. Mouse T cells purified with nylon wool columns were cultured in vitro for 6 d with irradiated APCs and either 20 μg wt or *dltA* WTA. CD4+ T cells were isolated from the co-culture with mouse CD4+ enrichment columns (R&D Systems), mixed with cytodex beads, and 3×10^5 T cells were injected s.c. into the flanks of mice. Control mice were injected with naïve T cells isolated from co-cultures with APCs and no stimulating antigen, APCs incubated with WTA (no T cells), or cytodex beads alone. Abscess formation was quantified by MPO activity.

Supporting Information

Figure S1 Characterization of *tagO* and *dltA* mutants. A) WTA content of the wt and *tagO* mutant as determined by phosphorous content of cell wall fractions in Newman and C) the isogenic CP5 mutant *cap5O*. The *tagO* mutants show only residual Pi, which indicates the lack of WTA. Growth was monitored in LB broth after inoculation from a pre culture grown to log-phase (B and D). E) WTA content of the Newman wt and *dltA* mutant as determined by the phosphorous content of cell wall fractions. WT and mutant had similar amounts of WTA. F) Cytochrome C binding to whole cells. Bacterial cells in PBS were incubated with 0.5 μg/ml cytochrome C. The positive charge conferred by the ester linked D-alanine in the wt WTA diminishes binding of the positively charged cytochrome C. This observed phenotype of the *dltA* mutant depends on the lack of D-alanine esters.

Figure S2 Abscess formation with purified WTA. 20 μg of wt WTA or *dltA* WTA was mixed with cytodex beads and injected s.c into the flanks of mice. After 48 h, the mice were euthanized and representative abscesses photographed (A). The abscesses were excised, fixed in formalin, embedded in paraffin, and stained with hematoxylin and eosin for histological analysis (B).

Acknowledgments

We thank Dr. Fikri Avri for performing the ^{1}H-nuclear magnetic resonance spectroscopy (NMR) and Drs. Timothy Meredith and Suzanne Walker for kindly providing the RN4220 *tagO::tet geh::tagO* strain.

Author Contributions

Conceived and designed the experiments: CW RMM JCL. Performed the experiments: CW. Analyzed the data: CW RMM JCL. Contributed reagents/materials/analysis tools: RMM. Wrote the paper: CW JCL.

References

1. Neuhaus FC, Baddiley J (2003) A continuum of anionic charge: structures and functions of D-alanyl-teichoic acids in gram-positive bacteria. Microbiol Mol Biol Rev 67: 686–723.
2. Baddiley J (1972) Teichoic acids in cell walls and membranes of bacteria. Essays Biochem 8: 35–77.
3. Hughes AH, Hancock IC, Baddiley J (1973) The function of teichoic acids in cation control in bacterial membranes. Biochem J 132: 83–93.
4. Tomasz A, Westphal M, Briles EB, Fletcher P (1975) On the physiological functions of teichoic acids. J Supramol Struct 3: 1–16.
5. Schlag M, Biswas R, Krismer B, Kohler T, Zoll S, et al. Role of staphylococcal wall teichoic acid in targeting the major autolysin Atl. Mol Microbiol.
6. Bernal P, Zloh M, Taylor PW (2009) Disruption of D-alanyl esterification of *Staphylococcus aureus* cell wall teichoic acid by the {beta}-lactam resistance modifier (-)-epicatechin gallate. J Antimicrob Chemother 63: 1156–1162.
7. Brown S, Zhang YH, Walker S (2008) A revised pathway proposed for *Staphylococcus aureus* wall teichoic acid biosynthesis based on in vitro reconstitution of the intracellular steps. Chem Biol 15: 12–21.
8. Koprivnjak T, Weidenmaier C, Peschel A, Weiss JP (2008) Wall teichoic acid deficiency in *Staphylococcus aureus* confers selective resistance to mammalian group IIA phospholipase A(2) and human beta-defensin 3. Infect Immun 76: 2169–2176.
9. Weidenmaier C, Kokai-Kun JF, Kristian SA, Chanturiya T, Kalbacher H, et al. (2004) Role of teichoic acids in *Staphylococcus aureus* nasal colonization, a major risk factor in nosocomial infections. Nat Med 10: 243–245.
10. Weidenmaier C, Peschel A, Xiong YQ, Kristian SA, Dietz K, et al. (2005) Lack of wall teichoic acids in *Staphylococcus aureus* leads to reduced interactions with endothelial cells and to attenuated virulence in a rabbit model of endocarditis. J Infect Dis 191: 1771–1777.

11. Weidenmaier C, Kokai-Kun JF, Kulauzovic E, Kohler T, Thumm G, et al. (2008) Differential roles of sortase-anchored surface proteins and wall teichoic acid in *Staphylococcus aureus* nasal colonization. Int J Med Microbiol 298: 505–513.
12. Tzianabos AO, Wang JY, Lee JC (2001) Structural rationale for the modulation of abscess formation by *Staphylococcus aureus* capsular polysaccharides. Proc Natl Acad Sci U S A 98: 9365–9370.
13. Peschel A, Otto M, Jack RW, Kalbacher H, Jung G, et al. (1999) Inactivation of the *dlt* operon in *Staphylococcus aureus* confers sensitivity to defensins, protegrins, and other antimicrobial peptides. J Biol Chem 274: 8405–8410.
14. Peschel A, Sahl HG (2006) The co-evolution of host cationic antimicrobial peptides and microbial resistance. Nat Rev Microbiol 4: 529–536.
15. Herbert S, Newell SW, Lee C, Wieland KP, Dassy B, et al. (2001) Regulation of *Staphylococcus aureus* type 5 and type 8 capsular polysaccharides by CO(2). J Bacteriol 183: 4609–4613.
16. Luong T, Sau S, Gomez M, Lee JC, Lee CY (2002) Regulation of *Staphylococcus aureus* capsular polysaccharide expression by *agr* and *sarA*. Infect Immun 70: 444–450.
17. O'Riordan K, Lee JC (2004) *Staphylococcus aureus* capsular polysaccharides. Clin Microbiol Rev 17: 218–234.
18. Cocchiaro JL, Gomez MI, Risley A, Solinga R, Sordelli DO, et al. (2006) Molecular characterization of the capsule locus from non-typeable *Staphylococcus aureus*. Mol Microbiol 59: 948–960.
19. Mazmanian SK, Kasper DL (2006) The love-hate relationship between bacterial polysaccharides and the host immune system. Nat Rev Immunol 6: 849–858.
20. Cobb BA, Kasper DL (2005) Zwitterionic capsular polysaccharides: the new MHCII-dependent antigens. Cell Microbiol 7: 1398–1403.
21. Kalka-Moll WM, Tzianabos AO, Bryant PW, Niemeyer M, Ploegh HL, et al. (2002) Zwitterionic polysaccharides stimulate T cells by MHC class II-dependent interactions. J Immunol 169: 6149–6153.
22. McLoughlin RM, Solinga RM, Rich J, Zaleski KJ, Cocchiaro JL, et al. (2006) CD4+ T cells and CXC chemokines modulate the pathogenesis of *Staphylococcus aureus* wound infections. Proc Natl Acad Sci U S A 103: 10408–10413.
23. Nilsson IM, Lee JC, Bremell T, Ryden C, Tarkowski A (1997) The role of staphylococcal polysaccharide microcapsule expression in septicemia and septic arthritis. Infect Immun 65: 4216–4221.
24. Thakker M, Park JS, Carey V, Lee JC (1998) *Staphylococcus aureus* serotype 5 capsular polysaccharide is antiphagocytic and enhances bacterial virulence in a murine bacteremia model. Infect Immun 66: 5183–5189.
25. Watts A, Ke D, Wang Q, Pillay A, Nicholson-Weller A, et al. (2005) *Staphylococcus aureus* strains that express serotype 5 or serotype 8 capsular polysaccharides differ in virulence. Infect Immun 73: 3502–3511.
26. McLoughlin RM, Lee JC, Kasper DL, Tzianabos AO (2008) IFN-gamma regulated chemokine production determines the outcome of *Staphylococcus aureus* infection. J Immunol 181: 1323–1332.
27. Stevens DL (2009) Treatments for skin and soft-tissue and surgical site infections due to MDR Gram-positive bacteria. J Infect 59 Suppl 1: S32–39.
28. Saxena S, Thompson P, Birger R, Bottle A, Spyridis N, et al. Increasing skin infections and *Staphylococcus aureus* complications in children, England, 1997-2006. Emerg Infect Dis 16: 530–533.
29. Tzianabos AO, Chandraker A, Kalka-Moll W, Stingele F, Dong VM, et al. (2000) Bacterial pathogens induce abscess formation by CD4(+) T-cell activation via the CD28-B7-2 costimulatory pathway. Infect Immun 68: 6650–6655.
30. Magnotti LJ, Upperman JS, Xu DZ, Lu Q, Deitch EA (1998) Gut-derived mesenteric lymph but not portal blood increases endothelial cell permeability and promotes lung injury after hemorrhagic shock. Ann Surg 228: 518–527.
31. van der Veen BS, de Winther MP, Heeringa P (2009) Myeloperoxidase: molecular mechanisms of action and their relevance to human health and disease. Antioxid Redox Signal 11: 2899–2937.
32. Moreillon P, Majcherczyk PA (2003) Proinflammatory activity of cell-wall constituents from gram-positive bacteria. Scand J Infect Dis 35: 632–641.
33. Lee JC, Takeda S, Livolsi PJ, Paoletti LC (1993) Effects of in vitro and in vivo growth conditions on expression of type 8 capsular polysaccharide by *Staphylococcus aureus*. Infect Immun 61: 1853–1858.
34. Burian M, Rautenberg M, Kohler T, Fritz M, Krismer B, et al. (2010) Temporal expression of adhesion factors and activity of global regulators during establishment of *Staphylococcus aureus* nasal colonization. J Infect Dis 201: 1414–1421.
35. Doss M, White MR, Tecle T, Hartshorn KL Human defensins and LL-37 in mucosal immunity. J Leukoc Biol 87: 79–92.
36. Cobb BA, Kasper DL (2008) Characteristics of carbohydrate antigen binding to the presentation protein HLA-DR. Glycobiology 18: 707–718.
37. Montgomery CP, Boyle-Vavra S, Adem PV, Lee JC, Husain AN, et al. (2008) Comparison of virulence in community-associated methicillin-resistant *Staphylococcus aureus* pulsotypes USA300 and USA400 in a rat model of pneumonia. J Infect Dis 198: 561–570.
38. Cho JS, Pietras EM, Garcia NC, Ramos RI, Farzam DM, et al. (2010) IL-17 is essential for host defense against cutaneous *Staphylococcus aureus* infection in mice. J Clin Invest 120: 1762–1773.
39. Cheng AG, Kim HK, Burts ML, Krausz T, Schneewind O, et al. (2009) Genetic requirements for *Staphylococcus aureus* abscess formation and persistence in host tissues. FASEB J 23: 3393–3404.
40. Bubeck Wardenburg J, Bae T, Otto M, Deleo FR, Schneewind O (2007) Poring over pores: alpha-hemolysin and Panton-Valentine leukocidin in *Staphylococcus aureus* pneumonia. Nat Med 13: 1405–1406.
41. Wang R, Braughton KR, Kretschmer D, Bach TH, Queck SY, et al. (2007) Identification of novel cytolytic peptides as key virulence determinants for community-associated MRSA. Nat Med 13: 1510–1514.
42. Kloos WE, Musselwhite MS (1975) Distribution and persistence of Staphylococcus and Micrococcus species and other aerobic bacteria on human skin. Appl Microbiol 30: 381–385.
43. Otto M (2009) *Staphylococcus epidermidis* – the 'accidental' pathogen. Nat Rev Microbiol 7: 555–567.
44. Iordanescu S, Surdeanu M (1976) Two restriction and modification systems in *Staphylococcus aureus* NCTC8325. J Gen Microbiol 96: 277–281.
45. Kraus D, Herbert S, Kristian SA, Khosravi A, Nizet V, et al. (2008) The GraRS regulatory system controls *Staphylococcus aureus* susceptibility to antimicrobial host defenses. BMC Microbiol 8: 85.
46. Pohlmann-Dietze P, Ulrich M, Kiser KB, Doring G, Lee JC, et al. (2000) Adherence of *Staphylococcus aureus* to endothelial cells: influence of capsular polysaccharide, global regulator *agr*, and bacterial growth phase. Infect Immun 68: 4865–4871.
47. Portoles M, Kiser KB, Bhasin N, Chan KH, Lee JC (2001) *Staphylococcus aureus* Cap5O has UDP-ManNAc dehydrogenase activity and is essential for capsule expression. Infect Immun 69: 917–923.
48. Mullane KM, Kraemer R, Smith B (1985) Myeloperoxidase activity as a quantitative assessment of neutrophil infiltration into ischemic myocardium. J Pharmacol Methods 14: 157–167.
49. Durr MC, Kristian SA, Otto M, Matteoli G, Margolis PS, et al. (2006) Neutrophil chemotaxis by pathogen-associated molecular patterns – formylated peptides are crucial but not the sole neutrophil attractants produced by *Staphylococcus aureus*. Cell Microbiol 8: 207–217.

13

Fish Tank Granuloma Caused by *Mycobacterium marinum*

Ting-Shu Wu[1,2], Cheng-Hsun Chiu[3], Chih-Hsun Yang[4], Hsieh-Shong Leu[1], Ching-Tai Huang[1], Yi-Chieh Chen[5], Tsu-Lan Wu[6,7], Pi-Yueh Chang[6,7,8], Lin-Hui Su[6,7], An-Jing Kuo[6,7], Ju-Hsin Chia[6,7,8], Chia-Chen Lu[9], Hsin-Chih Lai[7,8,10]*

1 Division of Infectious Diseases, Department of Internal Medicine, Chang Gung Memorial Hospital, Chang Gung University College of Medicine, Taoyuan, Taiwan, **2** Graduate Institute of Clinical Medical Sciences, Chang Gung University, Taoyuan, Taiwan, **3** Division of Infectious Diseases, Department of Pediatrics, Chang Gung Children's Hospital, Chang Gung Memorial Hospital, Chang Gung University College of Medicine, Taoyuan, Taiwan, **4** Department of Dermatology, Chang Gung Memorial Hospital, Chang Gung, Taoyuan, Taiwan, **5** Department of Plastic and Reconstructive Surgery, Chang Gung Memorial Hospital, Chang Gung University College of Medicine, Taoyuan, Taiwan, **6** Department of Laboratory Medicine, Chang Gung Memorial Hospital, Chang Gung University College of Medicine, Taoyuan, Taiwan, **7** Department of Medical Biotechnology and Laboratory Sciences, Chang Gung University, Taoyuan, Taiwan, **8** Graduate Institute of Medical Biotechnology and Laboratory Sciences, Chang Gung University, Taoyuan, Taiwan, **9** Department of Respiratory Therapy, Fu-Jen Catholic University, New Taipei, Taiwan, **10** Research Center for Pathogenic Bacteria, Chang Gung University, Taoyuan, Taiwan

Abstract

Introduction: *Mycobacterium marinum* causes skin and soft tissue, bone and joint, and rare disseminated infections. In this study, we aimed to investigate the relationship between treatment outcome and antimicrobial susceptibility patterns. A total of 27 patients with *M. marinum* infections were enrolled.

Methods: Data on clinical characteristics and therapeutic methods were collected and analyzed. We also determined the minimum inhibitory concentrations of 7 antibiotics against 30 isolates from these patients.

Results: Twenty-seven patients received antimycobacterial agents with or without surgical debridement. Eighteen patients were cured, 8 failed to respond to treatment, and one was lost to follow-up. The duration of clarithromycin (147 vs. 28; $p = 0.0297$), and rifampicin (201 vs. 91; $p = 0.0266$) treatment in the cured patients was longer than that in the others. Surgical debridement was performed in 10 out of the 18 cured patients, and in 1 of another group ($p = 0.0417$). All the 30 isolates were susceptible to clarithromycin, amikacin, and linezolid; 29 (96.7%) were susceptible to ethambutol; 28 (93.3%) were susceptible to sulfamethoxazole; and 26 (86.7%) were susceptible to rifampicin. However, only 1 (3.3%) isolate was susceptible to doxycycline.

Discussion: Early diagnosis of the infection and appropriate antimicrobial therapy with surgical debridement are the mainstays of successful treatment. Clarithromycin and rifampin are supposed to be more effective agents.

Editor: David M. Ojcius, University of California Merced, United States of America

Funding: This work was supported by the National Science Council (grant NSC99-2321-B-002-022-MY3), and Chang Gung Memorial Hospital (grant CMRPG381391). The funders had no role in study design, data collection and analysis, decision to publish or preparation of the manuscript.

Competing Interests: The authors have declared that no competing interests exist.

* E-mail: hclai@mail.cgu.edu.tw

Introduction

Mycobacterium marinum is a Runyon group I, slow-growing mycobacterium with an optimal growth temperature of 30°C [1]. It most frequently causes skin and soft tissue infections in the extremities [2]. Patients typically show clusters of nodules, ulcers, or verrucous plaques that may centripetally spread from the arms or legs in a sporotrichoid pattern; however, pulmonary infections, osteomyelitis, arthritis, and disseminated diseases are encountered to a lesser extent [3–6]. Many factors play important roles in causing *M. marinum* infections. These include prescription of local or systemic steroids or immunosuppressive agents, and structural lung diseases. Among these, the primary risk factor is exposure to aquatic environments or marine animals. Thus, *M. marinum* infection is also known as "fish tank granuloma" [7].

Currently, the most common regimens used for treating *M. marinum* infections are tetracycline, doxycycline (DOX), clarithromycin (CLR), and rifampicin (RIF) plus ethambutol (EMB) [8–10]. However, there are no standard regimens available for treating *M. marinum* infections; in addition, some unsatisfactory results were encountered with the available regimens [9–11]. The role of surgery is still a controversial issue [12]. So far, only 1 study has discussed the relationship between antimycobacterial agent selection and clinical outcomes on the basis of susceptibility testing results [9]. The aim of our study was to try to find the favorable therapeutic agents for *M. marinum* infection, evaluate the treatment benefits, and analyze factors influencing the treatment outcome.

Methods

Ethics statement

The study was approved by the Institutional Review Board of the Chang Gung Memorial Hospital Linkou Medical Center in December, 2009. Patients were requested to give written informed consent to store and use the data. No linkage of these data with other sources was done. No patient identifiers were included in the dataset used for this analysis. All bacterial strains were obtained from the Bacteria Bank, Department of Laboratory Medicine, Chang Gung Memorial Hospital.

Clinical review, case definition, and classification of outcomes

A subject was defined as a patient if he/she had a culture-positive *M. marinum* infection. We studied the records of 27 patients who were enrolled for treatment at at the Chang Gung Memorial Hospital, Taiwan between January 1, 1999 and December 31, 2010. We retrospectively analyze the patients' medical charts for demographic data, contact history, infection sites, comorbidities, histological results, antimycobacterial regimens, surgical history, and outcomes. Among the 27 patients, 24 had either skin or soft-tissue infections. 1 had arthritis, 1 had a corneal infection, and 1 had a pulmonary infection. Twenty-six patients received anti-mycobacterial therapy, and 1 patient received steroid inhalation therapy, because this patient was treated as hypersensitivity pneumonitis; 10 of these 27 patients underwent at least 1 episode of surgical debridement. The antimycobacterial regimens included the following: RIF 600 mg/day (for pediatric patients, 10–15 mg/kg), EMB 1200 mg/day (for pediatric patients, 15–25 mg/kg), CLR 500 mg twice a day, DOX 100 mg twice a day, co-trimoxazole (sulfamethoxazole-trimethoprim) (SXT) 800/160 mg twice a day, and amikacin (AMK) 7.5 mg/kg twice a day. The clinical outcomes were classified as follows: (i) successful: remission of lesions without any sequelae; (ii) unsuccessful: persistent symptoms and signs of infection, relapse, or recurrence of infection within 6 months after completion of therapy, or who was lost to follow-up.

Bacterial strains and chemicals

A total of 30 *M. marinum* isolates were collected. We isolated 3 strains from 1 patient, 2 strains from another, and 1 strain each from the remaining 25 patients. Bacteria were identified by traditional culture and biochemical methods [13]. The *hsp65* gene polymorphism analysis was performed to confirm the identification of *M. marinum*, as described by Telenti et al. [14]. All bacterial isolates were routinely maintained in skim milk collection tubes containing 50% glycerol and were refrigerated at −70°C before subcultivation. The reference strain *M. marinum* ATCC 927 was purchased from the American Type Cell Collection organization.

Acid-fast staining (AFS)

We followed the procedure described by Kent and Kubica [15]. Briefly, the specimens were stained with carbolfuchsin, decolorized by 3% acid-alcohol, and finally counter-stained with methylene blue. Results of the AFS smears were reported as follows: 1+, if 1–9 acid-fast bacilli (AFB) were observed per 100 oil power fields; 2+, if 1–9 AFB were observed per 10 oil power fields; 3+, if 1–9 AFB were observed per oil power field; and 4+, if ≥10 AFB were observed per oil power field.

Drug susceptibility test

The minimal inhibitory concentrations (MIC) of several antibiotics against *M. marinum* were studied by a microdilution assay, according to the methods described by Wallace and Brown et al. [16,17]. In brief, the drugs were 2-fold serially diluted in 7H9 broth with OADC enrichment. Each well of the 96-well plate contained 10^{-4} L drug-containing broth The final bacterial inocula had concentrations between 10^6 and 10^7 CFU/L. A 10^{-5} L bacterial suspension in Middlebrook solution that contained between 10 and 10^2 CFU was dispensed into each well, including the negative control wells. The following antibiotics were tested: RIF, EMB, CLR, AMK, sulfamethoxazole (SMX), linezolid (LZD), and DOX. CLR was provided by the Pharmaceutical Products Division, Abbott Laboratories, North Chicago, Ill., USA, and LZD was provided by Pfizer Inc., New York, N.Y., USA. The other antimicrobials were purchased from Sigma Chemical Co., St. Louis, Mo., USA. The MIC was determined as the antibiotic concentration of the last well that showed no microbial growth from a series of dilutions of the antibiotic in a 96-well plate. The exception was SMX, for which the end-point was the well with approximately 80% growth inhibition compared with the growth in the negative control well. Susceptibility and resistance breakpoints of *M. marinum* strains were determined according to the Clinical and Laboratory Standards Institute (CLSI) standards [18]. Drugs susceptibility was defined at the following concentrations: RIF≤1 mg/L, EMB≤5 mg/L, CLR≤16 mg/L, AMK≤32 mg/L, SMX≤32 mg/L, and DOX≤4 mg/L. The breakpoint of LZD against mycobacteria was proposed as ≤8 mg/L, as described by Rodríguez et al. [19].

Statistical analysis

Statistical analyses were performed using STATA version 11 (STATA Corporation, College Station, TX, USA). The Mann–Whitney *U* test was used for inter-group comparisons of continuous variables. Categorical variables were compared using the χ^2 test or Fisher's exact test as appropriate. A p-value of <0.05 was considered statistically significant.

Results

Demogaphic data and clinical characteristics

In this study, we enrolled 27 patients who showed culture-positive *M. marinum* infections. According to the previously described criteria for clinical outcomes, 18 patients' outcomes were defined as successful, and 9 were unsuccessful. As shown in table 1, in the successful group, the median age was 48 years (inter-quartiles ranges [IQR], 35–64 years). In the unsuccessful group, the median age was 62 years (IQR, 41–65 years). Of the 27 patients, 11 were women, and 16 were men. These patients had underlying diseases such as hypertension (HTN) (5), coronary arterial disease (CAD) (2), cardiac dysrhythmia (1), diabetes mellitus (DM) (5), and gout (3). Twelve patients were exposed to a fish tank or pursued fishing as a hobby; 2 patients were exposed to shrimps and 1 had played in a swimming pool. One patient had received an intra-articular steroid injection for osteoarthritis. Three patients had minor or superficial trauma on their extremities. Eight patients had no contact history. The median (IQR) period from the appearance of lesions to visiting a doctor was 3 (1–6) months. Two patients had no documentation of this period. Fifteen patients had skin and soft tissue lesions on the right extremity, and 11 patients had lesions on the left side. Twenty-two patients had lesions on the upper limb, while only 4 patients had lesions on the lower limb. One of the patients showed lesions on more than 1 limb.

Table 1. Demographic data and treatment of *Mycobacterium marinum* infected patients.

Characters	Successful (n = 18)	Unsuccessful (n = 9)	P value
Median age [years (IQR)]	48 (35–64)	62 (41–65)	0.6431**a**
Gender [female: male]	6: 12	5: 4	0.2770**a**
Antimicrobial agents [median days (IQR); n]**c**			
INH	191 (73–226); 7	91; 1	0.5102**a**
RIF	201 (154–247); 13	91 (21–134); 5	0.0266**a**
EMB	220 (154–247); 13	91; 1	0.1724**a**
DOX	50.5 (28–73); 3	18 (12–21); 5	0.0507**a**
SXT	52.5 (28–77); 2	16 (14–18); 2	0.1213**a**
CIP	70.5 (22–119); 2	21 (15–143); 3	0.5637**a**
CLR	147 (91–281); 11	28 (21–35); 2	0.0297**a**
E		134; 1	
Surgical debridement [n]	10	1	0.0417**b**

IQR: inter-quartiles ranges, INH: isoniazid, RIF: rifampicin, EMB: ethambutol, DOX: doxycycline, SXT: sulfamethoxazole-trimethoprim, CIP: ciprofloxacin, CLR: clarithromycin, E: erythromycin.
[a]) by Mann-Whitney *U* test.
[b]) by Fisher's exact test.
[c]) patients received one or more than one agent.

One patient had a right corneal lesion after a hook injury when finshing shrimps, and another patient had a rare lung infection during combination ribavirin and pegylated interferon therapy for her chronic C hepatitis.

These patients did not consult a doctor until the symptoms worsened; the duration from the onset of symptoms to visiting a doctor varied from 15 days to as long as 3 years. The most common presentations were tender, erythematous nodules or plaques (18/27). Seven of the 27 patients presented with ulcerative wounds with a purulent discharge (figure 1). One of these patients had corneal involvement and complained of right-eye pain and photophobia, and another patient had dyspnea.

Acid-fast staining and histopathological findings

Of the 27 acid-fast stained pus and tissue specimens, 9 (33.3%) were positive. Of these 5, 3, and 1 specimens scored 1+, 2+, 3+, respectively; 3 specimens had no AFS documentation. Samples from 23 patients were subjected to both histopathological examinations and bacterial culturing, while samples from 4 other patients underwent only culture. The most commonly documented pathological condition was suppurative granulomatous inflammation (8/23), followed by granulomatous inflammation (7/23), caseating granulomatous inflammation (2/23), and necrotizing granulomatous inflammation (2/23). Four specimens were reported to indicate chronic inflammation, rheumatoid nodule, focal alveolar damage, and corneal ulcer.

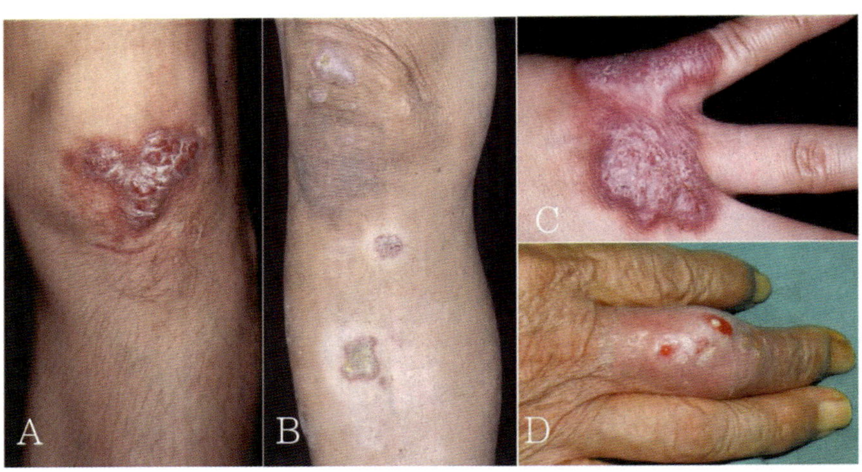

Figure 1. Cutaneous manifestations of *Mycobacterium marinum* infections. Footnote: *M. marinum* skin infections presented with (A) a solitary, or (B) multiple violaceous plaques with hyperkeratotic surface on limbs. The disease also presented as (C) a warty, verrucous plaque with an irregular border on hand, or (D) erythematous swelling of finger with pus discharge.

Antimicrobial susceptibilities

The quality control strain (*M. marinum* ATCC 927) was susceptible to all 7 drugs. The results of *in vitro* susceptibility testing indicated that *M. marinum* isolates were basically sensitive to the drugs used in the test, with a sensitivity rate ranging between 86.7% (RIF) to 100% (CLR, AMK, and LZD); the only exception was DOX, to which only 1 (3.3%) isolate was sensitive (table 2).

Treatment and outcome

Among these 27 patients, 25 patients got *M. marinum* skin and soft tissue infections, one had pulmonary infection, and the last had corneal infection. After medical treatment and/or surgical debridement, 18 were cured without any sequelae, 7 remained draining and unhealed wounds, 1 had complication of hypersensitivity pneumonitis, and one had right eye blindness.

For antimicrobial therapy, the median (IQR) duration of prescription (in days) for each antibiotic in the successful versus unsuccessful groups was as follows: CLR, 147 (91–281) vs. 28 (21–35) ($p=0.0297$); and RIF, 201 (154–247) vs. 91 (21–134) ($p=0.0266$). These figures indicate that the duration of prescription of CLR, and RIF was longer in the successful group than in the unsuccessful group. On the other hand, the median (IQR) duration of prescription for DOX was 50.5 (28–73) vs. 18 (12–21) ($p=0.0507$) in the successful versus unsuccessful group , respectively. This indicated there is a tendency to treatment failure for prescription of doxycycline. Furthermore, the median (IQR) duration of prescription of the following antibiotics in the successful versus unsuccessful groups was as follows: isoniazid (INH), 191 (73–226) vs. 91 ($p=0.5102$); EMB, 220 (154–247) vs. 91 ($p=0.1724$); SXT, 52.5 (28–77) vs. 16 (14–18) ($p=0.1213$); ciprofloxacin (CIP), 70.5 (22–119) vs. 21 (15–143) ($p=0.5637$); and erythromycin, 134, respectively. Besides, 10 patients in the successful group had received surgical debridement; whereas, only 1 patient in the unsuccessful group had received surgical debridement (Fisher's exact test; $p=0.0417$).

Eight patients received DOX treatment; of these, only 3 (37.5%) had successful results (table 3). In addition to the DOX therapy, 2 of these 3 patients further received adjuvant surgical debridement of the lesions, and the third patient received a combination of RIF and EMB treatment for 73 days, and consecutive prescription with CLR, RIF, and EMB for 147 days. Of the 5 patients who underwent unsuccessful DOX treatment, 1 received only local CIP treatment for corneal infection with sequela of right eye blindness, 1 had an overly short CLR and CIP treatment duration (21 days) with persistent nodules on her right hand,1 had an overly short RIF (21 days) and SXT (14 days) treatment duration with persistent plaques on his right hand, 1 further received SXT, CLR, CIP, and RIF, but had persistent nodules and relapsed 4 months after discontinuing the antibiotics, and the fifth unsuccessful patient became lost to follow-up.

Discussion

Efficiently treatment of *M. marinum* infection remains a challenge. One of the reasons that make diagnosis difficult is the patients' lack of awareness coupled with the fact that *M. marinum* infections progress slowly, with a median (IQR) progression time of 3 (1–6) months. As the patients did not consult the doctor until the clinical symptoms worsened, it was difficult to identify the relationship between *M. marinum* skin infections and previous trauma history. Besides, cutaneous lesions are generally nonspecific and are often initially misdiagnosed as pyoderma, furunculosis, or even sporotrichosis [20–22]. Regarding the clinical treatment, *M. marinum* infections are usually treated empirically with antituberculosis agents, and antibiotic-susceptibility testing is not routinely performed in many clinical laboratories. These issues make the treatment of *M. marinum* even more difficult. The results of this study presented the antibiotic susceptibility pattern of *M. marinum* and characterized the relationship between antimicrobial therapy, surgery, and treatment outcome in *M. marinum* infections in Taiwan. These results may thus be used as a reference for clinical treatment of *M. marinum* infections in other countries.

The CLSI report does not recommend routine susceptibility testing of this species. However, the test may be necessary for some patients whose samples are still culture positive after receiving several months of unsuccessful therapy [23]. The results of *in vitro* susceptibility in this study showed a high susceptibility rate (>90%) for CLR, LZD, AMK, or SMX, which was consistent with effective treatment results. It is suggested that each single agent can be considered for treating in superficial *M. marinum* infections. From the viewpoint of pharmacokinetics, LZD could be a good alternative oral agent, although there have been no clinical trials till date to support this hypothesis [24]. Despite some previous reports showing successful treatment of *M. marinum* infection with DOX or minocycline [25,26], the effectiveness of DOX treatment was still controversial due to several reports of treatment failure [11,26–28]. Our results showed that *M. marinum* strains showed only 3.3% (1/30) sensitivity to DOX. This may reflect the high rate of treatment failure encountered in our patients treated with DOX. The controversy over DOX therapy may be related to the regional drug resistance pattern of *M. marinum*. Thus, it is suggested that drug susceptibility testing of *M. marinum* should be

Table 2. *In vitro* susceptibilities of 30 *M. marinum* isolates.

Antimicrobial agents	MIC 50	MIC 90	Range	Modal MIC	Geometric mean MIC	95% CI	Sensitive rate (%)
Rifampicin	1	2	0.125–4	1	0.7	0.5–1	86.7
Ethambutol	0.25	4	0.25–16	0.5	1	0.5–1.5	96.7
Clarithromycin	4	6	0.125–8	4	3	2.2–4.1	100
Amikacin	2	8	0.125–16	8	2.3	1.4–3.9	100
Sulfamethoxazole	4	32	0.5–64	4	4.7	2.7–8.1	93.3
Linezolid	2	4	0.5–4	2	1.7	1.4–2.2	100
Doxycycline	16	32	4–32	16	14.9	12.0–18.6	3.3

MIC: minimum inhibitory concentrations, CI: confidence interval.

Table 3. Clincal manifestations of *M. marinum* infected patients who received doxycycline therapy.

Case	Age	Gender	Infection source	Site of lesions	Histology	Antibiotics (days)	Surgery	Outcome
1	41	M	Shrimp sting	Cornea	Ulcer	Topical DOX (12), topical CIP (15)	Keratectomy	Failed
2	50	F	Trauma	Right hand	Suppurative granulomatous inflammation	DOX (7), CLR (21), CIP (21)	None	Failed
3	65	M	Fish tank	Right hand	Suppurative granulomatous inflammation	DOX (21), RIF (21), SXT (14)	None	Failed
4	69	F	Fish tank	Right hand	Granulomatous inflammation	DOX (18), SXT (18), CLR (35), CIP (143), RIF (187)	None	Relapse
5	31	F	ND	Right hand	Suppurative granulomatous inflammation	DOX (21)	None	Lost to follow-up
6	39	M	ND	Right forearm	Suppurative granulomatous inflammation	DOX (ND)	Debridement	Successful
7	41	M	Fish tank	Right hand	Suppurative granulomatous inflammation	DOX (28)	Debridement	Successful
8	51	M	Fish	Left hand	ND	DOX (73), RIF (220), EMB (220), CLR (147)	None	Successful

F: female, M: male, CIP: ciprofloxacin, CLR: clarithromycin, DOX: doxycycline, EMB: ethambutol, RIF: rifampicin, SXT: co-trimoxazole, ND: not documented.

performed in patients whose treatment has failed and also in regions where the drug-resistance rate is high.

The potential reasons for the treatment failure/difficulty in *M. marinum* infections include delayed diagnosis and ineffective regimens in antimicrobial therapy. To date, there have been no comparative trials for treatment regimens in *M. marinum* skin and soft-tissue infections. A general approach is to treat patients with 2 active agents for 1–2 months after resolution of symptoms; the total treatment time is typically 3–4 months [9]. Furthermore, the duration of antimicrobial therapy in pulmonary or disseminated infections is also not standardized. Although, at present, there is no evidence indicating the superiority of combination therapy over monotherapy, there is a tendency to prescribe CLR plus EMB, or RIF plus EMB to treat a deep structure infection [9,29]. In deep structure infections, especially on the hands, early diagnosis and appropriate therapy may play a key role in preventing the loss of normal function [30]. In addition, our results indicated surgical debridement may contribute to favorable treatment outcome.

Among *M. marinum* infections, a rare case involving a pulmonary infection was observed. The patient was a middle-aged woman and received interferon and ribavirin therapy for chronic hepatitis C. She then acquired interstitial pneumonitis where the *M. marinum* strain was isolated. This strain was sensitive to all tested antibiotics except DOX. Due to the delayed diagnosis and the lack of antimicrobial therapy, she developed sequelae such as pulmonary fibrosis and rheumatoid arthritis-like disorders. In 2005, Lai et al. also reported a case of pulmonary infection in an immunocompetent patient [6]. The 2 cases indicated *M. marinum* causes superficial infections, in addition to disseminated or even pulmonary infections. It would be worth monitoring and investigating this phenomenon closely for a longer duration.

In conclusion, optimal antimicrobial therapy consisting of CLR and/or RIF plus ethambutol, and surgical debridement may have a high treatment success rate in *M. marinum* infection. In contrast, DOX prescription is not suitable for this purpose.

Acknowledgments

We wish to acknowledge Hui-Chin Liao for assistance with the laboratory work. We thank all of our colleagues at Chang Gung Memorial Hospital for the collection of clinical samples. Also, we thank Professor Chee-Jen Chang for the biostatistics consultation.

Author Contributions

Conceived and designed the experiments: TSW HCL. Performed the experiments: TSW HCL. Analyzed the data: CHC CHY HSL CTH YCC. Contributed reagents/materials/analysis tools: TLW PYC LHS AJK JHC CCL. Wrote the paper: TSW HCL CHC CHY.

References

1. Runyon EH (1981) Mycobacteria: an overview. Rev Infect Dis 3: 819–821.
2. Collins CH, Grange JM, Noble WC, Yates MD (1985) *Mycobacterium marinum* infections in man. J Hyg (Lond) 94: 135–149.
3. Sivan M, Bose D, Athanasou N, McNally M (2008) *Mycobacterium marinum* osteomyelitis of a long bone. Joint Bone Spine 75: 600–602.
4. Patel S, Duke O, Harland C (1995) Septic arthritis due to *Mycobacterium marinum*. J Rheumatol 22: 1607–1608.
5. Holmes GF, Harrington SM, Romagnoli MJ, Merz WG (1999) Recurrent, disseminated *Mycobacterium marinum* infection caused by the same genotypically defined strain in an immunocompromised patient. J Clin Microbiol 37: 3059–3061.
6. Lai CC, Lee LN, Chang YL, Lee YC, Ding LW, et al. (2005) Pulmonary infection due to *Mycobacterium marinum* in an immunocompetent patient. Clin Infect Dis 40: 206–208.
7. Swift S, Cohen H (1962) Granulomas of the skin due to *Mycobacterium balnei* after abrasions from a fish tank. N Engl J Med 267: 1244–1246.

8. Lewis FM, Marsh BJ, von Reyn CF (2003) Fish tank exposure and cutaneous infections due to *Mycobacterium marinum*: tuberculin skin testing, treatment, and prevention. Clin Infect Dis 37: 390–397.
9. Aubry A, Chosidow O, Caumes E, Robert J, Cambau E (2002) Sixty-three cases of *Mycobacterium marinum* infection: clinical features, treatment, and antibiotic susceptibility of causative isolates. Arch Intern Med 162: 1746–1752.
10. Wu TS, Chiu CH, Su LH, Chia JH, Lee MH, et al. (2002) *Mycobacterium marinum* infection in Taiwan. J Microbiol Immunol Infect 35: 42–46.
11. Ljungberg B, Christensson B, Grubb R (1987) Failure of doxycycline treatment in aquarium-associated *Mycobacterium marinum* infections. Scand J Infect Dis 19: 539–543.
12. Pang HN, Lee JY, Puhaindran ME, Tan SH, Tan AB, et al. (2007) *Mycobacterium marinum* as a cause of chronic granulomatous tenosynovitis in the hand. J Infect 54: 584–588.
13. Vincent V, Brown-Elliott BA, Jost KC Jr, Wallace RJ Jr (2003) *Mycobacterium*: Phenotypic and Genotypic Identification. In: Murray PR, Baron EJ, Jorgensen JH, Pfaller MA, Yolken RH, editors. Manual of Clinical Microbiology. 8th ed. Washington, D.C., USA: American Society for Microbiology Press. pp. 560–584.
14. Telenti A, Marchesi F, Balz M, Bally F, Böttger EC, et al. (1993) Rapid identification of mycobacteria to the species level by polymerase chain reaction and restriction enzyme analysis. J Clin Microbiol 31: 175–178.
15. Kent PT, Kubica GP (1985) Public health mycobacteriology: a guide for the level III laboratory . U.S. Department of Health and Human Services, Centers for Disease Control, Atlanta, Ga.
16. Wallace RJ Jr, Nash DR, Steele LC, Steingrube V (1986) Susceptibility testing of slowly growing mycobacteria by a microdilution MIC method with 7H9 broth. J Clin Microbiol 24: 976–981.
17. Brown BA, Wallace RJ Jr, Onyi GO (1992) Activities of clarithromycin against eight slowly growing species of nontuberculous mycobacteria, determined by using a broth microdilution MIC system. Antimicrob Agents Chemother 36: 1987–1990.
18. NCCLS (2003) Susceptibility Testing of Mycobacteria, Nocardiae, and Other Aerobic Actinomycetes: Approved Standard. Document M24-A. Wayne, PA: NCCLS.
19. Rodríguez JC, Ruiz M, López M, Royo G (2002) In vitro activity of moxifloxacin, levofloxacin, gatifloxacin and linezolid against *Mycobacterium tuberculosis*. Int J Antimicrob Agents 20: 464–467.
20. Madan V, Lear JT (2007) Sporotrichoid streptococcal pyoderma. J Eur Acad Dermatol Venereol 21: 572–573.
21. Feddersen A, Kunkel J, Jonas D, Engel V, Bhakdi S, et al. (1996) Infection of the upper extremity by *Mycobacterium marinum* in a 3-year-old boy - diagnosis by 16S-rDNA analysis. Infection 24: 47–48.
22. Adams RM, Remington JS, Steinberg J, Seibert JS (1970) Tropical fish aquariums. A source of *Mycobacterium marinum* infections resembling sporotrichosis. JAMA 211: 457–461.
23. Griffith DE, Aksamit T, Brown-Elliott BA, Catanzaro A, Daley C, et al. (2007) An official ATS/IDSA statement: diagnosis, treatment, and prevention of nontuberculous mycobacterial diseases. Am J Respir Crit Care Med 175: 367–416.
24. Dryden MS (2011) Linezolid pharmacokinetics and pharmacodynamics in clinical treatment. J Antimicrob Chemother 66 Suppl 4: iv7–iv15.
25. Osorio F, Magina S, Carvalho T, Goncalves MH, Azevedo F (2010) *Mycobacterium marinum* skin infection with tenosynovitis successfully treated with doxycycline. Dermatology Online Journal 16: 7.
26. Cummins DL, Delacerda D, Tausk FA (2005) *Mycobacterium marinum* with different responses to second-generation tetracyclines. Int J Dermatol 44: 518–520.
27. Schwendiman MN, Johnson RP, Henning JS (2009) Subcutaneous nodules with sporotrichoid spread. Dermatol Online J 15: 11.
28. Donta ST, Smith PW, Levitz RE, Quintiliani R (1986) Therapy of *Mycobacterium marinum* infections. Use of tetracyclines vs rifampin. Arch Intern Med 146: 902–904.
29. Rallis E, Koumantaki-Mathioudaki E (2007) Treatment of *Mycobacterium marinum* cutaneous infections. Expert Opin Pharmacother 8: 2965–2978.
30. Cheung JP, Fung B, Wong SS, Ip WY (2010) Review article: *Mycobacterium marinum* infection of the hand and wrist. J Orthop Surg (Hong Kong) 18: 98–103.

Changes in the Nasal Colonization with Methicillin-Resistant *Staphylococcus aureus* in Children: 2004-2009

Wen-Tsung Lo[1]*, Chih-Chien Wang[1], Wei-Jen Lin[1], Sheng-Ru Wang[2], Ching-Shen Teng[1], Ching-Feng Huang[1], Shyi-Jou Chen[1]

1 Department of Pediatrics, Tri-Service General Hospital, National Defense Medical Center, Taipei, Taiwan, **2** Department of Pediatrics, Wan Fang Hospital, Taipei, Taiwan

Abstract

Background: *Staphylococcus aureus* is an important cause of infection, particularly in persons colonized with this organism. This study compared the annual prevalence and microbiological characteristics of methicillin-resistant *S. aureus* (MRSA) nasal colonization in Taiwanese children from 2004 through 2009. Risk factors for MRSA were determined for the overall study period.

Methods: Children from birth to ≤14 years of age presenting for health maintenance visits or attending 1 of 57 kindergartens were recruited. Nasal swabs were obtained, and a questionnaire was administered. The prevalence and microbiological characteristics of MRSA colonization were also calculated for two 3-year periods: 2004–2006 and 2007–2009.

Results: Cultures of the anterior nares were positive for *S. aureus* in 824 (25.8%) of the 3,200 children, and MRSA colonization was found in 371 (11.6%) children. The prevalence of *S. aureus* colonization decreased from 28.1% in 2004–2006 to 23.3% in 2007–2009 ($p<0.01$), whereas the prevalence of MRSA colonization increased from 8.1% to 15.1% during this period ($p<0.0001$). Multivariate analysis revealed that the independent risk factors for MRSA carriage were different for male and female children, and also among age groups. Most MRSA isolates belonged to sequence type 59 (ST59) (86.3%); however, a multiresistant MRSA clone with ST338 background emerged in 2007–2009. Ten (62.5%) of the 16 MRSA isolates expressed the genotypic profile ST338/staphylococcal cassette chromosome *mec* V_T/Panton-Valentine leukocidin-positive/staphylococcal enterotoxin B-positive, and differed only in their antimicrobial susceptibility patterns.

Conclusion: The prevalence of nasal colonization by MRSA increased among healthy Taiwanese children from 2004–2006 to 2007–2009, despite an overall decrease in the prevalence of nasal colonization by *S. aureus*. A multiresistant MRSA clone characterized as ST338 was identified from these children.

Editor: Adam J. Ratner, Columbia University, United States of America

Funding: This study was supported by the National Science Council (grant NSC94-2314-B-016-029 and NSC95-2314-B-016-052) and Tri-Service General Hospital (grant TSGH-C94-12, TSGH-C95-11-S01, TSGH-C96-12-S01, TSGH-C97-21, TSGH-C98-19, TSGH-C98-20, TSGH-C99-23, and TSGH-C100-29). The funders had no role in study design, data collection and analysis, decision to publish, or preparation of the manuscript.

Competing Interests: The authors have declared that no competing interests exist.

* E-mail: drluoped@yahoo.com.tw

Introduction

Staphylococcus aureus is a common human pathogen of skin infections and invasive diseases in all age groups, such as pneumonia, osteomyelitis, and endocarditis, in healthcare and community settings [1]. Methicillin-resistant *S. aureus* (MRSA) isolates have been recognized as a source of healthcare-associated infections since the 1960s [2]. Over the past decade, the traditional notion of MRSA as a pathogen that is seemingly confined to the nosocomial arena has been challenged with the emergence of community-associated MRSA (CA-MRSA) in healthy individuals without conventional risk factors for MRSA acquisition, especially in the USA [3,4]. Reports of rapidly progressive fatal disease and serious complications resulting from virulent CA-MRSA infection including sepsis, necrotizing pneumonia, and necrotizing fasciitis have alerted medical professionals and the community alike to the need to face the increasing threat from community-based MRSA infections [5–8]. Initially, CA-MRSA strains were thought to lack an association with healthcare settings and to have unique microbiologic characteristics such as limited antibiotic resistance (except to β-lactam antimicrobial agents), different exotoxin gene profiles (e.g., Panton-Valentine leukocidin, PVL), and smaller staphylococcal cassette chromosome *mec* (SCC*mec*) type IV [9]. However, these epidemic strains have been shown to be transmitted in healthcare settings and to exhibit emerging resistance to non-β-lactam agents [10–12]. In Taiwan, MRSA strains of sequence type 59 (ST59), determined by multilocus sequence typing (MLST) and carrying type IV or a variant, type V_T SCC*mec* elements, were found to be the major strains of CA-MRSA [13–18].

S. aureus colonizes the anterior nares and other body sites, but the anterior nares are the most consistent site of colonization [19]. Carriage of *S. aureus*, including MRSA, is common in children, and genetic evidence supports a relationship between nasal carriage of *S. aureus* and MRSA and subsequent invasive staphylococcal infection [15,20–23]. Children could act as vectors for spreading *S.*

aureus and MRSA to both community and hospital environments [24]. In addition, day-care centers constitute reservoirs of MRSA where children are at increased risk of nasal colonization [15,25,26].

In Taiwan, the first island-wide prevalence survey of nasal colonization with *S. aureus* was conducted in 2005 and 2006, and it showed a measurable prevalence of colonization with MRSA in the community [27]. The objectives of the current study in children were to assess trends in the overall prevalence of nasal colonization by *S. aureus*, to identify the potential risk factors for MRSA nasal colonization, and to describe the evolving epidemiology of nasal colonization by *S. aureus* and by MRSA specifically.

Materials and Methods

Study design, population and location

This prospective observational study was conducted from 2004 to 2009 at Tri-Service General Hospital, a 1400-bed tertiary medical center in northern Taiwan. The study proposal was reviewed and approved by the National Defense Medical Center Institutional Review Board. Eligible children were 14 years of age or younger with no acute medical problem, who either presented for a health maintenance visit or attended one of 57 kindergartens in Taipei. Written informed consent was obtained from each child's parents or legal representative before nasal specimen collection or interviews. During the 6-year study period, all children who presented for health maintenance visits to our hospital were invited to participate in this study. In addition, the selection of the kindergartens from all kindergartens in Taipei was based on support for the surveillance study by the kindergartens' principals. The number of children sampled per kindergarten was proportional to the number of children attending each kindergarten. Based on a previous study [28], we estimated the rate of *S. aureus* colonization to be 30%. Therefore, we calculated that a sample size of 1100 children would be necessary to estimate risk factors for MRSA colonization, based on estimated prevalence ranging from 1% to 3%, with a 95% confidence interval ([CI] design effect, 1.5). Study participants were recruited sequentially until the estimated recruitment number was met.

Data collection

Individual variables, demographic characteristics of the family, and medical history over the preceding 12 months, including previous hospitalization, medication history prior to receiving the screening test, and any underlying diseases correlated with *S. aureus* colonization status were obtained by interviews with the guardians immediately after consent was obtained and before swabs were collected [29].

Nares cultures, bacterial strains and antimicrobial susceptibility testing

Nasal samples were obtained with a sterile cotton swab, placed in transport medium (Venturi Transystem, Copan Diagnostics, Corona, CA, USA), and then transported to and processed in the microbiology laboratory within 4 hours. Cotton swabs were plated on mannitol salt agar (MSA; BBL Microbiology Systems, Becton Dickinson, Company, Sparks, MD, U.S.A.). Each distinctive morphotype of mannitol-fermenting colony was selected from an MSA plate, subcultured to a trypticase soy agar plus 5% sheep blood agar plate (BAP; BBL Microbiology Systems, Becton Dickinson, Company, Sparks, MD, U.S.A.), and incubated at 37°C in a humidified incubator with 5% CO_2. Cultures on BAPs were screened using Slidex Staph Plus (bioMérieux, Marcy l'Etoile, France). MRSA identification and antimicrobial susceptibility testing were performed according to Clinical Laboratory Standards Institute (CLSI; formerly known as the NCCLS) guidelines [30,31]. Multidrug-resistant *S. aureus* isolates were defined as isolates resistant to three or more antimicrobial classes. All *S. aureus* isolates were frozen at −70°C for additional testing of organism characteristics.

Polymerase chain reaction

Chromosomal DNA from three to five isolated colonies was prepared using the Puregene DNA purification kit (Gentra, Minneapolis, Minnesota, USA) as recommended by the manufacturer, with lysostaphin at 2 mg/ml and RNase at 4 mg/ml for the lysis step. The presence of the *lukS-PV* and *lukF-PV* genes encoding PVL components was determined by a polymerase chain reaction (PCR)-based method with the primer pair and thermocycler conditions reported by Lina et al [32]. The presence of known macrolide-lincosamide-streptogramin resistance genes (*ermA*, *ermB*, *ermC* and *msrA*) was determined by PCR according to a previously described method [33,34]. Sequences specific for *sea* to *see*, *seg* to *sei*, *sek*, *seq*, *eta*, *etb*, and *tst*, encoding staphylococcal enterotoxins (SEA to SEE, SEG to SEI, SEK, and SEQ), exfoliative toxins (ETA and ETB), and toxic shock syndrome toxin-1, respectively, were detected using the methods described by Jarraud et al. and Diep et al [35,36]. SCC*mec* typing was performed using a multiplex PCR strategy with sets of region-specific primers as previously described [37]. Screening for SCC*mec* V_T was performed with the primer and thermocycler conditions reported by Boyle-Vavra et al. and Huang et al [14,27].

Genotyping

Pulsed-field gel electrophoresis (PFGE) was performed using the CHEF Mapper XA system (Bio-Rad Laboratories, Hercules, CA, USA) according to a published protocol [38]. Findings were interpreted on the basis of standard criteria [39]. To identify PFGE polymorphisms, band patterns were analyzed using Molecular Analyst Fingerprinting, Fingerprinting Plus and Fingerprinting DST software (Bio-Rad Laboratories, Richmond, CA, USA). The grouping method was used to deduce a dendrogram from the matrix by the unweighted pair group method using the arithmetic averages clustering technique after calculation of similarities using the Dice correlation coefficient between each pair of organisms; the PFGE patterns were distinguished at the 80% similarity level. Some isolates of representative PFGE patterns were subjected to MLST. MLST was performed by PCR amplification and sequencing of seven housekeeping genes using primers designed by Enright et al [40]. Each sequence was submitted to the MLST database website for assignment of the allelic profile and sequence type.

Statistical analysis

Data were entered into Microsoft Access XP software and exported into SPSS statistical software, version 10.0 (SPSS), which was used for data analyses. The categorical variables were compared using the chi-square test, Mantel-Haenszel test or Fisher's exact test. The trend in annual prevalence rates of colonization was examined using Poisson regression analysis. The prevalence and microbiological characteristics of colonization were also determined for two time periods (2004–2006 and 2007–2009) separately, to compare categorical variables between the two survey cycles. In addition, data from 2004 through 2009 were combined to provide more reliable estimates of the microbiological characteristics of and risk factors for MRSA colonization and to increase the study's power to detect statistically significant differences. To analyze the risk factors for carrying MRSA among male and female children in various age groups (<1 year, 1–5 years and >5 years of age), we used polytomous logistic regression to compare children with MRSA to those without *S. aureus* and children with MRSA to those with methicillin-susceptible *S. aureus* (MSSA). All parameters were initially determined by means of univariate analysis; those with p values of <0.05 and those being biologically meaningful were entered into the multivariate analysis. However, parameters with colinearity, tested by correlation matrices, were not simultaneously considered in the final model. In the multivariate analysis, stepwise model comparison was used to determine the best model. Risk factors were assessed using SAS 9.1.3 (SAS Institute, Inc., Cary, NC). All tests were two-tailed, and a p value of <0.05 was defined as statistically significant.

Results

Population characteristics

A total of 3200 children with ages ranging from 1 month to 14 years participated in this study: 1019 were recruited during health maintenance visits and 2181 were recruited from the 57 selected kindergartens. The median age of the participating children was 4.3 years, and 1602 (50.0%) were male.

Isolation of *S. aureus* from children

Of the 3200 nares specimens, 371 (11.6%) were positive for MRSA, 453 (14.2%) were positive for MSSA, and 2376 (74.2%) were culture negative for *S. aureus*. The percentage of MRSA isolates among all *S. aureus* isolates was 45.0%. From 2004–2006, a total of 1615 children were interviewed and examined; of these, 454 (28.1%) were culture-positive for *S. aureus*. Similarly, from 2007–2009, a total of 1585 children were interviewed and examined, and 370 (23.3%) of them were culture positive for *S. aureus*. The annual prevalence rates of MRSA and *S. aureus* nasal colonization are shown in the Figure 1. The prevalence of MRSA colonization significantly increased, at a rate of 25% per year ($p<0.0001$, test for trend), whereas the prevalence of *S. aureus* colonization decreased ($p=0.0006$, test for trend). Moreover, the prevalence of *S. aureus* nasal colonization decreased to 23.3% during 2007–2009 (95% CI, 21.2%–25.4%; $p<0.01$) from 28.1% during 2004–2006 (95% CI, 25.9%–30.3%) (Table 1). However, the prevalence of MRSA colonization increased to 15.1% (95% CI, 13.3%–16.8%) in 2007–2009 from 8.1% (95% CI, 6.8%–9.4%) in 2004–2006 ($p<0.0001$).

Tables 1 and 2 summarize the results of the surveillance for *S. aureus* and MRSA among children tested from 2004–2006 and 2007–2009. When prevalence was compared across surveys, a significant decrease in *S. aureus* nasal colonization occurred in children from kindergartens ($p<0.01$), in female children ($p<0.01$), and among children aged <1 year and >5 years ($p<0.0001$ and $p<0.01$, respectively). In addition, the prevalence of MRSA colonization increased in 2007–2009 among both male and female children ($p<0.0001$ and $p<0.001$, respectively), children attending both health maintenance visits and kindergartens ($p<0.0001$ and $p<0.001$, respectively), and children aged 1–5 years and >5 years ($p<0.001$ and $p<0.0001$, respectively).

Questionnaire data and statistical analysis

We used polytomous logistic regression to identify risk factors for MRSA colonization by comparing children with MRSA to those with MSSA and children with MRSA to those without carriage of *S. aureus*. The risk factors for MRSA colonization identified in the multivariate analysis are shown in Table 3. Overall, factors independently associated with an increased risk of MRSA colonization were different for male and female children and in various age groups. For male children, MRSA carriage was associated with antibiotic use in past 12 months ($p<0.05$, aged <1 year; $p<0.01$, aged 1–5 years; $p<0.0001$, aged >5 years), atopic dermatitis ($p<0.001$, aged <1 year; $p<0.0001$, aged 1–5 years and aged >5 years), and history of skin and soft tissue infection ($p<0.01$, aged <1 year and aged 1–5 years; $p<0.05$, aged >5 years). For male children aged <1 year only, chronic disease was associated with MRSA colonization ($p<0.05$). For male children aged 1–5 years, MRSA colonization was also associated with hospitalization in past 12 months ($p<0.0001$). For male children aged >5 years, household contact with hospital staff was associated with MRSA colonization ($p<0.001$).

The distribution of independent risk factors for MRSA carriage among female children in three different age groups was divergent. Among female children aged <1 year, household contact with hospital staff was associated with MRSA colonization ($p<0.01$). For female children aged 1–5 years, MRSA colonization was significantly associated with atopic dermatitis ($p<0.0001$), hospitalization in past 12 months ($p<0.0001$), history of skin and soft tissue infection ($p<0.0001$), and household contact with hospital staff ($p<0.01$). Among female children aged >5 years, antibiotic use in the past 12 months ($p<0.0001$), atopic dermatitis ($p<0.01$), and history of skin and soft tissue infection ($p<0.001$) were independently associated with MRSA colonization.

Microbiologic characteristics of MRSA colonizing isolates

The prevalence and distribution of isolates associated with community transmission among MRSA colonized children are shown in Table 4. The prevalence of PVL and SCC*mec* V_T among MRSA colonizing isolates did not vary significantly with source, sex or age. However, comparison of the prevalence across surveys revealed that a significant increase occurred in 2007–2009 ($p<0.0001$). Among the 371 children colonized with MRSA, the largest proportion, 86.3% (95% CI, 82.8%–89.8%), carried ST59 clonal type. ST338 clonal type, a single-locus variant of ST59 (1 nucleotide difference in the *gmk* locus), was the next most prevalent MLST type and was recovered from 4.3% (95% CI, 2.3%–6.4%) of children with MRSA colonization. Children aged >5 years were more likely to be colonized with ST59 clonal type than those aged <1 year and 1–5 years ($p<0.05$). In addition, colonization with ST338 clonal type was significantly more prevalent in 2007–2009 compared with 2004–2006 ($p<0.05$), but this difference was not evident in ST59 clonal type.

Except for an increase in the multidrug resistance rate in 2007–2009 ($p<0.05$), the resistance pattern, distribution of *erm* genotype and exotoxin profile of MRSA colonizing isolates did not vary significantly by source or survey period (Table 5 and Table 6). Although the resistance profile of ST59 clonal type did not change significantly during the study period (data not shown), isolates of ST338 clonal type expressed higher incidences of resistance to non-β-lactam antimicrobial agents (e.g., gentamicin and trimethoprim-sulfamethoxazole) and multiple drugs than isolates of ST59 clonal type ($p<0.0001$). Moreover, the combined results of molecular analyses showed that the majority (62.5%) of the 16 MRSA ST338 isolates expressed the genotypic profile ST338/SCC*mec* V_T/PVL-positive/SEB-positive.

Discussion

Several studies from the United States demonstrated that community-associated *S. aureus* infections among children and adults have increased rapidly in recent years and that MRSA is responsible for most of this increase [11,41]. In Taiwan, CA-MRSA infections in pediatric patients have been noted since 2002

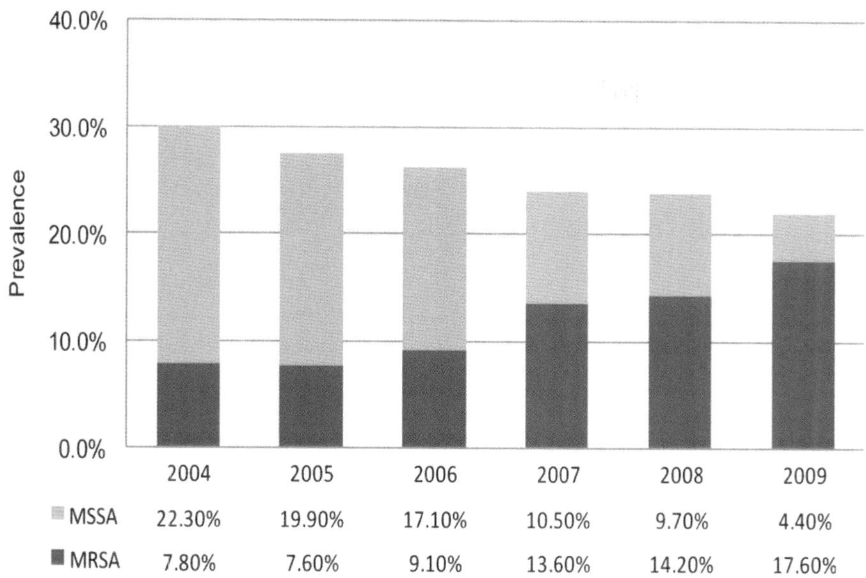

Figure 1. Annual prevalence of methicillin-resistant *Staphylococcus aureus* and methicillin-susceptible *S. aureus* nasal colonization in Taiwanese children, 2004–2009.

[13–16,18,42]. Subsequent to 2002, our pediatric infectious disease service has continued to see a dramatic increase in the number of pediatric consultations and evaluation for CA-MRSA infections in outpatient clinics, the pediatric emergency department and in pediatric wards. In addition, although the prevalence of MRSA colonization among children in the community has been extensively studied in Taiwan and the United States [14,27,43–48], few studies of MRSA colonization have examined the same population in a sequential manner [43]. In this study we attempted to characterize the MRSA colonization pool among children in the community served by our institute. Our results showed that the MRSA colonization rate among otherwise healthy children in community settings in Taiwan was 11.6% during the period from 2004 to 2009. The prevalence of *S. aureus* nasal colonization in this population was 25.8%, which is within the reported range and likely reflects that of the general population [43,45,48–52].

Between 2004–2006 and 2007–2009, the overall prevalence of *S. aureus* nasal colonization decreased, whereas the prevalence of MRSA colonization increased. These findings are consistent with a population-based study among people in the United States

Table 1. Prevalence of *Staphylococcus aureus* and methicillin-resistant *S. aureus* (MRSA) nasal colonization in children with different demographic characteristics, across surveys (2004–2006 vs. 2007–2009).

			Prevalence of nasal colonization, % (95% CI)			
	No. (%) of children		*S. aureus*		MRSA	
Category	2004–2006	2007–2009	2004–2006	2007–2009	2004–2006	2007–2009
All participants	1615 (50.5)	1585 (49.5)	28.1 (25.9–30.3)	23.3 (21.2–25.4)*	8.1 (6.8–9.4)	15.1 (13.3–16.8)**
Source						
Health maintenance visits	740 (45.8)	279 (17.6)	27.2 (24.0–30.4)	24.0 (19.0–29.0)	6.4 (4.6–8.1)	15.8 (11.5–20.1)**
Kindergartens	875 (54.2)	1306 (82.4)	28.9 (25.9–31.9)	23.2 (20.9–25.5)*	9.6 (7.7–11.6)	15.0 (13.1–16.9)***
Sex						
Male	822 (50.9)	780 (49.2)	28.2 (25.2–31.3)	25.6 (22.6–28.7)	8.3 (6.4–10.2)	16.7 (14.1–19.3)**
Female	793 (49.1)	805 (50.8)	28.0 (24.9–31.1)	21.1 (18.3–23.9)*	7.9 (6.1–9.8)	13.7 (11.3–16.0)***
Age, years						
<1	364 (22.5)	213 (13.5)	32.1 (27.4–36.9)	16.0 (11.0–20.9)**	6.9 (4.3–9.5)	9.4 (5.5–13.3)
1–5	720 (44.6)	503 (31.7)	23.2 (20.1–26.3)	24.7 (20.9–28.4)	7.6 (5.7–9.6)	13.5 (10.5–16.5)***
>5	531 (32.9)	869 (54.8)	32.0 (28.1–36.0)	24.4 (21.5–27.3)*	9.6 (7.1–12.1)	17.5 (15.0–20.0)**

CI, confidence interval.
*$p<0.01$,
**$p<0.0001$,
***$p<0.001$.

Table 2. Prevalence of *Staphylococcus aureus* and methicillin-resistant *S. aureus* (MRSA) nasal colonization in children with different demographic characteristics, 2004–2009.

			Prevalence of nasal colonization, % (95% CI)			
	No. (%) of children		*S. aureus*		MRSA	
Category	2004–2006	2007–2009	2004–2006	2007–2009	2004–2006	2007–2009
All participants	1615 (50.5)	1585 (49.5)	28.1 (25.9–30.3)	23.3 (21.2–25.4)	8.1 (6.8–9.4)	15.1 (13.3–16.8)
Source						
Health maintenance visits[a]	740 (45.8)	279 (17.6)	27.2 (24.0–30.4)	24.0 (19.0–29.0)	6.4 (4.6–8.1)	15.8 (11.5–20.1)
Kindergartens	875 (54.2)	1306 (82.4)	28.9 (25.9–31.9)	23.2 (20.9–25.5)	9.6 (7.7–11.6)*	15.0 (13.1–16.9)
Sex						
Male[a]	822 (50.9)	780 (49.2)	28.2 (25.2–31.3)	25.6 (22.6–28.7)	8.3 (6.4–10.2)	16.7 (14.1–19.3)
Female	793 (49.1)	805 (50.8)	28.0 (24.9–31.1)	21.1 (18.3–23.9)*	7.9 (6.1–9.8)	13.7 (11.3–16.0)
Age, years						
<1[a]	364 (22.5)	213 (13.5)	32.1 (27.4–36.9)	16.0 (11.0–20.9)	6.9 (4.3–9.5)	9.4 (5.5–13.3)
1–5	720 (44.6)	503 (31.7)	23.2 (20.1–26.3)**	24.7 (20.9–28.4)*	7.6 (5.7–9.6)	13.5 (10.5–16.5)
>5	531 (32.9)	869 (54.8)	32.0 (28.1–36.0)	24.4 (21.5–27.3)*	9.6 (7.1–12.1)	17.5 (15.0–20.0)***

CI, confidence interval.
[a]Reference group.
*$p<0.05$, for comparison with reference group within survey (2004–2006 or 2007–2009),
**$p<0.001$, for comparison with reference group within survey (2004–2006),
***$p<0.01$, for comparison with reference group within survey (2007–2009).

participating in the 2001 to 2004 National Health and Nutrition Examination Survey [49]. However, without additional surveillance it is impossible to determine whether these changes represent ongoing trends in the prevalence of colonization or are simply short-term modulations due to sampling variability or fluctuations in unmeasured variables including temperature and humidity [49].

Table 3. Risk factors associated with methicillin-resistant *Staphylococcus aureus* (MRSA) nasal colonization in children by multivariate analysis using polytomous logistic regression.

	MRSA Colonization, OR (95% CI)[a]					
	<1 year		1–5 years		>5 years	
	Male	Female	Male	Female	Male	Female
Risk factor	(n = 304)	(n = 273)	(n = 596)	(n = 627)	(n = 702)	(n = 698)
Personal risk factors						
Antibiotic use in past 12 months	4.1 (1.2–14.0)*		3.0 (1.5–6.1)**		12.3 (6.5–23.1)***	20.3 (10.1–40.8)***
Diagnosis of atopic dermatitis	7.6 (2.3–24.9)****		8.8 (4.0–19.5)***	9.7 (3.4–27.7)***	5.2 (2.4–11.3)***	5.0 (1.6–15.1)**
Chronic disease	23.0 (1.3–393.5)*					
Hospitalization in past 12 months			11.1 (5.5–22.3)***	5.9 (2.7–12.9)***		
History of skin/soft tissue infection	8.7 (1.7–44.4)**		3.1 (1.3–7.1)**	6.4 (2.6–15.5)***	1.9 (1.1–3.5)*	3.5 (1.8–6.8)****
Household risk factors						
Household contact with hospital staff		10.8 (2.0–58.3)**		4.4 (1.5–13.3)**	3.6 (1.7–7.7)****	

CI, confidence interval; OR, odds ratio.
[a]OR (95% CI) was presented as MRSA colonization vs. no. *S. aureus* colonization; *p* value of overall model was calculated by the Mantel-Haenszel test.
*$p<0.05$,
**$p<0.01$,
***$p<0.0001$,
****$p<0.001$.

Table 4. Prevalence of molecular traits among methicillin-resistant *Staphylococcus aureus* (MRSA) isolates recovered from MRSA-colonized children, by study variable, 2004-2009.

	Children colonized	No. (% [95% CI]) of isolates			
Variable	**with MRSA, no.**	**PVL present**	**SCC*mec* V_T present**	**ST59**	**ST338**
All participants	371	123 (33.2 [28.4–37.9])	101 (27.2 [22.7–31.8])	320 (86.3 [82.8–89.8])	16 (4.3 [2.3–6.4])
Source					
Health maintenance visits[a]	91	34 (37.4 [27.4–47.3])	29 (31.9 [22.3–41.4])	83 (91.2 [85.4–97.0])	5 (5.5 [0.8–10.2])
Kindergartens	280	89 (31.8 [26.3–37.2])	72 (25.7 [20.6–30.8])	237 (84.6 [80.4–88.9])	11 (3.9 [1.7–6.2])
Sex					
Male	198	65 (32.8 [26.3–39.4])	46 (23.2 [17.4–29.1])	169 (85.4 [80.4–90.3])	8 (4.0 [1.3–6.8])
Female[a]	173	58 (33.5 [24.5–40.6])	55 (31.8 [24.9–38.7])	151 (87.3 [82.3–92.3])	8 (4.6 [1.5–7.8])
Age, years					
<1[a]	45	18 (40.0 [25.7–54.3])	13 (28.9 [15.7–42.1])	34 (75.6 [63.0–88.1])	2 (4.4 [0.0–10.5])
1–5	123	42 (34.1 [25.8–42.5])	35 (28.5 [20.5–36.4])	102 (82.9 [76.3–89.6])	5 (4.1 [0.6–7.6])
>5	203	63 (31.0 [24.7–37.4])	53 (26.1 [20.1–32.2])	184 (90.6 [86.6–94.7]*)	9 (4.4 [1.6–7.3])
Survey					
2004–2006[a]	131	25 (19.1 [12.4–25.8])	14 (10.7 [5.4–16.0])	111 (84.7 [78.6–90.9])	1 (0.8 [0.0–2.3])
2007–2009	240	98 (40.8 [34.6–47.1]**)	87 (36.3 [30.2–42.3]**)	209 (87.1 [82.8–91.3])	15 (6.3 [3.2–9.3]*)

CI, confidence interval; PVL, Panton-Valentine leukocidin; SCC*mec*, staphylococcal cassette chromosome *mec*; ST, sequence type.
[a]Reference group.
*$p<0.05$,
**$p<0.0001$.

Results from this study indicate that the prevalence of MRSA colonization in our community pediatric population in northern Taiwan was 8.1% during the period of 2004–2006, which is within the reported range (4.8%–9.5%) compared with a different population of healthy Taiwanese children in 2005 and 2006 [27]. However, the nasal MRSA colonization prevalence of healthy Taiwanese children from the present study increased significantly, from 7.3% during 2005–2006 to 15.1% ($p<0.0001$, chi-square test) during 2007–2009 [27]. There may be two reasons for this difference. First, the prevalence of MRSA colonization

Table 5. Antimicrobial susceptibility for methicillin-resistant *Staphylococcus aureus* (MRSA) colonizing isolates in Taiwanese children, 2004-2009.

	Origin, no. (%)		Year, no. (%)		Clonal type, no. (%)		
Characteristic	**H**	**K**	**2004–2006**	**2007–2009**	**ST59**	**ST338**	***p*[a]**
Total isolates	91 (24.5)	280 (75.5)	131 (35.3)	240 (64.7)	320 (86.3)	16 (4.3)	
Resistance to							
Clindamycin	80 (87.9)	251 (89.6)	116 (88.5)	215 (89.6)	271 (84.7)	16 (100)	0.142
Erythromycin	82 (90.1)	259 (92.5)	121 (92.4)	220 (91.7)	288 (90.0)	16 (100)	0.380
Gentamicin	14 (15.4)	30 (10.7)	13 (9.9)	31 (12.9)	30 (9.4)	9 (56.3)	<0.0001
TMP-SMX	2 (2.2)	5 (1.8)	0 (0)	7 (2.9)	2 (0.6)	5 (31.3)	<0.0001
Ciprofloxacin	0 (0)	0 (0)	0 (0)	0 (0)	0 (0)	0 (0)	
Fusidic acid	0 (0)	0 (0)	0 (0)	0 (0)	0 (0)	0 (0)	
Mupirocin	1 (1.1)	0 (0)	0 (0)	1 (0.4)	1 (0.3)	0 (0)	0.999
Rifampin	1 (1.1)	2 (0.7)	0 (0)	3 (1.3)	3 (0.9)	0 (0)	0.999
Vancomycin	0 (0)	0 (0)	0 (0)	0 (0)	0 (0)	0 (0)	
Teicoplanin	0 (0)	0 (0)	0 (0)	0 (0)	0 (0)	0 (0)	
Multidrug[b]	14 (15.4)	36 (12.9)	11 (8.4)	39 (16.3)[c]	32 (10.0)	10 (62.5)	<0.0001

H, Health maintenance visits; K, Kindergartens; ST, sequence type; TMP-SMX, trimethoprim-sulfamethoxazole.
[a]*p* value derived from comparison of isolates of ST59 and ST338 clonal type (chi-square test, unless otherwise indicated).
[b]Multiresistance to at least 3 of the 10 non-β-lactam antimicrobial agents tested.
[c]$p<0.05$ across surveys (2004–2006 vs. 2007–2009, Fisher's exact test).

Table 6. Origin, year and clonal type-specific characteristics of methicillin-resistant *Staphylococcus aureus* (MRSA) colonizing isolates in Taiwanese children.

	Origin, no. (%)		Year, no. (%)		Clonal type, no. (%)		
Characteristic	**H**	**K**	**2004–2006**	**2007–2009**	**ST59**	**ST338**	**p[a]**
Total isolates	91 (24.5)	280 (75.5)	131 (35.3)	240 (64.7)	320 (86.3)	16 (4.3)	
erm genotype, no. of strains/total no. of strains tested (% of isolates)							
ermA	3/82 (3.7)	13/259 (5.0)	6/121 (5.0)	10/220 (4.5)	13/288 (4.5)	0/16 (0)	0.999
ermB	79/82 (96.3)	246/259 (95.0)	115/121 (95.0)	210/220 (95.5)	275/288 (95.5)	16/16 (100)	0.999
Virulence factor							
ETA	2 (2.2)	11 (3.9)	3 (2.3)	10 (4.2)	11 (3.4)	0 (0)	0.999
ETB	4 (4.4)	8 (2.9)	5 (3.8)	7 (2.9)	9 (2.8)	1 (6.3)	0.390
TSST-1	11 (12.1)	29 (10.4)	13 (9.9)	27 (11.3)	33 (10.3)	0 (0)	0.383
SEA	6 (6.6)	18 (6.4)	10 (7.6)	14 (5.8)	19 (5.9)	1 (6.3)	0.999
SEB	76 (83.5)	235 (83.9)	104 (79.4)	207 (86.3)	269 (84.1)	14 (87.5)	0.999
SEC	3 (3.3)	10 (3.6)	4 (3.1)	9 (3.8)	7 (2.2)	0 (0)	0.999
SED	1 (1.1)	7 (2.5)	2 (1.5)	6 (2.5)	5 (1.6)	0 (0)	0.999
SEE	0 (0)	3 (1.1)	1 (0.8)	2 (0.8)	2 (0.6)	0 (0)	0.999
SEG/SEI	27 (29.7)	76 (27.1)	35 (26.7)	68 (28.3)	88 (27.5)	4 (25.0)	0.999
SEH	0 (0)	2 (0.7)	2 (1.5)	0 (0)	1 (0.3)	0 (0)	0.999

ETA, exfoliative toxin A; ETB, exfoliative toxin B; H, Health maintenance visits; K, Kindergartens; SEA, staphylococcal enterotoxin A; SEB, staphylococcal enterotoxin B; SEC, staphylococcal enterotoxin C; SED, staphylococcal enterotoxin D; SEE, staphylococcal enterotoxin E; SEG, staphylococcal enterotoxin G; SEH, staphylococcal enterotoxin H; SEI, staphylococcal enterotoxin I; ST, sequence type; TMP-SMX, trimethoprim-sulfamethoxazole; SST-1, toxic shock syndrome toxin-1.
[a]*p* value derived from comparison of isolates of ST59 and ST338 clonal type.

among children in communities may be higher in the northern region than in other geographic areas of Taiwan [27]. Second, the present study was conducted 3 years after the previous study, so the difference may be due to an overall increase of MRSA colonization prevalence during this time. Furthermore, the increasing trend in the prevalence of nasal MRSA colonization might account for the increasing incidence of CA-MRSA infection in Taiwanese children [13,15,18,42,53,54].

Few studies have reported the determinants of MRSA colonization in community settings [55]. To the best of our knowledge, this is the first comprehensive survey of risk factors including personal and household risk factors for MRSA nasal carriage conducted in Taiwan, and it enrolled 3200 children including 2181 children attending 1 of 57 kindergartens in Taipei. Also, this is the first study in children to show that risk factors related to colonization with MRSA vary in terms of gender and age group. The multivariate analysis indicated that independent risk factors for MRSA colonization were use of antibiotics within the past year preceding sampling, diagnosis of atopic dermatitis, chronic disease, hospitalization in past 12 months, history of skin and soft tissue infection, and living with a family member who works in a hospital or clinic. These results have implications for pediatric infection control and clinical management strategies that are impacted by the different distribution of risk factors associated with an increase risk of MRSA colonization. For example, children with atopic dermatitis are more frequently colonized by MRSA in the anterior nares, which play a key role in the epidemiology and pathogenesis of concurrent skin and soft tissue infections [56].

It is well recognized that day care centers are efficient settings for the acquisition and transmission of pathogens and several determinants have been suggested, such as crowded conditions, frequent close physical contact, breakdown in appropriate hygiene and intensive exposure to antimicrobials [50]. Moreover, children with longer time periods of child care exposure are more prone to be colonized by MRSA than in children who are attending day care centers for the first time [24,26]. An increase in MRSA colonization among children attending kindergartens in our study was anticipated, however, a decrease in nasal colonization with *S. aureus* was unexpected. These findings might be explained, in part, by the previously reported excessive use of antibiotics in Taiwan [57,58], which highlights the importance of the problem of strong selective pressure from antimicrobial use in the community and may suppress MSSA and thus facilitate colonization by MRSA. In fact, it has been reported that Taiwanese physicians prescribe antibiotics to children under 16 years old for up to 45.5% of common colds [59]. We also found that the use of antibiotics was associated with MRSA colonization.

Previous studies throughout Taiwan found that ST59 MRSA isolates were the most common MLST type of MRSA causing CA-MRSA infections and nasal colonization [13–16,27,60]. Except in Western Australia and mainland China, however, ST59 MRSA isolates were rarely found in other Asian countries in recent large-scale studies [61–63]. In this study, molecular analysis indicated that the majority (90.6%) of MRSA colonizing isolates during the period 2004–2009 were clustered into minor variants of two clonal types, ST59 and ST338. Our results suggest that clonal spread of MRSA contributes to the high MRSA burden and that most colonized children acquired MRSA in the general community. The percentage of MRSA colonized children who carried ST59 with SCC*mec* IV/V_T was not significantly different between 2007–2009 (87.1%; 95% CI, 82.8%–91.3%) and 2004–2006 (84.7%; 95% CI, 78.6%–90.9%). Conversely, ST338 emerged in

2005 and accounted for 6.3% of MRSA colonizing isolates from 2007 to 2009 ($p<0.05$). More recently, PVL-positive CA-MRSA ST338 has been shown to be correlated with an increasing proportion of *S. aureus* infections among otherwise healthy children in the southern region of China and the majority of these clones belong to SCC*mec* V [63]. In the present study, most PVL-positive MRSA ST338 clones belonged to SCC*mec* V_T, which contains a ccrC recombinase gene variant (ccrC2) and *mec* complex C2 [14]. We did not find any SCC*mec* V isolates, which may indicate that the background of ST338 clones in Taiwan is different from mainland China. In antibiotic susceptibility testing, MRSA colonizing isolates expressed high incidences of resistance to non-β-lactam antibiotics and multiple drugs. In a previous longitudinal study of 257 MRSA bloodstream infections, Chen et al. reported that multiresistance may have provided an advantage for the CA-MRSA strains to easily enter and rapidly proliferate in healthcare facilities, with resulting blurring of the distinction between CA-MRSA and healthcare-associated MRSA [12]. Therefore, the apparent increase in the multidrug resistance and transmissibility of MRSA colonizing isolates is cause for concern. Further investigation is needed to determine whether colonization with these strains is becoming more prevalent.

Several study limitations merit consideration. First, the survey design was cross-sectional and children who were only intermittently colonized may not have been detected. Thus, the frequency of colonization with organisms might have been underestimated. Second, recall bias may have occurred when parents or guardians attempted to remember past events and exposures assessed by the questionnaire. In addition, the relatively small number of children less than 1 year of age with MRSA colonization might have limited the ability to detect all risk factors. Third, the persistence of MRSA colonization in the study subjects could not be determined and the incidence of subsequent MRSA infection could not be measured. Finally, this study was conducted at a single site and may not reflect colonization rates throughout the country.

In conclusion, this sequential, prospective observational study found the prevalence of MRSA nasal colonization increased in Taiwanese children from 2004–2006 to 2007–2009, despite a decrease in the overall prevalence of *S. aureus* colonization during the same period. Our investigation provides evidence of the constantly changing epidemiology of staphylococcal colonization in our community. Moreover, the detection of 16 isolates belonging to ST338, a multiresistant clone frequently associated with PVL genes, is of special concern in a young population as it has the potential to sharply limit therapeutic options should it become widespread.

Acknowledgments

We are grateful to L. K. Siu at the National Health Research Institute (Taipei, Taiwan) for laboratory support. We thank Shu-Ying Tsai for providing assistance with and maintaining the MRSA database.

Author Contributions

Conceived and designed the experiments: W-TL C-CW. Performed the experiments: W-TL C-CW W-JL S-RW C-ST. Analyzed the data: W-TL C-CW W-JL S-RW C-ST C-FH S-JC. Wrote the paper: W-TL.

References

1. Lowy FD (1998) *Staphylococcus aureus* infections. N Engl J Med 339: 520–532.
2. Barrett FF, McGehee RF, Jr., Finland M (1968) Methicillin-resistant *Staphylococcus aureus* at Boston City Hospital. Bacteriologic and epidemiologic observations. N Engl J Med 279: 441–448.
3. Herold BC, Immergluck LC, Maranan MC, Lauderdale DS, Gaskin RE, et al. (1998) Community-acquired methicillin-resistant *Staphylococcus aureus* in children with no identified predisposing risk. JAMA 279: 593–598.
4. Otter JA, French GL (2010) Molecular epidemiology of community-associated meticillin-resistant *Staphylococcus aureus* in Europe. Lancet Infect Dis 10: 227–239.
5. Adem PV, Montgomery CP, Husain AN, Koogler TK, Arangelovich V, et al. (2005) *Staphylococcus aureus* sepsis and the Waterhouse-Friderichsen syndrome in children. N Engl J Med 353: 1245–1251.
6. Mongkolrattanothai K, Boyle S, Kahana MD, Daum RS (2003) Severe *Staphylococcus aureus* infections caused by clonally related community-acquired methicillin-susceptible and methicillin-resistant isolates. Clin Infect Dis 37: 1050–1058.
7. Miller LG, Perdreau-Remington F, Rieg G, Mehdi S, Perlroth J, et al. (2005) Necrotizing fasciitis caused by community-associated methicillin-resistant *Staphylococcus aureus* in Los Angeles. N Engl J Med 352: 1445–1453.
8. Centers for Disease Control and Prevention (1999) Four pediatric deaths from community-acquired methicillin-resistant *Staphylococcus aureus*: Minnesota and North Dakota, 1997-1999. JAMA 282: 1123–1125.
9. Boyle-Vavra S, Daum RS (2007) Community-acquired methicillin-resistant *Staphylococcus aureus*: the role of Panton-Valentine leukocidin. Lab Invest 87: 3–9.
10. Seybold U, Kourbatova EV, Johnson JG, Halvosa SJ, Wang YF, et al. (2006) Emergence of community-associated methicillin-resistant *Staphylococcus aureus* USA300 genotype as a major cause of health care-associated blood stream infections. Clin Infect Dis 42: 647–656.
11. Kaplan SL, Hulten KG, Gonzalez BE, Hammerman WA, Lamberth L, et al. (2005) Three-year surveillance of community-acquired *Staphylococcus aureus* infections in children. Clin Infect Dis 40: 1785–1791.
12. Chen CJ, Hsueh PR, Su LH, Chiu CH, Lin TY, et al. (2009) Change in the molecular epidemiology of methicillin-resistant *Staphylococcus aureus* bloodstream infections in Taiwan. Diagn Microbiol Infect Dis 65: 199–201.
13. Wang CC, Lo WT, Chu ML, Siu LK (2004) Epidemiological typing of community-acquired methicillin-resistant *Staphylococcus aureus* isolates from children in Taiwan. Clin Infect Dis 39: 481–487.
14. Boyle-Vavra S, Ereshefsky B, Wang CC, Daum RS (2005) Successful multiresistant community-associated methicillin-resistant *Staphylococcus aureus* lineage from Taipei, Taiwan, that carries either the novel staphylococcal chromosome cassette *mec* (SCC*mec*) type V_T or SCC*mec* type IV. J Clin Microbiol 43: 4719–4730.
15. Lo WT, Lin WJ, Tseng MH, Wang SR, Chu ML, et al. (2006) Community-acquired methicillin-resistant *Staphylococcus aureus* in children, Taiwan. Emerg Infect Dis 12: 1267–1270.
16. Chen CJ, Su LH, Chiu CH, Lin TY, Wong KS, et al. (2007) Clinical features and molecular characteristics of invasive community-acquired methicillin-resistant *Staphylococcus aureus* infections in Taiwanese children. Diagn Microbiol Infect Dis 59: 287–293.
17. Takano T, Higuchi W, Otsuka T, Baranovich T, Enany S, et al. (2008) Novel characteristics of community-acquired methicillin-resistant *Staphylococcus aureus* strains belonging to multilocus sequence type 59 in Taiwan. Antimicrob Agents Chemother 52: 837–845.
18. Lo WT, Tang CS, Chen SJ, Huang CF, Tseng MH, et al. (2009) Panton-Valentine leukocidin is associated with exacerbated skin manifestations and inflammatory response in children with community-associated staphylococcal scarlet fever. Clin Infect Dis 49: e69–75.
19. Kluytmans J, van Belkum A, Verbrugh H (1997) Nasal carriage of *Staphylococcus aureus*: epidemiology, underlying mechanisms, and associated risks. Clin Microbiol Rev 10: 505–520.
20. Creech CB, 2nd, Talbot TR, Schaffner W (2006) Community-associated methicillin-resistant *Staphylococcus aureus*: the way to the wound is through the nose. J Infect Dis 193: 169–171.
21. Safdar N, Bradley EA (2008) The risk of infection after nasal colonization with *Staphylococcus aureus*. Am J Med 121: 310–315.
22. Teixeira LA, Resende CA, Ormonde LR, Rosenbaum R, Figueiredo AM, et al. (1995) Geographic spread of epidemic multiresistant *Staphylococcus aureus* clone in Brazil. J Clin Microbiol 33: 2400–2404.
23. von Eiff C, Becker K, Machka K, Stammer H, Peters G (2001) Nasal carriage as a source of *Staphylococcus aureus* bacteremia. Study Group. N Engl J Med 344: 11–16.
24. Hisata K, Kuwahara-Arai K, Yamanoto M, Ito T, Nakatomi Y, et al. (2005) Dissemination of methicillin-resistant staphylococci among healthy Japanese children. J Clin Microbiol 43: 3364–3372.
25. Masuda K, Masuda R, Nishi J, Tokuda K, Yoshinaga M, et al. (2002) Incidences of nasopharyngeal colonization of respiratory bacterial pathogens in Japanese children attending day-care centers. Pediatr Int 44: 376–380.
26. Lo WT, Lin WJ, Tseng MH, Lu JJ, Lee SY, et al. (2007) Nasal carriage of a single clone of community-acquired methicillin-resistant *Staphylococcus aureus* among kindergarten attendees in northern Taiwan. BMC Infect Dis 1: 51.
27. Huang YC, Hwang KP, Chen PY, Chen CJ, Lin TY (2007) Prevalence of methicillin-resistant *Staphylococcus aureus* nasal colonization among Taiwanese children in 2005 and 2006. J Clin Microbiol 45: 3992–3995.

28. Lu PL, Chin LC, Peng CF, Chiang YH, Chen TP, et al. (2005) Risk factors and molecular analysis of community methicillin-resistant *Staphylococcus aureus* carriage. J Clin Microbiol 43: 132–139.
29. Lo WT, Lin WJ, Tseng MH, Wang SR, Chu ML, et al. (2008) Risk factors and molecular analysis of Panton-Valentine leukocidin-positive methicillin-resistant *Staphylococcus aureus* colonization in healthy children. Pediatr Infect Dis J 27: 713–718.
30. Clinical and Laboratory Standards Institute (2009) Methods for disk diffusion: approved standard M02-A10 and M07-A8: performance standards for antimicrobial disk susceptibility tests. WaynePA: The Committee.
31. Clinical and Laboratory Standards Institute (2009) Performance standards for antimicrobial susceptibility testing: nineteenth informational supplement M100-S19. WaynePA: The Committee.
32. Lina G, Piémont Y, Godail-Gamot F, Bes M, Peter MO, et al. (1999) Involvement of Panton-Valentine leukocidin-producing *Staphylococcus aureus* in primary skin infections and pneumonia. Clin Infect Dis 29: 1128–1132.
33. Shortridge VD, Flamm RK, Ramer N, Beyer J, Tanaka SK (1996) Novel mechanism of macrolide resistance in *Streptococcus pneumoniae*. Diagn Microbiol Infect Dis 26: 73–78.
34. Almer LS, Shortridge VD, Nilius AM, Beyer JM, Soni NB, et al. (2002) Antimicrobial susceptibility and molecular characterization of community-acquired methicillin-resistant *Staphylococcus aureus*. Diagn Microbiol Infect Dis 43: 225–232.
35. Jarraud S, Cozon G, Vandenesch F, Bes M, Etienne J, et al. (1999) Involvement of enterotoxins G and I in staphylococcal toxic shock syndrome and staphylococcal scarlet fever. J Clin Microbiol 37: 2446–2449.
36. Diep BA, Carleton HA, Chang RF, Sensabaugh GF, Perdreau-Remington F (2006) Roles of 34 virulence genes in the evolution of hospital- and community-associated strains of methicillin-resistant *Staphylococcus aureus*. J Infect Dis 193: 1495–1503.
37. Oliveira DC, de Lencastre H (2002) Multiplex PCR strategy for rapid identification of structural types and variants of the *mec* element in methicillin-resistant *Staphylococcus aureus*. Antimicrob Agents Chemother 46: 2155–2161.
38. McDougal LK, Steward CD, Killgore GE, Chaitram JM, McAllister SK, et al. (2003) Pulsed-field gel electrophoresis typing of oxacillin-resistant *Staphylococcus aureus* isolates from the United States: establishing a national database. J Clin Microbiol 41: 5113–5120.
39. Tenover FC, Arbeit RD, Goering RV, Mickelsen PA, Murray BE, et al. (1995) Interpreting chromosomal DNA restriction patterns produced by pulsed-field gel electrophoresis: criteria for bacterial strain typing. J Clin Microbiol 33: 2233–2239.
40. Enright MC, Day NP, Davies CE, Peacock SJ, Spratt BG (2000) Multilocus sequence typing for characterization of methicillin-resistant and methicillin-susceptible clones of *Staphylococcus aureus*. J Clin Microbiol 38: 1008–1015.
41. Moran GJ, Krishnadasan A, Gorwitz RJ, Fosheim GE, McDougal LK, et al. (2006) Methicillin-resistant *S. aureus* infections among patients in the emergency department. N Engl J Med 355: 666–674.
42. Wu KC, Chiu HH, Wang JH, Lee NS, Lin HC, et al. (2002) Characteristics of community-acquired methicillin-resistant *Staphylococcus aureus* in infants and children without known risk factors. J Microbiol Immunol Infect 35: 53–56.
43. Creech CB, 2nd, Kernodle DS, Alsentzer A, Wilson C, Edwards KM (2005) Increasing rates of nasal carriage of methicillin-resistant *Staphylococcus aureus* in healthy children. Pediatr Infect Dis J 24: 617–621.
44. Huang YC, Su LH, Chen CJ, Lin TY (2005) Nasal carriage of methicillin-resistant *Staphylococcus aureus* in school children without identifiable risk factors in northern Taiwan. Pediatr Infect Dis J 24: 276–278.
45. Hussain FM, Boyle-Vavra S, Daum RS (2001) Community-acquired methicillin-resistant *Staphylococcus aureus* colonization in healthy children attending an outpatient pediatric clinic. Pediatr Infect Dis J 20: 763–767.
46. Nakamura MM, Rohling KL, Shashaty M, Lu H, Tang YW, et al. (2002) Prevalence of methicillin-resistant *Staphylococcus aureus* nasal carriage in the community pediatric population. Pediatr Infect Dis J 21: 917–922.
47. Shopsin B, Mathema B, Martinez J, Ha E, Campo ML, et al. (2000) Prevalence of methicillin-resistant and methicillin-susceptible *Staphylococcus aureus* in the community. J Infect Dis 182: 359–362.
48. Suggs AH, Maranan MC, Boyle-Vavra S, Daum RS (1999) Methicillin-resistant and borderline methicillin-resistant asymptomatic *Staphylococcus aureus* colonization in children without identifiable risk factors. Pediatr Infect Dis J 18: 410–414.
49. Gorwitz RJ, Kruszon-Moran D, McAllister SK, McQuillan G, McDougal LK, et al. (2008) Changes in the prevalence of nasal colonization with *Staphylococcus aureus* in the United States, 2001-2004. J Infect Dis 197: 1226–1234.
50. Lamaro-Cardoso J, de Lencastre H, Kipnis A, Pimenta FC, Oliveira LS, et al. (2009) Molecular epidemiology and risk factors for nasal carriage of *Staphylococcus aureus* and methicillin-resistant *S. aureus* in infants attending day care centers in Brazil. J Clin Microbiol 47: 3991–3997.
51. Fritz SA, Garbutt J, Elward A, Shannon W, Storch GA (2008) Prevalence of and risk factors for community-acquired methicillin-resistant and methicillin-sensitive *Staphylococcus aureus* colonization in children seen in a practice-based research network. Pediatrics 121: 1090–1098.
52. Miller M, Cook HA, Furuya EY, Bhat M, Lee MH, et al. (2009) *Staphylococcus aureus* in the community: colonization versus infection. PLoS ONE 4: e6708.
53. Chen CJ, Huang YC, Chiu CH, Su LH, Lin TY (2005) Clinical features and genotyping analysis of community-acquired methicillin-resistant *Staphylococcus aureus* infections in Taiwanese children. Pediatr Infect Dis J 24: 40–45.
54. Fang YH, Hsueh PR, Hu JJ, Lee PI, Chen JM, et al. (2004) Community-acquired methicillin-resistant *Staphylococcus aureus* in children in northern Taiwan. J Microbiol Immunol Infect 37: 29–34.
55. Graham PL, 3rd, Lin SX, Larson EL (2006) A U.S. population-based survey of *Staphylococcus aureus* colonization. Ann Intern Med 144: 318–325.
56. Lo WT, Wang SR, Tseng MH, Huang CF, Chen SJ, et al. (2010) Comparative molecular analysis of methicillin-resistant *Staphylococcus aureus* isolates from atopic dermatitis children and healthy subjects in Taiwan. Br J Dermatol 162: 1110–1116.
57. Liu YC, Huang WK, Huang TS, Kunin CM (1999) Extent of antibiotic use in Taiwan shown by antimicrobial activity in urine. Lancet 354: 1360.
58. Hsueh PR, Liu CY, Luh KT (2002) Current status of antimicrobial resistance in Taiwan. Emerg Infect Dis 8: 132–137.
59. Chang SC, Shiu MN, Chen TJ (2001) Antibiotic usage in primary care units in Taiwan after the institution of national health insurance. Diagn Microbiol Infect Dis 40: 137–143.
60. Wang JT, Liao CH, Fang CT, Chie WC, Lai MS, et al. (2009) Prevalence of and risk factors for colonization by methicillin-resistant *Staphylococcus aureus* among adults in community settings in Taiwan. J Clin Microbiol 47: 2957–2963.
61. Chongtrakool P, Ito T, Ma XX, Kondo Y, Trakulsomboon S, et al. (2006) Staphylococcal cassette chromosome *mec* (SCC*mec*) typing of methicillin-resistant *Staphylococcus aureus* strains isolated in 11 Asian countries: a proposal for a new nomenclature for SCC*mec* elements. Antimicrob Agents Chemother 50: 1001–1012.
62. Coombs GW, Monecke S, Ehricht R, Slickers P, Pearson JC, et al. (2010) Differentiation of clonal complex 59 community-associated methicillin-resistant *Staphylococcus aureus* in Western Australia. Antimicrob Agents Chemother 54: 1914–1921.
63. Geng W, Yang Y, Wu D, Huang G, Wang C, et al. (2010) Molecular characteristics of community-acquired methicillin-resistant *Staphylococcus aureus* isolated from Chinese children. FEMS Immunol Med Microbiol 58: 356–362.

A Novel Lipopeptide from Skin Commensal Activates TLR2/CD36-p38 MAPK Signaling to Increase Antibacterial Defense against Bacterial Infection

Dongqing Li, Hu Lei, Zhiheng Li, Hongquan Li, Yue Wang, Yuping Lai*

Shanghai Key Laboratory of Regulatory Biology, School of Life Sciences, East China Normal University, Shanghai, People's Republic of China

Abstract

Staphylococcus epidermidis (*S.epidermidis*) plays important protective roles by directly producing or by stimulating hosts to produce antimicrobial peptides (AMPs) against pathogenic infections. Although several AMPs from *S.epidermidis* have been identified, molecules that stimulate hosts to produce AMPs remain largly unknown. Here we demonstrate that a new lipopeptide (named LP01) purified from *S.epidermidis* culture media has a unique structure with heneicosanoic acid (21 carbons) binding to lysine^{11} of a peptide chain. *In vitro* LP01 increased the expression of β-defensin 2(hBD2) and hBD3 in neonatal human epidermal keratinocytes(NHEK), leading to increased capacity of cell lysates to inhibit the growth of *S.aureus*. *In vivo* LP01 induced the expression of mouse β-defensin 4(mBD4) to decrease the survival of local *S.aureus* in skin and systemic *S.aureus* survival in liver. The induction of beta-defensins by LP01 was dependent on TLR2 as *Tlr2*-deficient mice had decreased mBD4. Furthermore, knockdown of CD36 decreased the expression of hBD2 and hBD3, and p38 MAPK inhibitor significantly inhibited the expression of hBDs induced by LP01.Taken together, these findings demonstrate that lipopeptide LP01 from normal commensal *S.epidermidis* increases antimicrobial peptide hBD2 and hBD3 expression via the activation of TLR2/CD36-p38 MAPK, thus enhancing antimicrobial defense against pathogenic infections.

Editor: Bernhard Ryffel, French National Centre for Scientific Research, France

Funding: This work was supported by National Natural Science Foundation of China grants (NSFC) 81072422, 31222021&31170867, grants 11QA1401900, 12ZZ039 to Yuping Lai, NSFC grant 31100109 to Deming Jiang, Shanghai Natural science Foundation grant11ZR1409900 to Meiling Zhang, the program for professor of Special Appointment (Eastern Scholar) at Shanghai Institutions (Yuping Lai), and the Science and Technology Commission of Shanghai Municipality grant 11DZ2260300. Part of in-vitro studies was also supported by Johnson and Johnson. The funders had no role in study design, data collection and analysis, decision to publish, or preparation of the manuscript.

Competing Interests: Part of in-vitro studies was also supported by Johnson and Johnson. East China Normal University has applied for the pending Chinese patent for LP01 (Name: The preparation and application of lipopeptide 01 and its derivatives; Application Number: 201210138021.0; and date of patent: May 7, 2012)). There are no further patents, products in development or marketed products to declare.

* E-mail: yplai@bio.ecnu.edu.cn

Introduction

Skin, as a first line of defense, interfaces with the environment and is exposed to a myriad of microbes. Among these microbes, *Staphylococcus epidermidis* (*S.epidermidis*) is the most abundant bacterium that resides on skin and generally has a benign relationship with its host. Previously, we have gained considerable insights into beneficial roles of *S.epidermidis* by balancing inflammatory responses after skin injury. We discovered that lipoteichoic acid from *S.epidermidis* substantially attenuated keratinocyte response to skin injury through a TLR2-dependent inhibition of the TLR3 signaling via TNF receptor-associated factor 1 (TRAF1), thus suppressing unwanted inflammatory cytokine production [1]. Besides the regulation of inflammation in skin injury, other groups showed that *S.epidermidis* produced some antimicrobial molecules including Staphylococcin 1580 [2], Pep5 [3], PSMs [4] to benefit cutaneous immune defense by selectively inhibiting the survival of skin pathogens. We have also demonstrated that less than 10 kDa molecules from *S.epidermidis* culture media induced the production of β-defensins to enable the skin to mount an enhanced response to pathogens [5]. However, the identity of the molecule from *S.epidermidis* to induce β-defensins remains unknown.

Besides *S.epidermidis*, several other bacteria have been shown to produce lipopeptides to help hosts against pathogenic infections by disturbing gram-positive bacterial cell wall synthesis [6]. One of the most well-established lipopeptides with direct antimicrobial activity is daptomycin [6]. This lipopeptide can destruct the membrane of Gram-positive pathogens including Methicillin-resistant *Staphylococcus aureus*. In addition to daptomycin, other lipopeptides including Iturin A [7] and Fengycin [8] from *Bacillus subtilis*, polymyxins from *Paenibacillus polymyxa* [9] and fusaricidins from *Paenibacillus polymyxa* [10] have been identified to exert their direct antimicrobial activity. Besides direct antimicrobial activity, synthetic lipopeptides such as MALP-2 can induce antimicrobial peptide expression in several cell types such as keratinocytes [5]. These observations thereby raise the possibility that the molecule from *S.epidermidis* to induce AMP might be a lipopeptide.

Given that skin commensal bacteria increase host defense against pathogenic infections and lipopeptides from bacteria exert direct antimicrobial activity or induce host to produce antimicrobial peptides, we hypothesized that the molecule from *S.epidermidis* to induce β-defensins might be a kind of lipopeptide. In this study we successfully purified one novel lipopeptide from *S.epidermidis* culture media and further delineated the mechanism by which the

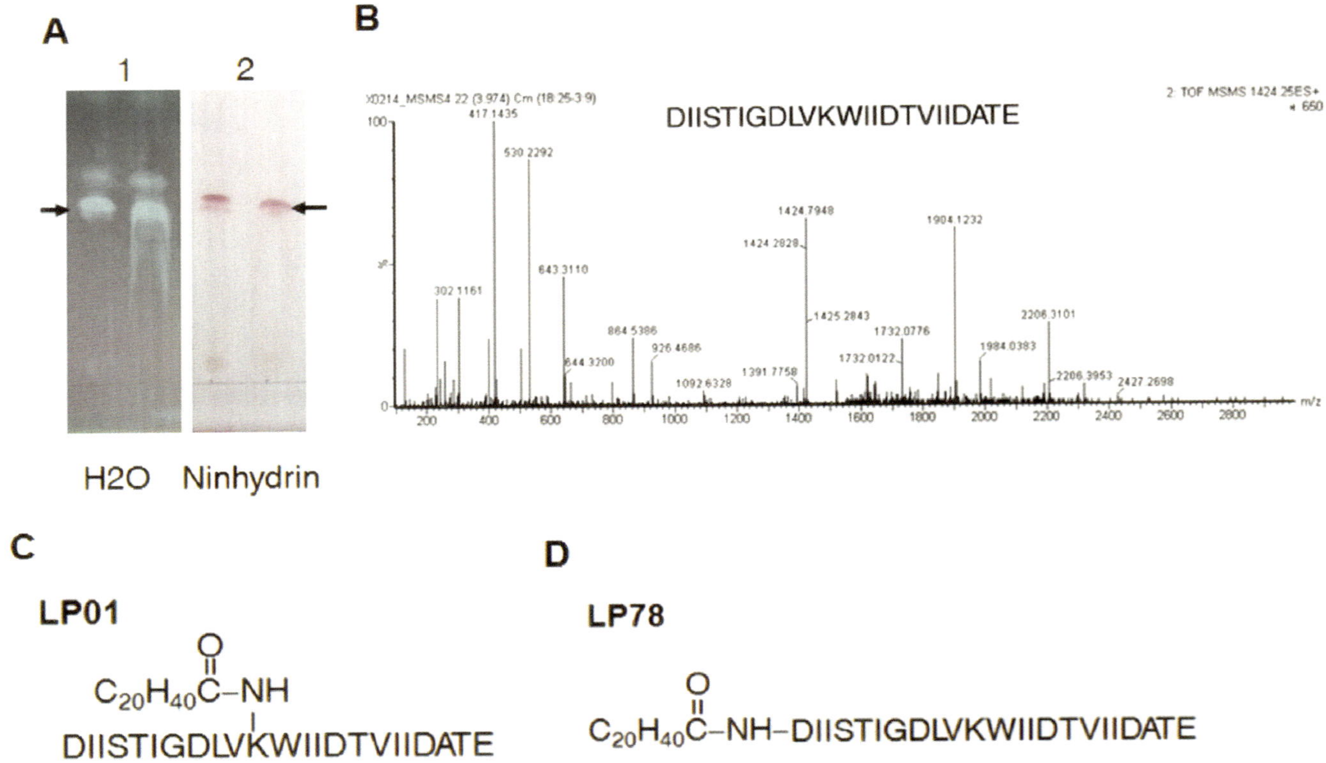

Figure 1. The identification of the lipopeptide from *Staphylococcus epidermidis*. A. The analysis of the lipopeptide from *S.epidermidis* by thin-layer chromatography. Duplicate samples were loaded on TLC plate and molecules with different hydrophobicity were separated. Water was used to show hydrophobicity of lipopeptides and ninhydrin was used to show that the lipopeptide contains amino acids. The arrows indicate LP01. **B.** Q-TOF MS/MS analysis of lipopeptide in positive-ion model. Q-TOF MS/MS analysis showed that the amino acid sequence of the lipopeptide was DIISTIGDLVKWIIDTVIIDATE. **C&D.** Two possible structures of the lipopeptide. Aspartic acid (D^1) at N-terminus and lysine (K^{11}) are two amino acids with free NH_3^+, and free -COOH of heneicosanoic acid might react with NH_3^+ to form CO–NH. Thereby heneicosanoic acid may bind to ^{1}D or ^{11}K of the peptide chain.

lipopeptide induced AMP against *S.aureus* infection. Our findings reveal the potential use of commensal bacterium-derived lipopeptides in treatment of skin infections.

Materials and Methods

Bacterial Strains and Mice

Staphylococcus epidermidis 1457, *Staphylococcus aureus*, *Escherichia coli DH5a* and *Propionibacterium acnes* were stored in our laboratory. *S.epidermidis* 1457 and *S.aureus* were cultured at 37°C for 16 h in Tryptic Soy Broth (TSB) medium (Sigma, St Louis, MO). *E.coli DH5a* was cultured at 37°C for 16 h in Lysogeny Broth (LB) medium. *P.acnes* was culture at 37°C in Reinforced Clostridial Medium in anaerobic pouch (MGC, JAPAN). All mice were kept under specific pathogen free conditions and maintained in accordance with the institutional guidelines. All animal experiments were approved by East China Normal University Animal Care and Use Committee.

Lipopeptide Purification and Identification

S.epidermidis 1457 was grown in TSB medium at 37°C for overnight. Next day, the overnight culture was diluted 1:100 into TSB and grown for another 16 hours. Bacterial supernatants were collected and filtered by 0.22 μm stericup. Bacterium-free culture supernatant was adjusted to pH = 2.0 and then stored at 4°C for overnight. Next day, the crude lipopeptide was extracted by methanol at 37°C for overnight and dried by rotary evaporation followed by loading on HPLC with a C18 column for further purification. The purified lipopeptide was analyzed by thin-layer chromatography (TLC) on silica-coated glass plates in solvent system (butyl alcohol: acetic acid: H2O = 4:2:1, v/v/v). Protein sequences were analyzed by Q-TOF MS/MS *de-novo* sequencing (Waters, ACQUITY™ UPLC&Q-TOF Premier). The structure of lipid of the lipopeptide was analyzed by GC/MS (Shimadzu, GC/MS-QP2010).

Real-time Quantitative RT-PCR

Total RNA was prepared using Trizol Reagent (TaKaRa, Japan) following the manufacturer's instructions. RNA was quantified by Thermo NANODROP 2000 spectrophotometer. Total RNA (1 μg) was reverse transcribed using PrimeScript® RT reagent Kit (TaKaRa, Japan) according to the manufacturer's instructions. Real-time RT-PCR was conducted on Mx3005P (Stratagene, USA) using SYBR® Premix ExTaq (TaKaRa, Japan). The quantification of gene expression was determined by the comparative $2\Delta\Delta C_T$ method. The primers used in this manuscriptare shown in the following: mBD4 forward: GGCTTCAGT-CAT GAGGATCCAT; mBD4 reverse: TTTGGGTAAAGGCTGCAAGTG; mBD14 forward: GTGGC CGGTGTGCTGTACT; mBD14 reverse: CGCTATTAGA ACATCGACCTATTTGT; hBD2 forward: CCAGCCAT-CAGCCATGAGGGT; hBD2 reverse: GGAGCCCTTTCT-

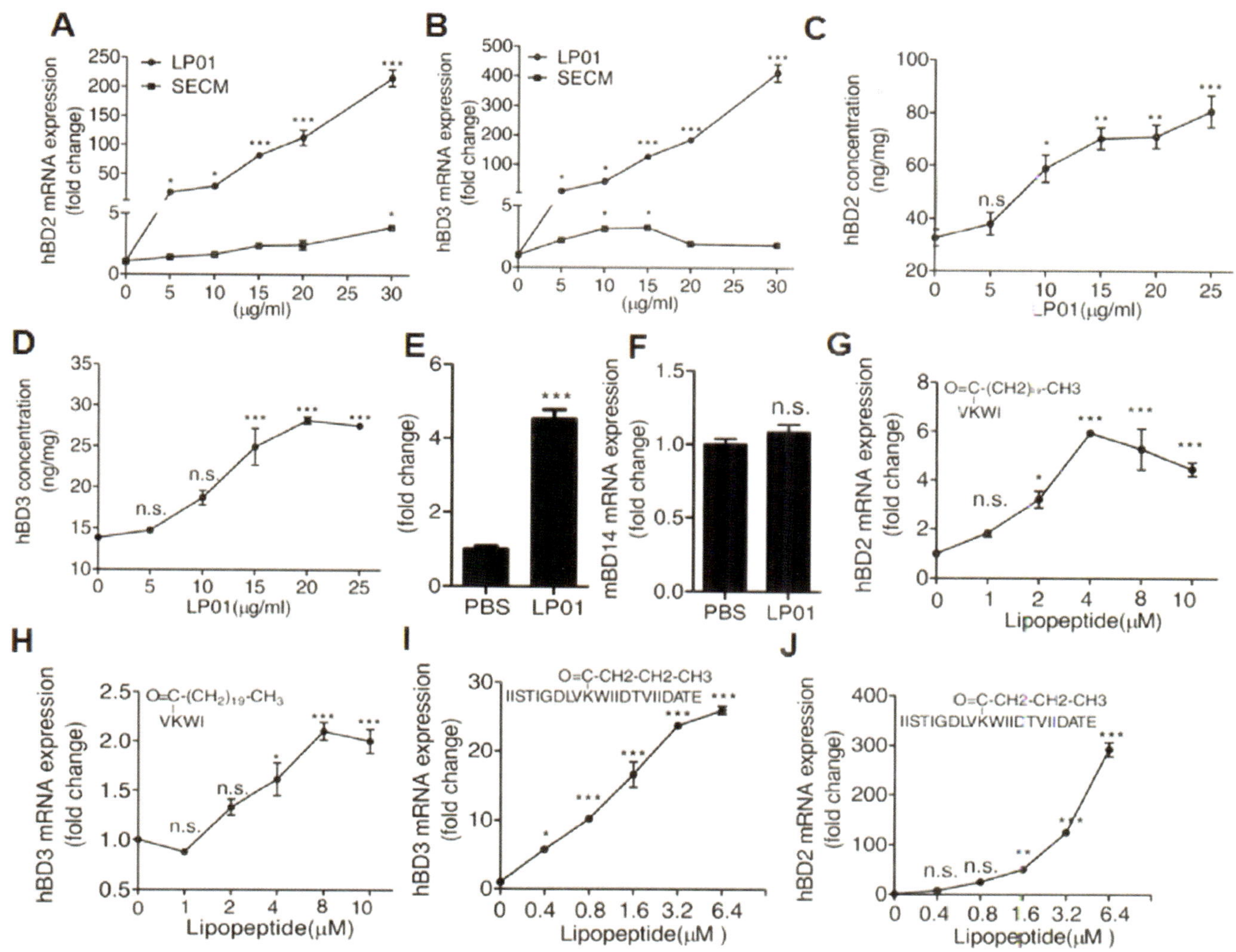

Figure 2. LP01 induces β-defensin expression in primary keratinocytes. A&B. Quantification of hBD2 and hBD3 mRNA expression in NHEKs treated with LP01 or SECM. **C&D.** hBD2 and hBD3 protein expression in cell lysates of NHEKs treated with LP01 by ELISA. **E&F.** Quantification of mBD4 and mBD14 mRNA expression stimulated with 15 μg/mL LP01 in primary murine keratinocytes. Primary murine keratinocytes were isolated from C57BL/6 mice. **G&H.** Quantification of hBD2 and hBD3 mRNA expression in NHEKs stimulated by LP01 with shortened peptide chain. **I&J.** Quantification of hBD2 and hBD3 mRNA expression in NHEKs stimulated by LP01 with shortened fatty acid chain. *$P<0.05$, **$P<0.01$ and ***$P<0.001$, n.s., no significance. P values were determined by one-way ANOVA or two-tailed t test. Data are the means ± SEM of $n=3$ and representative of two independent experiments.

GAATCCGCA; hBD3 forward: GCCTCTT CCAGGTGTTTTTG; hBD3 reverse: GAGACCACAGGTGC-CAATTT. The relative expression levels were determined by normalizing expression to 18s rRNA or glyceraldehyde 3-phosphate dehydrogenase (GAPDH). All the assays were performed in triplicate and repeated at least two times.

Primary Cell Culture and Stimulation by Lipopeptide

Neonatal human epidermal keratinocytes (Cascade Biologics, USA) were cultured in EpiLife medium supplemented with EDGS, 0.06 mM $CaCl_2$ (Cascade Biologics, USA) and Pen Strep(100 units/ml Penicillin and 100 μg/ml Sreptomycin). Murine primary keratinocytes were isolated from newborn skin by using dispase II (Sigma, St Louis, MO) and cultured in 154CF medium supplemented with HKGS and 0.2 mM $CaCl_2$ and Pen Strep(100 units/ml Penicillin and 100 μg/ml Sreptomycin) (Invitrogen, Shanghai). Keratinocytes were seeded in 6-, 12- or 24-well plates to grow to 70% confluence. To test whether the induction of hBDs by lipopeptide was in a dose-dependent manner, 2.5, 5, 10, 15, 20, 25, 30 μg/ml lipopeptide was used to stimulate NHEK cells. 15 μg/ml lipopeptide was used to stimulate murine primary keratinocytes. 24 h later, cells were harvested. The expression of genes was analyzed by using real-time RT-PCR and the protein levels of hBDs were determined by hBD2 and hBD3 ELISA Kit (Peprotech, Hamburg, Germany).

Bacterial Killing Assay

To test the capacity of NHEK cell lysate stimulated with LP01 in the inhibition of the growth of bacteria, NHEK cells were cultured in no P/S Epilife medium and then were treated with 15 μg/mL of LP01. After 24 hours, 100 μL of phosphate buffered saline (PBS) containing protease inhibitor cocktail was added into each well. Cells were collected by cell scraper and then sonicated on ice-cold water. After removed cell debris by centrifugation, the concentration of the lysates was determined by BCA™ Protein Assay Kit (Novagen, San Diego, CA). 10 μg of cell lysates was incubated with 1×10^6 CFU *P.acnes*, *S.aureus* or *S.epidermidis* at 37°C for 3 h. The bacterial were then serially diluted by 10-fold with PBS and plated on RCM agar plates (*P.acnes*), TSB agar plates (*S.aureus*, *S.epidermidis*) or LB agar plates (*E.coli DH5a*).

S.aureus Infection *in vivo*

The backs of 8-week adult mice were shaved and hair was removed by chemical depilation. 2 mg/kg of LP01 and PBS was intradermally injected into mouse back, respectively. Next day, 50 μL of live *S.aureus* ($OD_{600} = 0.7–0.8$) complexed with cytodex beads (Sigma, St Louis, MO) as carrier was intradermally injected 2 hours after injection of LP01. Lesional sizes caused by *S.aureus* infection were measured daily. At day 3, skin around the lesional sites, liver and spleen were taken and homogenized for *S.aureus* culture.

Inactivation of TLR2 or p38 MAPK

TLR2 inhibitor OxPAPC (InvivoGen, San Diego, CA) or p38 MAPK inhibitor SB202190(Sigma, St Louis, MO) was added 10 minutes before normal human keratinocytes or murine primary keratinocytes were treated with 15 μg/ml of LP01. 24 hours later, total RNA was extracted and cDNA synthesized by the PrimeScript® RT reagent Kit (TaKaRa, Japan). The level of gene expression was quantified by real-time RT-PCR by using Stratagene Mx3005P.

Immunoblotting

Normal human epidermal keratinocytes were treated with 15 μg/mL of LP01 for 1 hour in the presence or absence of inhibitors. Cells were lysed in the RIPA buffer (pH 7.4) containing protease inhibitor cocktail (Roche, Pleasanton, CA) after washed by ice-cold PBS for 3 times. Protein concentrations of the extracts were measured by BCA™ Protein Assay Kit (Novagen, San Diego, CA). 30 μg of total protein was used for western blot. The lysates were separated by 12% SDS-PAGE and analyzed by immunoblotting with phosphorylated p38 MAPK antibody or p38 MAPK antibody (Cell signaling, Danvers, MA), respectively. The membrane was scanned by Odyssey machine (Li-Cor Biosciences, Lincoln, NE).

Statistical Analysis

All data are present as mean±SEM. Two-tailed t-test was used to determine significances between two groups. The significances among multiple groups were determined by One-way or Two-way ANOVA with Bonferroni post test of GraphPad Prism Version 5 (San Diego, CA). For all statistical tests, we considered P values <0.05 to be statistically significant.

Results

The Structure of Lipopeptide 01 (LP01) from Skin Commensal *Staphylococcus epidermidis*

We have shown that less than 10 kDa molecules from *S.epidermidis* culture media induced the production of β-defensins and that one synthetic lipopeptide such as MALP-2 induced hBDs expression in keratinocytes [5], we thus hypothesized that the

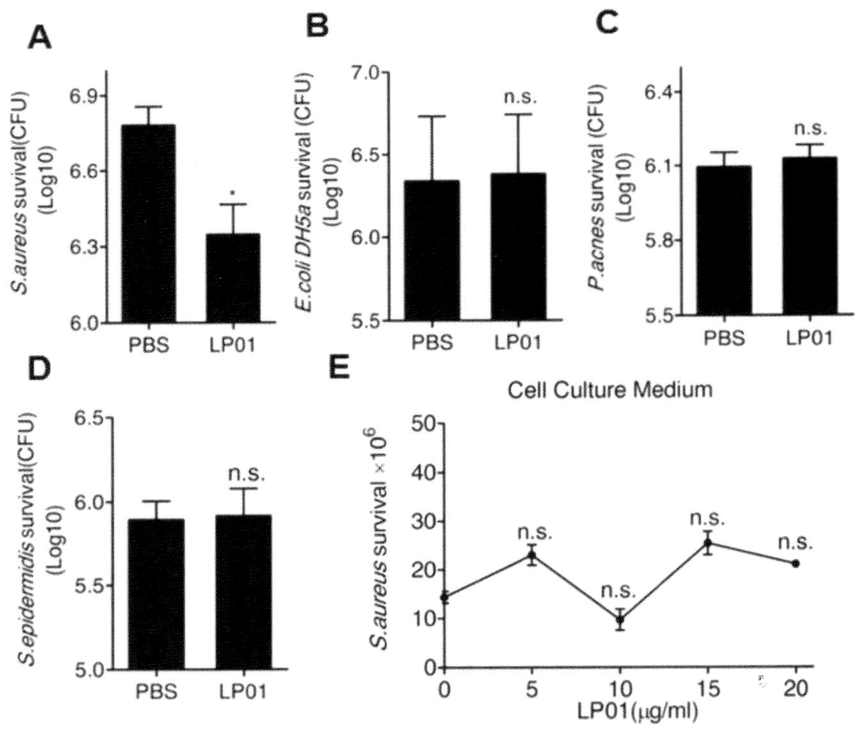

Figure 3. LP01 increases antibacterial activity of keratinocytes. The growth of *S.aureus* (**A**), *E.coli DH5a* (**B**), *P.acnes* (**C**) and *S.epidermidis* (**D**) after exposure to lysates of LP01-treated neonatal human epidermal keratinocytes or the growth of *S.aureus* after exposure to cell culture medium of LP01-treated NHEKs (**E**). The bacterial were serially diluted 10-fold with PBS and then counted by colony formation. *$P<0.05$; n.s., no significance. P values were determined by t-test. All data are representative of three independent experiments with $n=3$ and are means ± SEM.

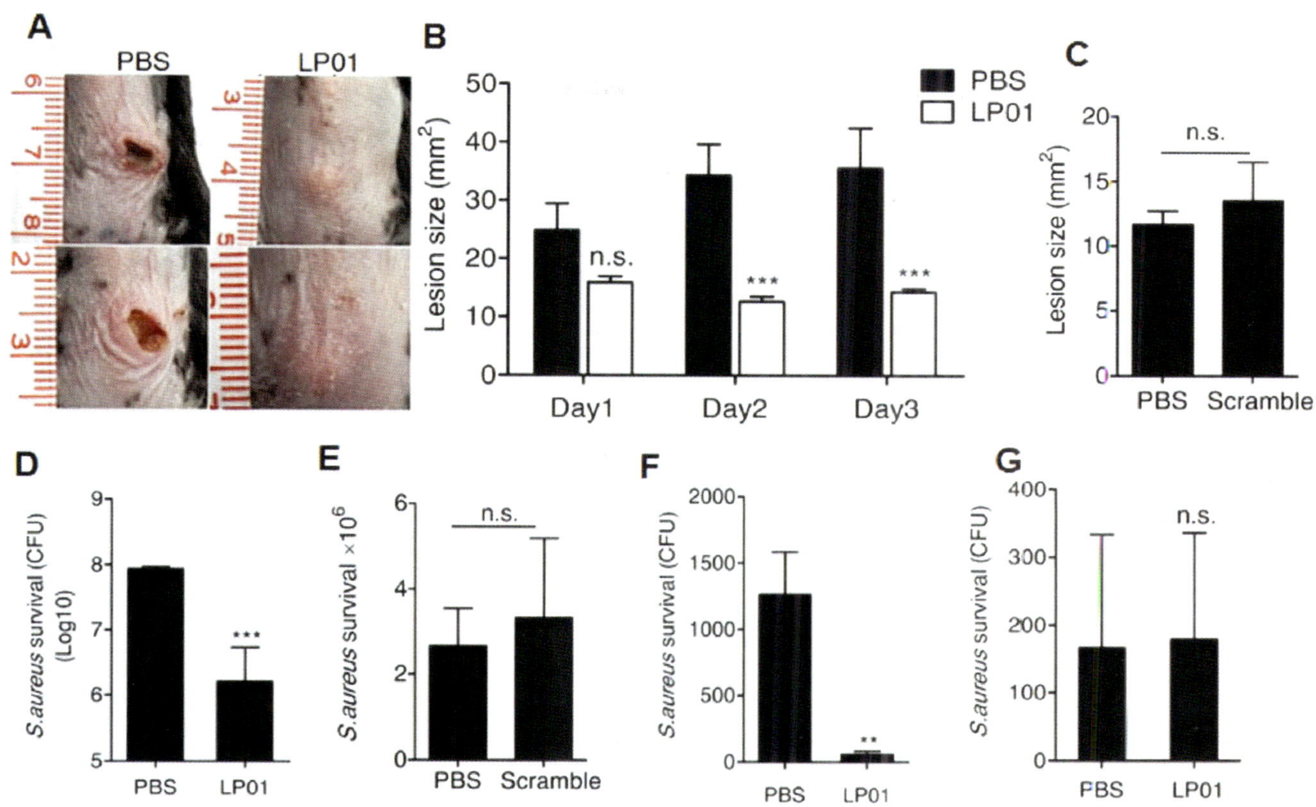

Figure 4. LP01 protects mice from *S.aureus* infection. A. Photograph of skin lesions caused by *S.aureus* at 3 days after *S.aureus* injection. **B.** ImageJ analysis of the lesional size of A. **C.** ImageJ analysis of the lesional size of PBS- or scrambled lipopeptide-treated mice. Local *S.aureus* survival in skin (**D and E**) and systemic *S.aureus* survival in liver (**F**) and spleen (**G**) of PBS- or scrambled lipopeptide- or LP01- pretreated mice. $^{**}P<0.01$; $^{***}P<0.001$. *P* values were determined by two-tailed t test or two-way ANOVA. All data are the means ± SEM of $n=6$ and representative of two independent experiments.

molecule from *Staphylococcus epidermidis* to induce β-defensins might be a lipopetide. To test this, we used methanol extraction, acid precipitation, thin-layer chromatography and high-performance liquid chromatography (HPLC) to isolate lipopeptides from the *S.epidermidis* culture media(Fig. 1) and confirmed that the lipopeptide we purified from *S.epidermidis* culture media had the capacity to induce huaman beta-defensin 2 (hBD2) and hBD3 expression in neonatal human epidermal keratinocytes (NHEKs)(-data not shown). The *de-novo* peptide sequencing showed that the peptide chain of the lipopeptide is DIISTIGDLVKWIIDTVIIDATE(Fig. 1B), and Gas chromatography mass spectrometry revealed that this lipopeptide contained one heneicosanoic acid $C_{20}H_{40}COOH$(Fig. 1C and 1D). The analysis of the peptide sequence showed that aspartic acid (D^1) at N-terminus and the amino acid at site 11 lysine (K^{11}) might be amino acids where heneicosanoic acid bound to the peptide chain. Therefore, structures of the lipopeptide might be as shown in Fig. 1C and Fig. 1D.

To determine the structure-function relationship of the lipopeptides, we synthesized the above two possible lipopeptides LP01 and LP78 and then evaluated their capacity to induce the expression of antimicrobial peptides. Compared to *S.epidermidis* culture media (SECM), synthetic LP01 significantly increased both mRNA and protein of hBD2 and hBD3 in NHEKs (Fig. 2A–2D) while synthetic LP78 did not (data not shown). In addition to NHEKs, LP01 significantly increased the expression of mouse beta-defensin 4 (mBD4, mouse homolog of human hBD2) but not mBD14 (mouse homolog of human hBD3) in primary murine keratinocytes (Fig. 2E and 2F). Furthermore, the capacity of LP01 to induce hBDs was more dependent on the intact peptide chain than the intact fatty acid. This was made evident by the fact that a shortened peptide chain with heneicosanoic acid markedly decreased hBDs induction while the intact peptide chain with shortened fatty acid slightly decreased hBDs induction (Fig. 2 G–J). These data suggest that LP01 with heneicosanoic acid binding to peptide chain (22 amino acids) is the lipopeptide from *S.epidermidis* to induce beta-defensins.

LP01 Increases Antibacterial Activity against *S.aureus* Infection

It is known that human hBD2 and hBD3 from epidermal keratinocytes exert bactericidal activity against *E.coli* and *S.aureus* infection [11,12]. Since LP01 significantly induced hBD2 and hBD3 protein expression in kerationcytes (Fig. 2A–2D) but not too much in cell culture media (data not shown), we next examined whether the induction of hBD2 and hBD3 by LP01 could increase the antibacterial capacity of keratinocytes *in vitro*. A cell lysate of undifferentiated NHEKs pretreated with 10 μg/ml of LP01 significantly inhibited the growth of *S.aureus* (Fig. 3A), but did not inhibit *E.coli* (Fig. 3B), *P.acnes* (Fig. 3C), and *S.epidermidis* itself (Fig. 3D). Moreover, due to the low secreted hBD2 and hBD3, cell

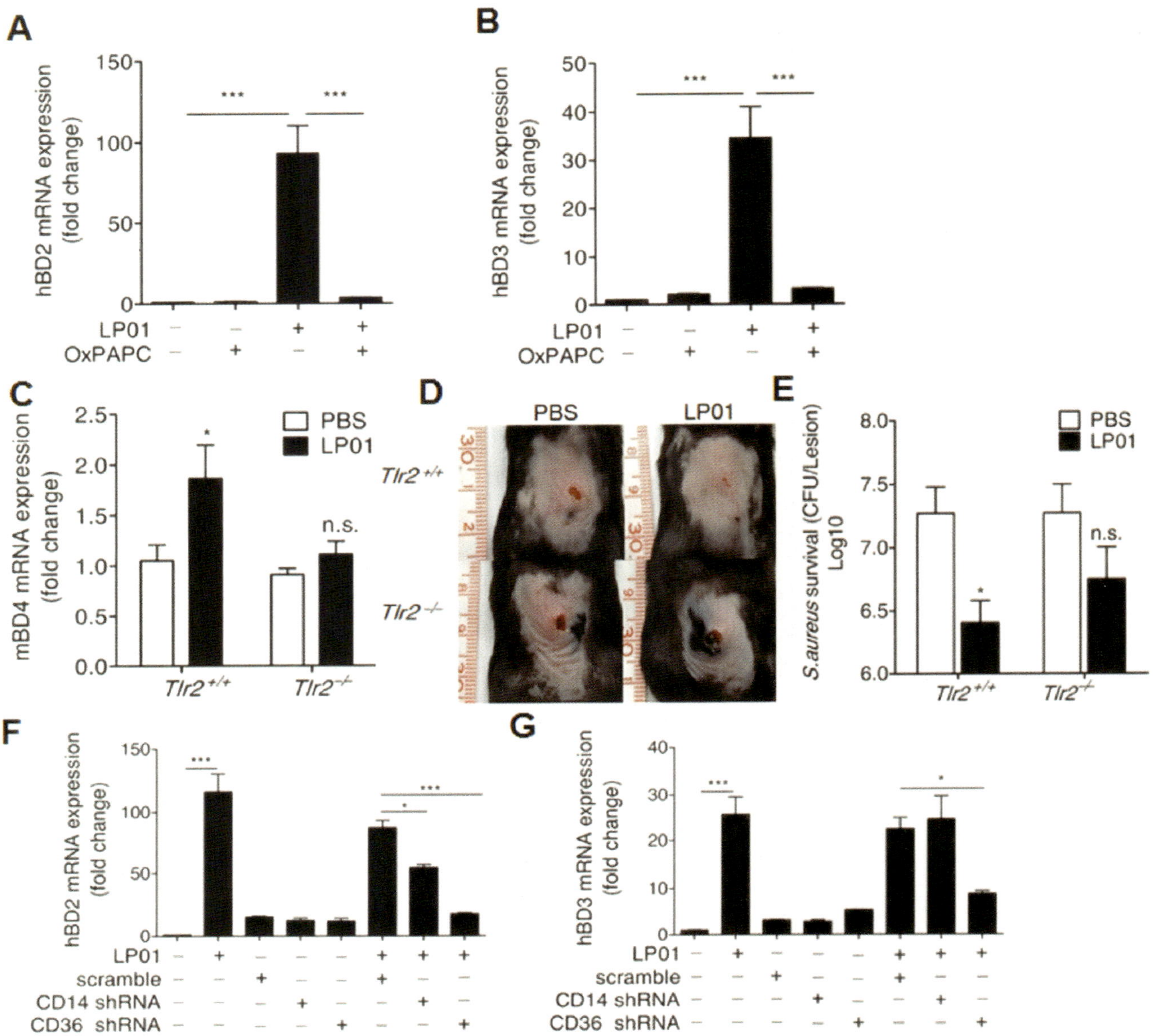

Figure 5. The induction of beta-defensins by LP01 is dependent on TLR2. A, B. The expression of hBD2 and hBD3 in NHEKs treated with 15 µg/mL of LP01 in the presence or absence of TLR2 inhibitor OxPAPC. **C.** mBD4 expression in mouse ears 24 h after injection by 2 mg/kg of LP01. **D.** Photograph of skin lesions caused by *S.aureus* at 3 days after *S.aureus* injection in *Tlr2*$^{+/+}$ and *Tlr2*$^{-/-}$ mice. **E.** *S.aureus* survival in skin of PBS- and LP01- pretreated *Tlr2*$^{+/+}$ and *Tlr2*$^{-/-}$ mice. **F–G.** Quantification of hBD2 and hBD3 expression in NHEK cells stimulated with LP01 after CD14 or CD36 was silenced. $^{*}P<0.05$, $^{***}P<0.001$. *P* values were determined by one-way or two-way ANOVA. All data are representative of two independent experiments with $n = 3–6$ and are the means ± SEM.

culture media of NHEKs treated with LP01 was not able to inhibit the growth of *S.aureus* (Fig. 3E).

To confirm that the induction of antimicrobial peptides in keratinocytes by LP01 would be relevant to protection against *S.aureus* infection *in vivo*, LP01 was intradermally injected into mice 24 and 2 hours before an infectious challenge at the site with *S.aureus*. LP01-treated mice showed significantly smaller infectious skin lesions when compared with control mice injected with PBS or scrambled lipopeptide (Fig. 4A–4C). Accompanied with smaller infectious lesions, the survival of *S.aureus* at the local site of infection was significantly decreased (Fig. 4D and 4E). In addition, the survival of *S.aureus* in liver, but not in spleen, was decreased (Fig. 4F and 4G). Taken together, these results demonstrate that the LP01 from *S. epidermidis* increases host defense aganist *S. aureus* infection.

The Induction of Beta-defensins by LP01 is Dependent on TLR2 and CD36

Having established the role of LP01 in *S.aureus* skin infection, we next sought to explore the mechanism by which LP01 regulates antimicrobial peptide expression. Since TLR2 is a well-known receptor on keratinocytes for lipopeptides [13,14], we assumed that the LP01 isolated from *S.epidrmidis* would activate TLR2 to induce antimicrobial peptide expression. To test this,

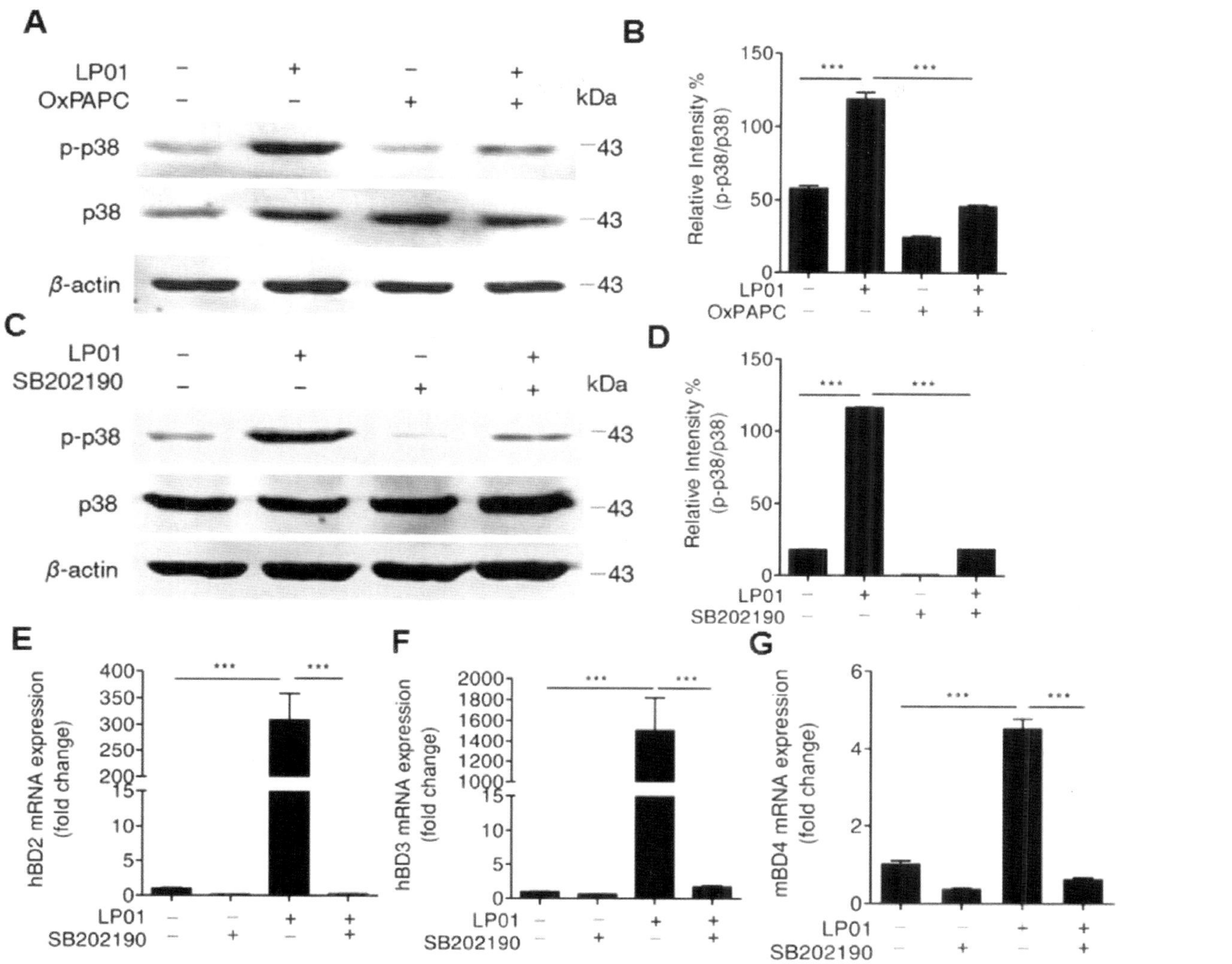

Figure 6. The activation of p38 MAPK is required for the induction of beta-defensins by LP01. A&B. TLR2 inhibitor OxPAPC inhibited p38 phosphorylation induced by 15 μg/mL of LP01 in NHEK cells. **C&D.** p38 MAPK inhibitor SB202190 inhibited p38 phosphorylation induced by 15 μg/mL of LP01 in NHEK cells. **E&F.** p38 MAPK inhibitor SB202190 completely inhibited hBD2 and hBD3 expression induced by 15 μg/mL of LP01 in NHEK cells. **G.** p38 MAPK inhibitor SB202190 completely inhibited mBD4 expression induced by 15 μg/mL of LP01 in murine primary keratinocytes. ***$P<0.001$. P values were determined by one-way ANOVA. Data are the means ± SEM of $n=3$ and representative of two to three independent experiments.

we first used the TLR2 inhibitor OxPAPC to block TLR2 activation. OxPAPC completely inhibited the expression of hBD2 and hBD3 induced by LP01 (Fig. 5A and 5B). Consistent with our *in vitro* observations, LP01 lost its capacity to induce the expression of mBD4 in *Tlr2*-deficient mice compared to wild-type mice (Fig. 5C). In addition, LP01 failed to protect mice from *S.aureus* infection in *Tlr2*-deficient mice as shown with bigger infectious skin lesions and increased surviving *S.aureus* (Fig. 5D and 5E). Furthermore, knockdown of a coreceptor for TLR2 heterodimer, CD36, significanlty decreased hBD2 and hBD3 expression induced by LP01 (Fig. 5F and 5G). However, knockdown of antoher coreceptor for TLR2 heterodimer, CD14, only significantly decreased LP01-induced hBD2 expression, but not hBD3 expression (Fig. 5F and 5G). Altogether, these data demonstrate that lipopeptide LP01 activates TLR2 and CD36 to induce hBD2 and hBD3 in skin.

The Activation of p38 MAPK is Required for the Induction of Beta-defensins by LP01

It has been reported that activation of TLR2 regulates multiple downstream molecules including NF-κB and mitogen-activated protein kinases(MAPKs) [15]. Specifically, p38 MAPK has been shown to play an important role in hBD2 and hBD3 production in epithelial cells such as keratinocytes [16,17]. We thus hypothesized that p38 MAPK might be the downstream molecule of TLR2 involved in the induction of hBDs by LP01. To test this hypothesis, we first checked if LP01 induced p38 MAPK phosphorylation after TLR2 was blocked. TLR2 inhibitor OxPAPC markedly decreased the phosphorylation of p38MAPK (Thr180/Tyr182) by LP01 (Fig. 6A and 6B). In addition to OxPAPC, p38 MAPK inhibitor, SB202190 completely inhibited p38 MAPK phosphorylation (Fig. 6C and 6D). Furthermore, the inhibition of p38 MAPK significantly decreased the expression of hBD2 and hBD3 in NHEKs (Fig. 6E and 6F) as well as mBD4 in primary murine keratinocytes (Fig. 6G). Taken together, these results demonstrate that p38 MAPK is the critical downstream molecule of TLR2 to induce hBD2 and hBD3 expression induced by LP01.

Discussion

To date, most studies on skin microbes have been conducted to analyze the type and diversity of microbes present on the skin by classic culture techniques or identified by sequencing surveys of 16s rRNA. However, sparse attention has been paid to the beneficial function of these microbes that inhabit on our skin. Here we have identified one new lipopeptide (LP01) from *S.epidermidis*, one of the most commonly isolated bacterial species from healthy human skin [18,19], and show that the lipopeptide activates TLR2/CD36-p38 MAPK to induce hBD2 and hBD3 expression, thus enabling the skin to mount an enhanced antimicrobial defense against pathogenic infections. Our results reveal that skin commensals play an important role in host antimicrobial defense and suggest that the preservation of these commensals on skin may be an effective way to achieve maintenance of healthy 'normal' skin function.

Epidemiologic and clinical studies indicate that the increased incidence of autoimmune and allergic diseases in developed countries is associated with reduced microbial exposure and alteration of microbial communities in various body sites [20]. Although high-throughput metabolomics analyses have been used to identify core microbial communities linked to the onset of pathologies, there is still a big challenging to define a 'normal healthy' microbiota of skin at the functional level [21,22,23]. Moreover, the molecular mechanisms underlying microbe-host interactions that shape host immune functions remain largely unknown. Previous work from Schittek and our group has demonstrated that skin commensals induce antimicrobial peptide RNase7 to amplify the innate immune response [24] and that *S.epidermidis* conditioned culture medium (SECM) increases antimicrobial peptide expression in keratinocytes [5]. Here we further advance our understanding of how skin commensal *S.epidermidis* regulates host immune responses against bacterial infections by defining the structure of lipopeptide LP01 from *S.epidermidis* and delineating the mechanism by which LP01 induces the expression of antimicrobial peptide hBD2 and hBD3.

In order to identify the structure of LP01, we used Q-TOF mass spectrometry *de-novo* sequencing technique to identify the amino acid sequence of the peptide chain and gas chromatography mass spectrometry technique to identify the fatty acid chain as priviously described [25,26]. According to the amino acid sequence of the lipopeptide, we found that there were two possiblities for fatty acid heneicosanoic acid binding to peptide chain. One possibility was that heneicosanoic acid bound to Lys^{11}, the other was that heneicosanoic acid bound to N-terminal amino acid Asp^{1}. To determine structure-function relationship, the above two possible lipopeptides were synthesized and their capacity to induce hBD2 and hBD3 expression was tested. Our results demonostrate that only the lipopeptide with heneicosanoic acid binding to Lys^{11} has the capacity to induce hBD2 and hBD3 expression, suggesting that Lys^{11} is the binding site of heneicosanoic acid. Furthermore, we have synthesized several derivatives of LP01 to prove that the intact peptide chain is essensial for the function of LP01 to induce AMPs. Our data show that heneicosanoic acid binding to shortened peptide chain completely lost its capacity to induce hBD2&3 while shortened fatty acid chain binding to the intact peptide chain kept its capacity to induce AMPs. These data suggest that the lipopeptide only with a unique structure has the capacity to induce AMPs.

Toll-like receptors (TLRs) have been reported to play an important role in host defense. They can recognize pathogen-associated molecular patterns (PAMPs) from microbes and damge-associated molecular patterns (DAMPs) from hosts. TLR2, as one of TLR family members, ususally works as TLR2/TLR1 or TLR2/TLR6 heterodimer and recognize a broad range of ligands, especially ligands of cell-wall componenets from gram-positive bacteria such as lipoteichoic acid (LTA) as well as peptidoglycan and lipoproteins [27]. LP01, as a lipopeptide from *S.epidermidis*, binds to TLR2 and then activates p38 MAPK to induce hBD2 and hBD3 expression. Furthrmore, we have shown that the coreceptor CD36 is also involved in the induction of hBD2 and hBD3 by LP01, which is consistent with previous observation that CD36 facilitates TLR2 recognition [28]. However, although it is reported that both CD36 and CD14 are required for TLR2 in response to LTA [29,30,31], in our system the silencing of CD14 only slightly decreased hBD2 expression but not hBD3 while knockdown of CD36 significantly reduced the expression of both hBD2 and hBD3. One explanation of this phenomenon is that CD36 and CD14 participate in different TLR2 signaling complex as CD36 is specifically involved in TLR2/TLR6-mediated response but not TLR2/TLR1-mediated response [29] while CD14 usually enhances signaling in respose to TLR2/TLR1 ligand Pam3CysSK4 [32]. The other explanation is that CD14 usually facilitates TLR2 ligands binding to TLR2 and NF-κB activation [32]. However, our data show that the induction of hBD2 and hBD3 requires p38 MAPK activation but not NF-κB activation. This is probably the reason that silencing of CD14 does not decrease the induction of hBD2 and hBD3 by LP01. Altogether, these data suggest that LP01, as a lipopeptide, activates TLR2/TLR6 signaling other than TLR2/TLR1 signaling. However, further investigation is needed.

In conclusion, these findings suggest that skin resident commensals are necessary for our protection from infections. Specifically, we find that lipopeptide LP01 from *S.epidermidis* exerts its effect by enhancing antimicrobial defense via the activation of TLR2/CD36-p38 MAPK signaling. Furthermore, our results indicate that identification of specific molecules from skin commensals to understand its roles in shaping host immune response is not only of primary importance for human health, but will also lead to the development of more rational antibacterial approaches. Our results also emphasize disadvantages of indiscriminate use of topical and systemic antibiotics to treat skin infections.

Acknowledgments

We thank Xi Li from Worldwide EM Innovation Center, Jonhson &Johnson China Ltd. for helpful discussion.

Author Contributions

Conceived and designed the experiments: YL DL. Performed the experiments: DL H. Lei ZL H. Li YW. Analyzed the data: DL H. Lei YL. Wrote the paper: YL DL.

References

1. Lai Y, Di Nardo A, Nakatsuji T, Leichtle A, Yang Y, et al. (2009) Commensal bacteria regulate Toll-like receptor 3-dependent inflammation after skin injury. Nat Med 15: 1377–1382.
2. Fitzgerald RJ, Morhart RE, Marquez C, Adams BO (1986) Inhibition of caries in hamsters treated with staphylococcin 1580. Infect Immun 54: 288–290.

3. Sahl HG, Ersfeld-Dressen H, Bierbaum G, Josten M, Kordel M, et al. (1987) Different mechanisms of insensitivity to the staphylococcin-like peptide Pep 5. Zentralbl Bakteriol Mikrobiol Hyg A 267: 173–185.
4. Cogen AL, Yamasaki K, Sanchez KM, Dorschner RA, Lai Y, et al. Selective antimicrobial action is provided by phenol-soluble modulins derived from Staphylococcus epidermidis, a normal resident of the skin. J Invest Dermatol 130: 192–200.
5. Lai Y, Cogen AL, Radek KA, Park HJ, Macleod DT, et al. (2010) Activation of TLR2 by a small molecule produced by Staphylococcus epidermidis increases antimicrobial defense against bacterial skin infections. J Invest Dermatol 130: 2211–2221.
6. Tally FP, DeBruin MF (2000) Development of daptomycin for gram-positive infections. J Antimicrob Chemother 46: 523–526.
7. Klich MA, Arthur KS, Lax AR, Bland JM (1994) Iturin A: a potential new fungicide for stored grains. Mycopathologia 127: 123–127.
8. Vanittanakom N, Loeffler W, Koch U, Jung G (1986) Fengycin–a novel antifungal lipopeptide antibiotic produced by Bacillus subtilis F-29-3. J Antibiot (Tokyo) 39: 888–901.
9. Dixon RA, Chopra I (1986) Polymyxin B and polymyxin B nonapeptide alter cytoplasmic membrane permeability in Escherichia coli. J Antimicrob Chemother 18: 557–563.
10. Li J, Jensen SE (2008) Nonribosomal biosynthesis of fusaricidins by Paenibacillus polymyxa PKB1 involves direct activation of a D-amino acid. Chem Biol 15: 118–127.
11. Harder J, Bartels J, Christophers E, Schroder JM (2001) Isolation and characterization of human beta -defensin-3, a novel human inducible peptide antibiotic. J Biol Chem 276: 5707–5713.
12. Harder J, Bartels J, Christophers E, Schroder JM (1997) A peptide antibiotic from human skin. Nature 387: 861.
13. Schroder NW, Morath S, Alexander C, Hamann L, Hartung T, et al. (2003) Lipoteichoic acid (LTA) of Streptococcus pneumoniae and Staphylococcus aureus activates immune cells via Toll-like receptor (TLR)-2, lipopolysaccharide-binding protein (LBP), and CD14, whereas TLR-4 and MD-2 are not involved. J Biol Chem 278: 15587–15594.
14. Sumikawa Y, Asada H, Hoshino K, Azukizawa H, Katayama I, et al. (2006) Induction of beta-defensin 3 in keratinocytes stimulated by bacterial lipopeptides through toll-like receptor 2. Microbes Infect 8: 1513–1521.
15. Vasselon T, Hanlon WA, Wright SD, Detmers PA (2002) Toll-like receptor 2 (TLR2) mediates activation of stress-activated MAP kinase p38. J Leukoc Biol 71: 503–510.
16. Kanda N, Watanabe S (2008) Leptin enhances human beta-defensin-2 production in human keratinocytes. Endocrinology 149: 5189–5198.
17. Lan CC, Wu CS, Huang SM, Kuo HY, Wu IH, et al. High-Glucose Environment Inhibits p38MAPK Signaling and Reduces Human beta-Defensin-3 Expression [corrected] in Keratinocytes. Mol Med 17: 771–779.
18. Evans CA, Smith WM, Johnston EA, Giblett ER (1950) Bacterial flora of the normal human skin. J Invest Dermatol 15: 305–324.
19. Marples MJ (1969) The normal flora of the human skin. Br J Dermatol 81: Suppl 1: 2–13.
20. Okada H, Kuhn C, Feillet H, Bach JF (2010) The 'hygiene hypothesis' for autoimmune and allergic diseases: an update. Clin Exp Immunol 160: 1–9.
21. Costello EK, Lauber CL, Hamady M, Fierer N, Gordon JI, et al. (2009) Bacterial community variation in human body habitats across space and time. Science 326: 1694–1697.
22. Qin J, Li R, Raes J, Arumugam M, Burgdorf KS, et al. (2010) A human gut microbial gene catalogue established by metagenomic sequencing. Nature 464: 59–65.
23. Hormannsperger G, Clavel T, Haller D (2012) Gut matters: microbe-host interactions in allergic diseases. J Allergy Clin Immunol 129: 1452–1459.
24. Wanke I, Steffen H, Christ C, Krismer B, Gotz F, et al. Skin commensals amplify the innate immune response to pathogens by activation of distinct signaling pathways. J Invest Dermatol 131: 382–390.
25. Guo Y, Huang E, Yuan C, Zhang L, Yousef AE Isolation of a Paenibacillus sp. strain and structural elucidation of its broad-spectrum lipopeptide antibiotic. Appl Environ Microbiol 78: 3156–3165.
26. Kim PI, Bai H, Bai D, Chae H, Chung S, et al. (2004) Purification and characterization of a lipopeptide produced by Bacillus thuringiensis CMB26. J Appl Microbiol 97: 942–949.
27. Baranova IN, Kurlander R, Bocharov AV, Vishnyakova TG, Chen Z, et al. (2008) Role of human CD36 in bacterial recognition, phagocytosis, and pathogen-induced JNK-mediated signaling. J Immunol 181: 7147–7156.
28. Bjorkbacka H (2006) Multiple roles of Toll-like receptor signaling in atherosclerosis. Curr Opin Lipidol 17: 527–533.
29. Hoebe K, Georgel P, Rutschmann S, Du X, Mudd S, et al. (2005) CD36 is a sensor of diacylglycerides. Nature 433: 523–527.
30. Stuart LM, Deng J, Silver JM, Takahashi K, Tseng AA, et al. (2005) Response to Staphylococcus aureus requires CD36-mediated phagocytosis triggered by the COOH-terminal cytoplasmic domain. J Cell Biol 170: 477–485.
31. Reed-Geaghan EG, Savage JC, Hise AG, Landreth GE (2009) CD14 and toll-like receptors 2 and 4 are required for fibrillar A{beta}-stimulated microglial activation. J Neurosci 29: 11982–11992.
32. Nilsen NJ, Deininger S, Nonstad U, Skjeldal F, Husebye H, et al. (2008) Cellular trafficking of lipoteichoic acid and Toll-like receptor 2 in relation to signaling: role of CD14 and CD36. J Leukoc Biol 84: 280–291.

16

Natural History of Cutaneous Human Papillomavirus (HPV) Infection in Men: The HIM Study

Shalaka S. Hampras[1], Anna R. Giuliano[1], Hui-Yi Lin[2], Kate J. Fisher[2], Martha E. Abrahamsen[1], Bradley A. Sirak[1], Michelle R. Iannacone[3], Tarik Gheit[4], Massimo Tommasino[4], Dana E. Rollison[1]*

1 Department of Cancer Epidemiology, Moffitt Cancer Center, Tampa, Florida, United States of America, **2** Department of Biostatistics, Moffitt Cancer Center, Tampa, Florida, United States of America, **3** QIMR Berghofer Medical Research Institute, Cancer and Population Studies, Royal Brisbane Hospital, Brisbane, Queensland, Australia, **4** Infections and Cancer Biology Group, International Agency for Research on Cancer-World Health Organization, Lyon, France

Abstract

Accumulating evidence suggests that cutaneous human papillomavirus (HPV) infection is associated with non-melanoma skin cancer (NMSC). Little is known about the natural history of cutaneous HPV. A sub-cohort of 209 men with no NMSC history, initially enrolled in the HPV infection in men (HIM) study, were followed for a median of 12.6 months. Epidemiological data were collected through self-administered questionnaires. Cutaneous HPV DNA was measured in normal skin swabs (SS) and eyebrow hairs (EB) for 25 and 16 HPV types in genera β and γ, respectively. Any β HPV infection was more prevalent in SS (67.3%) compared to EB (56.5%, $p = 0.04$). Incidence in SS was higher than 20 per 1,000 person-months for HPV types 4, 5, 23, 38 and 76. Median duration of persistence of β and γ HPV infection was 8.6 and 6.1 months in EB, respectively, and 11.3 months and 6.3 months, in SS, respectively. Older age (>44 years vs. 18-30 years) was significantly associated with prevalent (SS OR = 3.0, 95% CI = 1.2–7.0) and persistent β HPV infection (EB OR = 6.1, 95% CI = 2.6–14.1). History of blistering sunburn was associated with prevalent (OR = 2.8, 95% CI = 1.3–5.8) and persistent (OR = 2.3, 95% CI = 1.2–4.6) β HPV infection in SS. Cutaneous HPV is highly prevalent in men, with age and blistering sunburn being significant risk factors for cutaneous β HPV infection.

Editor: Robert D. Burk, Albert Einstein College of Medicine, United States of America

Funding: This work was supported by the National Cancer Institute at the National Institutes of Health (RO1CA098803 and R25 CA078447 to C.M. Nielson). The funders had no role in study design, data collection and analysis, decision to publish, or preparation of the manuscript.

Competing Interests: The authors have declared that no competing interests exist.

* Email: dana.rollison@moffitt.org

Introduction

Human papillomavirus (HPV) is a non-enveloped DNA virus, primarily infecting stratified epithelium [1,2]. HPV infections are broadly classified as mucosal (α genus) or cutaneous (α, β, γ, μ, Nv genera) [3]. An etiologic role for mucosal HPV infection has been established for several cancers, including penile [4] and cervical [5,6] as well as a subset of head and neck cancers [7]. In the majority of cervical cancers, viral DNA integrates into the host genome, further facilitating the transformation of infected cells [8,9]. Accumulating evidence suggests that, infection with cutaneous HPV types is associated with increased risk of non-melanoma skin cancer (NMSC), in both immunocompetent and immunocompromised individuals [10–12], perhaps through an indirect mechanism. For example, inhibition of ultraviolet radiation induced apoptosis has been suggested as a potential mechanism of carcinogenic activity of cutaneous HPV [13,14].

The earliest evidence for oncogenic potential of β HPV types came from studies by Jablonska and colleagues, in 1972, which demonstrated the presence of β HPV types in cutaneous lesions of patients suffering from Epidermodysplasia Verruciformis (EV) [15], a rare hereditary skin disease that often progresses to squamous cell carcinoma (SCC) of skin in solar exposed areas. Cutaneous HPV DNA has been detected in eyebrow hairs, normal skin samples as well as tumor tissues from NMSC cases [16]. Several studies have reported a positive association between cutaneous HPV DNA and/or seropositivity and NMSC [17–20]. Despite its potential role in the development of SCC, very little is known about the natural history of cutaneous HPV infection. This information is essential to further elucidate the role of cutaneous HPV in skin cancer and also to guide future preventive measures targeted at reducing the burden of cutaneous HPV infection.

Few studies have evaluated the prevalence and persistence of cutaneous HPV among healthy individuals. Cutaneous HPV is thought to be ubiquitous in skin, with hair follicles serving as the reservoirs of persistent HPV infection [21,22]. High prevalence of cutaneous HPV in skin of infants and young children, indicates that exposure to HPV occurs very early in life [23], with asymptomatic infection persisting for several years [24]. Prevalence rates ranging from 42% in African population to 70% in European and Asian populations have been reported among healthy adults [25]. Prevalence of over 90% have been reported among immunocompromised patients [22].

Table 1. Baseline characteristics of 209 male participants in the humanpapilloma virus infection (HIM) Study, Tampa, Florida.

Variable	n (%)
Age	
18–30	108 (51.7)
31–44	44 (21.0)
45+	57 (27.3)
Self-Identified Race	
White	155 (74.5)
Other	53 (25.5)
Spanish/Hispanic/Latino	
No	177 (84.7)
Yes	32 (15.3)
Marital status	
Single, Never Married or Divorced/Separated	148 (70.8)
Married or Cohabiting, Living Together	61 (29.2)
Highest level of education	
High school or below	38 (18.2)
Vocational school/Some college	110 (52.6)
Graduated college/Graduate school	61 (29.2)
Skin reaction to season's first sun exposure	
No change in skin color	37 (17.9)
Tan with no sunburn	53 (25.6)
Mild sunburn that becomes a tan	80 (38.6)
Sunburn	37 (17.9)
Ever had a blistering sunburn	
No	103 (49.7)
Yes	104 (50.2)
Lifetime number of blistering sunburns	
None	103 (49.7)
1	38 (18.3)
2	28 (13.5)
3+	38 (18.3)
Had an alcoholic beverage in the past month	
No	35 (16.7)
Yes	174 (83.3)
Number of days drank in past month	
0	35 (19.9)
1–8	81 (46.0)
9+	60 (34.1)
Current smoker	
No	176 (84.2)
Yes	33 (15.8)
Ever smoker	
No	123 (59.4)
Yes	84 (40.6)
Smoking status	
Never	123 (59.4)
Former	51 (24.6)
Current	33 (15.9)
Ever been diagnosed with an STD	
No	180 (86.1)
Yes	29 (13.9)

Table 1. Cont.

Variable	n (%)
Lifetime female vaginal sex partners	
0–1	42 (20.1)
2–9	61 (30.6)
10+	96 (48.2)
Female vaginal sex partners in past 6 months	
None	53 (25.6)
1	105 (50.7)
2+	49 (23.7)
Lifetime male anal-sex partners	
None	158 (90.3)
1+	17 (9.7)
Male anal-sex partners in the past 3 months	
None	182 (98.9)
1+	2 (1.09)

In this study, we describe the natural history of cutaneous HPV infection in a cohort of 209 healthy men in Tampa, Florida. We evaluated a spectrum of epidemiological measures including risk factors associated with prevalence, persistence and incidence across two genera of cutaneous HPV infection. We observed that cutaneous HPV is highly prevalent in men and that, age and blistering sunburn are significant risk factors for cutaneous β HPV infection in men.

Material and Methods

Study population

The study population for the current analysis comprises a sub-cohort of men who participated in the U.S. site of the HPV infection in men (HIM) study, a large, multi-national prospective cohort study of the natural history of HPV infection in men [26,27]. The HIM study methods have been described in detail previously [26,27]. Briefly, between July 2005 and September 2009, study participants were recruited to the HIM study in Tampa, Florida, through mass advertisement targeted to university students, faculty, staff and members of the general population. Inclusion criteria were: 1) men aged 18–70 years; 2) reside in Florida; 3) have had no prior diagnosis of penile or anal cancers; 4) have never been diagnosed with genital and/or anal warts; 5) have not participated in an HPV vaccine study; 6) have no prior diagnosis of HIV/AIDS; 7) have no current penile discharge or burning during urination; 8) were not currently being treated for an STD; 9) have not been imprisoned or homeless during last 6 months; and 10) had not been in a drug or alcohol treatment program over the last 6 months at enrollment. Between November 2008 and June 2010, 1,082 participants in the HIM study were invited to participate in a supplemental study of the natural history of cutaneous HPV infection, requiring additional biospecimen collection. In the parent HIM study, the participants were followed every six months up to four years of follow-up. Nine hundred and sixty seven men enrolled in the parent HIM study had at least one sample of eyebrow hair or skin swab at their baseline visit. Of these 967 men, 965 men (99.8%) had three samples (one sample of eyebrow hair and one skin swab sample each, from sun exposed and unexposed skin), at their baseline visit. 89.4% and 66.7% men had all three samples at two and three visits, respectively. In order to maximize our observation time and facilitate estimation of incidence and persistence, the sub-study was restricted to those men who had all three samples for at least 4 visits (n = 211). Of these, 209 men had viable samples and were included in the final analysis.

Ethics statement

Written informed consent was obtained from all participants in the parent study, and a separate addendum to the consent was completed by all participants in the sub-study. The parent study and sub-study protocols were approved by institutional review boards at each recruiting site, including the Human Subjects Committees of the University of South Florida, the Ludwig Institute for Cancer Research, São Paulo, Brazil, the Centro de Referencia e Tratamento de Doencas Sexualmente Transmissiveis e AIDS, Brazil, and the National Institute of Public Health of Mexico, as described previously [27].

Data collection

Questionnaires. At the enrollment visit, HIM study participants completed a comprehensive self-administered questionnaire with information on demographics (age, race, education, and marital status), socioeconomic status, medical history, smoking status, alcohol consumption, and sexual history. Additional questions on risk factors for skin cancer (skin's reaction to season's first sun exposure, history of blistering sunburn, etc.) were added to the cutaneous HPV sub-study.

Eyebrow hairs and swabs of normal skin. Although, in the parent HIM study, swabs from both sun exposed and unexposed skin were collected, only swabs from sun-exposed skin were used for HPV DNA measurement in the present sub-study due to limited funding. A 5×5 cm area of normal, sun exposed skin, from the top of forearm, was pre-wetted (0.9% NaCl) and swabbed back and forth five times using a cotton-tipped Dacron swab (Digene, Gaithersburg, MD, USA). All swabs were placed in a separate vial and preserved in 500 µl Digene Standard Transport Medium (STM) for HPV DNA testing. Three to four hairs were plucked from each eyebrow (6–8 eyebrow hairs per individual) using disposable tweezers. Hairs with attached follicles

Table 2. Prevalence, incidence and persistence of type-specific cutaneous HPV infection at baseline in eyebrow hairs and normal skin swabs of men residing in Tampa, Florida.

	Eyebrow hairs					Normal skin swabs				
HPV type	Prevalence n (%) HPV positive[a]	Incident Cases**	Incidence per 1000 person months	Persistent cases	Persistence[§§]%	Prevalence n (%) HPV positive[a]	Incident cases**	Incidence per 1000 person months	Persistent cases	Persistence§§ %
Any β*	118 (56.5)	40	37.49	71	48.3	105 (67.3)	50	85.01	95	63.8
β_1*	63 (30.1)	43	22.74	41	46.1	72 (46.2)	91	56.95	65	57.5
5*	16 (7.7)	17	6.39	10	43.5	27 (17.3)	42	22.02	21	47.7
8	14 (6.7)	6	2.2	8	42.1	7 (4.5)	21	9	5	62.5
12*	20 (9.6)	11	4.16	14	56.0	31 (19.9)	38	19.53	20	50.0
14	5 (2.4)	4	1.39	1	20.0	6 (3.8)	23	9.96	4	33.3
19	6 (2.9)	4	1.41	1	11.1	4 (2.6)	12	5.11	4	44.4
20	10 (4.8)	9	3.25	6	35.3	5 (3.2)	22	9.54	9	60.0
21*	7 (3.3)	6	2.13	4	33.3	12 (7.7)	27	12.43	13	52.0
24*	17 (8.1)	12	4.58	11	42.3	25 (16)	33	16.72	13	34.2
25	2 (1)	1	0.34	2	66.7	2 (1.3)	7	2.95	5	71.4
36	7 (3.3)	8	2.84	4	36.4	10 (6.4)	15	6.62	4	26.7
47	7 (3.3)	4	1.42	6	66.7	9 (5.8)	15	6.7	8	53.3
93	9 (4.3)	4	1.44	5	41.7	10 (6.4)	22	9.83	7	36.8
β_2	83 (39.7)	38	24.05	49	44.1	69 (44.2)	95	60.07	57	50.9
9	12 (5.7)	4	1.45	6	40.0	10 (6.4)	32	14.63	6	27.3
15	8 (3.8)	1	0.35	5	55.6	11 (7.1)	15	6.72	7	46.7
17	13 (6.2)	6	2.21	10	52.6	16 (10.3)	34	16.22	11	36.7
22	17 (8.1)	10	3.76	9	37.5	10 (6.4)	29	12.94	9	50.0
23	28 (13.4)	14	5.68	13	35.1	13 (8.3)	48	23.01	16	51.6
37	15 (7.2)	10	3.75	11	45.8	14 (9)	34	15.49	14	66.7
38	32 (15.3)	18	7.57	16	34.8	22 (14.1)	44	22.35	19	44.2
80	7 (3.3)	16	5.77	4	23.5	8 (5.1)	27	12.02	7	38.9
β_3	36 (17.2)	12	5.06	18	40.0	28 (17.9)	61	24.62	25	65.8
49	5 (2.4)	2	0.7	0	0.0	2 (1.3)	9	3.75	1	33.3
75	6 (2.9)	5	1.76	1	11.1	6 (3.8)	11	4.64	2	40.0
76	29 (13.9)	7	2.83	17	48.6	23 (14.7)	44	21.67	23	63.9
β_4 (92)	2 (1)	3	1.04	1	25.0	3 (1.9)	5	2.1	3	50.0
β_5 (96)	7 (3.3)	3	1.07	3	30.0	4 (2.6)	16	6.81	3	42.9
Any □[b]*	33(15.9)	30	13.02	16	30	56(26.8)	90	49.77	49	51
4*	13(6.2)	16	5.92	5	23	28(13.4)	65	28.49	24	45
48	1(0.5)	2	0.68	1	50	0(0)	14	4.96	2	50
50	13(6.2)	7	2.58	9	45	15(7.2)	32	12.54	15	52

Table 2. Cont.

HPV type	Eyebrow hairs					Normal skin swabs				
	Prevalence n (%) HPV positive[a]	Incident Cases**	Incidence per 1000 person months	Persistent cases	Persistence[§§]%	Prevalence n (%) HPV positive[a]	Incident cases**	Incidence per 1000 person months	Persistent cases	Persistence§§ %
60	0(0)	1	0.34	0	0	0(0)	1	0.35	0	-
65	3(1.4)	10	3.46	1	13	7(3.3)	32	11.94	6	35
88	2(1)	0	0	0	0	2(1)	2	0.71	0	-
95	1(0.5)	0	0	0	0	2(1)	1	0.35	0	-
108	0	0	0	0	-	0	3	1.05	1	100
112	2(1)	0	0	1	50	3(1.4)	7	2.52	4	50
116	0(0)	1	0.34	0	-	3(1.4)	2	0.71	0	-
121	3(1.4)	1	0.34	2	50	7(3.3)	5	1.81	3	38
123	4(1.9)	2	0.69	1	20	5(2.4)	26	9.51	2	18

[a]Total numbers of men with valid baseline samples that were tested for HPV: n = 209 and n = 208 eyebrow hairs for β and γ HPV testing, respectively, and n = 156 and n = 209 skin swabs from sun-exposed skin for β and γ HPV testing, respectively.
*Statistically significant difference based on McNemar's exact test ($p<0.05$).
[b]γ HPV types 101, 103, 108, 109 and 119 were measured in skin and eyebrow hairs but were not detected in our population at baseline.
**Only for men who tested negative for any or type-specific HPV infection at baseline.
[§§]out of men who were positive for any or type-specific HPV infection at the first of two or more consecutive visits. γ HPV types 101, 103, 109, 119 were not detected in skin and eyebrow hair. γ HPV types 88 and 95 were not detected in eyebrow hairs but were detected in skin swabs of 2 and 1 incident infections, respectively.

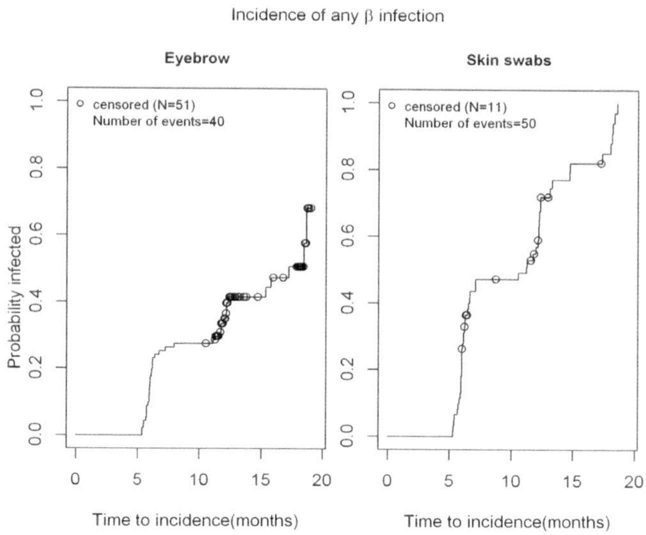

Figure 1. Time to incidence of β-HPV infection in normal skin swabs and eyebrow hairs of men. Kaplan Meier estimate for time to incidence of any β HPV infection in a sample of 209 men. Participants who were negative for all HPV types at baseline were included. Time was counted until their first visit with a HPV positive sample or until censored. The 'last observation carried forward' approach was taken when counting time to incidence (e.g. 0 NA 1 pattern of HPV positivity at consecutive visits, the NA was treated as '0' and the time was counted in the time to incidence.). This only affected skin swab samples since most people were β globin or HPV positive for eyebrows and thus their samples were not removed.

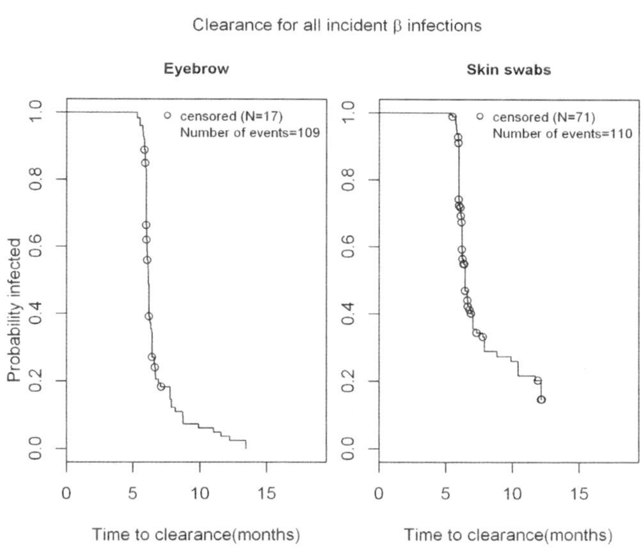

Figure 2. Time to clearance of β-HPV infection in normal skin swabs and eyebrow hairs of men. Kaplan Meier estimate for time to clearance for all type-specific incident infections a study participant (n = 209) had before their last visit with a valid sample. The 'last observation carried forward' approach was taken when counting time to clearance (e.g. for 0 1 NA 0 pattern of HPV positivity, the NA was treated as '1' and the time was counted towards the time to clearance). This only affected skin swab samples since most people were β globin or HPV positive for eyebrows and thus their samples were not removed.

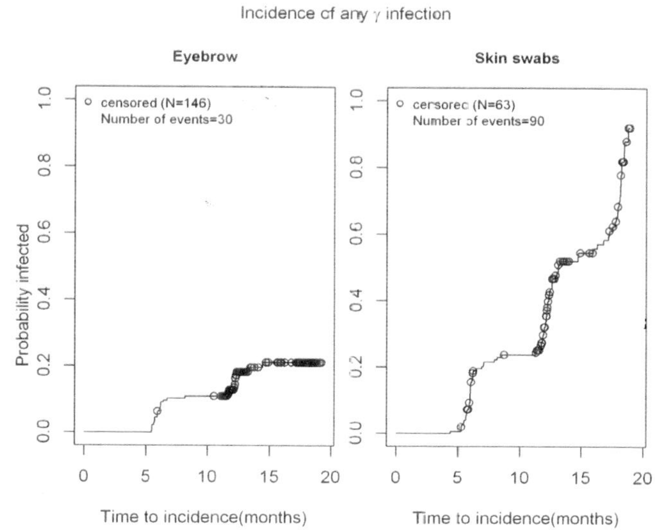

Figure 3. Time to incidence of γ-HPV infection in normal skin swabs and eyebrow hairs of men. Kaplan Meier estimate for time to incidence of any β HPV infection in a sample of 209 men. Participants who were negative for all HPV types at baseline were included. Time was counted until their first visit with a HPV positive sample or until censored. The 'last observation carried forward' approach was taken when counting time to incidence (e.g. 0 NA 1 pattern of HPV positivity at consecutive visits, the NA was treated as '0' and the time was counted in the time to incidence.).

were snap frozen in liquid nitrogen. All tissues were stored at −70°C until testing for cutaneous HPV DNA.

DNA extraction from skin swabs and eyebrow hair. DNA extraction was performed at the International

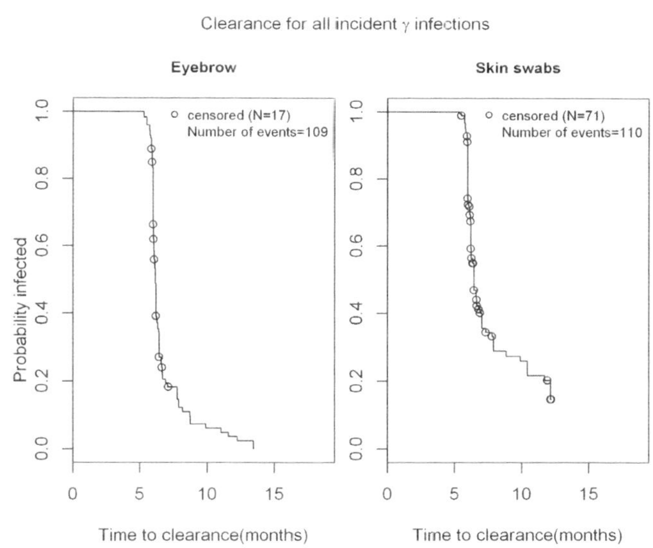

Figure 4. Time to clearance of γ-HPV infection in normal skin swabs and eyebrow hairs of men. Kaplan Meier estimate for time to clearance for all type-specific incident infections a study participant (n = 209) had before their last visit with a valid sample. The 'last observation carried forward' approach was taken when counting time to clearance (e.g. for 0 1 NA 0 pattern of HPV positivity, the NA was treated as '1' and the time was counted towards the time to clearance).

Table 3. Associations between baseline characteristics and genus β HPV prevalence in eyebrow hairs and normal skin swabs of men residing in Tampa, Florida.

	Eyebrow hairs			Normal skin swabs		
Variable	**Total (n = 209)**	**Any β infection (n = 118) n (%)**	**Age adjusted OR (95 %CI)**	**Total (n = 156)**	**Any β infection (n = 105) n (%)**	**Age adjusted OR (95 %CI)**
Age*						
18–30	108	52 (48.1)	1.0 (reference)	72	44 (61.1)	1.0 (reference)
31–44	44	27 (61.4)	1.7 (0.84–3.5)	33	19 (57.6)	0.9 (0.37–2)
>44	57	39 (68.4)	**2.3 (1.2–4.6)**	51	42 (82.4)	**3.0 (1.2–7.0)**
Race						
White	155	87 (56.1)	1.0 (reference)	115	78 (67.8)	1.0 (reference)
Other	53	30 (56.6)	1.1 (0.6–2.0)	40	26 (65.0)	0.9 (0.4–2.0)
Spanish/Hispanic/Latino						
No	177	99 (55.9)	1.0 (reference)	132	89 (67.4)	1.0 (reference)
Yes	32	19 (59.4)	1.3 (0.6–2.9)	24	16 (66.7)	1.2 (0.4–3.0)
Marital status						
Single, Never Married or Divorced/Separated	148	82 (55.4)	1.0 (reference)	106	66 (62.3)	1.0 (reference)
Married or Cohabiting, Living Together	61	36 (59)	0.9 (0.5–1.7)	50	39 (78)	1.9 (0.9–4.4)
Highest level of education						
High school or below	38	26 (68.4)	1.0 (reference)	28	17 (60.7)	1.0 (reference)
Vocational school/Some college	110	59 (53.6)	0.6 (0.3–1.4)	81	57 (70.4)	1.8 (0.7–4.5)
Graduated college/Graduate school	61	33 (54.1)	0.4 (0.9–1.0)	47	31 (66.0)	1.0 (0.4–2.8)
Skin reaction to season's first sun exposure						
No change in skin color	37	20 (54.1)	1.0 (reference)	30	24 (80)	1.0 (reference)
Tan with no sunburn	53	26 (49.1)	1.0 (0.4–2.2)	41	28 (68.3)	0.6 (0.2–1.9)
Mild sunburn that becomes a tan	80	46 (57.5)	1.2 (0.6–2.7)	62	36 (58.1)	0.4 (0.1–1.0)
Sunburn	37	25 (67.6)	1.7 (0.7–4.6)	21	17 (81)	0.9 (0.2–3.9)
Ever had a blistering sunburn						
No	103	54 (52.4)	1.0 (reference)	78	45 (57.7)	1.0 (reference)
Yes	104	63 (60.6)	1.3 (0.8–2.4)	76	60 (78.9)	**2.8 (1.3–5.8)**
Lifetime number of blistering sunburns						
None	103	54 (52.4)	1.0 (reference)	78	45 (57.7)	1.0 (reference)
1	38	24 (63.2)	1.7 (0.8–3.7)	27	21 (77.8)	3.0 (1.0–8.4)
2	28	16 (57.1)	1.2(0.5–2.9)	23	17 (73.9)	2.3 (0.8–6.8)
>2	38	23 (60.5)	1.1 (0.5–2.5)	26	22 (84.6)	3.2 (0.9–10.9)
Had an alcoholic beverage in the past month						
No	35	19 (54.3)	1.0 (reference)	27	18 (66.7)	1.0 (reference)
Yes	174	99 (56.9)	1.1(0.5–2.4)	129	87 (67.4)	1.2 (0.5–2.9)
Number of days drank alcohol in past month						
0	35	19 (54.3)	1.0 (reference)	27	18 (66.7)	1.0 (reference)
1–8	81	48 (59.3)	1.3 (0.6–3.0)	57	39 (68.4)	1.3 (0.4–3.6)
9+	60	31 (51.7)	0.9 (0.4–2.1)	43	30 (69.8)	1.4 (0.5–4.2)
Current smoker						
No	176	96 (54.5)	1.0 (reference)	131	89 (67.9)	1.0 (reference)
Yes	33	22 (66.7)	1.4 (0.6–3.1)	25	16 (64)	0.7(0.3–1.9)
Ever smoker						
No	123	64 (52)	1.0 (reference)	88	59 (67)	1.0 (reference)
Yes	84	53 (63.1)	1.2 (0.7–2.3)	67	45 (67.2)	0.7 (0.3–1.6)
Smoking status						
Never	123	64 (52)	1.0 (reference)	88	59 (67)	1.0 (reference)

Table 3. Cont.

	Eyebrow hairs			Normal skin swabs		
Variable	**Total (n = 209)**	**Any β infection (n = 118) n (%)**	**Age adjusted OR (95 %CI)**	**Total (n = 156)**	**Any β infection (n = 105) n (%)**	**Age adjusted OR (95 %CI)**
Former	51	31 (60.8)	1.1 (0.6–2.3)	42	29 (69)	0.8 (0.3–1.9)
Current	33	22 (66.7)	1.5 (0.6–3.4)	25	16 (64)	0.7 (0.2–1.9)
Ever been diagnosed with an STD						
No	180	98 (54.4)	1.0 (reference)	131	87 (66.4)	1.0 (reference)
Yes	29	20 (69)	1.4 (0.6–3.4)	25	18 (72)	0.9 (0.3–2.6)
Lifetime female vaginal sex partners						
0–1	42	23 (54.8)	1.0 (reference)	27	16 (59.3)	1.0 (reference)
2–9	61	37 (60.7)	1.1 (0.5–2.5)	40	29 (72.5)	1.6 (0.5–4.5)
10+	96	56 (58.3)	0.6 (0.2–1.4)	82	57 (69.5)	0.9 (0.3–2.7)
Female vaginal sex partners in past 6 months						
None	53	28 (52.8)	1.0 (reference)	38	27 (71.1)	1.0 (reference)
1	105	65 (61.9)	1.6 (0.8–3.2)	81	63 (77.8)	1.7 (0.7–4.1)
2+	49	25 (51)	1.2 (0.5–2.8)	35	15 (42.9)	0.4 (0.1–1.2)
Lifetime male anal-sex partners						
None	158	88 (55.7)	1.0 (reference)	118	81 (68.6)	1.0 (reference)
1+	17	12 (70.6)	1.7 (0.6–5.2)	14	10 (71.4)	1.1 (0.3–4.0)

OR = odds ratio, CI = confidence interval. *Unadjusted logistic regression. All analyses, except for age, were adjusted for age using logistic regression.

Agency for Research on Cancer in Lyon, France, using the Qiagen BioRobot EZ1 with the EZ1 DNA tissue kit according to the manufacturer's instructions (Qiagen, Hilden, Germany). Briefly, the Dacron swabs were carefully cut into an Eppendorf tube using scissors and incubated overnight in proteinase K and buffer G2 (Qiagen, Hilden, Germany) at 56°C. An EZ1 DNA Forensic protocol was used to extract the DNA from eyebrow hairs according to the manufacturer's instructions. To monitor the possible occurrence of cross-contamination between the different specimens during DNA extraction, tubes containing buffer only were also included (one tube with buffer every ten specimens).

Viral DNA detection using Multiplex PCR/Luminex assay. The detection of viral DNA was performed by a multiplex PCR/Luminex assay [28], followed by the HPV typing using Luminex beads coupled with β or γ HPV type-specific probes. The assay was performed using approximately 100 ng of total DNA and specific primers amplifying a part of the E7 gene for 25 HPV types in genus β (5, 8, 9, 12, 14, 15, 17, 19, 20, 21, 22, 23, 24, 25, 36, 37, 38, 47, 49, 75, 76, 80, 92, 93, 96) and 16 HPV types in genus γ (4,48,50, 60, 65, 88, 95, 101, 103,108,109, 112,116,119,121,123) [28,29]. Although, a large number of HPV types are being continually discovered, a limited coverage of HPV types was offered in the multiplex assay. Two primers for the amplification of β-globin were included in the assay to provide a positive control for the quality of the template DNA. The positivity of the assay was given by the intensity of the fluorescent signal detected by the Luminex apparatus and was expressed as the median fluorescence intensity (MFI) of at least 100 beads per bead set. The cutoff was calculated for each HPV-specific probe by considering the MFI values obtained with no respective PCR product. The cutoff was computed by adding 5 MFI to 1.1× the median background value, as described by Schmitt et al. [30]. All MFI values above the cut-off have been considered positive. PCR was performed with the QIAGEN multiplex PCR kit according to the instructions of the manufacturer. This multiplex PCR protocol is highly sensitive, being able to detect only 10 copies of the viral genome [28,29]. HPV genotyping was successfully repeated in a blind manner, three times in 10 individual subjects, demonstrating reliability of multiplex PCR for detection of specific HPV types [28]. Similar strategy was used for determining the sensitivity and specificity of γ HPV assay, showing features similar to those of the β HPV assay.

Following PCR amplification, 10 μL of each reaction was analyzed by multiplex genotyping using a Luminex based assay as described [31]. Results were expressed as the median fluorescence intensity (MFI) of at least 100 beads per bead set. Of the 1,385 samples, 1,234 (89%) were β-globin positive. Thirty (2%) β-globin negative and HPV positive samples were included, while 120 (9%) β-globin negative and HPV negative samples were excluded from the analyses. All the tubes containing buffer only were tested negative for HPV DNA and β globin.

Statistical analysis

Baseline characteristics, including demographics, skin cancer risk factors, lifestyle factors and history of sexually transmitted diseases, were summarized for the cohort using descriptive statistics. HPV prevalence in eyebrow hairs and normal skin swabs was estimated by phylogenetic species along with concurrent infections with other HPV types. Type-specific prevalence of HPV was defined as the proportion of men who were positive for a given HPV out of the baseline cohort with valid samples. Genus- and species-specific prevalence was defined as the proportion of men who were positive for at least one HPV type in the given genus or species. The statistical significance of differences in the prevalence of HPV infection between eyebrow hairs and normal skin swabs was tested using Fisher's exact test. Incidence (in

Table 4. Association between baseline characteristics and prevalence of species-specific HPV infection in men residing in Tampa, Florida.

	Eyebrow hairs		Skin swabs	
	β1 positive n = 63 Age Adjusted OR (95% CI)*	**β2 positive n = 83 Age Adjusted OR (95% CI)***	**β1 positive n = 72 Age Adjusted OR (95% CI)**	**β2 positive n = 69 Age Adjusted OR (95% CI)**
Age				
18–30	1.0(reference)	1.0(reference)	1.0(reference)	1.0(reference)
31–44	1.8 (0.8–4.1)	1.7 (0.8–3.8)	1.0 (0.4–2.4)	1 (0.4–2.5)
>44	**2.7 (1.3–6.0)**	**2.4 (1.2–5.0)**	**3.1 (1.2–7.7)**	**3.6 (1.4–9.0)**
Skin reaction to season's first sun exposure				
No change in skin color	-	-	1.0(reference)	1.0(reference)
Tan with no sunburn	-	-	0.7 (0.2–2.4)	0.4 (0.1–1.4)
Mild sunburn that becomes a tan	-	-	0.4(0.1–1.1)	0.4 (0.1–1.3)
Sunburn			1.0 (0.2–4.5)	0.8 (0.2–3.9)
Ever had a blistering sunburn				
No	1.0(reference)	1.0(reference)	1.0(reference)	1.0(reference)
Yes	1.3 (0.69–2.6)	1.3 (0.7–2.4)	**2.6 (1.2–5.7)**	**3.1 (1.4–7.0)**
Lifetime number of blistering sunburns				
None	1.0(reference)	1.0(reference)	1.0(reference)	1.0(reference)
1	1.6 (0.6–4.1)	1.4 (0.6–3.4)	2.5 (0.8–7.7)	2.7 (0.8–8.5)
2	1.9 (0.8–5.0)	1.0 (0.4–2.6)	2.6 (0.9–8.0)	2.3 (0.7–7.4)
>2	0.7 (0.2–2.0)	1.4 (0.6–3.1)	2.7 (0.7–10.0)	5.0 (1.4–17.7)
Female vaginal sex partners in past 6 months				
None	-	-	1.0(reference)	1.0(reference)
1	-	-	1.9 (0.7–5.1)	1.6(0.6–4.3)
2+	-	-	0.5 (0.1–1.4)	0.4 (0.1–1.2)

OR = odds ratio, CI = confidence interval. These factors were selected based on significance in the multinomial logistic regression models.

person-months) was determined for any HPV infection, as well as type-specific and species-specific HPV infections in normal skin swabs or eyebrow hairs. For analyses of incidence of any HPV infection, the participant had to be negative for all HPV types (genus β or γ) at baseline, and only the first incidence of any HPV infection was taken into account. Similarly, for species-specific and type-specific HPV infections, the participant had to be negative at baseline for that particular HPV species or type, respectively. Time to incidence of HPV infection was defined as interval, in months, between baseline visit and first visit with a positive HPV sample or time point being censored. Due to fewer events, median time to incidence of γ HPV infection in eyebrow hairs could not be estimated. Time to clearance of HPV infection was defined as interval (in months) between incident HPV infection and clearance of all type-specific HPV infections.

Persistence of any HPV (genus β or γ) or type-specific HPV was defined as any or type-specific HPV infection at ≥2 consecutive visits. For a given type of HPV persistence, only participants who were positive for the HPV genus or type and had at least one follow-up visit after that were included. Kappa coefficient (k) was used to determine the concordance of viral infections across eyebrow hairs and skin swabs for each β-HPV type. The kappa coefficients <0 indicates no agreement, 0–0.20 as slight, 0.21–0.40 as fair, 0.41–0.60 as moderate, 0.61–0.80 as substantial, and 0.81–1 as almost perfect agreement [32].

Logistic regression models were used to estimate age-adjusted odds ratios (OR) and 95% confidence intervals (CI) for the associations between risk factors and prevalence of overall and species-specific HPV infections (β1 and β2) (due to sample size constraints, risk factors associated with type-specific HPV infections were not examined.). Variables that were significantly associated with β HPV prevalence in an age-adjusted model were further evaluated after stratification by β HPV species. Logistic regression was conducted to estimate the association between risk factors and incidence as well as persistence of HPV infection, after adjusting for age. Logistic regression analyses were conducted separately for HPV infection in eyebrow hairs and normal skin swabs. Kaplan-Meier curves were derived for incidence and clearance of any HPV infection. An alpha level of 0.05 was considered statistically significant. Adjustment for multiple comparisons was not conducted. All analyses were conducted using SAS software, version 9.3 (SAS Institute Inc., Cary, NC, USA) and R software, version 2.13.1.

Results

The median follow up time was 12.6 months. As seen in Table 1, majority (74.5%) of men self-reported their race as White and was between 18 and 30 years of age (51.7%).

HPV DNA in eyebrow hair and normal skin

As seen in Table 2, cutaneous HPV prevalence was higher among normal skin swab samples than eyebrow hairs, particularly for any β HPV type (67.3% in normal skin swabs vs. 56.5% in

Table 5. Associations of baseline characteristics with incidence and persistence for any type of β HPV infection in men residing in Tampa, Florida.

	Incidence		Persistence	
	Eyebrow hairs Age Adjusted OR(95% CI) n=40	**Normal skin swabs Age Adjusted OR (95% CI) n=50**	**Eyebrow hairs Age Adjusted OR (95% CI) n=71**	**Normal skin swabs Age Adjusted OR(95% CI) n=95**
Age*				
18–30	1.0 (referent)	1.0 (referent)	1.0 (referent)	1.0 (referent)
31–44	0.9 (0.3–2.8)	0.5 (0.1–2.04)	2.0 (0.8–4.6)	2.4 (0.9–6.7)
>44	0.4 (0.1–1.3)	0.8 (0.1–4.6)	**6.1 (2.6–14.1)**	1.2 (0.6–2.4)
Self-Identified Race				
White	1.0 (referent)	1.0 (referent)	1.0 (referent)	1.0 (referent)
Other	1.3 (0.5–3.3)	0.3 (0.1–1.1)	0.58 (0.25–1.34)	0.44 (0.2–0.99)
Spanish/Hispanic/Latino				
No	1.0 (referent)	1.0 (referent)	1.0 (referent)	1.0 (referent)
Yes	0.6 (0.1–2.02)	2.6 (0.3–23.5)	1.04 (0.4–2.7)	0.8 (0.3–1.9)
Marital status				
Single, Never Married or Divorced/Separated	1.0 (referent)	1.0 (referent)	1.0 (referent)	1.0 (referent)
Married or Cohabiting, Living Together	1.6(0.6–4.4)	0.6 (0.1–2.7)	1.4 (0.6–3.0)	0.9 (0.4–1.8)
Highest level of education				
High school or below	1.0 (referent)	1.0 (referent)	1.0 (referent)	1.0 (referent)
Vocational school/Some college	4.01 (0.8–20.5)	3.05 (0.6–14.9)	1.5 (0.6–3.9)	1.7 (0.7–4.1)
Graduated college/Graduate school	5.9 (1.03–34.2)	1.6 (0.3–7.9)	1.7 (0.6–5.0)	1.2 (0.4–3.4)
Skin reaction to season's first sun exposure				
No change in skin color	1.0 (referent)	1.0 (referent)	1.0 (referent)	1.0 (referent)
Tan with no sunburn	0.8 (0.2–2.8)	3.1 (0.5–19.2)	0.8 (0.2–2.4)	1.1 (0.4–3.1)
Mild sunburn that becomes a tan	0.8 (0.2–2.5)	3 (0.6–14.9)	0.9 (0.3–2.6)	1.1 (0.4–2.9)
Sunburn	0.7 (0.2–3.5)	1.4 (0.2–12.02)	0.8 (0.2–2.5)	1.4 (0.4–4.5)
Ever had a blistering sunburn				
No	1.0 (referent)	1.0 (referent)	1.0 (referent)	1.0 (referent)
Yes	1.1 (0.5–2.7)	1.58 (0.43–5.89)	1.45 (0.72–2.93)	2.27 (1.13–4.54)
Lifetime number of blistering sunburns				
None	1.0 (referent)	1.0 (referent)	1.0 (referent)	1.0 (referent)
1	0.4 (0.1–1.7)	2.4 (0.2–23.3)	0.6 (0.2–1.7)	0.9 (0.4–2.2)
2	1.2 (0.3–4.3)	0.5 (0.1–2.5)	4.01 (1.3–12.2)	5.04 (1.3–18.9)
>2	2.7 (0.8–9.9)	Could not be estimated	1.5 (0.6–4.0)	5.5 (1.7–18.5)
Had an alcoholic beverage in the past month				
No	1.0 (referent)	1.0 (referent)	1.0 (referent)	1.0 (referent)
Yes	1.0 (0.3–2.9)	0.4 (0.04–3.1)	0.7(0.2–1.8)	0.6 (0.2–1.5)
Number of days drank in past month				
0	1.0 (referent)	1.0 (referent)	1.0 (referent)	1.0 (referent)
'1–8	1.1 (0.3–3.6)	0.4 (0.04–3.5)	0.5 (0.2–1.5)	0.4 (0.1–1.1)
9+	0.7 (0.2–2.6)	0.3 (0.03–3.9)	0.9 (0.3–2.9)	1.4 (0.5–4.2)
Current smoker				
No	1.0 (referent)	1.0 (referent)	1.0 (referent)	1.0 (referent)
Yes	0.5 (0.1–2.05)	0.8 (0.2–3.7)	0.9 (0.3–2.4)	0.4 (0.1–1.02)
Ever smoker				
No	1.0 (referent)	1.0 (referent)	1.0 (referent)	1.0 (referent)
Yes	0.7 (0.3–1.7)	0.7 (0.2–2.4)	1.06 (0.5–2.3)	1.0 (0.5–2.1)
Smoking status				
Never	1.0 (referent)	1.0 (referent)	1.0 (referent)	1.0 (referent)

Table 5. Cont.

	Incidence		Persistence	
	Eyebrow hairs Age Adjusted OR(95% CI) n = 40	**Normal skin swabs Age Adjusted OR (95% CI) n = 50**	**Eyebrow hairs Age Adjusted OR (95% CI) n = 71**	**Normal skin swabs Age Adjusted OR(95% CI) n = 95**
Former	0.8 (0.3–2.2)	0.7 (0.2–2.9)	1.1 (0.5–2.8)	1.7 (0.7–4.3)
Current	0.5 (0.1–2.02)	0.7 (0.1–3.5)	1.0 (0.3–2.7)	0.5 (0.2–1.3)
Ever been diagnosed with an STD				
No	1.0 (referent)	1.0 (referent)	1.0 (referent)	1.0 (referent)
Yes	2.1 (0.5–9.3)	1.3 (0.2–7.5)	0.9 (0.3–2.4)	0.5 (0.2–1.5)
Lifetime female vaginal sex partners				
0–1	1.0 (referent)	1.0 (referent)	1.0 (referent)	1.0 (referent)
2–9	0.7 (0.2–2.5)	1.9 (0.3–12.7)	1.4 (0.5–3.7)	0.8 (0.3–2.3)
10+	0.7 (0.2–2.2)	1.1 (0.2–5.2)	0.9 (0.3–2.6)	0.8 (0.2–2.4)
Female vaginal sex partners in past 6 months				
None	1.0 (referent)	1.0 (referent)	1.0 (referent)	1.0 (referent)
1	2.1 (0.7–6.2)	0.1 (0.01–1.3)	1.0 (0.4–2.4)	1.3 (0.6–3.03)
2+	1.5 (0.4–5.0)	0.3 (0.03–3.5)	0.9 (0.3–2.7)	1.5 (0.5–4.4)

OR = odds ratio, CI = confidence interval.
*Unadjusted logistic regression. All analyses, except for 'age' are adjusted for age.

eyebrow hairs). HPV types in genus β, species 1 (5, 12, 21 and 24) were the most highly prevalent in normal skin swabs and their prevalence in skin swabs was higher compared to that in eyebrow hairs (McNemar's $p = 0.004$). No significant difference was noted in the prevalence of β2 HPV types between the two sites of infection. Significantly higher prevalence of γ HPV infection was also observed in normal skin swabs (26.8%) compared to eyebrow hairs (15.9%, McNemar's $p = 0.002$). The concordance between HPV DNA in eyebrow hairs and normal skin swabs varied by HPV type, with kappa values ranging from no agreement ($k = -0.022$) for HPV type 123 to substantial agreement ($k = 0.80$) for types 47 in β1, 92 in β4 and 112 in γ HPV (data not shown).

As seen in Figure 1, the median time to incidence of cutaneous β-HPV infection was 17.3 months in eyebrow hairs with a slightly shorter time to incidence in normal skin swabs (11.2 months). Thus, at 12 months, 35% of men had newly acquired cutaneous β-HPV infection in eyebrow hairs while 57% men acquired new cutaneous β-HPV infection in skin swabs. The median time to clearance for any β HPV infection was 6.1 months in eyebrow hairs and 6.44 months in normal skin swabs (Figure 2). For γ HPV infection, the median time to incidence in normal skin swabs was 13.1 months (Figure 3), while the median time to clearance in both, eyebrow hairs and normal skin swabs, was 6.1 months and 6.4 months, respectively (Figure 4).

Incidence and persistence of cutaneous HPV are presented in Table 2. In general, incidence and persistence rates were higher in normal skin swabs compared to those in eyebrow hairs for β and γ HPV infection. The top five HPV types with highest incidence of infection in eyebrow hairs were 38 (β2), 5 (β1), 4 (γ), 80 (β2) and 23 (β2), ranging from 5.7 to 7.6 cases per 1000 person months; while in normal skin swabs these included 4 (γ), 23 (β2), 38 (β2), 5 (β1) and 76(β3), ranging from 21.7 to 28.5 cases per 1000 person months. More than 50% of men had persistence of HPV types 25, 47, 12, 15 and 17 in eyebrow hairs and persistence of HPV types 20, 21, 47, 23, 50, 108, 25, 37, 76 and 8 in skin swabs. Median duration of persistence of β and γ HPV infection was 8.6 and 6.1 months in eyebrow hairs, respectively and 11.3 months and 6.3 months, in skin swabs, respectively.

Risk factors associated with prevalence, incidence and persistence of HPV infection

Men aged >44 years were more than twice and thrice as likely to have prevalent baseline β HPV infection in eyebrow hairs and skin swabs, respectively, compared to men aged 18–30 years (Table 3). A positive history of blistering sunburn was associated with a more than two-fold increased prevalence of β HPV infection in normal skin swabs, although the association between frequency of sunburns and HPV prevalence did not reach statistical significance (Table 3). No other demographic, lifestyle or sexual history related factors were associated with prevalence of HPV.

Evaluation of species-specific β HPV prevalence indicated that men aged >44 years were twice more likely to harbor β1 and β2 types of HPV in eyebrow hairs and more than threefold likely to have β1 and β2 types of HPV infection in normal skin swabs (Table 4), compared to men ages 18–30 years. Similarly, a positive history of blistering skin burns was associated with more than two fold (OR = 2.6, 95% CI = 1.2–5.7) and more than threefold (OR = 3.1, 95% CI = 1.4–7.0) increased prevalence of β1 and β2 HPV in normal skin swabs, respectively. This association was stronger for β2 HPV infection in normal skin swabs (OR = 5.0, 95% CI = 1.4–17.7) among individuals with a history of more than 2 lifetime episodes of sunburns compared to those who reported none. Overall, while the association of these factors with β HPV infection did not vary significantly by HPV species, age and history of blistering sunburns appeared to have strong positive associations with β HPV infection, particularly in normal skin swabs.

No significant associations were seen between baseline factors and incident β HPV infection (Table 5) and prevalence or

Table 6. Association of baseline characteristics with prevalence, incidence and persistence of γ HPV infection in men residing in Tampa, Florida.

	Prevalence		Incidence		Persistence	
	Eyebrow hairs n = 33	**Normal skin swabs n = 56**	**Eyebrow hairs n = 30**	**Normal skin swabs n = 90**	**Eyebrow hairs n = 16**	**Normal skin swabs n = 49**
	Age Adjusted OR (95% CI)	**Age Adjusted OR(95% CI)**	**Unadjusted OR(95%CI)**	**Unadjusted OR(95%CI)**	**Unadjusted OR(95%CI)**	**Unadjusted OR(95%CI)**
Age						
18–30	1.0 (referent)	1.0 (referent)	1.0 (referent)	1.0 (referent)	1.0 (referent)	1.0 (referent)
31–44	0.6 (0.2–1.6)	0.7 (0.3–1.6)	0.3 (0.1–1.0)	0.3 (0.1–0.6)	2.1 (0.4–11.3)	0.5 (0.1–1.5)
>44	0.7 (0.29–1.7)	1.1 (0.5–2.2)	0.6 (0.2–1.4)	0.4 (0.2–0.9)	2.7 (0.7–10.3)	0.7 (0.3–1.8)
Self-Identified Race						
White	1.0 (referent)	1.0 (referent)	1.0 (referent)	1.0 (referent)	**	1.0 (referent)
Other	0.6 (0.2–1.6)	0.6 (0.3–1.2)	0.8 (0.3–2.01)	0.7 (0.4–1.5)		0.4 (0.2–1.2)
Spanish/Hispanic/Latino						
No	1.0 (referent)	1.0(referent)	1.0(referent)	1.0(referent)	1.0 referent)	1.0(referent)
Yes	0.7 (0.2–2.1)	0.9 (0.4–2.1)	1.4 (0.5–3.8)	0.8 (0.3–1.9)	1.2(0.2–7.4)	0.9 (0.3–3.2)
Marital status						
Single, Never Married or Divorced/ Separated	1.0(referent)	1.0(referent)	1.0(referent)	1.0(referent)	1.0(referent)	1.0(referent)
Married or Cohabiting, Living Together	0.5 (0.2–1.4)	0.6 (0.3–1.4)	0.6 (0.2–1.5)	1.0 (0.5–1.9)	1.5 (0.4–6.0)	0.5 (0.2–1.2)
Highest level of education						
High school or below	1.0(referent)	1.0(referent)	1.0(referent)	1.0(referent)	1.0(referent)	1.0(referent)
Vocational school/Some college	0.7 (0.3–1.8)	1.5 (0.633.8)	1.8 (0.6–5.9)	1.5 (0.6–3.5)	1.4 (0.3–6.1)	1.4 (0.5–4.1)
Graduated college/Graduate school	0.4 (0.1–1.4)	1.2 (0.4–3.1)	0.8 (0.2–3.1)	0.5 (0.2–1.2)	1.3 (0.2–8.4)	0.8 (0.2–3.05)
Skin reaction to season's first sun exposure						
No change in skin color	1.0(referent)	1.0(referent)	1.0(referent)	1.0(referent)	1.0(referent)	1.0(referent)
Tan with no sunburn	0.9 (0.3–3.2)	0.6 (0.2–1.7)	1.7 (0.5–5.5)	0.9 (0.3–2.6)	1.0 (0.1–7.4)	2.5 (0.7–9.0)
Mild sunburn that becomes a tan	1.3 (0.4–3.9)	1.45 (0.6–3.4)	1.3 (0.4–4.1)	0.8 (0.3–2.12)	0.8 (0.1–5.2)	2.2 (0.7–7.05)
Sunburn	1.5 (0.4–5.3)	0.73 (0.2–2.1)	0.2 (0.02–1.7)	0.3 (0.1–0.9)	2.5 (0.3–21.4)	3.2 (0.7–14.1)
Ever had a blistering sunburn						
No	1.0(referent)	1.0(referent)	1.0(referent)	1.0(referent)	1.0(referent)	1.0(referent)
Yes	0.9 (0.4–1.9)	1.1 (0.6–2.0)	0.6 (0.3–1.3)	1.0 (0.5–1.9)	3.2 (0.9–10.8)	0.8 (0.4–1.9)
Lifetime number of blistering sunburns						
None	1.0(referent)	1.0(referent)	1.0(referent)	1.0(referent)	1.0(referent)	1.0(referent)
1	0.7 (0.2–2.1)	1.5 (0.7–3.3)	0.2 (0.05–1.1)	1.2 (0.5–3.1)	1.7 (0.3–10.8)	0.5 (0.2–1.4)
2	0.6 (0.2–2.2)	0.9 (0.4–2.5)	0.5 (0.1–1.9)	1.7 (0.6–4.9)	6.2 (0.8–46.1)	1.0 (0.3–3.5)
>2	1.5 (0.6–4.05)	0.8 (0.3–2.02)	1.1 (0.4–3.1)	0.6 (0.2–1.3)	3.5 (0.8–15.3)	1.5 (0.5–4.7)
Had an alcoholic beverage in the past month						
No	1.0(referent)	1.0(referent)	1.0(referent)	1.0(referent)	1.0(referent)	1.0(referent)
Yes	0.6 (0.2–1.4)	1.3 (0.6–3.2)	0.9 (0.3–2.6)	0.5 (0.2–1.3)	0.7 (0.2–2.7)	1.4 (0.5–4.2)
Number of days drank in past month						
0	1.0(referent)	1.0(referent)	1.0(referent)	1.0(referent)	1.0(referent)	1.0(referent)
1–8	0.5 (0.2–1.5)	1.1 (0.4–2.8)	0.6 (0.2–2.1)	0.5 (0.2–1.3)	0.5 (0.1–2.8)	1.0 (0.3–3.4)
9+	0.9 (0.3–2.4)	1.4 (0.5–3.7)	1.5 (0.5–4.7)	0.8 (0.3–2.2)	0.8 (0.2–3.7)	2.4 (0.7–8.5)
Current smoker						
No	1.0(referent)	1.0(referent)	1.0(referent)	1.0(referent)	1.0(referent)	1.0(referent)
Yes	1.1 (0.4–3.2)	0.7 (0.3–1.85)	1.1 (0.4–3.1)	0.9 (0.4–2.2)	1.2 (0.3–5.7)	1.5 (0.5–4.7)
Ever smoker						
No	1.0(referent)	1.0(referent)	1.0(referent)	1.0(referent)	1.0(referent)	1.0(referent)
Yes	1.4 (0.6–3.2)	0.8 (0.4–1.6)	1.2 (0.5–2.6)	0.8 (0.4–1.6)	3.1 (0.9–10.4)	1.1 (0.5–2.5)
Smoking status						

Table 6. Cont.

	Prevalence		Incidence		Persistence	
	Eyebrow hairs n = 33	Normal skin swabs n = 56	Eyebrow hairs n = 30	Normal skin swabs n = 90	Eyebrow hairs n = 16	Normal skin swabs n = 49
	Age Adjusted OR (95% CI)	Age Adjusted OR(95% CI)	Unadjusted OR(95%CI)	Unadjusted OR(95%CI)	Unadjusted OR(95%CI)	Unadjusted OR(95%CI)
Never	1.0(referent)	1.0(referent)	1.00(referent)	1.00(referent)	1.0(referent)	1.0(referent)
Former	1.48 (0.6–3.7)	0.86 (0.4–1.9)	1.2 (0.5–3.1)	0.8 (0.4–1.7)	**4 (1.01–15.9)**	0.9 (0.3–2.4)
Current	1.31 (0.4–4.1)	0.7 (0.3–1.9)	1.1 (0.38–3.37)	0.9 (0.4–2.1)	2.0 (0.4–10.4)	1.5 (0.5–4.8)
Ever been diagnosed with an STD						
No	1.0(referent)	1.0(referent)	1.0(referent)	1.0(referent)	**	1.0(referent)
Yes	0.6 (0.2–2.4)	1.05 (0.41–2.6)	0.2 (0.02–1.3)	0.7 (0.3–1.9)		0.2 (0.04–0.9)
Lifetime female vaginal sex partners						
0–1	1.0(referent)	1.0(referent)	1.0(referent)	1.0(referent)	1.0(referent)	1.0(referent)
2–9	1.4 (0.5–3.9)	0.4 (0.2–1.1)	0.3 (0.1–1.1)	0.7 (0.3–1.9)	1.82 (0.4–9.3)	0.5 (0.1–1.6)
10+	0.6 (0.2–2.1)	1.0 (0.4–2.4)	0.6 (0.2–1.6)	0.6 (0.2–1.5)	1.7 (0.3–8.1)	0.4 (0.1–1.1)
Female vaginal sex partners in past 6 months						
None	1.0(referent)	1.0(referent)	1.0(referent)	1.0(referent)	1.0(referent)	1.0 (referent)
1	0.4 (0.2–1.0)	1.4 (0.6–3.0)	0.8 (0.3–2.1)	1.1 (0.5–2.3)	0.3 (0.1–1.1)	0.7(0.2–1.9)
2+	0.4 (0.2–1.3)	0.9 (0.4–2.4)	1.5 (0.5–4.3)	1.3 (0.5–3.1)	0.3 (0.05–1.4)	0.9 (0.3–2.8)

OR = odds ratio, CI = confidence interval.
**No subjects left in the 'Other' racial group and in the 'diagnosed with STD' group. The sample size was too small to conduct age-adjusted analyses of incidence and persistence of γ HPV infection.

incidence of γ HPV infection, in eyebrow hairs or normal skin swabs (Table 6).

Findings on factors associated with persistence of β HPV infection were similar to those of prevalent infections described above. Age>44 years was associated with a six fold (OR = 6.1, 95%CI = 2.6–14.2) increased persistence of infection with β HPV in eyebrow hairs (Table 5) but not in normal skin swabs. History of blistering skin burn was associated with persistence of β HPV in normal skin swabs (OR = 2.3, 95% CI = 1.2–4.6), with increasing frequency of sunburns showing stronger association (Table 5). When restricted to White men, history of blistering sunburns was associated with 2.7 times increased persistence of any HPV infection in normal skin swabs (OR = 2.73, 95% CI = 1.19–6.26), after adjusting for age (data not shown). As expected, this association was stronger than that observed for the overall population (OR = 2.3, 95% CI = 1.2–4.6) (Table 5). However, when analyses were restricted to White men and stratified by HPV species, there were no significant associations between history of blistering sunburns and persistence of β1 (OR = 0.87, 95% CI = 0.29–2.62) or β2 (OR = 1.33, 95% CI = 0.54–3.27) infection in normal skin swabs, after adjusting for age (data not shown).

No significant associations were observed between baseline characteristics and persistence of γ HPV except a significantly increased persistence (OR = 4.0, 95% CI = 1.0–15.9) in eyebrow hairs among former smokers compared to never smokers (Table 6).

Discussion

In this HIM study sub-cohort of 209 healthy men, we observed a high prevalence of cutaneous β HPV and γ HPV in normal skin swabs, higher than that in eyebrow hair samples. Although cutaneous HPV seroprevalence rates have been reported previously [33–35], seroreactivity is not a direct estimate of HPV infection. Hence, we attempted to directly measure type and species-specific HPV DNA in normal skin swabs and eyebrow hairs.

Results presented here contrast to that of other studies which reported a higher prevalence of cutaneous HPV in eyebrow hairs among individuals without a history of skin cancer [36,37] and lower prevalence (13–37%) in skin [37,38]. Tarmorshuizen et al. reported a prevalence of 54% in eyebrow hairs among healthy controls [39], which was similar to our findings. Differences across studies could be a reflection of variation in number of HPV types examined. For example, while we evaluated 41 HPV types (25 HPV types from genus β and 16 HPV types from genus γ), previous studies have evaluated fewer HPV types within each genus (6 to 28 HPV types overall across studies) [36–39]. Apart from this, methodological differences or even differences in geographical location of study populations may explain the inconsistencies in HPV prevalence across studies. Indeed, HPV prevalence rate has been shown to vary by country [25,36]. In our study, while we observed a strong association between history of blistering sunburn and both prevalence and persistence of β HPV, no association was seen between tanning ability and β HPV infection, indicating that exposure to ultraviolet (UV) radiation rather than host genetics may be more important determinants of cutaneous HPV infection. Thus, geographical variation in UV radiation might have contributed to variable prevalence estimates in the literature. While we were unable to measure HPV prevalence in sun-unexposed skin, our previous study of NMSC cases indicates that the prevalence of β-HPV is higher in sun-exposed skin swabs (100% prevalence) compared to sun-unexposed swabs (95% prevalence) among NMSC cases [16].

Older age and history of blistering sunburns were significantly associated with both prevalence and persistence of HPV but not with incidence of cutaneous HPV infection. Our findings are consistent with previous reports on the association between age and prevalence of HPV [36,39]. A positive history of blistering sunburn was associated with a more than two fold increased prevalence of β HPV infection in skin, with a stronger association for β2 HPV infection. While an inverse association between frequency of sunburns and β HPV seropositivity has been reported previously [33], we found a positive association between lifetime history of one blistering sunburn and prevalent β HPV infection in normal skin swabs. We also observed a strong association between frequency of blistering sunburns and persistence of β HPV infection, likely explaining the elevated prevalence observed here. UV exposure mediated immunosuppression may predispose individuals to a higher risk of cutaneous HPV persistence and hence prevalence [40]. Indeed, higher prevalence of cutaneous HPV has been observed among individuals who reported working outdoors for longer duration [41].

The findings of our study should be interpreted with caution. The external validity of these findings is limited to men. Future studies should include women, especially given the previously reported differences in seroprevalence of specific types of cutaneous HPV by gender [35]. Our findings are generalizable to non-Hispanic Whites only. However, our study population of Florida residents is at higher risk of NMSC compared to other U.S. states, corresponding to Florida's higher UV radiation index [42], and hence may represent a population that could be targeted for novel NMSC prevention measures. To maximize the sample size, persistence of HPV infection was determined using both incident and prevalent HPV infections. Therefore, the true duration of HPV infection is unknown, given the prevalent cases at baseline. Finally, we examined only 25 HPV types in genus β and 16 HPV types in genus γ. Given the large number of HPV types that are being continually discovered, our results on overall β and γ HPV infection may not reflect the true associations that can be affected by unexamined and unknown HPV types.

The study has several strengths. This is the first study to report HPV infection across a continuum of incidence, prevalence, persistence and clearance of cutaneous HPV across different genera, by type and species. We compared HPV infection in normal skin swabs as well as eyebrow hairs, thus providing a comprehensive report on natural history of HPV using biomarkers from two tissues. This is particularly important since concordance between HPV infection in normal skin swabs and eyebrow hairs was found to vary by HPV type. Along with rates of HPV infection, we also evaluated a range of epidemiological factors associated with HPV infection, overall and by species. Analyses were adjusted for potential confounders.

In conclusion, we observed high prevalence, incidence and persistence of cutaneous HPV infection among cancer-free men. Age and history of blistering sunburns were significantly associated with prevalence and persistence of β HPV. The association of blistering sunburns with both persistence of HPV infection, but not with incidence, suggests that sunlight exposure does not affect acquisition of new HPV infection but the duration of HPV infection could be affected by sunlight exposure through UV related immune dysregulation or actual promotion of HPV infection. Given the potential role of cutaneous β HPV in NMSC, the findings are valuable in defining a high risk population for development of novel preventive measures.

Acknowledgments

We thank the Donald A. Adam Comprehensive Melanoma Research Center at Moffitt Cancer Center for their support in conducting this study.

Author Contributions

Conceived and designed the experiments: DER TG MT ARG. Performed the experiments: TG MT. Analyzed the data: HL KJF MRI. Contributed reagents/materials/analysis tools: TG MT KJF HL. Contributed to the writing of the manuscript: SSH DER ARG HL KJF MEA TG MT. Coordination of the study: BAS MEA.

References

1. Braaten KP, Laufer MR (2008) Human Papillomavirus (HPV), HPV-Related Disease, and the HPV Vaccine. Rev Obstet Gynecol 1: 2–10.
2. Chiantore MV, Vannucchi S, Accardi R, Tommasino M, Percario ZA, et al. (2012) Interferon-beta induces cellular senescence in cutaneous human papilloma virus-transformed human keratinocytes by affecting p53 transactivating activity. PLoS One 7: 16.
3. Bzhalava D, Guan P, Franceschi S, Dillner J, Clifford G (2013) A systematic review of the prevalence of mucosal and cutaneous human papillomavirus types. Virology 445: 224–231.
4. Heideman DA, Waterboer T, Pawlita M, Delis-van Diemen P, Nindl I, et al. (2007) Human papillomavirus-16 is the predominant type etiologically involved in penile squamous cell carcinoma. J Clin Oncol 25: 4550–4556.
5. Smith JS, Lindsay L, Hoots B, Keys J, Franceschi S, et al. (2007) Human papillomavirus type distribution in invasive cervical cancer and high-grade cervical lesions: a meta-analysis update. Int J Cancer 121: 621–632.
6. Castellsague X, Pawlita M, Roura E, Margall N, Waterboer T, et al. (2013) Prospective seroepidemiologic study on the role of Human Papillomavirus and other infections in cervical carcinogenesis: Evidence from the EPIC cohort. Int J Cancer 13: 28665.
7. Michaud DS, Langevin SM, Eliot M, Nelson HH, Pawlita M, et al. (2014) High-risk HPV types and head and neck cancer. Int J Cancer 26: 28811.
8. Mansour M, Touka M, Hasan U, Bellopede A, Smet A, et al. (2007) E7 properties of mucosal human papillomavirus types 26, 53 and 66 correlate with their intermediate risk for cervical cancer development. Virology 367: 1–9.
9. Pecoraro G, Morgan D, Defendi V (1989) Differential effects of human papillomavirus type 6, 16, and 18 DNAs on immortalization and transformation of human cervical epithelial cells. Proc Natl Acad Sci U S A 86: 563–567.
10. Proby CM, Harwood CA, Neale RE, Green AC, Euvrard S, et al. (2011) A case-control study of betapapillomavirus infection and cutaneous squamous cell carcinoma in organ transplant recipients. Am J Transplant 11: 1498–1508.
11. Struijk L, Bouwes Bavinck JN, Wanningen P, van der Meijden E, Westendorp RG, et al. (2003) Presence of human papillomavirus DNA in plucked eyebrow hairs is associated with a history of cutaneous squamous cell carcinoma. J Invest Dermatol 121: 1531–1535.
12. Neale RE, Weissenborn S, Abeni D, Bavinck JNB, Euvrard S, et al. (2013) Human Papillomavirus Load in Eyebrow Hair Follicles and Risk of Cutaneous Squamous Cell Carcinoma. Cancer Epidemiology Biomarkers & Prevention 22: 719–727.
13. Jackson S, Storey A (2000) E6 proteins from diverse cutaneous HPV types inhibit apoptosis in response to UV damage. Oncogene 19: 592–598.
14. Muschik D, Braspenning-Wesch I, Stockfleth E, Rosl F, Hofmann TG, et al. (2011) Cutaneous HPV23 E6 prevents p53 phosphorylation through interaction with HIPK2. PLoS One 6: 16.
15. Jablonska S, Dabrowski J, Jakubowicz K (1972) Epidermodysplasia Verruciformis as a Model in Studies on the Role of Papovaviruses in Oncogenesis. Cancer Research 32: 583–589.
16. Rollison DE, Pawlita M, Giuliano AR, Iannacone MR, Sondak VK, et al. (2008) Measures of cutaneous human papillomavirus infection in normal tissues as biomarkers of HPV in corresponding nonmelanoma skin cancers. Int J Cancer 123: 2337–2342.
17. Farzan SF, Waterboer T, Gui J, Nelson HH, Li Z, et al. (2013) Cutaneous alpha, beta and gamma human papillomaviruses in relation to squamous cell carcinoma of the skin: A population-based study. Int J Cancer 28: 28176.
18. Iannacone MR, Gheit T, Waterboer T, Giuliano AR, Messina JL, et al. (2012) Case-control study of cutaneous human papillomaviruses in squamous cell carcinoma of the skin. Cancer Epidemiol Biomarkers Prev 21: 1303–1313.
19. Andersson K, Michael KM, Luostarinen T, Waterboer T, Gislefoss R, et al. (2012) Prospective study of human papillomavirus seropositivity and risk of nonmelanoma skin cancer. Am J Epidemiol 175: 685–695.
20. Iannacone MR, Gheit T, Waterboer T, Giuliano AR, Messina JL, et al. (2013) Case-control study of cutaneous human papillomavirus infection in Basal cell carcinoma of the skin. J Invest Dermatol 133: 1512–1520.
21. de Koning MN, Struijk L, Bavinck JN, Kleter B, ter Schegget J, et al. (2007) Betapapillomaviruses frequently persist in the skin of healthy individuals. J Gen Virol 88: 1489–1495.
22. Boxman IL, Berkhout RJ, Mulder LH, Wolkers MC, Bouwes Bavinck JN, et al. (1997) Detection of human papillomavirus DNA in plucked hairs from renal transplant recipients and healthy volunteers. J Invest Dermatol 108: 712–715.

23. Antonsson A, Karanfilovska S, Lindqvist PG, Hansson BG (2003) General acquisition of human papillomavirus infections of skin occurs in early infancy. J Clin Microbiol 41: 2509–2514.
24. Hsu JY, Chen AC, Keleher A, McMillan NA, Antonsson A (2009) Shared and persistent asymptomatic cutaneous human papillomavirus infections in healthy skin. J Med Virol 81: 1444–1449.
25. Antonsson A, Erfurt C, Hazard K, Holmgren V, Simon M, et al. (2003) Prevalence and type spectrum of human papillomaviruses in healthy skin samples collected in three continents. J Gen Virol 84: 1881–1886.
26. Anic GM, Lee J-H, Stockwell H, Rollison DE, Wu Y, et al. (2011) Incidence and human papillomavirus (HPV) type distribution of genital warts in a multinational cohort of men: the HPV in men study. Journal of Infectious Diseases 204: 1886–1892.
27. Giuliano AR, Lee JH, Fulp W, Villa LL, Lazcano E, et al. (2011) Incidence and clearance of genital human papillomavirus infection in men (HIM): a cohort study. Lancet 377: 932–940.
28. Gheit T, Billoud G, de Koning MN, Gemignani F, Forslund O, et al. (2007) Development of a sensitive and specific multiplex PCR method combined with DNA microarray primer extension to detect Betapapillomavirus types. J Clin Microbiol 45: 2537–2544.
29. Gheit T, Landi S, Gemignani F, Snijders PJ, Vaccarella S, et al. (2006) Development of a sensitive and specific assay combining multiplex PCR and DNA microarray primer extension to detect high-risk mucosal human papillomavirus types. J Clin Microbiol 44: 2025–2031.
30. Schmitt M, Dondog B, Waterboer T, Pawlita M, Tommasino M, et al. (2010) Abundance of Multiple High-Risk Human Papillomavirus (HPV) Infections Found in Cervical Cells Analyzed by Use of an Ultrasensitive HPV Genotyping Assay. Journal of Clinical Microbiology 48: 143–149.
31. Iannacone MR, Gheit T, Pfister H, Giuliano AR, Messina JL, et al. (2013) Case-control study of genus-beta human papillomaviruses in plucked eyebrow hairs and cutaneous squamous cell carcinoma. Int J Cancer 17: 28552.
32. Viera AJ, Garrett JM (2005) Understanding interobserver agreement: the kappa statistic. Fam Med 37: 360–363.
33. Sampogna F, Bavinck JNB, Pawlita M, Abeni D, Harwood CA, et al. (2012) Factors associated with the seroprevalence of 26 cutaneous and two genital human papillomavirus types in organ transplant patients. Journal of General Virology 93: 165–174.
34. Antonsson A, Green AC, Mallitt KA, O'Rourke PK, Pandeya N, et al. (2010) Prevalence and stability of antibodies to 37 human papillomavirus types—a population-based longitudinal study. Virology 407: 26–32.
35. Iannacone MR, Michael KM, Giuliano AR, Waterboer T, Pawlita M, et al. (2010) Risk factors for cutaneous human papillomavirus seroreactivity among patients undergoing skin cancer screening in Florida. Journal of Infectious Diseases 201: 760–769.
36. de Koning MNC, Weissenborn SJ, Abeni D, Bouwes Bavinck JN, Euvrard S, et al. (2009) Prevalence and associated factors of betapapillomavirus infections in individuals without cutaneous squamous cell carcinoma. Journal of General Virology 90: 1611–1621.
37. Schneider I, Lehmann MD, Kogosov V, Stockfleth E, Nindl I (2013) Eyebrow hairs from actinic keratosis patients harbor the highest number of cutaneous human papillomaviruses. BMC Infect Dis 13: 1471–2334.
38. Escutia B, Ledesma E, Serra-Guillen C, Gimeno C, Vilata JJ, et al. (2011) Detection of human papilloma virus in normal skin and in superficial and nodular basal cell carcinomas in immunocompetent subjects. Journal of the European Academy of Dermatology and Venereology 25: 832–838.
39. Termorshuizen F, Feltkamp MC, Struijk L, de Gruijl FR, Bavinck JN, et al. (2004) Sunlight exposure and (sero)prevalence of epidermodysplasia verruciformis-associated human papillomavirus. J Invest Dermatol 122: 1456–1462.
40. Iannacone MR, Wang W, Stockwell HG, O'Rourke K, Giuliano AR, et al. (2012) Sunlight Exposure and Cutaneous Human Papillomavirus Seroreactivity in Basal Cell and Squamous Cell Carcinomas of the Skin. Journal of Infectious Diseases 206: 399–406.
41. Chen AC, McMillan NA, Antonsson A (2008) Human papillomavirus type spectrum in normal skin of individuals with or without a history of frequent sun exposure. J Gen Virol 89: 2891–2897.
42. EPA UV Index: United States Environmental Protection Agency.

17

Evaluation of Genetically Inactivated Alpha Toxin for Protection in Multiple Mouse Models of *Staphylococcus aureus* Infection

Rebecca A. Brady[1], Christopher P. Mocca[1], Ranjani Prabhakara[1], Roger D. Plaut[1], Mark E. Shirtliff[2,3], Tod J. Merkel[1], Drusilla L. Burns[1]*

1 Center for Biologics Evaluation and Research, Food and Drug Administration, Bethesda, Maryland, United States of America, **2** Department of Microbial Pathogenesis, University of Maryland School of Dentistry, Baltimore, Maryland, United States of America, **3** Department of Microbiology and Immunology, University of Maryland School of Medicine, Baltimore, Maryland, United States of America

Abstract

Staphylococcus aureus is a major human pathogen and a leading cause of nosocomial and community-acquired infections. Development of a vaccine against this pathogen is an important goal. While *S. aureus* protective antigens have been identified in the literature, the majority have only been tested in a single animal model of disease. We wished to evaluate the ability of one *S. aureus* vaccine antigen to protect in multiple mouse models, thus assessing whether protection in one model translates to protection in other models encompassing the full breadth of infections the pathogen can cause. We chose to focus on genetically inactivated alpha toxin mutant HlaH35L. We evaluated the protection afforded by this antigen in three models of infection using the same vaccine dose, regimen, route of immunization, adjuvant, and challenge strain. When mice were immunized with HlaH35L and challenged via a skin and soft tissue infection model, HlaH35L immunization led to a less severe infection and decreased *S. aureus* levels at the challenge site when compared to controls. Challenge of HlaH35L-immunized mice using a systemic infection model resulted in a limited, but statistically significant decrease in bacterial colonization as compared to that observed with control mice. In contrast, in a prosthetic implant model of chronic biofilm infection, there was no significant difference in bacterial levels when compared to controls. These results demonstrate that vaccines may confer protection against one form of *S. aureus* disease without conferring protection against other disease presentations and thus underscore a significant challenge in *S. aureus* vaccine development.

Editor: Eliane Namie Miyaji, Instituto Butantan, Brazil

Funding: This work was supported by the Intramural Research Program of the Center for Biologics Evaluation and Research, Food and Drug Administration, and by the National Institute of Allergy and Infectious Diseases, National Institutes of Health (grants R01AI69568 and ARRA AI69568 to MES). The funders had no role in study design, data collection and analysis, decision to publish or preparation of the manuscript.

Competing Interests: The authors have declared that no competing interests exist.

* E-mail: drusilla.burns@fda.hhs.gov

Introduction

Staphylococcus aureus is a leading cause of both nosocomial and community-acquired infections in the United States [1,2]. *S. aureus* infections range from superficial skin infections to life-threatening, invasive illnesses such as sepsis, osteomyelitis, and endocarditis. This bacterium colonizes the anterior nares of approximately 28% of the population [3], and infections can be caused by the colonizing strain [4–6]. *S. aureus* features an extensive and highly redundant repertoire of virulence factors that allow it to colonize and damage the host, as well as evade host immune responses and cause a variety of diseases in multiple host compartments. The profile of expressed proteins exhibited by this pathogen can vary according to growth state (planktonic vs biofilm) [7–9]. Therefore, the potential exists for antigens expressed in one type of infection (e.g., acute infections such as sepsis) to not be present in other types of infection, such as chronic biofilm infections.

S. aureus infections are increasingly caused by antibiotic resistant isolates, including the well known methicillin resistant strains (MRSA). In the past decade, vancomycin resistant *S. aureus* (VRSA) has also been isolated, highlighting the ability of the bacterium to adapt to the current repertoire of therapies available and illustrating the importance of a prophylactic vaccine for *S. aureus*. A number of antigens have been tested for their ability to protect animals against various *S. aureus* infections, including adhesins [10–21], other surface proteins [22–29], secreted toxins [30–32], and polysaccharides [33–35]. However, to this point, no *S. aureus* vaccine exists.

For an *S. aureus* vaccine to be broadly applicable, it would need to protect against a variety of *S. aureus* infections. Thus far, however, most protective antigens identified in the literature were tested in one or only a few animal models of *S. aureus* disease that do not represent the full breadth of diseases caused by this organism. In this work, we wished to determine the protective capability of a single antigen in multiple models of *S. aureus* disease that encompass a broad spectrum of bacterial growth–from infection with planktonic *S. aureus* to biofilm infection, from acute to chronic disease, and from superficial infection limited to the skin to invasive systemic illness. For each model, we administered the antigen using the same dose, same dosing schedule, and same adjuvant in order to mimic how vaccines are actually formulated

Table 1. Primers used in this study.

Primer	Sequence (5′→3′)
Hla USOE	TATGGTCTCGGATCCAGCAGATTCTGATATTAACATTAAAACC
Hla USIE	TATGGTCTCGCATGCCATTTTCTTTATCATAAGTG
Hla DSOE	TATGGTCTCCTCGAGTTA*ATGATGATGATGATGATG*ATTTGTCATTTCTTCTTTTTCC
Hla DSIE	TATGGTCTCACATGCTCAAAAAAGTATTTTATAG

USOE: Upstream outer end; USIE: Upstream inner end; DSOE: Downstream outer end; DSIE: Downstream inner end. Upstream primers were used to generate a PCR product, and downstream primers were used separately to generate a second product. The two products were then ligated together. The codon change from histidine to leucine at position 35 is noted in DSIE (underlined). The six-histidine tag is indicated in DSOE (italics).

and used. We also used the same challenge strain in each model. For this study, we chose to use a genetically inactivated form of alpha hemolysin (HlaH35L) [36] as the vaccine antigen. Immunization with this antigen has previously been shown to decrease mortality and lung colonization in a mouse pneumonia model [32], decrease lesion size and lessen dermonecrosis in a murine skin infection model [30], and also lessen lethality in a peritonitis model [37]. A truncated Hla was very recently shown to elicit protection in both pneumonia and bacteremia models [38]. A heat-inactivated form of alpha-toxoid has also been shown to protect against corneal damage in a *S. aureus* keratitis model [39]. However, these studies used different antigen preparations, different dosing, and different adjuvants, which do not reflect the likely real world scenario in which a single vaccine formulation would be used and administered on a single dosing schedule.

In this study, we tested purified, recombinant HlaH35L in three mouse models of USA300 infection: systemic infection (IV), skin and soft tissue infection (SSTI), and chronic prosthetic implant infection (PII). Utilizing the same antigen, dosing regimen, route of immunization, adjuvant and the same bacterial challenge strain in all three models allowed for evaluation of potential variation in protective capability of the antigen against different disease forms. Results using these three divergent models indicated a differential ability of recombinant HlaH35L to protect against staphylococcal illnesses that are at different ends of the infection spectrum.

Materials and Methods

Ethics Statement

For all animal studies, protocols were reviewed and approved by the Institutional Animal Care and Use Committees (IACUC) of the Center for Biologics Evaluation and Research (Bethesda, MD; permit number 2010-04) or the University of Maryland School of Medicine (Baltimore, MD; permit number 09-07-02). All surgeries were performed under ketamine/xylazine anesthesia, and all efforts were made to minimize animal suffering. Animals were sacrificed at the time points indicated below using CO_2 inhalation.

Bacterial Strains, Plasmids, and Reagents

S. aureus USA300 strain NRS384 (NARSA) was used as a PCR template for cloning. PCR primers were generated by the CBER Core Facility (Bethesda, MD). Chemi-competent TOP10 *Escherichia coli* cells and the pTRChis2c expression plasmid were obtained from Invitrogen (Carlsbad, CA). Chemi-competent BL21 *E. coli* were generated in our laboratory as described by Mandel and Higa [40]. *S. aureus* strain SAP149, which is NRS384 expressing a modified *lux* operon from *Photorhabdus luminescens* on an integrated plasmid (unpublished data), was used for all challenge experiments. All reagents were obtained from ThermoFisher Scientific (Waltham, MA) unless noted.

Cloning, Expression, and Purification of HlaH35L

In order to generate non-toxic Hla, the gene was reconstructed by joining together PCR fragments of *hla* using BsaI as described by Stemmer and Morris [41]. The CAC codon at position 35 was altered to CTC to change histidine to leucine. The primers used are shown in Table 1, with the codon change indicated in the DSIE primer. A C-terminal six-histidine tag and stop codon were added in frame with the coding sequence. The PCR fragments were digested with BsaI and cloned into pTRChis2c (Invitrogen) downstream of the *lac* operon. Ligated vectors were then transformed into *E. coli* TOP10 cells. Positive transformants were selected in the presence of ampicillin, and mutants were confirmed by sequencing. Plasmids were then transformed into *E. coli* BL21 for gene expression.

For production and purification of recombinant HlaH35L, LB cultures were supplemented with 50 µg/ml ampicillin and inoculated 1:100 with an overnight growth of BL21/HlaH35L. Cultures were incubated at 37°C with shaking to an optical density at 600 nm (OD_{600}) of 0.5, and 1 mM IPTG was added. Incubation continued for four hours, at which point bacteria were harvested by centrifugation.

HlaH35L was purified through affinity chromatography. Briefly, bacterial pellets were resuspended in lysis buffer (50 mM NaH_2PO_4, 0.5 M NaCl, pH 8.0, supplemented with 1 mg/ml lysozyme) and incubated on ice for 30 minutes. Resuspended pellets were sonicated and cellular debris removed by centrifugation at 4000×*g* for 15 minutes. Lysates were then applied to Ni-NTA columns (His-Pur, ThermoFisher) and incubated on a rotator for 60 minutes. The column was washed four times with wash buffer (50 mM NaH_2PO_4, 0.5 M NaCl, 20 mM imidazole, pH 8.0), and recombinant protein was eluted with 50 mM NaH_2PO_4, 0.5 M NaCl, 250 mM imidazole, pH 8.0. The eluted protein was concentrated and diafiltered into 20 mM Tris, 50 mM NaCl, 2 mM EDTA, pH 8.0 using Amicon® Ultra 15 ml 10,000 MWCO Centrifugal Filters (ThermoFisher). Purity was confirmed by SDS-PAGE, and protein was quantified using BCA (Pierce, Rockford, IL) following the manufacturer's instructions. Recombinant HlaH35L was stored at −70°C until use.

Immunization

For all three challenge studies, animals were immunized in the following manner: Purified, recombinant HlaH35L was thawed and subsequently diafiltered into phosphate-buffered saline (PBS, Quality Biological, Gaithersburg, MD) using Amicon® Ultra 15 ml Centrifugal Filters (10,000 MWCO). HlaH35L was then quantified by BCA and resolved via SDS-PAGE to confirm concentration and purity before adsorption to Alhydrogel® for one hour on ice (Brenntag Biosector, Frederiksund, Denmark; 2 mg/ml final concentration) with added CpG (CBER Core Facility, Bethesda, MD; 150 µg/ml final concentration). Six week old, female mice were immunized subcutaneously in the flank with 20 µg HlaH35L, 200 µg Alhydrogel®, and 15 µg CpG in 100 µl total volume on days zero and 14. Control mice received the same concentration of Alhydrogel® and CpG without HlaH35L. All mice were bled prior to challenge on day 28.

Enzyme Linked Immunosorbant Assay (ELISA)

Ninety-six well plates (MaxiSorp, ThermoFisher) were coated with 1 µg/ml HlaH35L diluted in PBS by incubating the plates at 4°C overnight. The plates were washed three times with 0.9% NaCl, 0.05% Tween-20 and then blocked with 2% (w/v) nonfat dry milk in PBS for two hours at 37°C. The blocked plates were washed again, and sera from immunized or control mice were diluted serially in dilution buffer (PBS with 2% fetal bovine serum (Invitrogen) and 0.05% Tween-20), and incubated at RT for two hours. After washing, anti-mouse IgG conjugated to horseradish peroxidase (HRP; KPL Inc., Gaithersburg, MD) was diluted in dilution buffer, added to the plates, and incubated at RT for two hours. Plates were washed again and reactivity was analyzed by adding ABTS® ELISA HRP Substrate (KPL, Inc.) and incubating for ten minutes at RT. The reaction was stopped through the addition of ABTS® Stop Solution (KPL), and optical densities were read at 405 nm (OD_{405}) on a VersaMax Microplate Reader (Molecular Devices, Sunnyvale, CA). Data were plotted using GraphPad Prism software (Version 5, GraphPad Software, La Jolla, CA) with a 4-parameter logistic (4PL) curve fit of OD (Y axis) versus logarithm of the reciprocal serum dilution (X axis). Titers are defined as the effective dilution that gives 50% of the maximal absorbance (ED_{50}) for each sample.

Skin and Soft Tissue Challenge

On the day of challenge, an overnight growth of *S. aureus* SAP149 was used to inoculate four 50 ml aliquots of Tryptic Soy Broth (TSB; MP Biomedicals, Solon, OH), supplemented with 10 µg/ml chloramphenicol (Sigma Aldrich, St. Louis, MO), at a dilution of 1:50. The cultures were grown at 37°C with shaking until an OD_{600} of 0.8 was reached, and then centrifuged at 4000×*g* for 15 minutes. All four bacterial pellets were resuspended together in 50 ml PBS, and bacterial counts were obtained using a Petroff-Hausser Counting Chamber (Hausser Scientific Partnership, Horsham, PA). The bacteria were centrifuged again at 4000×*g* for 15 minutes and then resuspended in an appropriate volume of PBS to give a concentration of 1×10^{11} CFU/ml. The bacterial count was confirmed with serial dilution and plating on Tryptic Soy Agar (TSA; MP Biomedicals).

Immunized and control mice were anesthetized with 2 mg Ketamine (Ketaject, Phoenix Pharmaceutical, St. Joseph, MO) and 0.1 mg Xylazine (AnaSed, Akorn, Decatur, IL) administered IP. Images were obtained of each animal's left ear using a Nikon SMZ 745T dissecting microscope. Left ears were sterilized with 70% ethanol, and then 1×10^{9} CFU of *S. aureus* SAP149 were administered to the left ear of each mouse in a volume of 10 µl, using a Morrow Brown needle as described by Prabhakara *et al.* [42]. Subsets of animals were photographed on days four and seven following challenge and then sacrificed. The left ear was excised, minced, and homogenized in sterile PBS. Serial dilutions were plated on TSA. A second group of mice was imaged serially on days four, seven, and 14 in order to follow the infection progression over time in the same animals. These mice were sacrificed, and ears were harvested and plated, on day 14 post-challenge.

Intravenous (IV) Challenge

An overnight culture was started using a single hemolytic colony of *S. aureus* SAP149 from a one-day-old 5% blood agar plate (Becton Dickinson, Sparks, MD) containing 10 µg/ml chloramphenicol and incubated at 37°C overnight. On the day of the challenge experiment, TSB containing 10 µg/ml chloramphenicol was inoculated with a 1:100 dilution of the overnight growth. The culture was incubated at 37°C with shaking until the OD_{600} reached approximately 0.63. The cell concentration calculation is based on previous experimentation in which it was determined that at an OD_{600} of 0.63 the concentration of the growth is approximately 3.66×10^{8} CFU/ml (data not shown). The cells were then pelleted by centrifugation at 4000×*g* for 10 minutes. The pellet was re-suspended in 1X PBS (Quality Biological) and brought to a concentration of 3×10^{7} CFU/ml. The challenge dose concentration was verified by serial dilution and plating on TSA. BALB/c mice were challenged via the lateral tail vein with 100 µl of the bacterial suspension two weeks following the second immunization. Two weeks following challenge, the mice were euthanized and kidneys were harvested, homogenized in PBS, and plated on TSA.

Prosthetic Implant Infection

The prosthetic implant model was conducted in a manner similar to that previously described [43]. Briefly, on the day of challenge, an overnight culture of *S. aureus* SAP149 was centrifuged at 4000×*g* for 10 minutes. The pellet was washed with PBS, counted with a Petroff-Hausser Counting Chamber, and then resuspended to a concentration of 1×10^{6} CFU/ml. Ten C57BL/6 mice per experimental group received implants. Mice were anesthetized via IP injection of 100 mg/kg Ketamine (Ketaset®; Fort Dodge Laboratories, Inc., Fort Dodge, Iowa) and 10 mg/kg Xylazine (Rugby Laboratories, Inc., Rockville Center, NY). The left leg of each mouse was cleansed with povidone iodine and rinsed with 70% ethanol before surgical implantation of an autoclaved 0.25 mm insect pin into the tibia (Fine Science Tools, Foster City, CA) as described [43,44]. The implanted pin was then inoculated with 1 µl of the *S. aureus* SAP149 suspension. Three weeks following implantation, mice were sacrificed and the left tibiae were harvested, cut into small pieces, and placed in 300 µl of sterile 0.85% saline per 100 µg of bone. Bones were then homogenized using a Polytron PT 1200 handheld homogenizer (Kinematica, Bohemia, NY) at 25,000 rpm, and serial 10-fold dilutions of bone homogenates were plated on TSA II, 5% defibrinated sheep's blood agar plates to enumerate viable *S. aureus* per gram bone, as previously described [43].

Statistical Analysis

For all challenge experiments, CFU levels were compared between HlaH35L-immunized animals and adjuvant-only control animals using GraphPad Prism. Differences in CFU levels were evaluated using the untailed Student's *t* test. For IV challenge experiments, the data from two identical experiments run on separate days were combined. ELISA titers were defined as the ED_{50} for sera pooled within a group from each experiment. ED_{50} values were compared across challenge experiments using ANOVA.

Results

HlaH35L Immunization Decreases Disease Severity and Bacterial Colonization in a Skin and Soft Tissue Infection Model of *S. aureus* Infection

In order to evaluate the effect of HlaH35L immunization in an SSTI model of *S. aureus* infection, we challenged immunized or control mice with 1×10^9 CFU *S. aureus* SAP149 in the left ear two weeks after the second immunization. This model was developed by Prabhakara *et al.* [42] and leads to a self-limited, localized infection that generates a necrotic lesion. The challenge was conducted using a Morrow Brown needle such that the bacteria do not penetrate past the upper epidermal layer of the skin. We followed several animals over time in order to monitor lesion formation and subsequent tissue damage (Figure 1). In control animals that received Alhydrogel® and CpG adjuvant without antigen, we saw that mice lost large portions of the affected ears as the infection progressed. However, in HlaH35L-immunized animals, tissue loss was minimal or did not occur (Figure 1). Animals were euthanized at days four and seven post-challenge and serial dilutions of the homogenized, affected ears were plated. Animals receiving HlaH35L with Alhydrogel® and CpG had significantly lower levels of *S. aureus* SAP149 present in the challenged ears than did control mice receiving adjuvant alone at both time points (Figure 2A and 2B). By day 14 post-challenge, all animals had colonization levels approaching the limit of detection (Figure 2C); this result is not unexpected, as this SSTI model is self-limiting [42]. These results were reproducible over two independent experiments. These data indicate that HlaH35L immunization leads to a lesser infection with lower bacterial levels and nominal tissue damage when compared to controls.

HlaH35L Immunization Decreases Bacterial Colonization of Kidneys in a Systemic Model of *S. aureus* Infection

To test whether HlaH35L immunization lessens *S. aureus* systemic infection, mice were immunized with HlaH35L adjuvanted with Alhydrogel® and CpG, or adjuvant alone as a control. Mice were then challenged with 3×10^6 CFU of *S. aureus* SAP149 via the lateral tail vein, resulting in bacteria being introduced directly into the bloodstream. When kidneys were harvested two weeks following challenge, we noted a decrease in bacterial levels in the immunized mice. The experiment was run twice; one experiment yielded statistically significant results, whereas the other did not (Figure 3). Combining data from the two experiments to increase effective sample size and therefore increase statistical power demonstrated that immunization with HlaH35L significantly reduced kidney colonization after IV challenge when compared to controls ($P=0.006$).

HlaH35L Immunization does not Lessen Bacterial Colonization of Infected Tibiae in a Model of Chronic Biofilm Infection

In order to determine if HlaH35L immunization is able to decrease levels of *S. aureus* in a model of chronic biofilm infection, we challenged immunized and control mice by introducing a metal implant and then inoculating the implant with 1×10^3 CFU *S. aureus* SAP149. Twenty-one days post-challenge, levels of *S. aureus* in the tibiae of immunized mice were determined and compared to that of mice having received Alhydrogel® and CpG alone. The experiment was performed in duplicate. There was no significant difference in bacterial colonization of affected tibiae observed between groups (Figure 4A and B) in either experiment. These data suggest that HlaH35L immunization does not lessen severity of chronic *S. aureus* biofilm infection.

We should note that this model utilizes C57BL/6 mice instead of BALB/c mice, because BALB/c mice, unlike what is seen in clinical cases of *S. aureus* prosthetic implant infection, can spontaneously clear the infection even if a biofilm is first grown on the pin prior to implantation. In order to determine the importance of mouse strain in the other models, we performed ELISA on pools of sera from immunized mice for each of the three challenge models used in this study. We found no significant difference between the antibody titers (expressed as ED_{50}s) for HlaH35L-immunized animals from the three model groups (data not shown; $P=0.874$, ANOVA). Moreover, we also performed *S. aureus* SSTI challenge using C57BL/6 mice and found that

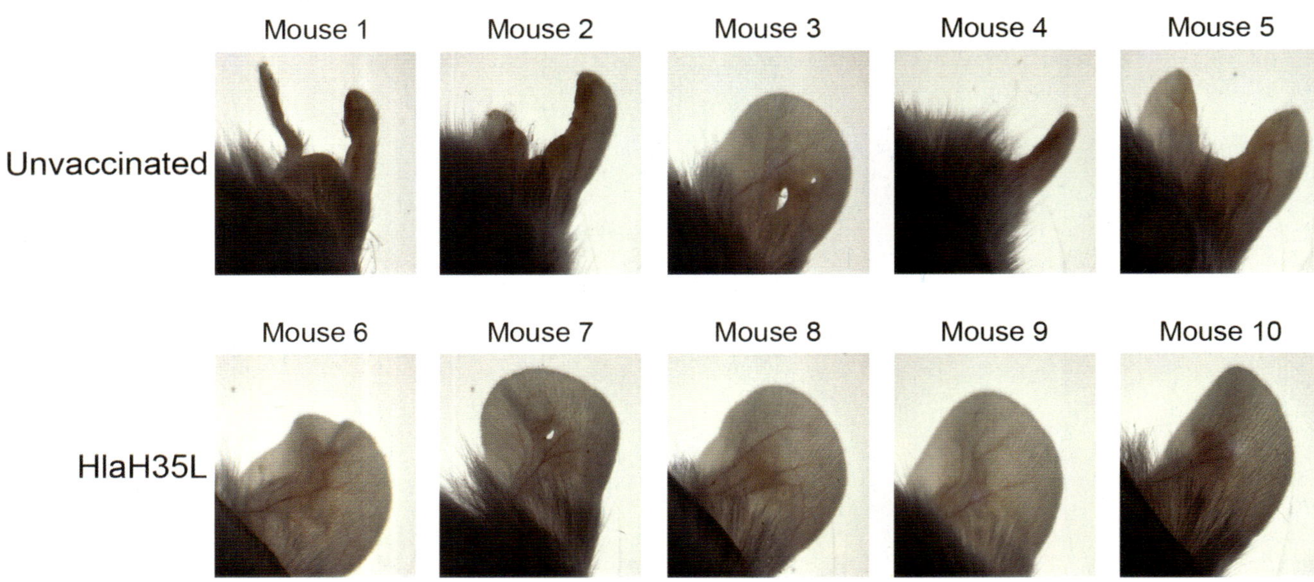

Figure 1. Assessment of tissue damage from SSTI in control vs HlaH35L-immunized mice. Photographs were taken on day 14 post-challenge.

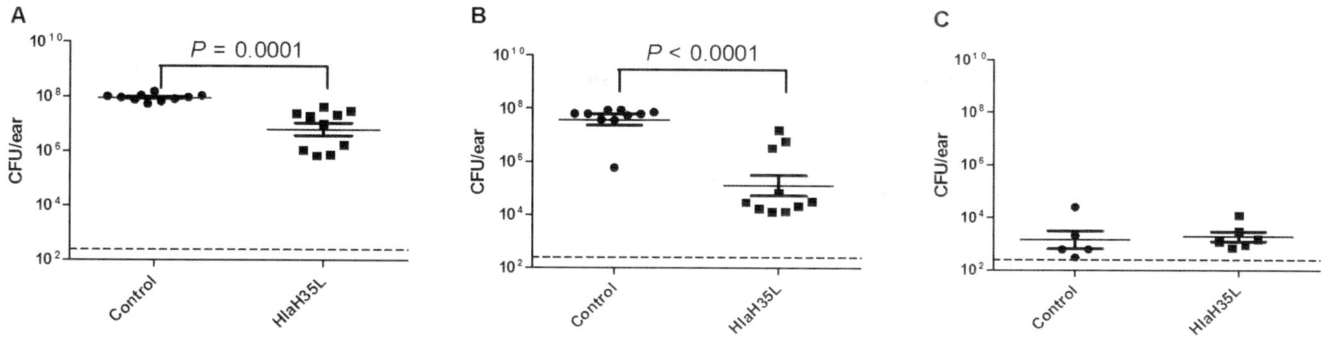

Figure 2. Analysis of HlaH35L in a skin and soft tissue infection model of *S. aureus* infection. Control animals receiving aluminum hydroxide/CpG adjuvant (●) and animals receiving HlaH35L with adjuvant (■) were compared at days four (A), seven (B), and fourteen (C) post-challenge. The CFU per ear are plotted, with the mean +/− SEM indicated for each group and *P* value calculated by two-tailed Student's t test. The dashed line indicates the limit of detection.

significantly lower infection levels were obtained in mice immunized with HlaH35L as compared to control mice (data not shown), similar to the results obtained with BALB/c mice. These results indicate that HlaH35L can elicit protection in the skin and soft tissue infection model regardless of whether BALB/c or C57BL/6 mice are used.

Discussion

While a good deal of research into potential *S. aureus* vaccine candidates has been conducted, the vast majority of publications detailing such investigations have described testing in a single animal model of infection. While an antigen may elicit protection against single, or even similar, disease types, broad protection against the wide variety of infections that a dynamic pathogen such as *S. aureus* causes may be difficult to achieve. Therefore, testing potential candidates in animal models that encompass both acute infections, e.g. skin and soft tissue infections or sepsis, and chronic infections such as osteomyelitis, would be informative.

In this study, we undertook the evaluation of a single protein antigen that has been published in several works to generate a protective response in animals against *S. aureus* infection and that has been included in *S. aureus* vaccines in clinical trials [45]. Inactivated alpha toxin has been shown to reduce bacterial populations and/or protect mice from lethality against pneumonia [32], skin infection [30], and, recently, sepsis [38] and peritoneal abscess models [37]. However, the toxin has not been tested against chronic, biofilm-associated infections. Moreover, those studies used different dosing regimens, adjuvants, and challenge strains. For this work, we eliminated potential laboratory-to-laboratory variability by using the same protein preparation for immunizations and the same challenge strain for protection studies. We also used a single dosing regimen and the same adjuvant for all studies to better mimic how a vaccine would actually be used. We found that HlaH35L combined with Alhydrogel® and CpG administered to mice that were then subjected to *S. aureus* SSTI or systemic challenge led to lower infection levels than did adjuvant alone. The difference between vaccine and control groups was statistically robust in the SSTI model. The difference between the two groups for the systemic infection model, while statistically significant when data from two experiments were combined, was less robust. Possibly, HlaH35L is only marginally protective in our systemic infection model, and the more moderate level of protection required a greater number of animals to reach statistical significance.

We found that the same immunization strategy did not elicit protection in a prosthetic implant infection model. This model was developed by Prabhakara *et al.* to recapitulate what is seen in humans with biofilm infections: The infection remains localized,

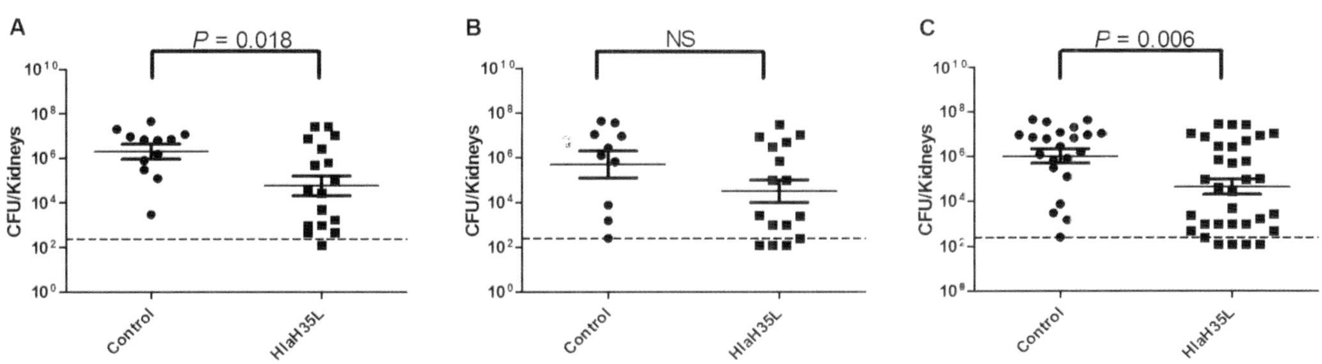

Figure 3. Analysis of HlaH35L in a systemic infection model of *S. aureus* infection. Control animals receiving aluminum hydroxide/CpG adjuvant (●) and animals receiving HlaH35L with adjuvant (■) were compared in an IV challenge model with 3×10^6 CFU SAP149 as the challenge dose. Shown are the data for two individual experiments performed identically (A and B) and the combined data (C). The CFU per pair of kidneys are plotted, with the mean +/− SEM indicated for each group and the *P* value determined by two-tailed Student's t-test. The dashed line indicates the limit of detection.

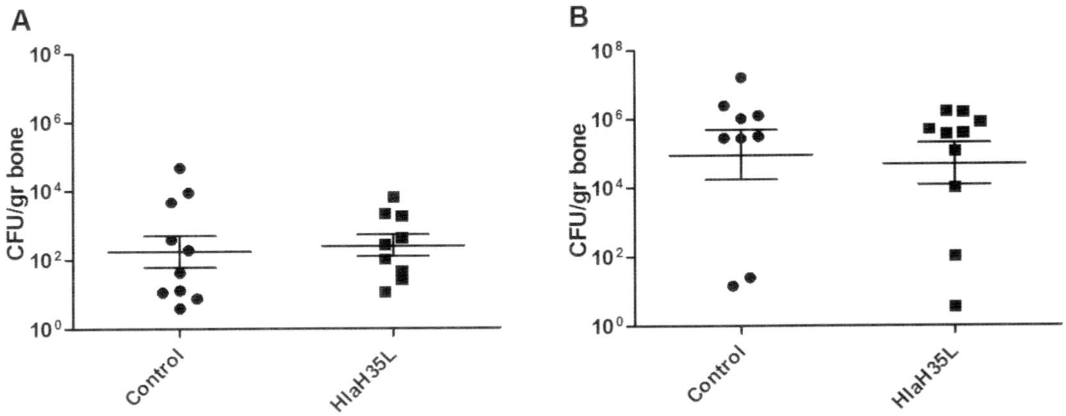

Figure 4. Analysis of HlaH35L in a prosthetic implant model of *S. aureus* infection. Control animals receiving aluminum hydroxide with CpG adjuvant (●) and animals receiving HlaH35L with adjuvant (■) were compared. Shown are the results for two experiments performed identically (A and B). The CFU per gram of bone are plotted, with the mean +/− SEM indicated for each group.

with bacterial levels constant after seven days. The infection also persists long term (>49 days), and is unable to be cleared by antibiotics or the host immune response [43]. We found that there was no significant difference in the level of *S. aureus* in infected tibiae from either HlaH35L-immunized or control mice. This finding may not be surprising, as microarray analyses have indicated that *hla* is down-regulated during biofilm growth [7,46]. It is also possible that alpha toxin may be present at some level within the mature biofilm, but that it plays no role in such an environment; alternatively, alpha toxin may not affect biofilm development or bacterial colonization of bone. In these cases, antibodies capable of toxin neutralization would not be expected to be effective in clearing the biofilm-associated bacteria. Regardless of the underlying reason why an HlaH35L vaccine was not protective in this model, this failure indicates that antigens that are chosen based on their effectiveness in other types of staphylococcal infection, such as systemic disease, may not be useful in the case of chronic, biofilm-associated infections.

Because expressed virulence factors vary among different manifestations of *S. aureus* disease, it is important to determine if a vaccine antigen may be broadly protective. To our knowledge, no group has described testing of individual *S. aureus* antigens in both acute and chronic infection models, within a laboratory using the same protein preparation, same dosing regimen, same adjuvant and the same challenge strain. Our work indicates that an antigen that is protective against one disease form may not be protective against other forms. In particular, protection against acute infection may not be predictive of protection against chronic biofilm-associated *S. aureus* disease. These results demonstrate that if a single antigen is to be used, care should be taken to ensure that the antigen is universally expressed, accessible to the host immune response, and necessary for bacterial persistence under all *S. aureus* growth conditions. An alternate strategy might be to formulate a vaccine that includes multiple protective antigens that play critical roles in both acute and chronic forms of infection. In either case, robust testing in multiple animal models may provide useful information regarding the potential of a vaccine to protect against a dynamic pathogen such as *S. aureus*.

Acknowledgments

Strain NRS384 was obtained through the Network on Antimicrobial Resistance in Staphylococcus aureus (NARSA), supported under NIAID, NIH Contract No. N01-AI-95359.

Author Contributions

Conceived and designed the experiments: RAB CPM R. Prabhakara R. Plaut MES TJM DLB. Performed the experiments: RAB CPM R. Prabhakara MES. Analyzed the data: RAB CPM DLB. Contributed reagents/materials/analysis tools: RAB CPM R. Prabhakara MES TJM DLB. Wrote the paper: RAB CPM R. Prabhakara R. Plaut MES TJM DLB.

References

1. Krespi YP, Kizhner V (2012) Laser-assisted nasal decolonization of *Staphylococcus aureus*, including methicillin-resistant *Staphylococcus aureus*. Am J Otolaryngol 33: 572–575.
2. Klevens RM, Morrison MA, Nadle J, Petit S, Gershman K, et al. (2007) Invasive Methicillin-Resistant *Staphylococcus aureus* Infections in the United States. JAMA 298: 1763–1771.
3. Gorwitz RJ, Kruszon-Moran D, McAllister SK, McQuillan G, McDougal LK, et al. (2008) Changes in the prevalence of nasal colonization with *Staphylococcus aureus* in the United States, 2001–2004. J Infect Dis 197: 1226–1234.
4. Peacock SJ, de Silva I, Lowy FD (2001) What determines nasal carriage of *Staphylococcus aureus*? Trends Microbiol 9: 605–610.
5. von Eiff C, Becker K, Machka K, Stammer H, Peters G (2001) Nasal carriage as a source of *Staphylococcus aureus* bacteremia. Study Group. N Engl J Med 344: 11–16.
6. Foster TJ (2004) The *Staphylococcus aureus* "superbug". J Clin Invest 114: 1693–1696.
7. Resch A, Rosenstein R, Nerz C, Gotz F (2005) Differential gene expression profiling of *Staphylococcus aureus* cultivated under biofilm and planktonic conditions. Appl Environ Microbiol 71: 2663–2676.
8. Beenken KE, Dunman PM, McAleese F, Macapagal D, Murphy E, et al. (2004) Global gene expression in *Staphylococcus aureus* biofilms. J Bacteriol 186: 4665–4684.
9. Resch A, Leicht S, Saric M, Pasztor L, Jakob A, et al. (2006) Comparative proteome analysis of *Staphylococcus aureus* biofilm and planktonic cells and correlation with transcriptome profiling. Proteomics 6: 1867–1877.
10. Arrecubieta C, Matsunaga I, Asai T, Naka Y, Deng MC, et al. (2008) Vaccination with clumping factor A and fibronectin binding protein A to prevent *Staphylococcus aureus* infection of an aortic patch in mice. J Infect Dis 198: 571–575.
11. Brouillette E, Lacasse P, Shkreta L, Belanger J, Grondin G, et al. (2002) DNA immunization against the clumping factor A (ClfA) of *Staphylococcus aureus*. Vaccine 20: 2348–2357.
12. Cheng AG, McAdow M, Kim HK, Bae T, Missiakas DM, et al. (2010) Contribution of coagulases towards *Staphylococcus aureus* disease and protective immunity. PLoS Pathog 6: e1001036.
13. Gong R, Hu C, Xu H, Guo A, Chen H, et al. (2010) Evaluation of clumping factor A binding region A in a subunit vaccine against *Staphylococcus aureus*-induced mastitis in mice. Clin Vaccine Immunol 17: 1746–1752.

14. Hu DL, Narita K, Hyodo M, Hayakawa Y, Nakane A, et al. (2009) c-di-GMP as a vaccine adjuvant enhances protection against systemic methicillin-resistant *Staphylococcus aureus* (MRSA) infection. Vaccine 27: 4867–4873.
15. Josefsson E, Hartford O, O'Brien L, Patti JM, Foster T (2001) Protection against experimental *Staphylococcus aureus* arthritis by vaccination with clumping factor A, a novel virulence determinant. J Infect Dis 184: 1572–1580.
16. Josefsson E, Higgins J, Foster TJ, Tarkowski A (2008) Fibrinogen binding sites P336 and Y338 of clumping factor A are crucial for *Staphylococcus aureus* virulence. PLoS One 3: e2206.
17. Mamo W, Boden M, Flock JI (1994) Vaccination with *Staphylococcus aureus* fibrinogen binding proteins (FgBPs) reduces colonisation of *S. aureus* in a mouse mastitis model. FEMS Immunol Med Microbiol 10: 47–53.
18. Schaffer AC, Solinga RM, Cocchiaro J, Portoles M, Kiser KB, et al. (2006) Immunization with *Staphylococcus aureus* clumping factor B, a major determinant in nasal carriage, reduces nasal colonization in a murine model. Infect Immun 74: 2145–2153.
19. Shannon O, Uekotter A, Flock JI (2006) The neutralizing effects of hyperimmune antibodies against extracellular fibrinogen-binding protein, Efb, from *Staphylococcus aureus*. Scand J Immunol 63: 184–190.
20. Shkreta L, Talbot BG, Diarra MS, Lacasse P (2004) Immune responses to a DNA/protein vaccination strategy against *Staphylococcus aureus* induced mastitis in dairy cows. Vaccine 23: 114–126.
21. Zhou H, Xiong ZY, Li HP, Zheng YL, Jiang YQ (2006) An immunogenicity study of a newly fusion protein Cna-FnBP vaccinated against *Staphylococcus aureus* infections in a mice model. Vaccine 24: 4830–4837.
22. Anderson AS, Scully IL, Timofeyeva Y, Murphy E, McNeil LK, et al. (2012) *Staphylococcus aureus* transporter MntC is a highly conserved cell surface protein that elicits protective immunity against both *S. aureus* and *Staphylococcus epidermidis*. J Infect Dis 205: 1688–1696.
23. Brady RA, O'May GA, Leid JG, Prior ML, Costerton JW, et al. (2011) Resolution of *Staphylococcus aureus* biofilm infection using vaccination and antibiotic treatment. Infect Immun 79: 1797–1803.
24. Clarke SR, Brummell KJ, Horsburgh MJ, McDowell PW, Mohamad SA, et al. (2006) Identification of in vivo-expressed antigens of *Staphylococcus aureus* and their use in vaccinations for protection against nasal carriage. J Infect Dis 193: 1098–1108.
25. Glowalla E, Tosetti B, Kronke M, Krut O (2009) Proteomics-based identification of anchorless cell wall proteins as vaccine candidates against *Staphylococcus aureus*. Infect Immun 77: 2719–2729.
26. Ster C, Beaudoin F, Diarra MS, Jacques M, Malouin F, et al. (2010) Evaluation of some *Staphylococcus aureus* iron-regulated proteins as vaccine targets. Vet Immunol Immunopathol 136: 311–318.
27. Stranger-Jones YK, Bae T, Schneewind O (2006) Vaccine assembly from surface proteins of *Staphylococcus aureus*. Proceedings of the National Academy of Sciences 103: 16942–16947.
28. Joshi A, Pancari G, Cope L, Bowman E, Cua D, et al. (2012) Immunization with *Staphylococcus aureus* iron regulated surface determinant B (IsdB) confers protection via Th17/IL17 pathway in a murine sepsis model. Hum Vaccin Immunother 8: 336–346.
29. Kim HK, Cheng AG, Kim HY, Missiakas DM, Schneewind O (2010) Nontoxigenic protein A vaccine for methicillin-resistant *Staphylococcus aureus* infections in mice. J Exp Med 207: 1863–1870.
30. Kennedy AD, Bubeck Wardenburg J, Gardner DJ, Long D, Whitney AR, et al. (2010) Targeting of alpha-hemolysin by active or passive immunization decreases severity of USA300 skin infection in a mouse model. J Infect Dis 202: 1050–1058.
31. Narita K, Hu DL, Tsuji T, Nakane A (2008) Intranasal immunization of mutant toxic shock syndrome toxin 1 elicits systemic and mucosal immune response against *Staphylococcus aureus* infection. FEMS Immunol Med Microbiol 52: 389–396.
32. Bubeck Wardenburg J, Schneewind O (2008) Vaccine protection against *Staphylococcus aureus* pneumonia. J Exp Med 205: 287–294.
33. Gening ML, Maira-Litran T, Kropec A, Skurnik D, Grout M, et al. (2010) Synthetic {beta}-(1->6)-linked N-acetylated and nonacetylated oligoglucosamines used to produce conjugate vaccines for bacterial pathogens. Infect Immun 78: 764–772.
34. Cook J, Hepler R, Pancari G, Kuklin N, Fan H, et al. (2009) *Staphylococcus aureus* capsule type 8 antibodies provide inconsistent efficacy in murine models of staphylococcal infection. Hum Vaccin 5: 254–263.
35. Ho MM, Bolgiano B, Martino A, Kairo SK, Corbel MJ (2006) Preclinical laboratory evaluation of a bivalent *Staphylococcus aureus* saccharide-exotoxin A protein conjugate vaccine. Hum Vaccin 2: 89–98.
36. Menzies BE, Kernodle DS (1994) Site-directed mutagenesis of the alpha-toxin gene of *Staphylococcus aureus*: role of histidines in toxin activity in vitro and in a murine model. Infect Immun 62: 1843–1847.
37. Rauch S, Dedent AG, Kim HK, Bubeck Wardenburg J, Missiakas DM, et al. (2012) Abscess formation and alpha-hemolysin induced toxicity in a mouse model of *Staphylococcus aureus* peritoneal infection. Infect Immun 80: 3721–3732.
38. Adhikari RP, Karauzum H, Sarwar J, Abaandou L, Mahmoudieh M, et al. (2012) Novel Structurally Designed Vaccine for *S. aureus* alpha-Hemolysin: Protection against Bacteremia and Pneumonia. PLoS One 7: e38567.
39. Hume EB, Dajcs JJ, Moreau JM, O'Callaghan RJ (2000) Immunization with alpha-toxin toxoid protects the cornea against tissue damage during experimental *Staphylococcus aureus* keratitis. Infect Immun 68: 6052–6055.
40. Mandel M, Higa A (1970) Calcium-dependent bacteriophage DNA infection. J Mol Biol 53: 159–162.
41. Stemmer WP, Morris SK (1992) Enzymatic inverse PCR: a restriction site independent, single-fragment method for high-efficiency, site-directed mutagenesis. Biotechniques 13: 214–220.
42. Prabhakara R, Foreman O, De Pascalis R, Lee GM, Plaut RD, et al. (2013) An Epicutaneous Model of Community-Acquired *Staphylococcus aureus* Skin Infections. Infect Immun: Epub 4 Feb 2013.
43. Prabhakara R, Harro JM, Leid JG, Harris M, Shirtliff ME (2011) Murine immune response to a chronic Staphylococcus aureus biofilm infection. Infect Immun 79: 1789–1796.
44. Li D, Gromov K, Soballe K, Puzas JE, O'Keefe RJ, et al. (2008) Quantitative mouse model of implant-associated osteomyelitis and the kinetics of microbial growth, osteolysis, and humoral immunity. J Orthop Res 26: 96–105.
45. Ohlsen K, Lorenz U (2010) Immunotherapeutic strategies to combat staphylococcal infections. Int J Med Microbiol 300: 402–410.
46. Brady RA, Leid JG, Camper AK, Costerton JW, Shirtliff ME (2006) Identification of *Staphylococcus aureus* proteins recognized by the antibody-mediated immune response to a biofilm infection. Infect Immun 74: 3415–3426.

Nasal Carriage of *Staphylococcus aureus* in Botucatu, Brazil: A Population-Based Survey

Fabiana Venegas Pires[1], Maria de Lourdes Ribeiro de Souza da Cunha[2], Lígia Maria Abraão[1], Patrícia Y. F. Martins[2], Carlos Henrique Camargo[2], Carlos Magno Castelo Branco Fortaleza[1]*

1 Departamento de Doenças Tropicais, Faculdade de Medicina de Botucatu, Universidade Estadual Paulista, Botucatu, Brazil, **2** Departamento de Microbiologia e Imunologia, Instituto de Biociências de Botucatu, Universidade Estadual Paulista, Botucatu, Brazil

Abstract

Recent increases in the incidence and severity of staphylococcal infections renewed interest in studies that assess the burden of asymptomatic carriage of *Staphylococcus aureus* in the community setting. We conducted a population-based survey in the city of Botucatu, Brazil (122,000 inhabitants), in order to identify the prevalence of nasal carriage of *Staphylococcus aureus* (including methicillin-resistant strains). Nasal swabs were obtained from 686 persons over one year of age. Resistance to methicillin was assessed through phenotypic methods, identification of the *mec*A gene and typing of the Staphylococcal Chromosome Cassette *mec* (SCC*mec*). Methicillin-resistant *S. aureus* (MRSA) isolates were characterized using Pulsed-Field Gel Electrophoresis (PFGE), Multilocus Sequence Typing (MLST) and *spa* typing. Polymerase chain reaction was applied to identify genes coding for Panton-Valentine Leukocidin (PVL) in isolates. The prevalence of overall *S. aureus* carriage was 32.7% (95%CI, 29.2%–36.2%). Carriers were significantly younger (mean age, 28.1 versus 36.3 for non-carriers; OR for age, 0.98; 95%CI, 0.97–0.99) and likely to report recent skin infection (OR, 1.85; 95%CI, 1.03–3.34). Carriage of methicillin-resistant *S. aureus* (MRSA) was found in 0.9% of study subjects (95%CI, 0.4%–1.8%). All MRSA isolates harbored SCC*mec* type IV, and belonged to *spa* types t002 or t021, but none among them harbored genes coding for PLV. In MLST, most isolates belonged to clones ST5 or ST1776. However, we found one subject who carried a novel clone, ST2594. Two out of six MRSA carriers had household contacts colonized with isolates similar to theirs. Our study pointed to dissemination of community-associated MRSA among the Brazilian population.

Editor: Holger Rohde, Universitätsklinikum Hamburg-Eppendorf, Germany

Funding: This work was supported by "Fundação de Amparo à Pesquisa do Estado de São Paulo" (FAPESP, grant #2011/06988-2, www.fapesp.br). The funder had no role in study design, data collection and analysis, decision to publish, or preparation of the manuscript.

Competing Interests: The authors have declared that no competing interests exist.

* E-mail: cmfortaleza@uol.com.br

Introduction

Recent reports point out to an increase in incidence and severity of staphylococcal infections arising in the community [1,2]. The emergence and worldwide spread of community-associated methicillin-resistant *Staphylococcus aureus* (CA-MRSA) worsened this picture [3]. Most CA-MRSA strains are genetically unrelated to hospital-acquired clones. Also, they have been implicated in the etiology of severe diseases, such as necrotizing pneumonia and skin and soft tissue infection. The severity of CA-MRSA infections has been linked to a major virulence factor, the Panton-Valentine Leukocidin (PVL) [4].

This phenomenon renewed interest in research focusing on the epidemiology of *S. aureus* as a whole and MRSA, both in the community and in healthcare settings. Some studies were directed towards identifying the burden of MRSA infections. Klevens et al. reported that, among 8,987 invasive MRSA infections from 9 sites in the United States (U.S.), 13.7% could be classified as community-associated [5]. From a different perspective, studies from Europe reported MRSA accounting for 6% to 30% of *S. aureus* infections in outpatients [6]. In Asian countries that proportion ranged from 2.5% to 39% [7]. One study conducted in five major African towns, including 542 patients with *S. aureus* infections, identified 86 MRSA isolates, of which 9 were classified as CA-MRSA [8]. Those cases accounted for 11.5% of community-associated *S. aureus* infections, though data may be biased due to criteria for collecting cultures [9].

There is strong evidence of continuous increase in the incidence of CA-MRSA disease during the past decade, at least in the U.S. [10]. Even though data from Europe suggest that the threat posed by CA-MRSA is lower when compared to the U.S., cases of invasive infections are regularly reported in several countries [6,11,12]. Reports of CA-MRSA infections in Africa [8] and Asia [7,13] confirm the worldwide importance of this pathogen.

In order to identify the sources and dynamics of CA-MRSA in the general population, some epidemiological studies addressed the prevalence and determinants of asymptomatic carriage (also termed "colonization") of *S. aureus* and MRSA in the community setting. Those studies are based on the evidence that colonization represents a reservoir for pathogenic strains and/or a pre-infectious stage [14,15]. In the U.S., the nasal carriage of *S. aureus* was assessed in 9,622 persons as part of the National Health and Nutrition Examination Survey (NHANES) in 2001–2002. The study found prevalence of 32.4% and 0.8% for *S. aureus* and MRSA, respectively [16,17]. In the following years, there was a slight decrease in the overall prevalence of *S. aureus* colonization, while the carriage of MRSA almost doubled [18].

Even though extensive research has focused on the global epidemiology of *S. aureus* and MRSA, there are significant gaps of information for regions in Asia, Africa and South America [19]. In Brazil, reports of CA-MRSA infections are scarce, and all data and strains were obtained from patients in university hospitals from highly populated cities [20–22].

Our study was designed to fill this gap, providing population-based data about *S. aureus* and MRSA colonization in a small city in inner Brazil. We also aimed to identify factors associated to colonization and the molecular epidemiology of colonizing strains.

Materials and Methods

Ethical issues

This study was conducted according to the principles expressed in the Declaration of Helsinki. It was approved by the reference Committee for Ethics in Research ("Comitê de Ética em Pesquisa" from "Faculdade de Medicina de Botucatu". City of Botucatu, São Paulo State, Brazil). A written informed consent was obtained from all study subjects or their legal guardians.

Study design and population

We conducted a cross-sectional study in order to identify the prevalence of carriage *S. aureus* among urban population in the city of Botucatu, Brazil (22°53′09″S, 48°26′42″W). The city is located in São Paulo State, in Southeastern Brazil. It has approximately 122,000 inhabitants, 95% of whom live in urban areas. The survey was conducted during the year 2011.

The sample size was estimated in OpenEpi software (Emory University, Atlanta, GA) using the following parameters: city population, 122,000; anticipated *S. aureus* prevalence, 32.4%; confidence limits, 5%; design effect, 2. We estimated the inclusion of 672 subjects. The sample size was later extended for 686, for operational reasons.

The sample was stratified for age and gender, according to the 2010 census data. Subjects with less than one year of age were excluded. Households and subjects from the urban area of Botucatu were selected from an updated version of the database used in the São Paulo State Health Survey [23].

Collection of swabs and microbiologic methods

Nasal swabs were obtained from the selected subjects. Humidified swabs were inserted in both nares as deeply as possible, until the subjects reported discomfort. Specimens were transported in Stuart medium and cultured in Baird Parker agar. Species identification was performed as follows: The isolates obtained were stained by the Gram method for the determination of purity and observation of morphology and specific staining. After confirmation of these characteristics, the strains were submitted to catalase and coagulase tests. Fermentation tests of maltose, trehalose and mannitol were performed to differentiate *S. aureus* from other coagulase-positive staphylococci [24]. The isolates were also submitted to genotypic identification by Polymerase Chain Reaction (PCR), using primers for amplification of chromosomal DNA fragment which is specific for *S. aureus* (442-bp fragment). We followed the protocol described by Martineau et al. [25] and used primers *Sa442*-1 (5′-AAT CTT TGT CGG TAC ACG ATA TTC TTC ACG-3′) and *Sa442*-2 (5′-CGT AAT GAG ATT TCA GTA GAT AAT ACA ACA-3′).

Susceptibility tests followed guidelines from the Clinical Laboratory Standards Institute (CLSI), using disks for oxacillin and cefoxitin [26].

Molecular detection and characterization of SCC*mec*

For the purposes of our study, *S. aureus* isolates were classified as MRSA when they harbored the *mecA* gene, which is responsible for methicillin-resistance. PCR for detection of *mecA* was performed as described by Murakami et al. [27]. All reactions included positive (*S. aureus* ATCC 33591) and negative (*S. aureus* ATCC 25923) controls. The multiplex-PCR protocol described by Milheiriço et al [28] was used for the characterization of the staphylococcal cassette chromosome *mec* (SCC*mec*).

Molecular strain typing

All MRSA isolates were submitted to strain typing. For Pulsed-Field Gel Electrophoresis (PFGE), we used a protocol modified from McDoughal et al. [29], based on DNA digestion with the restriction enzyme *Sma*I. The analysis of similarity was performed using the Dice coefficient. Clusters were defined on the basis of similarity values over 80%. Dendrograms were drawn based on Unweighted Pair Group Method Using Arithmetic Averages (UPGMA) in the BioNumerics 6.1 software (Applied Maths, Belgium). Several MRSA isolates originated from different countries were included as controls in the dendrogram.

Multilocus sequence typing (MLST) was subsequently performed, amplifying and sequencing genes *arcC, aroE, glpF, gmk, pta, tpi* and *yqiL*, as described by Enright et al. [30]. Analysis of results focused on the consensus sequence, according to data from *S. aureus* official MLST site (http://saureus.mlst.net).

spa typing was performed according to the protocol described by Shopsin et al [31]. PCR was performed using primers 1095F (5′-AGACGATCCTTCGGTGAGC-3′) e 1517R (5′-GCTTTTGCAATGTCATTTACTG-3′). The amplified product was purified and sequenced. The analysis of repetitions was carried out in the software Bionumerics (Applied Maths, Belgium), which assessed (through specific plugin) the database from Ridom Spa Server (http://www.spaserver.ridom.de).

Detection of genes coding for PVL

All *S. aureus* isolates were tested for the presence of genes coding for PVL (*lukS-PV, lukF-PV*). We used a PCR protocol, as previously described [32].

Epidemiological analysis

A questionnaire was applied to all study subjects. Several issues were assessed, including demographics, practice of sports, behavioral factors and comorbidities. Subjects were also questioned about infectious diseases, use of antimicrobials and exposure to healthcare settings during the previous year.

All collected data were stored in database in EPI INFO 3.5 (Centers for Disease Control and Prevention, Atlanta, GA, USA) and analyzed using SPSS 19.0 (IBM, Armonk, NY, USA). Analysis was performed separately for two outcomes: (a) overall *S. aureus* carriage and (b) carriage of MRSA.

All data were initially submitted to bivariate analysis. Dichotomous variables were analyzed using the Chi-square or Fisher Exact test. For continuous variables, we used Student's T or the Mann-Whitney U test. Multivariate analysis was performed using logistic regression models. A "change-in-estimate" approach use used for selection of variables [33]. In the first step, logistic regression included all variables with $p<0.1$ in the bivariate analysis. New models included all the other variables, one at a time. Variables that changed the Odds Ratio of significant factors in more than 10% were kept in the final model. As counterproof, we performed the multivariate analysis using forward and backward strategies for variable selection, and obtained similar results. P<0.05 was used for definition of statistical significance in all steps of statystical analysis.

Results

The overall prevalence of nasal carriage of *S. aureus* was 32.7% (95%CI, 29.2%–36.2%). The bivariate analysis of factors associated with carriage is presented in **Table 1**. **Table 2** displays the final multivariate logistic regression model. Briefly, persons carrying *S. aureus* were significantly younger than non-carriers, and more likely to report recent skin infection. Genes coding for PVL were found in five out of 224 isolates (2.2%), all of which were methicillin-susceptible. It is worth noting that only one out of five subjects carrying PVL-positive isolates reported recent skin infection. Given the small number of subjects, the incidence of skin infections in the previous year for carriers of PVL-positive (20%) and PVL-negative (11%) isolates was not statistically significant (p = 0.5).

On the other hand, MRSA isolates were found colonizing the nares of 0.9% of the study subjects (95%CI, 0.4%–1.8%). None of the six MRSA-colonized subjects reported recent exposure to healthcare settings. All their household contacts (15 persons) were screened, and carriage of MRSA was found in two of them.

All MRSA isolates harbored SCC*mec* type IV, but none of them carried genes coding for PVL. There was a major PFGE cluster grouping isolates from four out of six MRSA-positive subjects, plus one household contact (**Figure 1**). The isolates in that cluster were characterized as *spa* type t002. In MLST, most belonged to ST5. However, one isolated differed in the allele for the gene *glpF*. The data were submitted to the MSLT homepage (http://saureus.mlst.net), and a novel number was attributed to that allele (320). The isolated was characterized as a novel clone (ST 2594).

The two remaining subjects carried MRSA isolates that presented different PFGE patterns and *spa* types (t002 and t021), but belonged to ST1176. One of them had a household contact colonized with an isolate that was similar to hers in all typing methods.

Discussion

Several recent studies have assessed *S. aureus* asymptomatic colonization among non-hospitalized persons. Many among them focused on special populations, such as sportsmen [34], military [35], prison inmates [36] or remote communities [37,38]. Others enrolled specific age groups, such as children [39,40,41] and elderly persons [41]. While these studies are of great interest, it is still necessary to estimate the burden of *S. aureus* and MRSA carriage among general population from different countries. Our study aimed to contribute to this issue.

This was the first study to focus *S. aureus* colonization in Brazil using a population-based approach. Our findings point out to a prevalence of both *S. aureus* and MRSA colonization similar to that reported in the 2001–2002 NHANES reports [16,17] and in minor studies from the U.S. [42,43]. We found that about one third of the population of Botucatu carries *S. aureus* on their nares. On the other hand, the spread of MRSA in the community is limited. Still, we can estimate more than 1,000 persons carrying MRSA in the city of Botucatu at the time when the study was conducted. This is in contrast with results from two studies that focused on asymptomatic *S. aureus* carriage in Europe. The Tromso Staph and Skin Study enrolled 2,279 subjects, finding prevalence of *S. aureus* nasal colonization of 26.2% for healthcare workers and 26.0% for the general population [44]. Pooled results from Dutch surveys reported colonization in 34.9% of 3,198 children and 27.1% of 3,851 adults over 55 years of age [41]. Despite their sample size, neither studies from Norway or Netherlands found any case of MRSA colonization. At the other end of the epidemiological spectrum in Europe, one study from Malta reported MRSA nasal colonization in 8.8% of 329 healthy individuals [45].

The comparison of our results with data from other countries or continents is difficult, due to differences in the target populations and sites of collection of cultures. Still, it is worth reporting that surveys in African countries found asymptomatic colonization with *S. aureus* and a whole and MRSA in 33% and 9% of 120 persons from the Niger delta (Nigeria) [46] and in 29% and 1% of 500 subjects from rural and semi-urban areas in Lambaréné, Gabon [47]. One study from Queensland (Australia) enrolled 396 patients presenting to general practice and 303 randomly selected volunteers. The prevalence rates of methicillin-susceptible *S. aureus* and MRSA nasal colonization were 28% and 0.7% [48].

Hamdan-Partida et al. [49] investigated 1,243 healthy volunteers from Mexico, finding *S. aureus* and MRSA in 59.8% and 8.6% of study subjects. Those authors followed subjects for 6-years in order to characterize persistent carriage, which occurred in 13.0% of colonized persons. Cultures from nares and throat were performed, and this strategy increased the detection of *S. aureus*. However, the study subjects were selected on the basis of the possibility of long term follow up. Therefore, the sample was not stratified in order to reflect the demographic distribution of Mexican population.

In a study from India, the reported prevalence rates among 1,000 subjects were 22.5% for *S. aureus* and 16.6% for MRSA [50]. A comparison of these results with ours is hindered by the fact that researchers also screened subjects for colonization in body sites other than the nares: namely, forearms and palms. Once again, the approach used for selection of subjects is unclear. Several groups were enrolled, including people from different economic classes, healthcare workers and inpatients. The latter two groups seem overrepresented, so one may doubt the validity of the results as estimates of the colonization burden in the general population.

In our study, we found an inverse association between age and *S. aureus* colonization. This finding has been consistently reported in other studies [16,18]. Indeed, research that specifically focused on children identified high rates of both *S. aureus* and MRSA colonization [51,52]. Interestingly, a survey conducted among Pygmies from Gabon identified peek colonization rates among teenagers [38].

In our study, *S. aureus* colonization was associated with the report of skin infections in the past year. In fact, incidence of skin infections during that period was 11.2% for carriers of *S. aureus*. Also, those infections affected two out of six MRSA-colonized subjects. An interesting result is obtained when we reanalyze our database, selecting skin infection as an outcome, and including alternatively colonization with *S. aureus* as a whole or MRSA in multivariate logistic regression models. In this analysis, the previous history of skin infections is independently associated both with the carriage of *S. aureus* (OR, 2.04; 95%CI, 1.11–3.73; p = 0.02) and of MRSA (OR, 9.19; 95%CI, 1.158–53.47; p = 0.01). On the other hand, the presence of PVL genes was not associated to skin infections, possibly due to the small number of isolates harboring those genes.

The association of nasal colonization with *S. aureus* and skin or soft tissue infections was reported as early as the 1960s [53]. In the following decades, studies related colonization with chronic furunculosis and surgical site infections [54,55,56,57]. Based on those results, decolonization with mupirocin has been advised for preventing recurrent skin infections [55,57].

Table 1. Bivariate analysis of factors associated with nasal carriage of *Staphylococcus aureus* among persons living in the city of Botucatu, Brazil, alongside with data from six MRSA carriers in that population.

Factors	*S. aureus* (224)	Controls (462)	OR (95%CI)	*P*	MRSA (6)
Demographic data					
Male gender	**119 (53.3)**	**185 (40.0)**	**1.70 (1.23–2.34)**	**0.001**	3 (50.0)
Age, mean (range)	**28.1 (1–90)**	**36.3 (1–87)**	**...**	**<0.001**	43.7 (20–56)
Student	**94 (42.0)**	**130 (28.2)**	**1.84 (1.32–2.57)**	**<0.001**	1 (16.7)
Less than fundamental schooling*	106 (47.3)	187 (41.3)	1.23 (0.93–1.76)	0.13	1 (16.7)
Employed	74 (33.0)	178 (38.5)	0.79 (0.56–1.10)	0.16	4 (66.7)
Family income, median (range) in US dollars**	800 (200–6,000)	750 (350–8,000)	...	0.92	700 (300–2,500)
Child attending a crèche	**16 (7.1)**	**22 (4.8)**	**1.84 (0.79–2.99)**	**0.02**	0 (0.0)
Military	0 (0.0)	1 (0.2)	0.0 (...)	1.00	0 (0.0)
Has been in a prison	0 (0.0)	1 (0.2)	0.0 (...)	1.00	0 (0.0)
Has been in a nursing home	1 (0.4)	1 (0.2)	2.07 (0.13–33.20)	0.55	0 (0.0)
Behavioral factors					
Smoking	20 (8.9)	56 (12.1)	0.71 (0.42–1.22)	0.21	0 (0.0)
Alcoholism***	30 (13.4)	64 (13.9)	0.96 (0.60–1.53)	0.87	0 (0.0)
Use of illegal drugs (inhaled)	0	1 (0.2)	0.0 (...)	1.00	0 (0.0)
Use of illegal drugs (intravenous)	0 (0.0)	2 (0.4)	0.0 (...)	1.00	0 (0.0)
Regular practice of sports	**61 (27.2)**	**86 (18.6)**	**1.64 (1.12–2.38)**	**0.01**	
Use of earrings	**76 (33.9)**	**206 (44.6)**	**0.64 (0.46–0.89)**	**0.008**	0 (0.0)
Use of piercing	7 (3.1)	24 (5.2)	0.59 (0.25–1.38)	0.22	0 (0.0)
Tatoo	18 (8.0)	47 (10.2)	0.77 (0.44–1.36)	0.37	0 (0.0)
Comorbidities and health-related factors					
Heart disease	5 (2.2)	15 (3.2)			0 (0.0)
Lung disease	14 (6.3)	17 (3.7)	1.75 (0.84–3.61)	0.13	1 (16.7)
Renal disease	0 (0.0)	3 (0.6)	0.0 (...)	0.23	0 (0.0)
Central Nervous System Disease	5 (2.2)	13 (2.8)	0.79 (0.28–2.24)	0.66	0 (0.0)
Diabetes mellitus	**4 (1.8)**	**13 (2.8)**	**0.35 (0.12–0.95)**	**0.04**	0 (0.0)
Solid malignancy	2 (0.4)	5 (1.1)	0.83 (0.16–3.30)	1.0	0 (0.0)
Pressure ulcer	2 (0.4)	9 (1.9)	0.45 (0.10–2.12)	1.0	0 (0.0)
Recent skin infection****	25 (11.2)	27 (5.8)	2.02 (1.15–3.56)	0.01	2 (33.3)
Recent pneumonia****	3 (1.3)	11 (2.4)	0.56 (0.15–2.02)	0.57	0 (0.0)
Use of antimicrobials****	56 (25.0)	93 (20.1)	1.32 (0.91–1.93)	0.15	2 (33.3)
Use of steroids****	4 (1.8)	6 (1.3)	1.38 (0.39–4.95)	0.74	0 (0.0)
Admission to a hospital****	14 (6.3)	20 (4.3)	1.47 (0.73–2.97)	0.28	0 (0.0)
Surgery****	8 (3.6)	13 (2.8)	1.28 (0.52–3.13)	0.59	0 (0.0)

Note. All data presented in number(%), unless otherwise specified. Statistically significant results presented in boldface. OR Odds Ratio; CI, Confidence interval.
*Less than eight years of schooling.
** Data represent the family monthly income. Based on November 2012 exchange parameters (1 dollar is approximately equal to 2 'reais" [Brazilian currency]).
***Regular consumption of alcoholic beverages more than two times a week.
****Events from the past year.

However, this issue remains controversial [58]. Some studies reported association of *S. aureus* or MRSA colonization with several non-infectious skin diseases [59,60,61]. High prevalence of MRSA (of community or healthcare origin) carriage was found in the nares and skin of patients from a dermatology outpatient service [62]. On the other hand, nasal decolonization has failed to prevent recurrent skin infections [63]. Finally, studies focusing on the association of skin infections with colonization of patients and their households reported conflicting results [64,65,66].

In regard to our results, as well as those reported in the papers discussed above, one must remember that data obtained from cross-section studies are ambiguous in regard to causality. It is therefore possible that carriage of *S. aureus* led to the development of infection, or that colonization just remained after the infectious syndrome was controlled.

Though limited, our data on MRSA colonization suggest that there are few clones spreading in the community, possibly through social contact. All isolates harbored SCC*mec* type IV, and belonged to Clonal Complex 5 (ST5, ST1176 or ST2594) on

Table 2. Final model of multivariate analysis of factors associated with nasal carriage of *Staphylococcus aureus* among persons living in the city of Botucatu, Brazil.

Factors	OR (95%CI)	P
Age	**0.98 (0.97–0.99)**	**0.01**
Male gender	1.26 (0.82–1.96)	0.3
Student	1.11 (0.71–1.75)	0.6
Attends a crèche	1.03 (0.50–2.12)	0.9
Practice of sports	1.26 (0.84–1.89)	0.3
Use of earrings	0.74 (0.47–1.16)	0.2
Diabetes mellitus	0.56 (0.19–1.68)	0.3
Recent skin infection*	**1.85 (1.03–3.34)**	**0.04**

Note. Significant results are presented in boldface. OR, Odds Ratio. CI, Confidence interval.
* In the past year.

MLST. Most of them belonged to the same *spa* type (t002). Finally, a major PFGE cluster comprised isolates from four out of six subjects. Interestingly, two MRSA carriers (subjects #103 and #106) lived on the same street, and their isolates had 100% electrophoretic similarity. Also, two household contacts were colonized with strains similar to those found in their related subjects.

Those findings are noteworthy. Clonal complex 5 is widely spread through America, Europe, Asia and Australia [67]. ST1176 was recently described on clinical cultures from patients admitted to hospitals in the city of São Paulo, 140 miles apart from Botucatu [68]. ST2594 is a novel clone, identified in our survey, and belongs to Clonal complex 5. In summary, our study found evidence of clonal spread on regional and household levels.

The routes of *S. aureus* spread in the community are yet to be elucidated. The same is true for CA-MRSA clones, in spite of extensive research applying methods from classic and molecular epidemiology [19]. It has been suggested that methodological approaches based on social networks may help in filling gaps in our current knowledge. An interesting study addressed this issue focusing on the most basic social network: the household [64]. Analysis of determinants and clonality of *S. aureus* colonization was performed both on individual and aggregate levels. The authors found evidence for transmission within the household, but also for continuous introduction of new strains into households.

Another interesting result concerns PVL. Genes coding for this virulence factor were found in few *S. aureus* isolates, all of which were methicillin-susceptible. The absence of PVL in MRSA isolates colonizing asymptomatic persons is not surprising. In fact, PVL was not an effective marker for CA-MRSA in all studies [69]. Besides, it is expected that PVL-harboring clones are more prevalent among people with active infections.

Our study has several limitations. Most are inherent to the cross-sectional design, which did not allow us to assess the acquisition of *S. aureus* and MRSA over time. Also, new evidence pointed out that relying only on nasal samples may have underestimated the colonization prevalence [49]. The scarcity of subjects with the outcome cast doubt on the validity of the analysis of determinants of MRSA colonization. Finally, authors have questioned the role of nasal colonization as a major issue in CA-MRSA epidemiology [70]. Analyzing data from outbreak reports, they conclude that skin-skin and skin-fomite contact may provide an efficient route for cross-transmission, even in the absence of colonization.

Despite all those limitations, our study has several strengths. First, subjects were selected so as to provide a representative sample of the urban population of the city of Botucatu. Several potential determinants of colonization, including previous contact with healthcare settings, were assessed in the questionnaire. The analysis was extensive, and mixed classical epidemiological and molecular methods to provide the first data on population carriage of *S. aureus* and MRSA in Brazil. Our findings are particularly relevant at a time when CA-MRSA reaches the status of a public health threat. There are lots of issues to be addressed, including policies for screening patients upon admission to hospitals and guidelines for treating suspected staphylococcal infections. Also, surveillance for CA-MRSA infection should be implemented on a nation-wide basis, in order to make sure if data from asymptomatic MRSA carriage correlate with the etiology of skin and soft-tissue infections. It is worth reporting that one adolescent with CA-MRSA cellulitis that started after trauma in a soccer match and

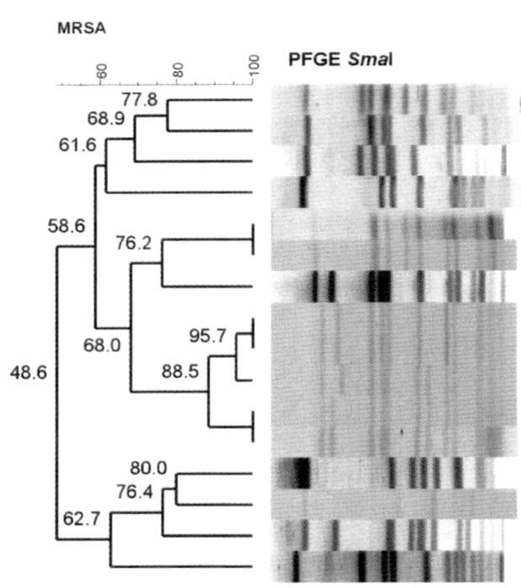

Strain	Source	Age/Sex	SCC*mec*	Sector	*spa*	ST	*arcC*	*aroE*	*glp*	*gmk*	*pta*	*tpi*	*yqi*
NCTC8325	Control		IV			8	3	3	1	1	4	4	3
USA800	Control		IV			5	1	4	1	4	12	1	10
USA300	Control		IV			8	3	3	1	1	4	4	3
OSPC	Control		IV			30	2	2	2	2	6	3	2
610 (Contact)	Nasal Carriage	19/M	IV	113	t002	1176	1	4	1	4	12	1	130
610	Nasal Carriage	39/F	IV	113	t002	1176	1	4	1	4	12	1	130
JCSC4469	Control		IV										
103	Nasal Carriage	56/F	IV	171	t002	5	1	4	1	4	12	1	10
106	Nasal Carriage	43/F	IV	171	t002	5	1	4	1	4	12	1	10
251	Nasal Carriage	49/M	IV	182	t002	5	1	4	1	4	12	1	10
251 (Contact)	Nasal Carriage	77/F	IV	182	t002	5	1	4	1	4	12	1	10
661	Nasal Carriage	55/F	IV	200	t002	2594	1	4	320	4	12	1	10
EMRSA15	Control		IV			22	164	72	50	43	49	67	59
341	Nasal Carriage	20/M	IV	89	t021	1176	1	4	1	4	12	1	130
JCSC1968	Control		IV			91	1	26	28	18	59	54	50
MR108	Control		IV			74	2	2	2	19	6	3	2

Figure 1. Dendrogram showing Pulsed Field Gel Electrophoresis typing of the study isolates, alongside with results from Multilocus Sequence Typing and *spa* typing. International SCCmec type IV clones are included as controls. Note. Data on age/gender and urban area typing are included. Control strains were kindly provided by Dr. Antonio Carlos Campos Pignatari (Universidade Federal de São Paulo, City of São Paulo, São Paulo State, Brazil) and Dr. Agnes Marie Sá Figueiredo (Universidade Federal do Rio de Janeiro, City of Rio de Janeiro, Rio de Janeiro State, Brazil).

progressed to severe sepsis was diagnosed in Bofete, a small town neighboring Botucatu. The isolate belonged to ST5, spa type 311, and harbored PVL genes [71]. As with our results, this occurrence demonstrates the circulation of CA-MRSA in regions distant from major urban centers, and reinforces the necessity of including CA-MRSA in the agenda of public health offices in Brazil.

In conclusion, we found that prevalence rates of *S. aureus* and MRSA colonization in a small city in inner Brazil were similar to those reported in nationwide US surveys. There is evidence of low-level (but consistent) spread CA-MRSA clones, a finding that deserves further investigation. Our results demonstrate the importance of including CA-MRSA among pathogens of interest for public health surveillance at the regional level.

Acknowledgments

Disclaimer: Partial results were presented at ID week (joint Meeting of IDSA, SHEA, HIVMA, and PIDS) in San Diego, 2012.

Author Contributions

Conceived and designed the experiments: CMCBF MLRSC FVP. Performed the experiments: FVP LMA PYFM CHC. Analyzed the data: CMCBF MLRSC CHC. Contributed reagents/materials/analysis tools: PYFM CHC LMA. Wrote the paper: CMCBF MLRSC FVP.

References

1. Hayward A, Knott F, Petersen I, Livermore DM, Duckworth G, et al. (2008) Increasing hospitalizations and general practice prescriptions for community-onset staphylococcal disease, England. Emerg Infect Dis 14: 720–726.
2. Saxena S, Thompson P, Birger R, Bottle A, Spyridis N, et al. (2010) Increasing skin infections and *Staphylococcus aureus* complications in children, England, 1997–2006. Emerg Infect Dis 16: 530–533.
3. Grundmann H, Aires-de-Sousa M, Boyce J, Tiemersma E (2006) Emergence and resurgence of meticillin-resistant *Staphylococcus aureus* as a public-health threat. Lancet 368: 874–885.
4. Bassetti M, Nicco E, Mikulska M (2009) Why is community-associated MRSA spreading across the world and how will it change clinical practice? Int J Antimicrob. Agents 34 (Suppl 1): S15–S19.
5. Klevens RM, Morrison MA, Nadle J, Petit S, Gershman K, et al. (2007) MRSA Investigators. Invasive methicillin-resistant *Staphylococcus aureus* infections in the United States. JAMA 298: 1763–1771.
6. Köck R, Becker K, Cookson B, van Gemert-Pijnen JE, Harbarth S, et al. (2010) Methicillin-resistant *Staphylococcus aureus* (MRSA): burden of disease and control challenges in Europe. Euro Surveill 15: 19688.
7. Chuang YY, Huang YC (2013) Molecular epidemiology of community-associated meticillin-resistant *Staphylococcus aureus* in Asia. Lancet Infect Dis 13: 698–708.
8. Breurec S, Zriouil SB, Fall C, Boisier P, Brisse S, et al. (2011) Epidemiology of methicillin-resistant *Staphylococcus aureus* lineages in five major African towns: emergence and spread of atypical clones. Clin Microbiol Infect 17: 160–165.
9. Breurec S, Fall C, Pouillot R, Boisier P, Brisse S, et al. (2011) Epidemiology of methicillin-susceptible *Staphylococcus aureus* lineages in five major African towns: high prevalence of Panton-Valentine leukocidin genes. Clin Microbiol Infect 17: 633–639.
10. Casey JA, Cosgrove SE, Stewart WF, Pollak J, Schwartz BS (2013) A population-based study of the epidemiology and clinical features of methicillin-resistant *Staphylococcus aureus* infection in Pennsylvania, 2001–2010. Epidemiol Infect 141: 1166–1179.
11. Johnson AP (2011) Methicillin-resistant *Staphylococcus aureus*: the European landscape. J Antimicrob. Chemother. 66 (Suppl 4): iv43–iv48.
12. Mithoe D, Rijnders MI, Roede BM, Stobberingh E, Möller AV (2012) Prevalence of community-associated meticillin-resistant *Staphylococcus aureus* and Panton-Valentine leucocidin-positive *S. aureus* in general practice patients with skin and soft tissue infections in the northern and southern regions of The Netherlands. Eur J Clin Microbiol Infect Dis 31: 349–56.
13. Wu D, Wang Q, Yang Y, Geng W, Wang Q, et al. (2010) Epidemiology and molecular characteristics of community-associated methicillin-resistant and methicillin-susceptible *Staphylococcus aureus* from skin/soft tissue infections in a children's hospital in Beijing, China. Diagn Microbiol Infect Dis 67: 1–8.
14. Kluytmans J, van Belkum A, Verbrugh H (1997) Nasal carriage of *Staphylococcus aureus*: epidemiology, underlying mechanisms, and associated risks. Clin Microbiol Rev 10: 505–520.
15. Safdar N, Bradley EA (2008) The risk of infection after nasal colonization with Staphylococcus aureus. Am J Med 121: 310–315.
16. Kuehnert MJ, Kruszon-Moran D, Hill HA, McQuillan G, McAllister SK, et al. (2006) Prevalence of *Staphylococcus aureus* nasal colonization in the United States, 2001–2002. J Infect Dis 193: 172–179.
17. Graham PL 3rd, Lin SX, Larson EL (2006) A U.S. population-based survey of Staphylococcus aureus colonization. Ann Intern Med 144: 318–325.
18. Gorwitz RJ, Kruszon-Moran D, McAllister SK, McQuillan G, McDougal LK, et al. (2008) Changes in the prevalence of nasal colonization with *Staphylococcus aureus* in the United States, 2001–2004. J Infect Dis 197: 1226–1234.
19. Mediavilla JR, Chen L, Mathema B, Kreiswirth BN (2012) Global epidemiology of community-associated methicillin resistant *Staphylococcus aureus* (CA-MRSA). Curr Opin Microbiol 15: 588–595.
20. Ribeiro A, Coronado AZ, Silva-Carvalho MC, Ferreira-Carvalho BT, Dias C, et al. (2007) Detection and characterization of international community-acquired infections by methicillin-resistant *Staphylococcus aureus* clones in Rio de Janeiro and Porto Alegre cities causing both community- and hospital-associated diseases. Diagn Microbiol Infect Dis 59: 339–345.
21. Silva-Carvalho MC, Bonelli RR, Souza RR, Moreira S, dos Santos LC, et al. (2009) Emergence of multiresistant variants of the community-acquired methicillin-resistant *Staphylococcus aureus* lineage ST1-SCCmecIV in 2 hospitals in Rio de Janeiro, Brazil. Diagn Microbiol Infect Dis 65: 300–305.
22. Reinert C, McCulloch JA, Watanabe S, Ito T, Hiramatsu K, et al. (2008) Type IV SCCmec found in decade old Brazilian MRSA isolates. Braz J Infect Dis 12: 213–236.
23. Cesar CL, Carandina L, Alves MC, Barros MB, Goldbaum M (2005) Saúde e condição de vida em São Paulo. Inquérito multicêntrico de saúde no estado de São Paulo – ISA/SP. São Paulo, Brazil: Universidade de São Paulo, Faculdade de Saúde Pública. 212 p.
24. Winn Jr WM, Allen S, Janda W, Koneman E, Procop G, et al (2005) Koneman's Color Atlas and Textbook of Diagnostic Microbiology, 6th Ed. Philadelphia: Lippincott Williams & Wilkins. 1,736p.
25. Martineau F, Picard FJ, Roy PH Ouellette M, Bergeron MG (1998) Species-specific and ubiquitous-DNA-based assays for rapid identification of Staphylococcus aureus. J Clin Microbiol. 6: 618–23.
26. Clinical and Laboratory Standards Institute (2009) Performance standards for antimicrobial disk susceptibility tests; approved standard, tenth edition (M02-A10). Wayne, PA: CLSI. 76 p.
27. Murakami K, Minamide K, Wada K, Nakamura E, Teraoka H, et al. (1991) Identification of methicillin-resistant strains of staphylococci by polymerase chain reaction. J Clin Microbiol 29: 2240–2244.
28. Milheiriço C, Oliveira DC, de Lencastre H (2007) Update to the multiplex PCR strategy for assignment of mec element types in *Staphylococcus aureus*. Antimicrob. Agents Chemother 51: 3374–3377.
29. McDougal LK, Steward CD, Killgore GE, Chaitram JM, McAllister SK, et al. (2003) Pulsed-field gel electrophoresis typing of oxacillin-resistant *Staphylococcus aureus* isolates from the United States: establishing a national database. J Clin Microbiol. 41: 5113–5120.
30. Enright MC, Day NP, Davies CE, Peacock SJ, Spratt BG (2000) Multilocus sequence typing for characterization of methicillin- resistant and methicillin-susceptible clones of *Staphylococcus aureus*. J Clin Microbiol 38: 1008–1015.
31. Shopsin B, Gomes M, Montomery SO, Smith DH, Waddington M, et al. (1999) Evaluation of Protein A Gene Polymorphic Region DNA Sequencing for Typing of *Staphylococcus aureus* Strains. J Clin Microbiol 37: 3556–3563.
32. Lina G, Piémont Y, Godail-Gamot F, Bes M, Peter MO, et al. (1999) Involvement of Panton-Valentine leukocidin-producing *Staphylococcus aureus* in primary skin infections and pneumonia. Clin Infect Dis 29: 1128–1132.
33. Greenland S (1989) Modeling and variable selection in epidemiologic analysis. Am J Public Health 79: 340–349.
34. Lear A, McCord G, Peiffer J, Watkins RR, Parikh A, et al. (2011) Incidence of *Staphylococcus aureus* nasal colonization and soft tissue infection among high school football players. J Am Board Fam Med 24: 429–435.
35. Qu F, Cui E, Guo T, Li H, Chen S, et al. (2010) Nasal colonization of and clonal transmission of methicillin-susceptible *Staphylococcus aureus* among Chinese military volunteers. J Clin Microbiol 48: 64–69.
36. Lee CJ, Sankaran S, Mukherjee DV, Apa ZL, Hafer CA, et al. (2011) *Staphylococcus aureus* oropharyngeal carriage in a prison population. Clin Infect Dis 52: 775–778.
37. O'Brien FG, Coombs GW, Pearman JW, Gracey M, Moss F, et al. (2009) Population dynamics of methicillin-susceptible and -resistant *Staphylococcus aureus* in remote communities. J Antimicrob Chemother 64: 684–693.
38. Schaumburg F, Köck R, Friedrich AW, Soulanoudjingar S, Ngoa UA, et al. (2011). Population structure of *Staphylococcus aureus* from remote African Babongo Pygmies. PLoS Negl Trop Dis 5: e1150.
39. Tavares DA, Sá-Leão R, Miragaia M, de Lencastre H (2010) Large screening of CA-MRSA among *Staphylococcus aureus* colonizing healthy young children living in two areas (urban and rural) of Portugal. BMC Infect Dis 10: 110.

40. Chen CJ, Hsu KH, Lin TY, Hwang KP, Chen PY, et al. (2011). Factors associated with nasal colonization of methicillin-resistant *Staphylococcus aureus* among healthy children in Taiwan. J Clin Microbiol. 49: 131–137.
41. Melles DC, Tenover FC, Kuehnert MJ, Witsenboer H, Peeters JK, et al. (2008) Overlapping population structures of nasal isolates of *Staphylococcus aureus* from healthy Dutch and American individuals. J Clin Microbiol. 46: 235–241.
42. Rim JY, Bacon AE 3rd (2007) Prevalence of community-acquired methicillin-resistant *Staphylococcus aureus* colonization in a random sample of healthy individuals. Infect Control Hosp Epidemiol 28: 1044–6.
43. Malik S, Vranken P, Silio M, Ratard R, Van Dyke R (2009) Prevalence of community-associated methicillin-resistant *Staphylococcus aureus* colonization outside the healthcare environment. Epidemiol Infect 137: 1237–1241.
44. Olsen K, Sangvik M, Simonsen GS, Sollid JU, Sundsfjord A, et al. (2013) Prevalence and population structure of *Staphylococcus aureus* nasal carriage in healthcare workers in a general population. The Tromsø Staph and Skin Study. Epidemiol Infect 141: 143–152.
45. Scerri J, Monecke S, Borg MA (2013) Prevalence and characteristics of community carriage of methicillin-resistant *Staphylococcus aureus* in Malta. J Epidemiol Glob Health 3: 165–173.
46. Onanuga A, Temedie TC (2011) Nasal carriage of multi-drug resistant *Staphylococcus aureus* in healthy inhabitants of Amassoma in Niger delta region of Nigeria. Afr Health Sci 11: 176–181.
47. Ateba Ngoa U, Schaumburg F, Adegnika AA, Kösters K, Möller T, et al. (2012) Epidemiology and population structure of *Staphylococcus aureus* in various population groups from a rural and semi urban area in Gabon, Central Africa. Acta Trop 124: 42–47.
48. Munckhof WJ, Nimmo GR, Schooneveldt JM, Schlebusch S, Stephens AJ, et al. (2009) Nasal carriage of *Staphylococcus aureus*, including community-associated methicillin-resistant strains, in Queensland adults. Clin Microbiol Infect 15: 149–55.
49. Hamdan-Partida A, Sainz-Espuñes T, Bustos-Martínez (2010) Characterization and persistence of *Staphylococcus aureus* strains isolated from the anterior nares and throats of healthy carriers in a Mexican community. J Clin Microbiol 48: 1701–1705.
50. Goud R, Gupta S, Neogi U, Agarwal D, Naidu K, et al. (2011) Community prevalence of methicillin and vancomycin resistant *Staphylococcus aureus* in and around Bangalore, southern India. Rev Soc Bras Med Trop 44: 309–312.
51. Gardella N, Murzicato S, Di Gregorio S, Cuirolo A, Desse J, et al. (2011). Prevalence and characterization of methicillin-resistant *Staphylococcus aureus* among healthy children in a city of Argentina. Infect Genet Evol 11: 1066–71.
52. Adler A, Givon-Lavi N, Moses AE, Block C, Dagan R (2010) Carriage of community-associated methicillin-resistant *Staphylococcus aureus* in a cohort of infants in southern Israel: risk factors and molecular features. J Clin Microbiol 48: 531–8.
53. Williams RE (1963) Healthy carriage of *Staphylococcus aureus*: its prevalence and importance. Bacteriol Rev 27: 56–71.
54. Weems JJ, Beck LB (2002) Nasal Carriage of *Staphylococcus aureus* As a Risk Factor for Skin and Soft Tissue Infections. Curr Infect Dis Rep 4: 420–425.
55. Durupt F, Mayor L, Bes M, Reverdy ME, Vandenesch F, et al. (2007) Prevalence of *Staphylococcus aureus* toxins and nasal carriage in furuncles and impetigo. Br J Dermatol 157: 1161–1167.
56. Fritz SA, Epplin EK, Garbutt J, Storch GA (2009) Skin infection in children colonized with community-associated methicillin-resistant *Staphylococcus aureus*. J Infect 59: 394–401.
57. Demos M, McLeod MP, Nouri K (2012) Recurrent furunculosis: a review of the literature. Br J Dermatol 167: 725–732.
58. Smith CH, Goldman RD (2012) *Staphylococcus aureus* decolonization for recurrent skin and soft tissue infections in children. Can Fam Physician 58: 1350–1352.
59. Ertam I, Biyikli SE, Yazkan FA, Aytimur D, Alper S (2007) The frequency of nasal carriage in chronic urticaria patients. J Eur Acad Dermatol Venereol 21: 777–780.
60. Talpur R, Bassett R, Duvic M (2008) Prevalence and treatment of Staphylococcus aureus colonization in patients with mycosis fungoides and Sézary syndrome. Br J Dermatol 159: 105–112
61. Petry V, Lipnharski C, Bessa GR, Silveira VB, Weber MB, et al. (2013). Prevalence of community-acquired methicillin-resistant *Staphylococcus aureus* and antibiotic resistance in patients with atopic dermatitis in Porto Alegre, Brazil. Int J Dermatol. E-pub ahead of print. doi:10.1111/ijd.12020
62. Pacheco RL, Lobo RD, Oliveira MS, Farina EF, Santos CR, et al. (2011) Methicillin-resistant *Staphylococcus aureus* (MRSA) carriage in a dermatology unit. Clinics (Sao Paulo) 66: 2071–2077.
63. Rahimian J, Khan R, LaScalea KA (2007) Does nasal colonization or mupirocin treatment affect recurrence of methicillin-resistant *Staphylococcus aureus* skin and skin structure infections? Infect Control Hosp Epidemiol 28:1415–1416.
64. Miller M, Cook HA, Furuya EY, Bhat M, Lee MH, et al. (2009) *Staphylococcus aureus* in the community: colonization versus infection. PLoS One 4: e6708.
65. Fritz SA, Hogan PG, Hayek G, Eisenstein KA, Rodriguez M, et al. (2012) *Staphylococcus aureus* colonization in children with community-associated Staphylococcus aureus skin infections and their household contacts. Arch Pediatr Adolesc Med 166: 551–557.
66. Fritz SA, Hogan PG, Hayek G, Eisenstein KA, Rodriguez M, et al. (2012) Household versus individual approaches to eradication of community-associated *Staphylococcus aureus* in children: a randomized trial. Clin Infect Dis 54: 743–51.
67. Monecke S, Coombs G, Shore AC, Coleman DC, Akpaka P, et al. (2011) A field guide to pandemic, epidemic and sporadic clones of methicillin-resistant *Staphylococcus aureus*. PLoS One 6: e17936.
68. Carmo MS, Inoue F, Andrade SS, Paschoal L, Silva FM, et al. (2011) New multilocus sequence typing of MRSA in São Paulo, Brazil. Braz J Med Biol Res 44: 1013–1017.
69. Rossney AS, Shore AC, Morgan PM, Fitzgibbon MM, O'Connell B, et al. (2007) The emergence and importation of diverse genotypes of methicillin-resistant *Staphylococcus aureus* (MRSA) harboring the Panton-Valentine leukocidin gene (pvl) reveal that pvl is a poor marker for community-acquired MRSA strains in Ireland. J Clin Microbiol 45: 2554–2563.
70. Miller LG, Diep BA (2008) Clinical practice: colonization, fomites, and virulence: rethinking the pathogenesis of community-associated methicillin-resistant *Staphylococcus aureus* infection. Clin Infect Dis 46: 752–760.
71. Camargo CH, da Cunha M de L, Bonesso MF, da Cunha FP, Barbosa AN, et al. (2013) Systemic CA-MRSA infection following trauma during soccer match in inner Brazil: clinical and molecular characterization. Diagn Microbiol Infect Dis 76: 372–374.

Skin and Soft Tissue Infections and Associated Complications among Commercially Insured Patients Aged 0–64 Years with and without Diabetes in the U.S.

Jose A. Suaya[1*¶], Debra F. Eisenberg[2¶], Christy Fang[2], Loren G. Miller[3,4¶]

1 GlaxoSmithKlineVaccines, Philadelphia, Pennsylvania, United States of America, 2 HealthCore, Inc., Wilmington, Delaware United States of America, 3 Los Angeles BioMedical Research Center at Harbor-UCLA, Division of Infectious Diseases, Harbor-UCLA Medical Center, Torrance, California, United States of America, 4 David Geffen School of Medicine at UCLA, Los Angeles, California, United States of America

Abstract

Introduction: Skin and soft tissue infections (SSTIs) are common infections occurring in ambulatory and inpatient settings. The extent of complications associated with these infections by diabetes status is not well established

Methods: Using a very large repository database, we examined medical and pharmacy claims of individuals aged 0–64 between 2005 and 2010 enrolled in U.S. health plans. Diabetes, SSTIs, and SSTI-associated complications were identified by ICD-9 codes. SSTIs were stratified by clinical category and setting of initial diagnosis.

Results: We identified 2,227,401 SSTI episodes, 10% of which occurred in diabetic individuals. Most SSTIs were initially diagnosed in ambulatory settings independent from diabetes status. Abscess/cellulitis was the more common SSTI group in diabetic and non-diabetic individuals (66% and 59%, respectively). There were differences in the frequencies of SSTI categories between diabetic and non-diabetic individuals ($p<0.01$). Among SSTIs diagnosed in ambulatory settings, the SSTI-associated complication rate was over five times higher in people with diabetes than in people without diabetes (4.9% vs. 0.8%, $p<0.01$) and SSTI-associated hospitalizations were 4.9% and 1.1% in patients with and without diabetes, respectively. Among SSTIs diagnosed in the inpatient setting, bacteremia/endocarditis/septicemia/sepsis was the most common associated complication occurring in 25% and 16% of SSTIs in patients with and without diabetes, respectively ($p<0.01$).

Conclusions: Among persons with SSTIs, we found SSTI-associated complications were five times higher and SSTI-associated hospitalizations were four times higher, in patients with diabetes compared to those without diabetes. SSTI prevention efforts in individuals with diabetes may have significant impact on morbidity and healthcare resource utilization.

Editor: Nasia Safdar, UW Medical School, United States of America

Funding: This observational study has been sponsored by GlaxoSmithKline (GSK). This original research is a collaboration among researchers from HealthCore, Los Angeles BioMedical Research Institute at Harbor-UCLA Medical Center (LA BioMed) and GSK. While J.A.S. is a GSK employee, decisions on study design, data collection and analysis, decision where to publish, and preparation of the manuscript were done solely and collectively by the authors and not by the funder.

Competing Interests: This observational study has been sponsored by GlaxoSmithKline. J.A.S. is employed by the GlaxoSmithKline group of companies. At the time of this study, J.A.S. worked at GSK Vaccines. D.E. is an employee of HealthCore, which has received funds for GSK for performing research. C.F. was an employee of HealthCore at the time of this research. L.M. has received consulting fees for this study from GSK. L.M. has also received consulting fees from GSK, Pfizer, and Cubist for other research projects. Decisions on study design, data collection and analysis, decision where to publish and preparation of the manuscript were done solely and collectively by the authors.

* E-mail: Jose.2.Suaya@GSK.com

¶ These authors contributed equally to this work.

Introduction

Skin and soft-tissue infections (SSTIs) are common reasons to seek medical care in the inpatient and outpatient settings. There were an estimated 869,800 hospital admissions in the United States (U.S.) for SSTIs in 2004.[1] Several investigations have noted that the incidence of SSTIs is increasing in both the inpatient and outpatient settings in the U.S. during the first decade of the 21st Century, with increases of 29% in the inpatient setting over a 4-year period [1] and 50% in the outpatient setting over an 8-year period [2]. These SSTI incidence increases are typically attributed to the rise of community-associated methicillin resistant *Staphylococcus aureus* (CA-MRSA) as an emerging cause of SSTIs [1–3].

There are data suggesting patients with diabetes are at increased risk for skin infection [4]. Although one investigation reported no association between diabetes and lower limb cellulites [5], another found that individuals with diabetes were more than one and a half times more likely to develop cellulitis compared with those without diabetes [6]. In another investigation, those with type 1 and type 2 diabetes were 1.6 and 1.3 times more likely to develop an SSTI, respectively, than non-diabetic individuals [7]. Further, a Dutch investigation of more than 7,000 individuals with diabetes and 18,000 without diabetes reported that bacterial skin and mucous membrane infections were more common in those with diabetes [7]. Other studies have evaluated the incidence and severity of SSTI in people with diabetes caused by specific pathogens; however, a comparator group was not included in those investigations [5,8–10].

SSTIs can be associated with serious complications such as gangrene, osteomyelitis, bacteremia, and sepsis [11–14]. No study, to our knowledge, has compared SSTI complication rates between individuals with and without diabetes. To address this issue, we sought to estimate rates of SSTI-associated complications in a very large cohort of patients with and without diabetes.

Methods

Ethics statement

All data were handled in compliance with the Health Insurance Portability and Accountability Act (HIPAA) of 1996, and a limited dataset was used for the analyses. The limited dataset contained the fields of interest specific to the study, including eligibility, medical, and pharmacy information for the specified cohort during the study period, and limited the amount of protected health information (PHI) in the dataset. The study was approved by the institutional review board at the Los Angeles BioMedical Research Institute at Harbor-UCLA Medical Center.

Study design and data source

We performed an observational, retrospective cohort study utilizing administrative claims data consolidated in the HealthCore Integrated Research Database (HIRD). The HIRD consists of monthly eligibility status and medical and pharmacy claims from 14 health plans in the U.S. These plans include health maintenance, point-of-service, preferred provider organizations, and indemnity plans located across the Northeastern, Southeastern, mid-Atlantic, Midwestern, and Western regions. The HIRD has been used previously in multiple incidence cost studies [15–18].

Study population and unit of analysis

We identified individuals aged 0–64 years in the HIRD database with at least one claim for SSTI during the period 01/01/2005 through 12/31/2010. During that study period, there were approximately 35 million lives documented in the HIRD database. We excluded individuals aged 65 and older due to limited data capture of persons of this age within commercial insurance plans because they usually have Medicare coverage. No exclusion criteria were applied to the cohort and all patients had at least one day of eligibility prior to the first SSTI episode. Only individuals with at least one SSTI claim remained in the database to be used for study analyses.

Skin and soft-tissue infections (SSTIs)

We identified SSTIs by any of their specific International Classification of Diseases, Ninth Revision, Clinical Modification [ICD-9] clinical codes among any of the diagnoses reported in medical claims from ambulatory, emergency room, or inpatient settings for services that occurred during the study period. An SSTI episode was defined by at least one medical claim of an ICD-9 code outlined in Table 1. These codes are consistent with previous investigations using administrative data to identify SSTIs [1,3,7].

Table 1. Skin and soft tissue infections (SSTI) by group, clinical condition, and ICD-9 code.

SSTI Groups	ICD-9 Codes
Abscess/Cellulitis[a]	681.x-682.x, 035.x
Decubitus Ulcer[b]	707x
Surgical site infection & Device or Graft	
Surgical site infection	998.5x, 999.3x
Non-healing surgical wound[b]	998.83
Infection due to device or graft	996.6x
Folliculitis, Impetigo, Furuncle, Mastitis & Other SSTIs	
Folliculitis	704.8x
Impetigo	684.x
Carbuncle and furuncle	680.x
Mastitis	611.0x, 771.5x
"Other" skin and subcutaneous tissue infections	686.x

[a]This group also includes Erysipelas (ICD-9 code: 035.x).
[b]In this study, decubitus ulcer and non-healing surgical wound is considered as having an active infection if: a) clinical diagnosis is associated with prescription of any of the following antibiotics: dicloxacillin, vancomycin, cefalexin, cefazolin, linezolid, daptomycin, clindamycin, trimethoprim-sulfamethoxazole, doxycycline, minocycline, quinupristin-dalfopristin within ±10 days of the index diagnosis; and b) if there is no other concomitant clinical diagnosed infection.

The date of the earliest claim with an SSTI diagnosis was defined as the index date of the SSTI. Any two claims for SSTIs or associated complications within 30 days of each other were considered part of the same SSTI episode. After an index infection episode, any subsequent SSTI episode had to be preceded by at least 30 days without an SSTI claim to qualify as a distinct episode.

Diabetes status

Diabetes was defined as at least one medical claim with the ICD-9 code for diabetes [250.xx] during the study period. For the purpose of this investigation we did not distinguish type 1 diabetes from type 2 diabetes due to limited accuracy in administrative data. An identified SSTI infection was attributed to a diabetic patient only if the diabetes was diagnosed before or at the time of the first SSTI episode claim.

Classification of SSTI episodes

We categorized SSTI episodes three different ways: (1) clinical SSTI category (e.g., cellulitis, impetigo); (2) ambulatory versus inpatient onset; and (3) presence or absence of SSTI-associated complication during the episode.

Clinical SSTI categories

Based on the ICD-9 codes for SSTI (Table 1), we categorized SSTIs into four mutually exclusive clinical groups of increasing severity based on these authors' clinical judgment. These categories of SSTIs (starting with the least severe) are as follows: (1) folliculitis, impetigo, furuncle, mastitis, and other SSTIs; (2) abscess/cellulitis; (3) decubitus ulcer; and (4) surgical site infection, device or graft, and non-healing surgical wound. If an SSTI episode had claims with multiple SSTI clinical categories, as defined above, the most severe diagnosis was used to define the episode. Because decubitus ulcers and non-healing surgical wounds may not be infected, we only considered these diagnoses as representing an SSTI if the clinical diagnosis was associated with ≥1 prescription within 10 days of the diagnosis of any of the following antibiotics: dicloxacillin, vancomycin, cefalexin, cefazolin, linezolid, daptomycin, clindamycin, trimethoprim-sulfamethoxazole, doxycycline, minocycline, or quinupristin-dalfopristin.

SSTI by place of service of initial diagnosis

We used the place of service on the ICD-9 code claim for the first SSTI claim to classify each SSTI episode as occurring either in the ambulatory or inpatient setting. In addition, for ambulatory-onset SSTI infections, we calculated the proportion of episodes that resulted in an SSTI-related hospitalization. An SSTI-related hospitalization was defined as such if it met three conditions: (1) it was preceded by an ambulatory-onset SSTI diagnosis; (2) it contained any clinical diagnosis of an SSTI or an associated complication as one of the hospital discharge diagnoses; and (3) it occurred within the infection episode time frame. Similarly, for inpatient-onset SSTIs, we calculated re-hospitalizations as the proportion of infections resulting in an SSTI-related subsequent hospital admission. A re-hospitalization was defined as such if the SSTI, or an associated complication, was contained in any of the clinical diagnoses of the hospital discharge and if the hospitalization was within the episode infection timeframe.

SSTI-associated complications

We also identified complications, or sequelae, typically associated with SSTIs. These complications included lymphadenitis, myositis/necrotizing fasciitis, gangrene, osteomyelitis, bacteremia, endocarditis, septicemia, or sepsis. Due to overlapping clinical spectrum, the latter four were combined into one complication group. An SSTI episode was considered to have an SSTI-associated complication if the ICD-9-based complication diagnosis occurred during the index infection timeframe. ICD-9 codes for these complications are outlined in Table 1. In our analysis, an SSTI episode could have had multiple associated complications, as complications are not mutually exclusive. Based on clinical experience, we considered osteomyelitis to be associated with an SSTI episode even if it occurred up to 90 days from the beginning of the SSTI infection (index date).

Statistical Analyses

The unit of analysis was a SSTI episode. We evaluated overall SSTI-associated complication and hospitalization rates within the infection timeframe associated with each SSTI group by place of service of initial diagnosis stratified by diabetes status. We then estimated specific SSTI-associated complication rates for each SSTI category. We used the two-proportion z-test to obtain p-values. All analyses were performed using SAS® 9.2 (SAS Institute Inc, Cary, NC) and an alpha level of significance of 0.05 was used.

Results

SSTIs by diabetes status and age group

During the study period of 2005 to 2010, we identified 140,652 diabetic patients and 1,539,692 non-diabetic patients aged 0–64 years with at least one SSTI episode. There were 2,227,401 SSTI episodes, 10.0% of which occurred in patients with diabetes (Table 2). There were differences in the age group distribution of SSTIs between patients with and without diabetes ($p<0.01$). About three quarters (75.6%) of all SSTIs in patients with diabetes were in those aged 45–64 years. Most of the remaining SSTIs (22.8%) in diabetic patients occurred in individuals aged 18–44 years. In contrast, many (43.2%) of the SSTIs in patients without diabetes occurred in individuals aged 18–44 years. The remaining 25.5% and 31.3% of the SSTIs were in individuals aged 0–17 years and 45–64 years, respectively. Fewer SSTI episodes were initially diagnosed in ambulatory settings in patient with diabetes (88.7%) than in those without diabetes (96.2%, $p<0.01$). This association was similar across all age groups.

SSTI categories by place of service of initial diagnosis

There were differences in the frequency distribution of group of SSTIs between patients with and without diabetes ($p<0.01$) within place of initial diagnosis. Among SSTIs initially diagnosed in ambulatory settings, abscess and cellulitis represented 65.6% and 59.3% of all the SSTI episodes in patients with and without diabetes, respectively (Table 3). The SSTI category of folliculitis, impetigo, furuncle, mastitis, and other SSTIs was the second largest group of SSTIs in both patients with and without diabetes (22.6% vs. 37.8%). About 8.1% and 0.9% of SSTIs episodes in patients with and without diabetes were decubitus ulcers.

Similar to the ambulatory setting, among SSTIs initially diagnosed in inpatient settings, abscess and cellulitis was the most common SSTI category, accounting for about 50.5% and 54.5% of SSTIs in patients with and without diabetes, respectively (Table 3). However, the group of surgical site, device or graft infections was more common in inpatient settings than outpatient settings, representing 29.7% and 35.5% of SSTIs in patients with and without diabetes, respectively. Decubitus ulcers represented 15.2% and 3.2% of the SSTIs initially diagnosed in inpatient settings in patients with and without diabetes, respectively.

SSTI-associated complications

For each SSTI category, higher complication rates were observed in SSTIs occurring in patients with diabetes than without diabetes (Table 3). Among SSTIs initially diagnosed in ambulatory settings, the SSTI-associated complication rate was more than five times higher in patients with diabetes than without diabetes (4.9% vs. 0.8%, $p<0.01$). Similarly, SSTI-associated complication rates among SSTIs initially diagnosed in inpatient settings were over one and half times higher in diabetic than in non-diabetic individuals (36.7% vs. 21.7%, $p<0.01$). SSTI-associated complication rates were highest in decubitus ulcers and the combined category of surgical site infections/device or graft infection. For example, 32% and 13% of the decubitus ulcers initially diagnosed in an ambulatory setting were associated with complications in patients with and without diabetes, respectively. SSTI-associated complication rates were the lowest in the clinical group of folliculitis, impetigo, furuncle, mastitis, and other SSTIs, observed in 2.4% and 0.8% of the episodes in patients with and without diabetes, respectively.

SSTI-related hospitalizations

Among SSTIs diagnosed in the ambulatory care setting, SSTI-associated hospitalizations were 4.9% in patients with diabetes and 1.1% in non-diabetic patients, respectively (Table 3). Among SSTIs diagnosed in the inpatient care setting, SSTI-associated subsequent (re)hospitalizations were 15.1% and 7.8% in patients with and without diabetes, respectively (Table 3). For SSTIs diagnosed in the ambulatory setting, SSTI-related hospitalizations rates varied by the SSTI category, ranging from 0.4% in the

Table 2. Distribution of skin and soft tissue infection by diabetes status and age group from 2005 through 2010.

	SSTI Episodes*					
	In Diabetic Individuals			In Non-diabetic Individuals		
Age group	All SSTIs	As % of all	% of SSTIs in age group diagnosed in ambulatory settings	All SSTIs	As % of all	% of SSTIs in age group diagnosed in ambulatory settings
0–17 years	3,602	1.6%	94.1%	512,420	25.5%	98.0%
18–44 years	50,497	22.8%	90.2%	866,098	43.2%	96.7%
45–64 years	167,546	75.6%	88.1%	627,238	31.3%	94.1%
0–64 years	221,645	100.0%	88.7%	2,005,756	100.0%	96.2%

*Difference in frequency distribution of SSTIs by age group between individuals with and without diabetes was statistically significant ($p<.01$).

folliculitis group in non-diabetic individuals to 23.1% in decubitus ulcers in diabetic individuals. For SSTIs diagnosed in inpatient setting, SSTI-related subsequent hospitalizations also varied by the SSTI clinical category, ranging from 5.5% in the abscess/cellulitis group in non-diabetic patients to 27.9% in decubitus ulcers in diabetic patients. Again, for each group (except the folliculitis group), SSTIs in patients with diabetes were associated with significantly higher subsequent hospitalization rates than those patients without diabetes.

SSTI-specific complications

Specific SSTI-associated complications are outlined in Tables 4 and 5. Among patients with SSTIs initially diagnosed in ambulatory settings, osteomyelitis was the most commonly associated complication, occurring in 3.3% and 0.4% of patients with and without diabetes, respectively ($p<0.01$ for difference in proportions). Among SSTIs initially diagnosed in inpatient settings, bacteremia/endocarditis/septicemia/sepsis was the most common SSTI-associated complication occurring in 25% and 16% of patients with and without diabetes, respectively ($p<0.01$ for difference of proportions).

Conclusions

In our investigation of more than 2 million SSTIs from people with and without diabetes in a large database of commercially insured persons in the U.S., we found several novel observations about SSTIs. First, the majority of SSTIs were diagnosed in ambulatory settings for patients with and without diabetes, but significantly more infections were diagnosed in inpatient settings for patients with diabetes compared to patients without diabetes. Second, in both inpatient and ambulatory settings, for both patient groups, abscess and cellulitis were the most commonly diagnosed infections, although these were more common among those with diabetes compared with people without diabetes. Third, SSTI-associated complications were five-fold and one and a half-fold more common in individuals with diabetes than without diabetes for SSTIs initially diagnosed in ambulatory and inpatient setting, respectively. Finally, SSTI-related subsequent hospitalizations were more common in patients with diabetes in both the inpatient and outpatient settings.

There are many reasons why persons with diabetes are felt to be at increased risk for bacterial infections, such as SSTIs. These include impaired leukocyte chemotaxis, adherence, and intracellular bacterial killing [19]. Additionally, antigen-specific cell-mediated immunity and impaired proliferative responses to certain pathogens, such as *S. aureus*, the most commonly recognized cause of skin infection, has been described [19]. Despite descriptions of impaired immunity, clinical data supporting the association between diabetes and increased infection are very limited. While there are data suggesting that diabetic individuals are associated with higher risk of SSTIs [6,7], this is the first study, to our knowledge, to investigate the morbidity associated with SSTIs, and evaluate the differences in type and complications between patients with and without diabetes.

Shah, et al. found that individuals with diabetes have a 1.21 increased risk ratio (RR) for all infectious diseases compared with individuals without diabetes [6], They also observed that diabetic individuals were at higher risk for specific infectious diseases, for example, upper respiratory tract infections (RR 1.18), pneumonia (RR 1.46), and cystitis (RR 1.39). They did examine the risk of one skin infection, cellulitis, and found an increased risk in those with diabetes (RR 1.81) and also found an increased risk of osteomyelitis (RR 4.39). However, they did not examine other categories of skin infections, SSTI-associated hospitalizations, or SSTI-associated complications. Muller et al. also found type 1 and type 2 diabetic patients were at increased risk of bacterial skin and mucous membrane infections (ORs 1.59 and 1.33, respectively) [7]. However, they did not examine specific skin infections or their complications. Study populations in both studies were extremely small compared to the population examined in the current investigation.

In our population, not surprisingly, the relatively less severe SSTIs – folliculitis, impetigo, furuncles, and mastitis – were associated with relatively low rates of associated complications (1.6% and 0.4% in patients with and without diabetes, respectively) and hospitalizations (1.7% and 0.4%, respectively). Decubitus ulcers were the SSTI category with the highest proportions of associated complications (32.4% and 13.3%) and hospitalizations (23.1% and 8.6%). Surgical site infections/device or graft also had relatively high proportions of associated complications (10.4% and 5.0%) and hospitalizations (12.2% and 6.3%). These findings are consistent with our anecdotal clinical observations that more serious SSTIs are associated with higher likelihoods of complications and subsequent hospitalization.

We found SSTI-associated complications were generally uncommon in ambulatory onset SSTIs, occurring in less than 4% of SSTIs. The most common associated complication was osteomyelitis, which occurred in 3.2% and 0.4% of SSTIs in patients with and without diabetes, respectively. All other SSTI-associated complications were relatively uncommon occurring ≤1.0% of the time. As expected, SSTI-associated complications rates in the inpatient setting were higher than in SSTIs initially

Table 3. Skin and soft tissue infection-associated complication and hospitalization rates by diabetes status, major initial clinical diagnosis, and setting from 2005 through 2010.

	SSTI Episodes[a]				Any SSTI-associated Complication					SSTI-associated Subsequent Hospitalization[b]				
	In Diabetic Individuals		In Non-diabetic Individuals		In Diabetic Individuals		In Non-diabetic Individuals		Differ-ence	In Diabetic Individuals		In Non-diabetic Individuals		Differ-ence
Initial diagnosis setting and group of SSTIs	**N**	**As a % by setting**	**N**	**As a % by setting**	**N**	**%**	**N**	**%**	**p-value**	**N**	**%**	**N**	**%**	**p-value**
Initially Diagnosed in Ambulatory Settings														
Abscess/Cellulitis	129,006	65.6	1,144,576	59.3	3,048	2.36	9,047	0.79	<.01	4,310	3.34	14,377	1.21	<.01
Decubitus Ulcer	15,976	8.1	17,663	0.9	5,175	32.39	2,357	13.34	<.01	3,697	23.14	1,825	8.64	<.01
Surgical Site Infection & Device or Graft	7,097	3.6	37,334	1.9	736	10.37	1,861	4.98	<.01	867	12.22	2,475	6.26	<.01
Folliculitis, Impetigo, Furuncle, Mastitis & Other SSTIs	44,494	22.6	730,194	37.8	702	1.58	3,138	0.43	<.01	736	1.65	2,796	0.37	<.01
All SSTIs in subgroup	196,573	100.0	1,929,767	100.0	9,661	4.91	16,403	0.85	<.01	9,610	4.89	21,473	1.05	<.01
Initially Diagnosed in Inpatient Settings														
Abscess/Cellulitis	12,656	50.5	41,389	54.5	3,335	26.35	6,297	15.21	<.01	1,380	10.90	2,458	5.52	<.01
Decubitus Ulcer	3,802	15.2	2,403	3.2	2,397	63.05	1,236	51.44	<.01	1,059	27.85	566	22.39	<.01
Surgical Site Infection & Device or Graft	7,438	29.7	26,939	35.5	3,159	42.47	8,225	30.53	<.01	1,200	16.13	2,937	10.31	<.01
Folliculitis, Impetigo, Furuncle, Mastitis & Other SSTIs	1,176	4.7	5,258	6.9	310	26.36	754	14.34	<.01	146	12.41	421	7.59	<.01
All SSTIs in subgroup	25,072	100.0	75,989	100.0	9,201	36.70	16,512	21.73	<.01	3,785	15.10	6,382	7.84	<.01

[a]Difference in the frequency distribution of SSTI clinical groups between patients with and without diabetes was statistically significant ($p<.01$) in both those diagnosed in ambulatory settings and those diagnosed in inpatient settings.

[b]For patients with an initial diagnosis in the inpatient setting, this counts as a re-hospitalization.

Table 4. Complications of Lymphadenitis and Myositis/Necrotizing Fasciitis by diabetes status, major initial clinical diagnosis, and setting from 2005 through 2010.

			Type of SSTI-associated Complication[a]					
	SSTI Episodes		Lymphadenitis			Myositis/Necrotizing Fasciitis		
	In Diabetic Individuals	In Non-diabetic Individuals	In Diabetic Individuals	In Non-diabetic Individuals	Differ-ence	In Diabetic Individuals	In Non-diabetic Individuals	Differ-ence
Initial Diagnosis Setting and group of SSTIs	**N**	**N**	**N (%)**	**N (%)**	**p-value**	**N (%)**	**N (%)**	**p-value**
Initially Diagnosed in Ambulatory Settings								
Abscess/Cellulitis	129,006	1,144,576	110 (0.09%)	1,605 (0.14%)	<.01	106 (0.08%)	279 (0.02%)	<.01
Decubitus Ulcer	15,976	17,663	12 (0.08%)	10 (0.06%)	.26	78 (0.49%)	63 (0.36%)	.03
Surgical site infection & Device or Graft	7,097	37,334	3 (0.04%)	29 (0.08%)	.11	10 (0.14%)	24 (0.06%)	.05
Folliculitis, Impetigo, Furuncle, Mastitis & Other SSTIs	44,494	730,194	39 (0.09%)	692 (0.09%)	.31	27 (0.06%)	79 (0.01%)	<.01
All SSTIs in subgroup	196,573	1,929,767	164 (0.08%)	2,336 (0.12%)	<.01	221 (0.11%)	445 (0.02%)	<.01
Initially Diagnosed in Inpatient Setting								
Abscess/Cellulitis	12,656	41,389	34 (0.27%)	559 (1.35%)	<.01	294 (2.32%)	505 (1.22%)	<.01
Decubitus Ulcer	3,802	2,403	4 (0.11%)	3 (0.12%)	.41	88 (2.31%)	31 (1.29%)	<.01
Surgical site infection & Device or Graft	7,438	26,939	2 (0.03%)	31 (0.12%)	<.01	49 (0.66%)	106 (0.39%)	<.01
Folliculitis, Impetigo, Furuncle, Mastitis & Other SSTIs	1,176	5,258	1 (0.09%)	9 (0.17%)	.20	17 (1.45%)	40 (0.76%)	.03
All SSTIs in subgroup	25,072	75,989	41 (0.16%)	602 (0.79%)	<.01	431 (1.72%)	682 (0.90%)	<.01

[a]Complications are not mutually exclusive.

Table 5. Complications of gangrene, osteomyelitis, and bacteremia/endocarditis/septicemia/sepsis by diabetes status, major initial clinical diagnosis, and setting from 2005 through 2010.

	Type of SSTI-associated complication[a]								
	Gangrene			Osteomyelitis			Bacteremia/Endocarditis/Septicemia/Sepsis		
	In Diabetic Individuals	In Non-diabetic Individuals	Differ-ence	In Diabetic Individuals	In Non-diabetic Individuals	Differ-ence	In Diabetic Individuals	In Non-diabetic Individuals	Differ-ence
Initial Diagnosis Setting and group of SSTIs	**N (%)**	**N (%)**	**p-value**	**N (%)**	**N (%)**	**p-value**	**N (%)**	**N (%)**	**p-value**
Initially Diagnosed in Ambulatory Settings									
Abscess/Cellulitis	551 (0.43%)	432 (0.04%)	<.01	1,783 (1.38%)	3,995 (0.35%)	<.01	1,050 (0.81%)	3,161 (0.28%)	<.01
Decubitus Ulcer	1,239 (7.76%)	372 (2.11%)	<.01	4,014 (25.13%)	1,522 (8.62%)	<.01	1,273 (7.97%)	735 (4.16%)	<.01
Surgical site infection & Device or Graft	33 (0.46%)	52 (0.14%)	<.01	241 (3.40%)	972 (2.60%)	<.01	525 (7.40%)	909 (2.43%)	<.01
Folliculitis, Impetigo, Furuncle, Mastitis & Other SSTIs	113 (0.25%)	159 (0.02%)	<.01	344 (0.77%)	1,005 (0.14%)	<.01	269 (0.60%)	1,309 (0.18%)	<.01
All SSTIs in subgroup	1,936 (0.98%)	1,015 (0.05%)	<.01	6,382 (3.25%)	7,494 (0.39%)	<.01	3,117 (1.59%)	6,114 (0.32%)	<.01
Initially Diagnosed in Inpatient Setting									
Abscess/Cellulitis	669 (5.29%)	358 (0.86%)	<.01	1,183 (9.35%)	1,535 (3.71%)	<.01	2,139 (16.90%)	4,244 (10.25%)	<.01
Decubitus Ulcer	803 (21.12%)	172 (7.16%)	<.01	1,429 (37.59%)	393 (16.35%)	<.01	1,116 (29.35%)	861 (35.83%)	<.01
Surgical site infection & Device or Graft	123 (1.65%)	137 (0.51%)	<.01	598 (8.04%)	1,812 (6.73%)	<.01	2,747 (36.93%)	6,752 (25.06%)	<.01
Folliculitis, Impetigo, Furuncle, Mastitis & Other SSTIs	76 (6.46%)	62 (1.18%)	<.01	115 (9.78%)	217 (4.13%)	<.01	189 (16.07%)	510 (9.70%)	<.01
All SSTIs in subgroup	1,671 (6.66%)	729 (0.96%)	<.01	3,325 (13.26%)	3,957 (5.21%)	<.01	6,191 (24.69%)	12,367 (16.27%)	<.01

[a]Complications are not mutually exclusive.

diagnosed in ambulatory settings, with bacteremia/endocarditis/septicemia/sepsis group being the most common, occurring in 24.7% and 16.3% of those SSTIs in patients with and without diabetes, respectively.

Our investigation has limitations. First, our study employed administrative claims data. While cellulitis and abscesses are different clinical entities, ICD-9 codes group them together, and the accuracy of SSTI diagnosis from administrative claims data has not been fully validated. Thus, we may have overestimated or underestimated the true number and groups of SSTIs compared with medical records review. Second, our study included only persons aged 0–64, as persons over 65 years were uncommon in our database. It is likely that SSTIs and their associated complications were more common in the population aged 65 years and older [20–22]. A third limitation is that we do not have microbiologic correlation with SSTIs. Such data may lead to insights as to which pathogens may disproportionally affect individuals with diabetes. However, the HIRD databases do not contain inpatient microbiology data. Even if microbiologic data were available, it may be of limited utility given many SSTIs, such as cellulitis without abscess, cannot be easily cultured, or clinicians often choose not to perform bacterial cultures in persons with SSTIs [23]. Fourth, subsequent hospitalizations were assumed to be related to SSTIs, however it is possible that patients were hospitalized for other reasons and that the skin infection remained ongoing. Fifth, our study population consisted of individuals commercially insured and thus our findings may not be generalizable to uninsured or patients with Medicaid. Another limitation of our study was our inability to distinguish risk of SSTI between type 1 and type 2 diabetics. Administrative data has been found to be a poor means to distinguish these two diabetic types in children and younger adults in which both types are relatively prevalent [24]. Finally, as our unit of analysis was an SSTI episode and its complication rates, this study did not focus in estimating SSTI incidence among persons at risk stratified by diabetes status. Such an analysis would have broadened the understanding of the role of diabetes in not only the risk of complications associated with SSTIs but also in the risk of SSTIs themselves.

There are strengths to our study. First, we employed an extremely large database of the commercially insured U.S. population. Second, the population under study was geographically diverse, representing insured adults and children throughout the U.S. In addition, we employed a comprehensive approach to SSTIs, examining both ambulatory- and inpatient-onset SSTIs, whereas almost all other investigations of SSTIs have focused on one setting only. Finally, despite our lack of microbiologic information, our results are contemporary and reflect SSTIs that occur in the era of CA-MRSA, which has changed the epidemiology of skin infections in the first decade of the 21st century [25–26].

In summary, we found that diabetic patients with SSTIs have higher rates of both SSTI-associated complications and subsequent hospitalizations. Therefore, successful preventive interventions for SSTIs may have the greatest impact among persons with diabetes.

Acknowledgments

Authors would like to thank Margaret Kelly (GSK) and Betsy Marks (HealthCore) for their contributions to the style of the manuscript and Ashley Giambrone (GSK internship) and Ella Nkhoma (HealthCore) for statistical support. JAS, DFE and LGM, the guarantors of this publications, i.e., take full responsibility for the work as a whole, including the study design, access to data, and the decision to submit and publish the manuscript.

Author Contributions

Conceived and designed the experiments: JAS DFE LGM. Analyzed the data: JAS DFE CF LGM. Wrote the paper: JAS DFE CF LGM.

References

1. Edelsberg J, Taneja C, Zervos M, Haque N, Moore C, et al. (2009) Trends in US hospital admissions for skin and soft tissue infections. Emerg Infect Dis 15: 1516–1518.
2. Hersh AL, Chambers HF, Maselli JH, Gonzalez R (2008) National trends in ambulatory visits and antibiotic prescribing for skin and soft-tissue infections. Arch Intern Med 168: 1585–1591.
3. Pallin DJ, Egan DJ, Pelletier AJ, Espinola JA, Hooper DC, et al. (2008) Increased US emergency department visits for skin and soft tissue infections, and changes in antibiotic choices, during the emergence of community-associated methicillin-resistant Staphylococcus aureus. Ann Emerg Med 51: 291–298.
4. Jackson L (2005) Evaluating diabetes mellitus as a risk factor for community-acquired infections. Clin Infect Dis 41: 289–290.
5. Björnsdóttir S, Gottfredsson M, Thórisdóttir AS, Gunnarsson GB, Ríkardsdóttir H, et al. (2005). Risk factors for acute cellulitis of the lower limb: a prospective case-control study. Clin Infect Dis 41: 1416–1422.
6. Shah BR, Hux JE (2003) Quantifying the risk of infectious diseases for people with diabetes. Diabetes Care 26: 510–513.
7. Muller L, Gorter KJ, Hak E, Goudzwaard WL, Schellevis FG, et al. (2005) Increased risk of common infections in patients with type 1 and type 2 diabetes mellitus. Clin Infect Dis 41: 281–288.
8. Kao LS, Knight MT, Lally KP, Mercer DW (2005) The impact of diabetes in patients with necrotizing soft tissue infections. Surg Infect (Larchmt) 6: 427–438.
9. Nather A, Bee CS, Huak CY, Chew JL, Lin CB, et al. (2008) Epidemiology of diabetic foot problems and predictive factors for limb loss. J Diabet Compl 22: 77–82.
10. Dang CN, Prasad YD, Boulton AJ, Jude EB (2003) Methicillin resistant *Staphylococcus aureus* in the diabetic foot clinic: a worsening problem. Diabet Med 20: 159–161.
11. Wilson J, Guy R, Elgohari S, Sheridan E, Davies J, et al. (2011) Trends in sources of methicillin-resistant Staphylococcus aureus (MRSA) bacteraemia: data from the national mandatory surveillance of MRSA bacteraemia in England, 2006–2009. J Hosp Infect 79: 211–217.
12. Sreeramoju P, Porbandarwalla NS, Arango J, Latham K, Dent DL, et al. (2011) Recurrent skin and soft tissue infections due to methicillin-resistant Staphylococcus aureus requiring operative debridement. Am J Surg 201: 216–220.
13. Bhavan KP, Marschall J, Olsen MA, Fraser VJ, Wright NM, et al. (2010) The epidemiology of hematogenous vertebral osteomyelitis: a cohort study in a tertiary care hospital. BMC Infect Dis 10: 158.
14. Aragon-Sanchez J, Quintana-Marrero Y, Lazaro-Martinez JL, Hernández-Herrero MJ, García-Morales E, et al. (2009) Necrotizing soft-tissue infections in the feet of patients with diabetes: outcome of surgical treatment and factors associated with limb loss and mortality. Int J Lower Extremity Wounds 8: 141–146.
15. Kessler RC, Coulouvrat C, Hajak G, Lakoma MD, Roth T, et al. (2010) Reliability and validity of the brief insomnia questionnaire in the America Insomnia Survey. Sleep 33: 1539–1549.
16. Kim SY, Schneeweiss S, Liu J, Daniel GW, Chang CL, et al. (2010) Risk of osteoporotic fracture in a large population-based cohort study of patients with rheumatoid arthritis. Arthritis Res Ther 12: R154.
17. Lee TA, Chang C-L, Stephenson JJ, Sajjan SG, Maiese EM, et al. (2010) Impact of asthma controller medications on medical and economic resource utilization in adult asthma patients. Curr Med Res Opin 26: 2851–2860.
18. Ulcickas Yood M, Delorenze GN, Quesenberry CP Jr, Tsai AL, Phillips S, et al. (2010) Epidemiologic study of aripiprazole use and the incidence of suicide events. Pharmacoepidemiol Drug Saf 19: 1124–1130.
19. Rajagopalan S (2005) Serious infections in elderly patients with diabetes mellitus. Clin Infect Dis 40: 990–996.
20. Stevens DL, Bisno AL, Chambers HF, Everett ED, Dellinger P, et al. (2005) Practice guidelines for the diagnosis and management of skin and soft-tissue infections. Clin Infect Dis 41: 1373–1406.
21. Capitano B, Leshem OA, Nightingale CH, Nicolau DP (2003) Cost effect of managing methicillin-resistant *Staphylococcus aureus* in a long-term care facility. J Am Geriatr Soc 51: 10–16.
22. Chong C, Street PR (2008) Pneumonia in the elderly: a review of the epidemiology, pathogenesis, microbiology, and clinical features. South Med J 101: 1141–1145.
23. Chira S, Miller LG (2010) Staphylococcus aureus is the most common identified cause of cellulitis: a systematic review. Epidemiol Infect 138(3): 313–317.

Staphylococcus aureus Keratinocyte Invasion Is Dependent upon Multiple High-Affinity Fibronectin-Binding Repeats within FnBPA

Andrew M. Edwards[1]*, Ursula Potter[2], Nicola A. G. Meenan[3], Jennifer R. Potts[3,4], Ruth C. Massey[1]

1 Department of Biology and Biochemistry, University of Bath, Bath, United Kingdom, **2** Microscopic Analysis Suite, University of Bath, Bath, United Kingdom, **3** Department of Biology, University of York, York, United Kingdom, **4** Department of Chemistry, University of York, York, United Kingdom

Abstract

Staphylococcus aureus is a commensal organism and a frequent cause of skin and soft tissue infections, which can progress to serious invasive disease. This bacterium uses its fibronectin binding proteins (FnBPs) to invade host cells and it has been hypothesised that this provides a protected niche from host antimicrobial defences, allows access to deeper tissues and provides a reservoir for persistent or recurring infections. FnBPs contain multiple tandem fibronectin-binding repeats (FnBRs) which bind fibronectin with varying affinity but it is unclear what selects for this configuration. Since both colonisation and skin infection are dependent upon the interaction of *S. aureus* with keratinocytes we hypothesised that this might select for FnBP function and thus composition of the FnBR region. Initial experiments revealed that *S. aureus* attachment to keratinocytes is rapid but does not require FnBRs. By contrast, invasion of keratinocytes was dependent upon the FnBR region and occurred via similar cellular processes to those described for endothelial cells. Despite this, keratinocyte invasion was relatively inefficient and appeared to include a lag phase, most likely due to very weak expression of $\alpha_5\beta_1$ integrins. Molecular dissection of the role of the FnBR region revealed that efficient invasion of keratinocytes was dependent on the presence of at least three high-affinity (but not low-affinity) FnBRs. Over-expression of a single high-affinity or three low-affinity repeats promoted invasion but not to the same levels as *S. aureus* expressing an FnBPA variant containing three high-affinity repeats. In summary, invasion of keratinocytes by *S. aureus* requires multiple high-affinity FnBRs within FnBPA, and given the importance of the interaction between these cell types and *S. aureus* for both colonisation and infection, may have provided the selective pressure for the multiple binding repeats within FnBPA.

Editor: Malcolm James Horsburgh, University of Liverpool, United Kingdom

Funding: JRP acknowledges the British Heart Foundation (http://www.bhf.org.uk/) for a Senior Basic Science Research Fellowship. This work was funded by the Wellcome Trust (http://www.wellcome.ac.uk/), grant number WT 079588. The funders had no role in study design, data collection and analysis, decision to publish, or preparation of the manuscript.

Competing Interests: The authors have declared that no competing interests exist.

* E-mail: ae248@bath.ac.uk

Introduction

Staphylococcus aureus is a bacterium responsible for a wide range of superficial and invasive infections ranging in severity from mild to fatal [1]. In addition to causing severe morbidity and mortality in the healthcare environment, *S. aureus* is a growing problem in the community, causing serious infections in otherwise healthy people [2,3]. Treatment of *S. aureus* infections is often complicated by the high prevalence of antibiotic resistant strains [4,5]. Despite the ability of this organism to cause serious illness, *S. aureus* is primarily a commensal organism, residing within the nares and on the skin of 20–60% of the population either permanently or transiently [6]. Colonisation of the skin can lead to a number of persistent or recurring infections including, folliculitis, scalded skin syndrome, impetigo, colonisation of indwelling medical devices and wound infections [1,7,8].

Although originally considered an extracellular pathogen, there is both *in vitro* and *in vivo* evidence that *S. aureus* invades host cells. Although the role of invasion in colonisation and infection is unclear, it is hypothesised to facilitate evasion of immune surveillance, traversal of cellular barriers, evasion of antimicrobial therapy and to enable persistent infection [9–17]. Indeed, there is evidence that *S. aureus* is able to dramatically alter its phenotype (to the small colony variant phenotype) to enhance survival within host cells, which is associated with persistent infections [14,15].

The primary mechanism by which *S. aureus* enters host cells is well characterised; staphylococcal fibronectin binding proteins (FnBPs) interact with cell surface $\alpha_5\beta_1$ integrins via a fibronectin bridge [18–20]. It appears that FnBPA alone is sufficient for invasion since heterologous expression on the surface of otherwise non-invasive *Lactococcus lactis* or *Staphylococcus carnosus* confers the ability to invade host cells [19]. The indirect interaction of FnBPA with $\alpha_5\beta_1$ integrins leads to cell signalling events, actin rearrangement and internalization of the bacterium via a mechanism that is entirely dependent on host-cell processes [11,18,21].

FnBPs are multifunctional proteins, comprised of distinct regions with variable binding activity. The N-terminal domain binds both fibrinogen and elastin and is implicated in biofilm formation [22,23]. This region is followed by 11 (FnBPA) or 10 (FnBPB) non-identical fibronectin-binding repeats (FnBRs), with either high or low-affinity for fibronectin [24]. These multiple repeats enable a single FnBPA molecule to bind multiple fibronectin molecules [25–27]. It has been hypothesised that this facilitates bacterial interactions with multiple integrins, triggering cell signalling processes, actin rearrangement and bacterial internalisation [27–29]. We have previously shown that this region is essential for triggering bacterial invasion of endothelial cells [17,30]. In addition to its role in adhesion, invasion and biofilm formation, the high prevalence of *fnb* genes amongst *S. aureus* strains suggest that FnBPs might be important for colonisation; analysis of a panel of 163 clinical isolates revealed that 22% encoded just *fnb*A, 1% just *fnb*B and 77% encoded both genes [31].

We recently investigated how the composition of the FnBR region of FnBPA affected the invasion of endothelial cells and virulence in a murine bacteremia model [17]. This study demonstrated that a single high-affinity FnBR was sufficient to trigger invasion, although this was less efficient than FnBPA variants containing multiple FnBRs [17]. Multiple FnBRs were required for virulence, enhancing bacterial dissemination into the kidneys, as well as leading to significant weight loss and death [17]. Although it is important that we understand how this protein contributes to invasive infection, this is a relatively rare event. It is more likely that the frequent interactions that occur between *S. aureus* and keratinocytes, involved in colonisation and infection of both nasal and skin surfaces [12,13,32], are responsible for selection of FnBPA function. We therefore investigated the role of the FnBR-region in the adhesion to, and invasion of, keratinocytes.

Methods

Bacterial strains and growth conditions

A detailed list of the strains used in this study is presented in Table 1. *S. aureus* 8325.4 strains were cultured in Tryptic Soy Broth (TSB, Oxoid) at 37°C in air with shaking for 16 h. *S. aureus* CFU were quantified on Tryptic Soy Agar (TSA, Oxoid) plates incubated overnight at 37°C in air. *L. lactis* strains were cultured in M17 broth (supplemented with 0.5% w/v glucose) for 16 h at 30°C in air (with the indicated concentration of nisin). As required, bacteria were incubated in the presence of the following antibiotics: Chloramphenicol 10 μg ml^{-1} (*S. aureus*) or Erythomycin 5 μg ml^{-1} (*L. lactis*) or 250 μg ml^{-1} (*E. coli*).

S. aureus 8325.4-derived Δ*fnb*A/B expressing *fnb*A variants from a plasmid have been characterised previously [17] to establish equal surface expression levels between strains expressing each construct. All constructs have identical N-terminal and C-terminal domains, varying only in the composition of the FnBR-region.

Recombinant FnBR expression

A polypeptide corresponding to high-affinity repeats FnBR9,10 (FnBPA residues 763–838; Swiss-Prot entry P14738) was expressed and purified in a manner similar to that previously described for

Table 1. Strains and plasmids used in this study.

Species/strain/plasmid	Relevant characteristics	Source/Reference
E. coli		
(pMSP7517)	Nisin-inducible vector containing the *prg*B gene of *Enterococcus faecalis*	[51]
K12 ER2925	Cloning host	New England Biolabs
BL21	Recombinant peptide expression host	
pGEX-6P-2	Expresses GST-tagged FnBR9,10 peptide	This study
Staphylococcus aureus		
DU5883	*fnbA- fnbp-* isogenic mutant of 8325.4	[52]
DU5883 (pFnBA4)		
(referred to here as pFnBPR1–11)	*fnbp* - strain complemented with the plasmid pFnBA4 expressing full-length FnBPA: FnBPR1–11	
pFnBPR0	Expresses FnBPA variant containing no Fn-binding repeats: FnBPR0	[17]
pFnBPR1	Expresses FnBPA variant containing Fn-binding repeat 1 only: FnBPR1	
pFnBPR11	Expresses FnBPA variant containing Fn-binding repeat 11 only: FnBPR11	
pFnBPR10,11	Expresses FnBPA variant containing Fn-binding repeats 10 & 11: FnBPR10& 11	
pFnBPR1,10,11	Expresses FnBPA variant containing Fn-binding repeats 1, 10 & 11: FnBPR1, 10, 11	
pFnBPR9–11	Expresses FnBPA variant containing Fn-binding repeats 9–11: FnBPR9–11	
pFnBPR2	Expresses FnBPA variant containing Fn-binding repeat 2 only: FnBPR2	
pFnBPR8	Expresses FnBPA variant containing Fn-binding repeat 8 only: FnBPR8	
pFnBPR7,8	Expresses FnBPA variant containing Fn-binding repeats 7 & 8: FnBPR7,8	
pFnBPR6–8	Expresses FnBPA variant containing Fn-binding repeats 6–8: FnBPR6–8	
Lactococcus lactis		
L. lactis NZ9800	*nis*A defective isogenic mutant of NZ9700 (*fnb-*)	[53]
pMFnBPR1–11	Nisin controlled expression of FnBPA containing repeats 1–11: FnBPR1–11	[17]
pMFnBPR1	Nisin controlled expression of FnBPA containing repeat 1: FnBPR1	
pMFnBPR1,10,11	Nisin controlled expression of FnBPA containing repeats 1,10,11: FnBPR1,10,11	
pMFnBPR6–8	Nisin controlled expression of FnBPA containing repeats 6–8: FnBPR6–8	This study

single FnBRs [24]. The GST-tag was removed using 3C protease and FnBR9,10 was further purified by reversed-phase HPLC.

Construction and controlled expression of FnBPA variants in *L. lactis*

Expression levels of FnBPA variants in *S. aureus* and *L. lactis* have been determined previously [17]. With the exception of the pMR6-8 construct, all nisin-inducible FnBPA constructs have been described previously [17]. The pMR6-8 construct was made as described previously using standard molecular biology techniques [17,33]. Briefly, the enitre R6-8 *fnb*A variant was amplified from pFnBPR6-8 using primers containing NcoI and XhoI sites (AAACCATGGAGGAGGTATTATAGTGAAAAACAATCT-TAGG) (AAACTCGAGCTAACTTTATCTCTCAGTTCGT-TATC) and ligated into similarly digested pMSP7517 plasmid. Ligated constructs were transformed into $CaCl_2$ treated *E. coli* K12 ER2925. Plasmids were recovered from the *E. coli* transformants (the DNA sequence was confirmed) and transformed into *L. lactis* NZ9800. As all constructs contained the A domain (Table 1), expression was confirmed by assessment of fibrinogen binding [17]. Previous work has determined that nisin controlled expression of FnBPA variants in *L. lactis* using this system produces equal expression levels between strains at identical nisin concentrations [17].

Cell culture

The spontaneously immortalised keratinocyte cell line HaCat was used because it closely resembles primary keratinocyte cells and has been used previously in studies of *S. aureus*-keratinocyte interactions [34–37]. All cells were cultured in Dulbecco's modified Eagle's medium (Invitrogen), with calcium adjusted to 2.8 mM and supplemented with FBS (10%) and L-glutamine (2 mM) at 37°C and 5% CO_2, conditions that support differentiation, keratinization and tight-junction formation [38].

Cells were cultured in T75 flasks to approximately 95% confluency, liberated with trypsin-EDTA, resuspended in culture medium and added to 24-well plates containing thermanox glass coverslips [30]. Plates were incubated for 48 h as described above before the coverslips were removed, dip washed in (phosphate buffered saline)PBS and added to new 24-well plates containing fresh medium and bacteria [30]. For experiments using inhibitors of cell function, these were incubated with the cells 60 min prior to the addition of bacteria and concentrations maintained during the assay; Genistein (200 µM), Wortmannin (20 nM), cytochalasin D (50 µM), PP2 (10 µM), cholchicine (1 µM), cycloheximide (25 µM) and methyl-β-cyclodextrin (2 mM) [17]. EA.Hy926 cells were cultured and prepared as previously described [17].

Cell attachment and invasion assays

Attachment and invasion assays were performed as described before [17]. Cultured cells were dissociated from plastic flasks using trypsin-EDTA solution (Invitrogen) and approximately 5×10^5 (in 0.5 ml medium) were seeded into each well of 24-well plates (Nunc) containing 13 mm plastic Thermanox™ cover slips (Fisher) and allowed to attach for 48 h (37°C, 5% CO_2). Coverslips were dip-washed once in PBS and placed in the well of a new 24-well plate containing 490 µl of DMEM containing 10% FBS. To each well, 10 µl of washed bacteria were added (approximately 1×10^7 CFU *S. aureus* and 5×10^7 *L. lactis*) and incubated for 15–90 minutes at 37°C in 5% CO_2.

To measure the total number of bacteria associated with the cells (adherent and internalized – referred to in the text and figures as adhesion), coverslips were dip-washed three times in PBS and added to wells containing 500 µl 0.5% Triton X-100. Wells containing coverslips were agitated by pippetting to fully lyse the cells and CFU were enumerated by serial dilution and plating onto TSA agar plates and incubation overnight at 37°C.

For invasion assays, the bacterial suspension was removed and replaced with 500 µl DMEM/10% FBS supplemented with 200 µg ml^{-1} gentamicin and incubated at 37°C in 5% CO_2 for 60 min. Coverslips were washed three times in PBS, lysed and plated for CFU as described for the adhesion assay above. In assays where metabolic inhibitors were used, these were added to cell monolayers for 60 min prior to the experiment and concentrations maintained during incubation with bacteria.

Determination of $\alpha_5\beta_1$ integrin expression by keratinocytes and endothelial cells

HaCat Keratincoytes and EA. Hy926 endothelial cells were cultured in T75 flasks to approximately 95% confluency, as described above. Cells were liberated from the flasks by the use of non-enzymatic cell dissociation solution (4 ml, Sigma) and collected by centrifugation (2,000× g, 10 min). Cells were subsequently resuspended in lysis buffer (1% TX-100, 100 units ml^{-1} DNase, protease inhibitor cocktail (Sigma) in PBS) and incubated for 20 min at 37°C. Insoluble debris was pelleted by centrifugation and the supernatant recovered. Total protein was determined using the Bradford assay and 20 µl aliquots containing 10 µg protein mixed with Laemmli sample buffer [33] before boiling for 5 min. Samples were then subjected to SDS-PAGE on duplicate 10% acrylamide gels. Total protein was detected by the use of EZ-blue protein detection reagent (Sigma). Alternatively, proteins were transfered to nitrocellulose membrane using a Bio-Rad semi-dry blotter. The membrane was subsequently blocked in PBS containing 10% skimmed milk powder for 1 hr at room temperature. The protein bands corresponding to α_5 or β_1 integrin subunits were detected using rabbit polyclonal anti-integrin α_5 (H-104) or β_1 (M-106, both from Santa Cruz Biotechnology) antibodies and then HRP-conjugated protein A (Sigma). Bound antibody/protein A was detected using enhanced chemiluminescence reagent (GE Healthcare).

Scanning electron microscopy

S. aureus was incubated with keratinocytes or endothelial cells as above for invasion assays for 15–90 minutes. Coverslips were then washed twice with serum-free DMEM before fixation with DMEM containing 2.5% gluteraldehyde and 10 mg ml^{-1} potassium ferrocynaide for 2 hr at 37°C in 5% CO_2. Cells were postfixed in a solution of 1% osmium tetroxide and 1% potassium ferrocyanide for 1 hr in air at room temperature. Coverslips were washed twice in distilled water over 10 mins before staining with 2% uranyl acetate for 1 hr in the dark. Cells were subsequently dehydrated in increasing concentrations of acetone (50–100%) followed by 1:1 acetone: hexamethyldisilazane and finally 100% hexamethyldisilazane, which was allowed to evaporate over 1–2 hrs in air. Samples were then examined using a JEOL JSM6480LV scanning electron microscope.

Statistics

For adhesion and invasion assays, statistical analyses were performed with Student's *t* test using the Bonferroni correction for multiple comparisons [17]. Values that were statistically significantly different from controls are indicated by asterisks in the figures. Error bars indicate the mean average ± standard deviation of multiple independent experiments (indicated in the figure legend).

Results

S. aureus 8325.4 adhesion to keratinocytes is similar to endothelial cells but invasion levels are significantly lower

S. aureus attachment to the skin is the precursor to colonisation and infection. Invasion is also likely to play an important role, particularly in maintaining persistent or recurring infection [13]. We employed the well-characterised keratinocyte cell line HaCat as a model to study the role of FnBPA in bacterial adhesion to, and invasion of, the skin and nares. To determine the kinetics of keratinocyte-*S. aureus* interactions, we measured adhesion to and invasion of HaCat keratinocytes over time, until saturation levels were observed (Fig. 1). Adhesion occurred rapidly, with approximately 3×10^5 CFU (~3% inoculum) *S. aureus* attached after 15 minutes (Fig. 1). This number did not change significantly over time (up to 90 mins), suggesting that all available binding sites on the host cells were occupied (Fig. 1). Invasion, by contrast, occurred more slowly. After 15 mins $<10^3$ CFU *S. aureus* had internalised, despite the high number of adherent bacteria and there was no significant increase up to 30 mins, indicating that the invasion process includes a lag-phase (Fig. 1). However, between 30 and 45 mins this number increased >10-fold to $\sim10^4$ CFU (~0.1% inoculum). There was no further increase in the number of internalised *S. aureus* up to 90 minutes, indicating that maximal invasion levels had been reached (Fig. 1).

To compare how invasion of keratinocytes compared to endothelial cells we also examined the adhesion to and invasion of EA. hy926 endothelial cells over the same time period (Fig. 1). *S. aureus* adhesion to endothelial cells was identical to that of keratinocytes after 15 minutes (Fig. 1). Adhesion to the endothelial cells increased over time and was significantly greater than HaCat cells after 45 mins. *S. aureus* invasion of endothelial cells was, however, 16-fold greater than that of keratinocytes after 15 minutes (Fig. 1). Endothelial cell invasion continued to increase until reaching saturation at 45–60 mins, at which point it was still approximately 6-fold greater than that seen with keratinocytes.

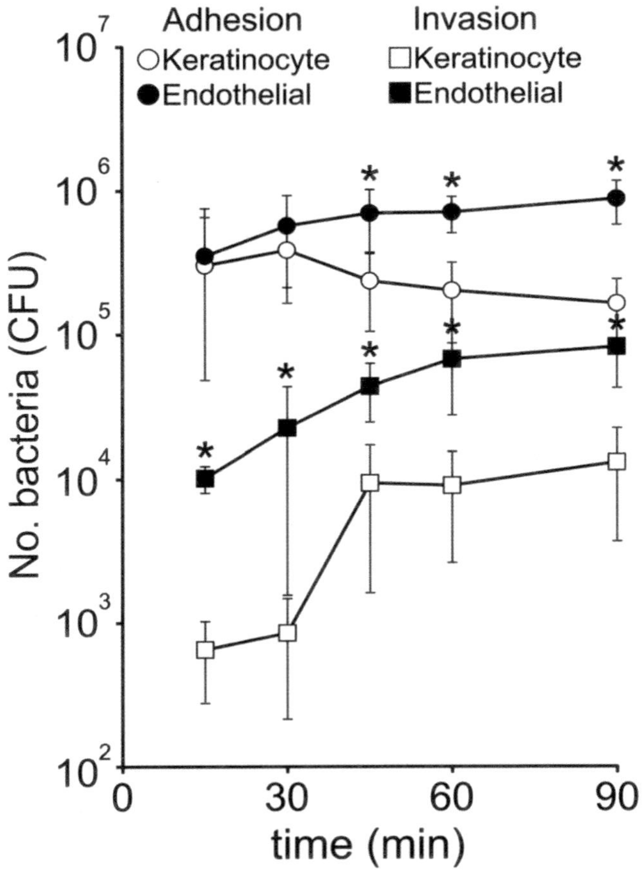

Figure 1. *S. aureus* adhesion to, and invasion of, keratinocyte and endothelial cells over time. The total number of *S. aureus* 8325.4 (DU5883 Δ*fnb*A/B pFnBA4 expressing full length FnBPA) associated (adherent and internalized; circles) and internalized (squares) with each cell type was determined over a period of 90 minutes. Values for adhesion to, and invasion of, endothelial cells that are statistically significantly different from those obtained with HaCat cells are denoted (*). Experiments were performed 3 times in duplicate. Multiplicity of infection (MOI) = 20. Error bars represent the standard deviation of the mean.

Low level keratinocyte invasion is not due to different invasion processes being utilised by S. aureus

Although several different pathogenic bacteria utilize integrins to trigger invasion, the cellular mechanisms involved can vary significantly. For example, *Streptococcus pyogenes* can invade via both caveolae and membrane ruffling depending on the invasin [39,40]. To examine whether the difference in efficiency of invasion of keratinocytes when compared to endothelial cells is due to the bacteria utilizing a different cellular process, we measured the internalisation of *S. aureus* FnBPR1–11 by HaCat cells pre-treated with inhibitors of cell function used previously in studies with endothelial cells [17]. Disruption of host cell actin rearrangement (cytochalasin D), PI3K signalling (wortmannin), Src kinase signalling (PP2) or microtubule function (colchicine) all significantly inhibited *S. aureus* invasion, albeit to differing degrees (Fig. 2). By contrast, inhibition of tyrosine kinases (genistein), de novo protein synthesis (cycloheximide) or depletion of cholesterol (methyl-β-cyclodextrin) did not significantly affect invasion (Fig. 2). This was identical to that found when endothelial cells were studied [17], demonstrating that differences in these cellular process were not responsible for the difference in cell invasion efficiency observed.

To confirm the role of cellular processes in invasion, we examined *S. aureus*-keratinocyte interactions using scanning electron microscopy (Fig. 3). After 15 minutes' incubation with *S. aureus* FnBPR1–11, there were significant numbers of attached bacteria but there were no visible changes in the host cell surface (Fig. 3A). After 30 minutes, a few adherent bacteria were associated with host-cell membrane alterations consistent with actin rearrangement (Fig. 3B–E). These morphological changes in the host cell membrane were consistent and we did not observe other types of changes, such as the formation of caveolae.

By 90 minutes post inoculation, a number of fully internalised bacteria could be observed within the keratinocytes (Fig. 3F,G). By contrast to *S. aureus* FnBPR1–11, *S. aureus* FnBPR0 did not induce any membrane alterations after 90 mins (Fig. 3H). We also examined the interaction of *S. aureus* FnBPR1–11 with EA. Hy926 cells. After 30 mins adherent bacteria were associated with membrane ruffles, similar to those observed with keratinocytes (Fig. 3I,J).

The composition of the FnBR region significantly affects invasion of keratinocytes

In a previous study we showed that a single high-affinity Fn binding repeat (FnBR) in FnBPA was sufficient for invasion of endothelial cells [17]. To assess the role of FnBPA, and in

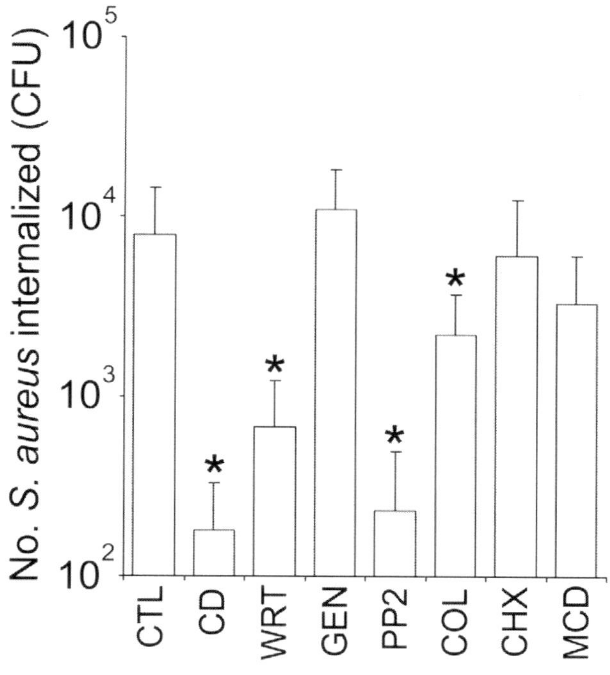

Figure 2. Keratinocyte invasion occurs via a similar mechanism to endothelial cells. HaCat cells were pre-incubated (60 min) with inhibitors of cell function before the addition of *S. aureus* FnBPAR1–11 (DU5883 Δ*fnb*A/B pFnBA4) and invasion determined after 90 mins. Inhibitors used were cytochalasin D (CD, inhibits actin polymerization), wortmannin (WRT, inhibits PI3-Kinase activity), genistein (GEN, inhibits tyrosine kinase activity), PP2 (PP2, Src kinase inhibitor), colchicine (COL, interferes with microtubule organisation), cycloheximide (CHX, inhibits eukaryotic protein synthesis) and methyl-β-cyclodextrine (MCD, depletes membrane cholesterol). Inhibitor-free medium was used as a positive control (CTL). Experiments were performed three times in duplicate. MOI = 20. Error bars represent the standard deviation of the mean. Values that are significantly different ($p = < 0.05$) from control are indicated (*).

particular the FnBR region, we examined adhesion to and invasion of HaCat cells by *S. aureus* expressing full length FnBPA: FnBPR1–11, a Δ*fnb*A/B mutant and *S. aureus* pFnBPR0 (which lacks the FnBR region) after 90 minutes (Fig. 4). Adhesion of *S. aureus* to HaCat cells was unaffected by the presence or absence of FnBPA (data not shown). Invasion, however, was dependent on the presence of FnBPA; *S. aureus* lacking FnBPs invaded at levels 15 times lower than *S. aureus* FnBPR1–11 (Fig. 5). FnBPA-triggered invasion was entirely dependent of the presence of the FnBR region; *S. aureus* FnBPR0 invaded HaCat cells at levels identical to *S. aureus* Δ*fnb*A/B (Fig. 5).

To examine how the composition of the FnBR region modulates invasion, we measured internalisation of *S. aureus* expressing FnBPA variants containing various numbers of high- or low-affinity tandem repeats (Fig. 4). Previous work has demonstrated that these variants are expressed on the surface of *S. aureus* at equal levels and characterised the fibronectin-binding of each construct [17]. Although *S. aureus* FnBPR1 or FnBPR11 invaded at levels significantly higher than *S. aureus* FnBPR0 this was >12-fold less than *S. aureus* FnBPR1–11 (Fig. 5). The presence of a second high affinity repeat (FnBPR10,11) was required to enhance internalisation to levels that were similar to that of *S. aureus* FnBPR1–11 (Fig. 5). Three high-affinity repeats (FnBPR1,10,11 and FnBPR9–11) also triggered invasion at similar levels to FnBPR1–11 (Fig. 5).

In contrast to the FnBPA variants with high-affinity repeats, *S. aureus* expressing FnBPA variants containing a single (FnBPR2 or FnBPR8) or two (FnBPR7,8) low-affinity repeats did not invade at levels that were significantly greater than FnBPR0 (Fig. 5). *S. aureus* expressing a FnBPA variant with three tandem low-affinity repeats (FnBPR6–8) did invade at levels above that of FnBPR0 but these were approximately 12-fold lower than *S. aureus* FnBPR1–11 (Fig. 5).

Over-expression of FnBPR1 or FnBPR6–8 fails to confer maximal invasion

We have shown previously that FnBPA-mediated invasion of endothelial cells is dependent on the total number of FnBRs on the bacterial cell surface, rather than the number within an individual FnBPA molecule [17]. As such, high-level expression of FnBPR1 can trigger endothelial cell invasion to similar levels as *S. aureus* expressing FnBPR1–11. To determine whether maximal invasion of keratinocytes (FnBPR1–11 levels) could be triggered by over-expression of otherwise weakly-invasive FnBPR1 or FnBPR6–8 constructs, or whether invasion is absolutely dependent on multiple FnBRs within FnBPA, we employed a nisin-inducible system to control and over-express FnBPA variants on the surface of *L. lactis* [17]. Previous work [17] has demonstrated that, at identical concentrations of nisin, expression levels of FnBPA variants on the surface of *L. lactis* are equal. *L. lactis* expressing each FnBPA construct at three surface expression levels (by inducing expression at three concentrations of nisin; 0, 10 or 100 ng ml^{-1}) were assessed for invasion of HaCat cells (Fig. 6). At the lowest level of expression (0 ng ml^{-1} nisin, at which low-level expression occurs due to a leaky promoter) there were only negligible levels of invasion by *L. lactis* expressing each of the FnBPA variants (Fig. 6). Induction of FnBPR1–11 expression (10 ng ml^{-1} nisin) increased invasion 80-fold to levels similar to those seen with *S. aureus* FnBPR1–11 (Figures 1 and 5). Greater induction of FnBPR1–11 expression (100 ng ml^{-1}) did not increase internalisation suggesting that maximal invasion levels had been reached (Fig. 6). Invasion of *L. lactis* FnBPR1,10,11 also increased dramatically when induced at 10 ng ml^{-1} nisin (relative to no induction), but at significantly lower levels than *L. lactis* FnBPR1–11 (Fig. 6). However, at the highest level of expression, *L. lactis* R1,10,11 was internalised at the same level as FnBPR1–11 (Fig. 6), mimicking the data obtained with *S. aureus* expressing FnBPA variants (Fig. 5). Induction of FnBPR1 or FnBPR6–8 expression (10 ng ml^{-1} nisin) promoted *L. lactis* invasion but at levels >30-fold lower than *L. lactis* FnBPR1–11 (Fig. 6). Further induction of FnBPR1 or FnBPR6–8 expression (100 ng ml^{-1} nisin) further increased invasion, but this was still 4-fold lower than that seen for *L. lactis* FnBPR1–11 at the same level of induction (Fig. 6).

Inefficient invasion of keratinocytes may be due to weak $\alpha_5\beta_1$ integrin expression

Although invasion processes do not seem to vary between endothelial cells and keratinocytes, a higher number of high affinity FnBRs are required for efficient invasion of keratinocytes. As such we hypothesised that the difference between the invasion efficiency of keratinocytes and endothelial cells may be due to differences in the density of the host cell ligand, the cell surface $\alpha_5\beta_1$ integrin. To test this, we compared the expression of the α_5 and β_1 integrin subunits in keratinocytes and endothelial cells by performing a Western-immunoblot of whole-cell protein extracts. This revealed that $\alpha_5\beta_1$ integrin expression levels were significantly higher in endothelial cells than keratinocytes (Fig. 7). This is consistent with studies of human skin [41], and may explain the differences in invasion levels between the two cells types.

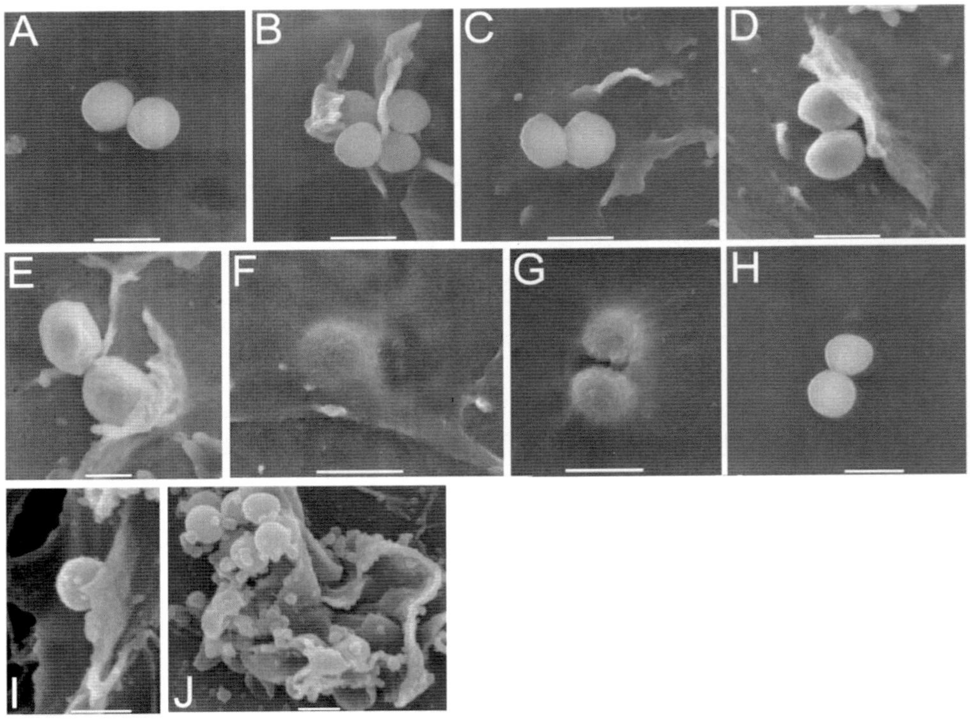

Figure 3. *S. aureus* FnBPR1–11 induces membrane ruffling and invasion of keratinocytes. *S. aureus* FnBPR1–11 (DU5883 Δ*fnb*A/B pFnBA4) was incubated with keratinocytes for 15 (A), 30 (B–E) or 90 mins (F,G) before washing, fixation, processing and examination by scanning electron microscopy. As a negative control, *S. aureus* FnBPR0 was also examined after 90 mins (H). As a comparison, the interaction of *S. aureus* FnBPR1–11 with EA. Hy926 endothelial cells after 30 mins was also visualised (I–J). In each case the bar represents 1 μm. MOI = 20.

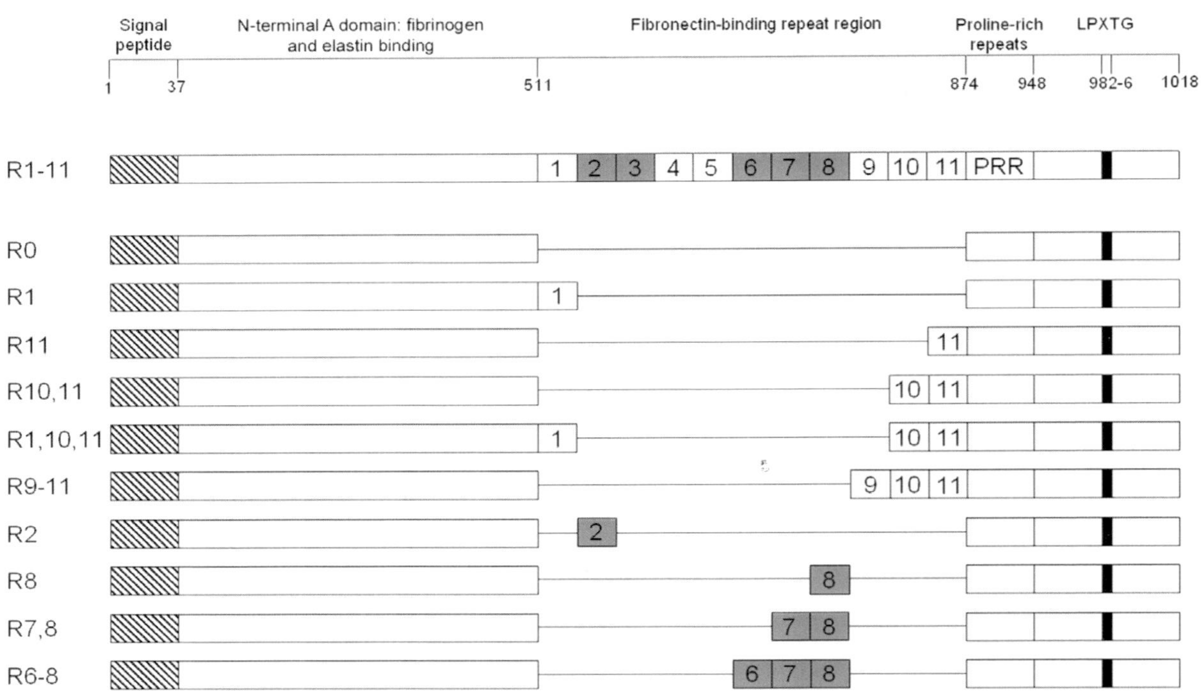

Figure 4. Diagrammatic representations of FnBPA and the variant constructs used in this study. The relative positions of each of the major functional domains of FnBPA from *S. aureus* 8325.4 (SWISS-Prot P14738) (not to scale) are indicated, along with a schematic of each of the FnBPA variant constructs used in this study, which vary only in the composition of the FnBR domain. Low-affinity FnBRs are shaded.

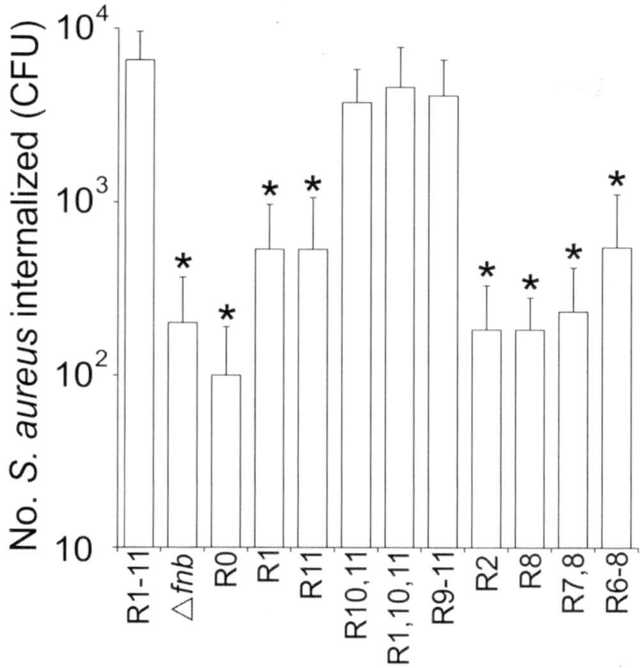

Figure 5. The composition of the FnBR domain of FnBPA modulates host cell invasion. Keratinocytes were incubated with either *S. aureus* DU5883 Δ*fnb*A/B (Δ*fnb*) or *S. aureus* Δ*fnb* expressing one of the FnBPA variant constructs detailed in figure 4 for 90 minutes and the number of internalized bacteria determined. Experiments were performed 3 times in duplicate. Error bars represent the standard deviation of the mean. MOI = 20. Values that are significantly different (p = <0.05) from *S. aureus* Δ*fnb* are indicated (*).

A FnBR peptide inhibits *S. aureus* invasion of keratinocytes

The rise in antibiotic resistance has prompted the search for novel approaches to preventing bacterial colonisation and infection. As there seems to be a critical ratio of FnBR and host ligand needed to invade cells ([17] Fig. 5 and 6), we hypothesized that an FnBR peptide might be sufficient to outcompete FnBPA and prevent *S. aureus* invasion. A tagless recombinantly-expressed peptide corresponding to FnBR9,10 (two high-affinity repeats) was used in an assay to examine its potential to block adhesion and invasion (Fig. 8). The peptide reduced adhesion approximately two-fold at the very highest concentration, despite FnBPA not being required for attachment of keratinocytes (Fig. 8, data not shown). By contrast, the peptide significantly inhibited *S. aureus* invasion at concentration of 1 nM (>2-fold reduction), which was even more pronounced at 2 nM (>5-fold) (Fig. 8). As such, this peptide may warrant further study as a potential novel prophylactic agent.

Discussion

S. aureus is able to colonise and infect skin, causing a wide spectrum of infections ranging from superficial to invasive, acute to chronic [1]. Infection can occur in healthy individuals as well as those with broken skin due to wounds, inserted medical devices or chronic skin conditions such as psoriasis [8]. Central to colonisation and infection is the interaction of *S. aureus* with keratinocytes, which form an important barrier between the internal organs and external environment. Adhesion of *S. aureus* to

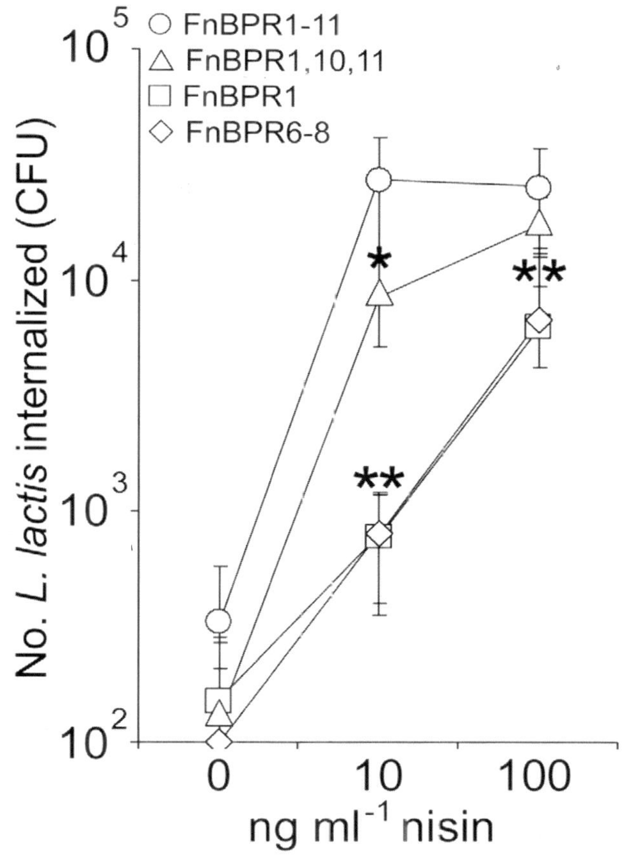

Figure 6. Over-expression of FnBPR1 or FnBPR6–8 fails to trigger maximal invasion of Keratinocytes. Expression of FnBPA variant constructs on the surface of *L. lactis* was performed using a nisin-inducible system. Invasion of *L. lactis* expressing FnBPAR1–11 (circles), FnBPAR1,10,11 (triangles), FnBPAR1 (squares) or FnBPAR6–8 (diamonds) was determined at 3 different levels of induction (0, 10 or 100 ng ml^{-1} nisin). Experiments were performed 3 times in duplicate. Error bars represent the standard deviation of the mean. MOI = 100. Values that are significantly different (p = <0.05) from *L. lactis* FnBPAR1–11 at identical nisin concentrations are indicated (*).

keratinocytes results in inflammatory cytokine release and stimulates secretion of several antimicrobial peptides, of which β-defensin 3 reaches levels sufficient to kill *S. aureus* [42,43]. Cellular invasion is apparently not necessary to trigger these responses but internalised bacteria cause necrotic and apoptotic cell death [37]. Interestingly, *S. aureus* adhesion to endothelial cells was equal to that of keratinocytes after 15 minutes, but was significantly greater after 90 minutes. This may reflect a decrease in keratinocyte-attached CFU due to the release of antimicrobial peptides by the HaCat cells.

Although the role of cellular invasion in colonisation and pathogenesis is unclear, previous work has shown that *S. aureus* can persist within keratinocytes for extended periods and it is possible that invasion provides shelter from the host antimicrobial arsenal. Intracellular *S. aureus* has been identified in chronic infections where it could form a protected reservoir as well as a mechanism of cellular dissemination and penetration of deeper tissues [14,15].

We have shown previously that endothelial cell invasion is dependent upon the surface density of the FnBRs within FnBPA. The presence of multiple repeats within FnBPA is equivalent to

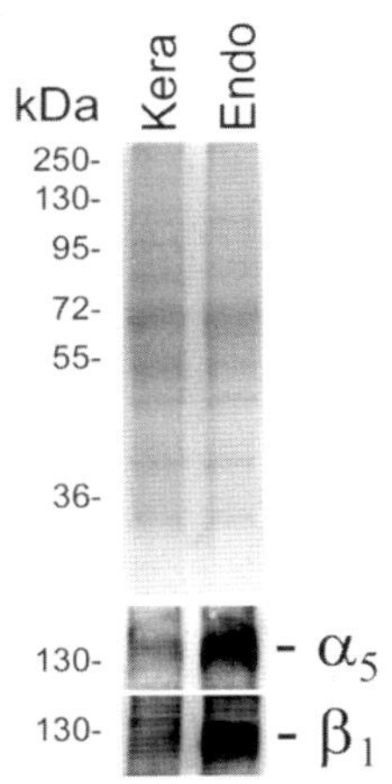

Figure 7. Keratinocyte expression of α_5 and β_1 integrins is lower than endothelial cells. HaCat keratinocytes (Kera) or EA. Hy926 endothelial (Endo) cells were harvested from flasks, lysed and the lysate examined by SDS-PAGE and Western-immunoblot to determine relative α_5 or β_1 integrin expression levels.

multiple invasins in a single molecule, significantly enhancing efficiency and reducing immune exposure [17].

As the interaction of *S. aureus* with keratinocytes is a considerably more common event than with endothelial cells, we hypothesized that it likely provides the main selective pressure for the composition of FnBPs. The lack of a role for FnBPA in adhesion to HaCat keratinocyte cells is not surprising since *S. aureus* encodes a large number of adhesins. Indeed, at least five different *S. aureus* surface proteins are implicated in attachment to nasal epithelial cells, including ClfB, IsdA, SdrC, SdrD and SasG, as well as wall teichoic acid, which is essential for nasal colonisation [44–47]. By contrast, invasion of HaCat keratinocytes was FnBPA-dependent and, in keeping with previous work [17], the FnBR region was essential. Previous work has shown that a single high-affinity, or three low-affinity repeats were sufficient to trigger maximal invasion of endothelial cells [17]. By contrast, our data indicate that keratinocyte invasion requires much higher surface densities of FnBRs than for invasion of endothelial cells. This may be a result of the significantly lower level of $\alpha_5\beta_1$ integrin expression by the keratinocyte cells, which is in keeping with *in vivo* analysis of normal human skin [41]. It is therefore possible that the difference in the speed of invasion is due to the increased length of time required for *S. aureus* to engage with sufficient $\alpha_5\beta_1$ integrins on the keratinocyte cell surface and for subsequent cell-signalling events to occur. Additionally, the presence of multiple FnBRs within FnBPA may increase the efficiency of Fn binding through cooperative binding to arrays of FnBRs as observed recently for a Fn-binding protein from *Streptococcus pyogenes* [48]. It is also possible that delayed entry of *S. aureus* into keratinocytes is desirable for the bacterium. A previous report [49] indicated that *S. aureus* delays uptake into endothelial cells in order to have sufficient time to prepare for intracellular life via up-regulation of e.g. toxin genes. It is possible that *S. aureus* employs a similar strategy for keratinocytes.

Although *S. aureus* invaded the endothelial cells more readily than the keratinocytes, the mechanism used appears to be the same (Figure 2 and [17]). Using identical concentrations of cell-function inhibitors used previously to study endothelial cell invasion [17], entry of *S. aureus* into HaCat cells was also found to involve PI3 and Src-kinases as well as actin rearrangement.

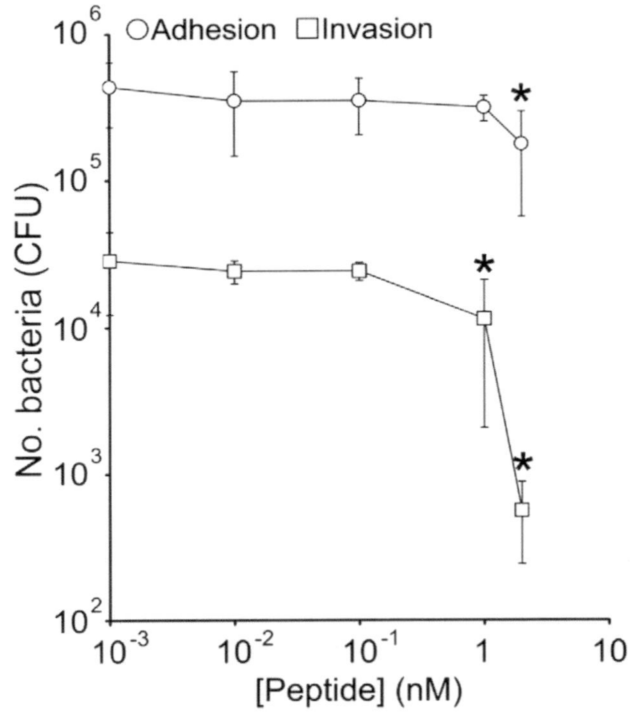

Figure 8. A recombinantly-expressed FnBR peptide inhibits *S. aureus* invasion. The adhesion to (circles), and invasion (squares) of, keratinocytes by *S. aureus* FnBPR1–11 (DU5883 Δ*fnbA/B* pFnBA4) in the presence of various concentrations of recombinant FnBPA peptide (R9,10). Values that statistically significantly difference from those obtained in the absence of peptide are indicated (*). MOI = 20. Experiments were performed 3 times in duplicate. Error bars represent the standard deviation of the mean.

Whilst one might expect genistein to have a similar effect to PP2, our data are not the first to suggest that genistein does not inhibit all the targets of PP2. Indeed, this phenomenon has been observed previously in studies of invasion mediated by fibronectin-binding protein invasins of *S. pyogenes*. Wang et al. [50] showed that invasion of epithelial cells by *L. lactis* expressing M-protein could be inhibited by PP2 but not by genistein. Conversely, invasion by *L. lactis* expressing the invasin SfbI was inhibited by genistein but not PP2. Interestingly, SfbI-mediated invasion relies on caveolae whilst M-protein mediated invasion does not, which ties in with our data showing no inhibition by methyl-β-cyclodextrin. It appears that, using our model system, FnBPA-mediated invasion is highly similar to that of *S. pyogenes* M-protein, rather than the structurally similar SfbI.

In summary, keratinocytes are significantly less amenable to invasion by *S. aureus* than endothelial cells, and require multiple repeats within FnBPA for invasion. As such, *S. aureus* interactions with keratinocytes and similar cells may provide the selection pressure for the multiple FnBRs within FnBPs. The poor penetration of many antibiotics into cells means that intracellular *S. aureus* could represent a reservoir for persistent infection [13,14]. Our data, in keeping with previous reports [18,30], strongly suggest that FnBR peptides are highly effective at reducing *S. aureus* invasion and might form a novel prophylactic approach to reducing carriage and/or the development of chronic infections. Such an approach may have the added benefit of preventing invasion by other skin colonising pathogens such as *S. pyogenes*, which employ similar mechanisms of internalisation [11].

Acknowledgments

We thank Timothy Foster (Trinity College Dublin) for providing strains and the pFNBA4 vector. Garry Dunny (University of Minnesota) and Michiel Kleerebezem (Wageningen University) are thanked for the pMSP7517 vector and Howard Jenkinson (University of Bristol) for *L. lactis* NZ9800. HaCat keratinocytes were kindly provided by Angela Nobbs (University of Bristol).

Author Contributions

Conceived and designed the experiments: AME JRP RCM. Performed the experiments: AME UP NAGM. Analyzed the data AME UP NAGM JRP RCM. Contributed reagents/materials/analysis tools: AME UP NAGM JRP RCM. Wrote the paper: AME UP NAGM JRP RCM.

References

1. Lowy FD (1998) *Staphylococcus aureus* infections. N Engl J Med 339: 520–532.
2. David MZ, Daum RS (2010) Community-associated methicillin-resistant *Staphylococcus aureus*: epidemiology and clinical consequences of an emerging epidemic. Clin Microbiol Rev 23: 616–687.
3. Deleo FR, Otto M, Kreiswirth BN, Chambers HF (2010) Community-associated meticillin-resistant *Staphylococcus aureus*. Lancet 375: 1557–1568.
4. Chambers HF, Deleo FR (2009) Waves of resistance: *Staphylococcus aureus* in the antibiotic era. Nat Rev Microbiol 7: 629–641.
5. DeLeo FR, Chambers HF (2009) Reemergence of antibiotic-resistant *Staphylococcus aureus* in the genomics era. J Clin Invest 119: 2464–2474.
6. Kluytmans J, van Belkum A, Verbrugh H (1997) Nasal carriage of *Staphylococcus aureus*: epidemiology, underlying mechanisms, and associated risks. Clin Microbiol Rev 10: 505–520.
7. Chiller K, Selkin BA, Murakawa GJ (2001) Skin microflora and bacterial infections of the skin. J Investig Dermatol Symp Proc 6: 170–174.
8. Brook I (2002) Secondary bacterial infections complicating skin lesions. J Med Microbiol 51: 808–812.
9. Lowy FD (2000) Is *Staphylococcus aureus* an intracellular pathogen? Trends Microbiol 8: 341–343.
10. Clement S, Vaudaux P, Francois P, Schrenzel J, Huggler E, et al. (2005) Evidence of an intracellular reservoir in the nasal mucosa of patients with recurrent *Staphylococcus aureus* rhinosinusitis. J Infect Dis 192: 1023–1028.
11. Sinha B, Herrmann M (2005) Mechanism and consequences of invasion of endothelial cells by *Staphylococcus aureus*. Thromb Haemost 94: 266–277.
12. Plouin-Gaudon I, Clement S, Huggler E, Chaponnier C, François P, et al. (2006) Intracellular residency is frequently associated with recurrent *Staphylococcus aureus* rhinosinusitis. Rhinology 44: 249–254.
13. von Eiff C, Peters G, Becker K (2006) The small colony variant (SCV) concept – the role of staphylococcal SCVs in persistent infections. Injury 37: S26–33.
14. Garzoni C, Kelley WL (2009) *Staphylococcus aureus*: new evidence for intracellular persistence. Trends Microbiol 17: 59–65.
15. Sendi P, Proctor RA (2009) *Staphylococcus aureus* as an intracellular pathogen: the role of small colony variants. Trends Microbiol 17: 54–58.
16. Zautner AE, Krause M, Stropahl G, Holtfreter S, Frickmann H, et al. (2010) Intracellular persisting *Staphylococcus aureus* is the major pathogen in recurrent tonsillitis. PLoS One 5: e9452.
17. Edwards AM, Potts JR, Josefsson E, Massey RC (2010) *Staphylococcus aureus* host cell invasion and virulence in sepsis is facilitated by the multiple repeats within FnBPA. PLoS Pathog 6: e1000964.
18. Sinha B, François PP, Nüsse O, Foti M, Hartford OM, Vaudaux P, et al. (1999) Fibronectin-binding protein acts as *Staphylococcus aureus* invasin via fibronectin bridging to integrin $\alpha_5\beta_1$. Cell Microbiol 1: 101–117.
19. Sinha B, Francois P, Que YA, Hussain M, Heilmann C, et al. (2000) Heterologously expressed *Staphylococcus aureus* fibronectin-binding proteins are sufficient for invasion of host cells. Infect Immun 68: 6871–6878.
20. Fowler T, Wann ER, Joh D, Johansson S, Foster TJ, Höök M (2000) Cellular invasion by *Staphylococcus aureus* involves a fibronectin bridge between the bacterial fibronectin-binding MSCRAMMs and host cell beta1 integrins. Eur J Cell Biol 79: 672–629.
21. Nitsche-Schmitz DP, Rohde M, Chhatwal GS (2007) Invasion mechanisms of Gram-positive pathogenic cocci. Thomb Haemost 98: 488–496.
22. Keane FM, Loughman A, Valtulina V, Brennan M, Speziale P, Foster TJ (2007) Fibrinogen and elastin bind to the same region within the A domain of fibronectin binding protein A, an MSCRAMM of *Staphylococcus aureus*. Mol Microbiol 63: 711–723.
23. O'Neill E, Pozzi C, Houston P, Humphreys H, Robinson DA, et al. (2008) A novel *Staphylococcus aureus* biofilm phenotype mediated by the fibronectin-binding proteins, FnBPA and FnBPB. J Bacteriol 190: 3835–3850.
24. Meenan NA, Visai L, Valtulina V, Schwarz-Linek U, Norris NC, et al. (2007) The tandem beta-zipper model defines high affinity fibronectin-binding repeats within *Staphylococcus aureus* FnBPA. J Biol Chem 282: 25893–25902.
25. Fröman G, Switalski LM, Speziale P, Höök MJ (1987) Isolation and characterization of a fibronectin receptor from *Staphylococcus aureus*. Biol Chem 262: 6564–6571.
26. Ingham KC, Brew S, Vaz D, Sauder DN, McGavin MJ (2004) Interaction of *Staphylococcus aureus* fibronectin-binding protein with fibronectin: affinity, stoichiometry, and modular requirements. J Biol Chem 279: 42945–42953.
27. Bingham RJ, Rudiño-Piñera E, Meenan NA, Schwarz-Linek U, Turkenburg JP, et al. (2008) Crystal structures of fibronectin-binding sites from *Staphylococcus aureus* FnBPA in complex with Fn domains. Proc Natl Acad Sci U S A 105: 12254–12258.
28. Ozeri V, Rosenshine I, Ben-Ze'Ev A, Bokoch GM, Jou TS, Hanski E (2001) *De novo* formation of focal complex-like structures in host cells by invading Streptococci. Mol Microbiol 41: 561–573.
29. Schwarz-Linek U, Höök M, Potts JR (2006) Fibronectin-binding proteins of gram-positive cocci. Microbes Infect 8: 2291–2298.
30. Massey RC, Kantzanou MN, Fowler T, Day NP, Schofield K, et al. (2001) Fibronectin-binding protein A of *Staphylococcus aureus* has multiple, substituting, binding regions that mediate adherence to Fn and invasion of endothelial cells. Cell Microbiol 3: 839–851.
31. Peacock SJ, Day NP, Thomas MG, Berendt AR, Foster TJ (2000) Clinical isolates of *Staphylococcus aureus* exhibit diversity in *fnb* genes and adhesion to human fibronectin. J Infect 41: 23–31.
32. von Eiff C, Becker K, Metze D, Lubritz G, Hockmann J, et al. (2001) Intracellular persistence of *Staphylococcus aureus* small-colony variants within keratinocytes: a cause for antibiotic treatment failure in a patient with darier's disease. Clin Infect Dis 32: 1643–1647.
33. Sambrook J, Fritsch EF, Maniatis T (1989) Molecular Cloning: a Laboratory Manual, 2nd edn. Cold Spring HarborNew York: Cold Spring Harbor Laboratory press.
34. Boukamp P, Dzarlieva-Petrusevska RT, Breitkreuz D, Hornung J, Markham A, Fusenig NE (1988) Normal keratinization in a spontaneously immortalized aneuploid human keratinocyte cell line. J Cell Biol 106: 761–771.
35. Boukamp P, Popp S, Altmeyer S, Hülsen A, Fasching, et al. (1997) Sustained nontumorigenic phenotype correlates with a largely stable chromosome content during long-term culture of the human keratinocyte line HaCat. Gene Chromosome Canc 19: 201–214.
36. Mempel M, Schmidt T, Weidinger S, Schnopp C, Foster T, et al. (1998) Role of *Staphylococcus aureus* surface-associated proteins in the attachment to cultured HaCaT keratinocytes in a new adhesion assay. J Invest Dermatol 111: 452–456.
37. Mempel M, Schnopp C, Hojka M, Fesq H, Weidinger S, et al. (2002) Invasion of human keratinocytes by *Staphylococcus aureus* and intracellular bacterial persistence represent haemolysin-independent virulence mechanisms that are followed by features of necrotic and apoptotic keratinocyte cell death. Br J Dermatol 146: 943–951.
38. Deyrieux AF, Wilson VG (2007) *In vitro* culture conditions to study keratinocyte differentiation using the HaCaT cell line. Cytotechnology 54: 77–83.
39. Dombek PE, Cue D, Sedgewick J, Lam H, Finlay BB, Cleary PP (1999) High-frequency intracellular invasion of epithelial cells by serotype M1 group A streptococci: M1 protein-mediated invasion and cytoskeletal rearrangements. Mol Microbiol 31: 859–870.
40. Rohde M, Muller E, Chhatwal GS, Talay SR (2003) Host cell caveolae act as an entry-port for group A streptococci. Cell Microbiol 5: 323–342.
41. Pellegrini G, De Luca M, Orecchia G, Balzac F, Cremona O, et al. (1992) Expression, topography, and function of integrin receptors are severely altered in keratinocytes from involved and uninvolved psoriatic skin. J Clin Invest 89: 1783–1795.
42. Aufiero B, Guo M, Young C, Duanmu Z, Talwar H, et al. (2007) *Staphylococcus aureus* induces the expression of tumor necrosis factor-alpha in primary human keratinocytes. Int J Dermatol 46: 687–694.
43. Kisich KO, Howell MD, Boguniewicz M, Heizer HR, Watson NU, Leung DY (2007) The constitutive capacity of human keratinocytes to kill *Staphylococcus aureus* is dependent on beta-defensin 3. J Invest Dermatol 127: 2368–2380.
44. Roche FM, Meehan M, Foster TJ (2003) The *Staphylococcus aureus* surface protein SasG and its homologues promote bacterial adherence to human desquamated nasal epithelial cells. Microbiology 149: 2759–2767.
45. Corrigan RM, Miajlovic H, Foster TJ (2009) Surface proteins that promote adherence of *Staphylococcus aureus* to human desquamated nasal epithelial cells. BMC Microbiol 30: 22.
46. Weidenmaier C, Kokai-Kun JF, Kristian SA, Chanturiya T, Kalbacher H, et al. (2004) Role of teichoic acids in *Staphylococcus aureus* nasal colonization, a major risk factor in nosocomial infections. Nat Med 10: 243–245.
47. Clarke SR, Brummell KJ, Horsburgh MJ, McDowell PW, Mohamad SA, et al. (2006) Identification of in vivo-expressed antigens of *Staphylococcus aureus* and their use in vaccinations for protection against nasal carriage. J Infect Dis 193: 1098–1108.
48. Marjenberg ZR, Ellis IR, Hagan RM, Prabhakaran S, Hook M, et al. (2010) Cooperative binding and activation of fibronectin by a bacterial surface protein. J Biol Chem 286: 1884–1894.
49. Schröder A, Schröder B, Roppenser B, Linder S, Sinha B, et al. (2006) *Staphylococcus aureus* fibronectin binding protein-A induces motile attachment sites

and complex actin remodeling in living endothelial cells. Mol Biol Cell 17: 5198–5210.

50. Wang B, Li S, Dedhar S, Cleary PP (2007) Paxillin phosphorylation: bifurcation point downstream of integrin-linked kinase (ILK) in streptococcal invasion. Cell microbial 9: 1519–1528.
51. Hirt H, Erlandsen SL, Dunny GM (2000) Heterologous inducible expression of *Enterococcus faecalis* pCF10 aggregation substance asc10 in *Lactococcus lactis* and *Streptococcus gordonii* contributes to cell hydrophobicity and adhesion to fibrin. J Bacteriol 182: 2299–2306.
52. Greene C, McDevitt D, Francois P, Vaudaux PE, Lew DP, Foster TJ (1995) Adhesion properties of mutants of *Staphylococcus aureus* defective in fibronectin-binding proteins and studies on the expression of *fnb* genes. Mol Microbiol 17: 1143–1152.
53. Kuipers OP, Beerthuyzen MM, Siezen RJ, De Vos WM (1993) Characterization of the nisin gene cluster *nis*ABTCIPR of *Lactococcus lactis*. Requirement of expression of the *nis*A and *nis*I genes for development of immunity. Eur J Biochem 216: 281–291.

Impact of Inhibitors and L2 Antibodies upon the Infectivity of Diverse Alpha and Beta Human Papillomavirus Types

Kihyuck Kwak[1], Rosie Jiang[1], Joshua W. Wang[1], Subhashini Jagu[1], Reinhard Kirnbauer[4], Richard B. S. Roden[1,2,3]*

1 Department of Pathology, The Johns Hopkins University, Baltimore, Maryland, United States of America, **2** Department of Gynecology and Obstetrics, The Johns Hopkins University, Baltimore, Maryland, United States of America, **3** Department of Oncology, The Johns Hopkins University, Baltimore, Maryland, United States of America, **4** Laboratory of Viral Oncology, Division of Immunology, Allergy and Infectious Diseases, Department of Dermatology, Medical University Vienna (MUW), Vienna, Austria

Abstract

The licensed human papillomavirus (HPV) vaccines elicit type-restricted immunity but do not target cutaneous HPV types of the beta genus that are associated with non-melanoma skin cancer in immune-compromised patients, and it is unclear if these diverse types share a common mechanism of infection. Residues 11-88 of minor capsid protein L2 contain cross-protective epitopes, and vaccination with concatamers of this region derived from as many as eight alpha HPV (L2 α11-88x8) is being developed as an alternative prophylactic vaccine with potentially broader efficacy. There is also interest in developing broadly protective topical microbicides, such as carrageenan or heparin that block HPV receptor interactions, or small molecule inhibitors of infection. Here we have examined several inhibitors of HPV infection and antisera to L2 α11-88x8 for their breadth of activity against infection by 34 HPV types from within both the alpha and beta families using pseudovirions (PsV) carrying a luciferase reporter as surrogates for native virus. We observed that both heparin and carrageenan prevented infection by mucosatropic HPV types, but surprisingly PsV of several epidermotropic alpha4 and beta HPV types exhibited increased infectivity especially at low inhibitor concentrations. Furin and γ-secretase inhibitors and L2 α11-88x8 antiserum blocked infection by all HPV PsV types tested. These findings suggest that the distinct tropism of mucosal and cutaneous HPV may reflect distinct cell surface receptor interactions, but a common uptake mechanism dependent upon furin and γ-secretase proteolytic activities. Carrageenan, which is being tested as a vaginal microbicide, broadly inhibited infection by the high-risk mucosatropic HPV PsV, but not most skin tropic alpha and beta HPV. Vaccination with an L2 multimer derived exclusively from alpha papillomavirus sequences induced antibodies that broadly neutralized PsV of all 34 HPVs from within both the alpha and beta families, suggesting each displays conserved L2 neutralizing epitopes.

Editor: Zhi-Ming Zheng, National Institute of Health - National Cancer Institute, United States of America

Funding: The study was funded by Public Health Service grant P50 CA098252, RO1 CA133749, and CA118790, the V Foundation, the Austrian Science Foundation (P18990B13) and the Vienna Science and Technology Fund (WWTF) (Life Science Call 2011) (LS11-006) as well as commercial funding from Sanofi Pasteur. The funders had no role in study design, data collection and analysis, decision to publish, or preparation of the manuscript.

Competing Interests: This study was partly funded by Sanofi Pasteur. Subhashini Jagu and Richard Roden are co-inventors on L2 patents (20090047301 Papillomavirus L2 N-Terminal Peptides for the Induction of Broadly Cross-Neutralizing Antibodies and 20100297144 MULTITYPE HPV PEPTIDE COMPOSITIONS AND METHODS FOR TREATMENT OR PREVENTION OF HUMAN PAPILLOMAVIRUS INFECTION), licensed to Shantha Biotechnics Ltd., GlaxoSmithKline, PaxVax, Inc., and Acambis, Inc., and have received research funding from Shantha Biotechnics Ltd., Sanofi Pasteur and GlaxoSmithKline. Richard Roden is a founder of Papivax LLC. The terms of these arrangements are managed by Johns Hopkins University in accordance with its conflict of interest policies. Reinhard Kirnbauer is a co-inventor on patent (7,361,356 Self-assembling recombinant papillomavirus capsid proteins), licensed to GlaxoSmithKline (GSK) and Merck (MSD).

* E-mail: roden@jhmi.edu

Introduction

Human papillomaviruses (HPV) comprise a family of at least 120 non-enveloped epitheliotropic viruses which contain a double-stranded circular DNA genome and are phylogenetically classified into five genera; alpha, beta, gamma, mu and nu [1]. Papillomavirus infections generally produce benign papillomas or warts of either skin or mucosa, such as condylomata accuminata (anogenital warts) associated with 'low-risk' types HPV6 and 11. However, the sexually transmitted 'high-risk' members of the alpha genus mucosal HPVs are essential etiological agents in cervical cancer, and also in a significant fraction of anal, penile, vaginal, vulval and oropharyngeal cancers [2,3]. HPV16 and HPV18 are the most impactful high-risk HPV types, together causing 70% of cervical cancer, with a dozen or so other alpha HPVs associated with the remaining cases [4,5], although it is important to recognize that the majority of infections are cleared by patients. The beta HPVs infect skin beginning early in childhood and are associated with non-melanoma skin cancer in sun-exposed areas of immunocompromised patients or those with the rare hereditary disease epidermodysplasia verruciformis (EDV), notably HPV5 and HPV8 [6]. Conversely, beta HPV infections are generally clinically inapparent in immune competent patients, but may cooperate with UV-induced DNA damage in the development of cutaneous squamous cell cancers [6]. Infections with HPV of the gamma, mu and nu genera typically produce benign and self-limiting skin warts [1].

Papillomavirus virions have a non-enveloped 60 nm diameter capsid with $T = 7d$ iscosahedral symmetry [7]. The capsid is formed from 360 molecules of the major capsid protein L1 via assembly of 72 star-shaped capsomers or pentamers, each comprising five L1 molecules. The capsid also contains as many as 72 molecules of the minor capsid protein L2 and, while its location is not totally clear, at least a portion of L2 is buried at the base of central cavity at the center of each capsomer [8]. Five surface loops of L1 with high variation in amino acid sequence among different types contain the immunodominant neutralization epitopes and act as domain linkers for the conserved internal jelly roll structure [9].

Recombinant expression of L1 is sufficient to form virus-like particles (VLP) that mimic native virus morphologically and immunologically. Similar to infectious virions, VLP can bind to heparan sulfate proteoglycans (HSPG) on the cell surface, and HSPG mimetics such as soluble heparan sulphate or carrageenan compete this interaction [10,11,12,13,14,15,16]. Indeed, consistent use of the carrageenan-based vaginal microbicide, Carraguard, with condoms was negatively associated with the acquisition of high-risk HPV infections in a randomized, double-blind and placebo controlled trial [17]. L2 facilitates viral genome encapsidation during virion assembly and is critical for infection [18,19]. At the initiation of infection, virions undergo a conformational change that reveals the amino terminus of L2 on the capsid surface such that it is cleaved by the cellular protease furin [20,21]. Furin cuts L2 at residue 11 in HPV16 and this cleavage is required for infection [20]. L2 interacts with several cellular components, including cyclophilin, annexin, syntaxin-18 and sorting nexin 17, believed to contribute to infectious cell entry, although the mechanisms are not fully elucidated [22,23,24,25]. L2 also enables virion egress from the endosome and translocates with the viral genome to the nucleus to establish infection [26]. The regulated intra-membrane protease γ-secretase is required for endosomal escape, but its cellular target remains to be defined [27,28].

The licensed HPV vaccines, Cervarix and Gardasil, were both developed to prevent HPV16- and HPV18-associated persistent anogenital infection and disease, in particular epithelial dysplasias and cancers, and Gardasil to also prevent benign genital warts associated with HPV6 and HPV11 [29]. Vaccination elicits type-restricted neutralizing antibodies and protection due to immunodominant epitopes formed by hyper-variable surface loops of the L1 VLP antigens [9]. Both vaccines provide limited cross-protection, particularly toward HPV31 or HPV45, close phylogenetic relatives ofHPV16 and HPV18, respectively [30,31,32]. However the duration of cross-protection is unclear, and is weak to ineffective for more distantly related types [33]. A nonavalent L1 VLP vaccine is currently in development to broaden protection among the high-risk mucosal alpha HPV types (http://clinicaltrials.gov/show/NCT00543543). Another approach is vaccination with the amino terminus of L2 including residues 11-88 [34,35,36]. This region of L2 is well conserved and can elicit broadly neutralizing antibodies, although at lower titer than L1 VLP, because L2 does not form an immunogenic VLP structure. However, because L2 protective epioptes are linear, those derived from multiple HPV types can be concatenated into a single antigen, e.g. α11-88x8 that compromises a fusion of the 11-88 region of the eight medically significant alpha HPV types 6, 16, 18, 31, 39, 51, 56 and 73. Vaccination with L2 α11-88x8, or passive transfer of its antiserum, provides broad immunity against vaginal challenge with alpha HPV, but its activity against other genera has not been examined [35].

Our mechanistic understanding of papillomavirus infectious process(es) is based on studies generally performed with only a few HPV types. Here we examine if medically significant HPV types of different genera, carcinogenic potential and tropism share a common infection mechanism. As the known inhibitors and vaccines have also been tested predominantly against a limited number of HPV types, their breadth of activity cannot be fully appreciated. Further, several studies indicate differences in receptor usage and uptake pathways by different HPV types [14,37,38]. Because of the technical difficulties of culturing and measuring the infectivity of papillomaviruses *in vitro*, PsV are used as surrogates for biologic studies of native virions, particularly given their capacity to deliver a reporter construct upon its encapsidation by over-expression of L1 and L2 [39]. In light of this, we generated PsV for 34 HPV types from the alpha and beta genera to better understand the commonalities and differences in the infectious pathway of diverse HPV types with distinct biology.

Materials and Methods

Pseudovirion (PsV) production

L1/L2 expression plasmids were provided by Martin Müller and Lutz Gissmann (DKFZ, Heidelberg, Germany), Christopher Buck and John Schiller (NCI, Bethesda, MD), and Helena Faust (Lund University, Malmö, Sweden) and Joakim Dillner (Karolinska Institutet, Stockholm, Sweden). Additional constructs were synthesized by Biobasic (Table S1). Briefly, the L1 and L2 genes for individual isolates of HPV genotypes documented in Genbank were codon-optimized for expression in human cells and cloned with a 5′ Kozak sequence (GCCACC) and two 3′ stop codons (TAATAG) into the mammalian double expression vector pVITRO1-neo-mcs (InvivoGen) as listed in Table S1. The L1 gene flanked by BamHI-XbaI was cloned into the BglII-NheI region of MCS2, followed by the L2 gene flanked by BamHI-XbaI which was cloned into the BamHI-AvrII region of MCS1. All HPV PsV were produced as described in http://home.ccr.cancer.gov/Lco/pseudovirusproduction.htm. Briefly, plasmids containing L1 and L2 late genes of different HPV types were transfected with plasmid expressing luciferase reporter gene into 293TT cells utilizing TransIT-2020 transfection reagent. Cells were incubated for 48 h at 37°C, harvested, washed with DPBS-Mg (DPBS supplemented with 9.5 mM $MgCl_2$), and lysed with equal volume of lysis buffer (DPBS supplemented with 0.5% w/v Brij58 and 0.2% v/v benzonase). For PsV maturation, cell lysates were incubated for 24 h at 37°C and adjusted to 850 mM NaCl. For extraction lysates were centrifuged at $10{,}000 \times g$ for 10 min, and clarified supernatants loaded onto a 12 mL step gradient of Optiprep (39, 33, 27% *w/v*), and spun at 40,000 rpm in a SW40 rotor for 15 h at 16°C. After centrifugation, 1 mL fractions were collected from the top layer and the fraction demonstrating the highest infectivity was selected for further experiments.

HPV Infectivity assays

1.5×10^4 293TT, HeLaT or HaCaT cells in 100 μL DMEM-10 or KH-SV cells in 100 μL KSFM were infected with 250, 500, 1000, or 2000 million particles of each HPV types in 100 μL medium in triplicate and incubated for 72 h at 37°C. Luciferase activity was measured as described in inhibition assays. All experiments were performed in triplicate.

HPV Inhibition assays

293TT cells were seeded at 1.5×10^4 cells in 100 μL 10% FBS DMEM (DMEM-10) per well in 96-well plates and allowed to attach overnight. For heparin and carrageenan inhibition studies, heparin (Sigma H-4784) and carrageenan (Sigma C1138) were serially diluted in DMEM-10 and incubated with 250 million PsV particles of different HPV types in 100 μL DMEM-10 for 1 h at 37°C. Mixtures were added to 293TT cells and incubated at concentrations of 64, 128, 256, 512 μg/mL of heparin or carrageenan for 72 h at 37°C. For furin inhibition studies, furin inhibitor 1 (Decanoyl-RVKR-CMK) was mixed with 250 million particles of each HPV type in 100 μL DMEM-10 and the mixtures were immediately transferred to 293TT cells and incubated at 20 μM concentration of furin inhibitor 1 for 72 h at 37°C. For γ-secretase inhibition studies, XXI was mixed with 250 million particles of each HPV type in 100 μL DMEM-10 and the mixtures were immediately transferred to 293TT cells and incubated at a final concentration of 500 nM XXI for 72 h at 37°C. As a positive control, 4 μL of L1 antiserum from mice vaccinated i.m. with L1 DNA utilizing electroporation in 50 μL of culture medium was mixed with 250 million particles of each HPV type in 50 μL. Mixtures were transferred to 293TT cells and incubated for 72 h at 37°C. Following infection cells were washed with 1× PBS, and lysed with 30 μL of Cell Culture Lysis Reagent on rocking shaker for 15 min at room temperature. Lysates were transferred to 96-well black plate and luciferase activity was measured by GloMax-Multi Detection System after adding 50 μL of luciferin substrate to each well. All experiments were performed in triplicate.

Neutralization assay

293TT cells were pre-plated at 1.5×10^4 cells per well in 96-well plate and incubated 24 h at 37°C. 4 μL of rabbit L2 α11-88x8 antiserum [35] was serially diluted two-fold in 50 μL of culture medium. As a negative control, pre-immune serum was applied. 250 million particles of each HPV type in 50 μL of culture medium were mixed with serially diluted serum in triplicate and then transferred to pre-plated 293TT cells and cultured for 72 h at 37°C. Luciferase activity was measured as described above.

SDS-PAGE and Western blotting

Each HPV PsV preparation was normalized by the amount of L1 protein. Samples were boiled for 5 min with reducing gel sample buffer, subjected to SDS-PAGE analysis using 4-20% Tris-HCl gels, and proteins were transferred to PVDF membrane. The membrane was blocked with 5% non-fat milk in PBST (PBS containing 0.1% Tween-20) at room temperature for 1 hour, incubated with a rabbit L2 α11-88x8 antiserum at room temperature for 1 hour and binding detected with HRP-conjugated goat anti-rabbit IgG secondary antiserum.

Quantitative real time PCR measurement of luciferase reporter plasmid

Reporter plasmid was extracted from 20 μL of each HPV PsV preparation using PureLink Viral RNA/DNA extraction kits. The real time PCR was performed with 25 μL of universal PCR Master Mix, 900 nM of forward and reverse primers (TTG ACC GCC TGA AGT CTC TGA and ACA CCT GCG TCG AAG ATG TTG), 250 nM of TaqMan probe (6FAM-CCG CTG AAT TGG AAT CCA TCT TGC TC-TAMRA), and 5 μL of extracted reporter plasmid in 50 μL final volume using an I-Cycler IQ (Bio-Rad). Each sample was conducted in duplicate.

Data analysis and statistics

To calculate the neutralization titer value (the reciprocal of the dilution that causes 50% reduction in luciferase activity), the non-linear model Y = Bottom + (Top-Bottom) /(1+10^((LogEC50-X)*HillSlope)) was fitted to the $\log_{10}$ transformed neutralization data using Graphpad Prism 6 and the estimated EC50 [with 95% confidence intervals] is reported as the titer. Comparisons between the infectivity of members of papillomavirus species was determined by the Mann Whitney test, and means ± standard error are presented graphically using Graphpad Prism 6.

Results

Generation and characterization of 34 HPV PsV types

PsV are useful surrogates for biologic studies of native virions, particularly given their capacity to recapitulate early events of papillomavirus infection and neutralization, deliver a reporter gene of choice and their relative ease of production [39]. Here we encapsidated a vector expressing firefly luciferase (pY-luc) into HPV PsV because of this reporter's low background, high sensitivity and utility in the mouse challenge model [35]. Recombinant mammalian expression of papillomavirus capsid genes is dramatically enhanced by their codon modification [40,41], presumably reflecting the disruption of negative regulatory sequences [42]. Several PsV vectors have been previously described [39,43,44,45,46] and we generated constructs for additional HPV types that were not previously available (Sequences in Table S1 and constructs may be obtained from Addgene (www.addgene.com)). HPV PsV were prepared by co-transfection of 293TT cells with pY-luc and the L1/L2 expression vectors per standard methodology [39].

We first tested infectivity of each HPV PsV type normalized to 250 million particles (as estimated based on L1 concentration) by measuring luciferase activity (relative light units, RLU) 72 h post-infection in 293TT cells. The HPV PsV infected cells showed dramatic differences in reporter expression (Figure 1A). Overall, the cutaneous HPV type PsV showed lower infectivity compared to mucosal tropic types ($p<0.0001$), and the PsVs derived from alpha species HPV showed greater infectivity that those derived from beta HPV types ($p = 0.01$). However, even for the weakest PsV types, the signal observed was still more than 100-fold higher than background signal. Furthermore, pre-incubation of the PsV with rabbit antiserum raised against the cognate L1 VLP prevented reporter delivery, consistent with antibody-mediated neutralization of an infection rather than a non-specific transfection. Rabbit antiserum to L1 VLP was not available for a number of HPV types. Instead, sera was harvested from mice two weeks after electroporation i.m. three times at two week intervals with the an HPV L1 expression vector [47]. Pre-incubation of the HPV PsV with these mouse antisera similarly inhibited reporter transfer (Figure S1).

It is possible that the weak infectivity of the PsV derived from cutaneous HPV types reflects use of 293TT cells a target cell line, rather than one derived from skin cells. Therefore we also tested infectivity of diverse alpha and beta HPV PsV in HeLaT clone 4 cells, a human cervical cancer line transduced with SV40 large T antigen [48], as well as in the spontaneous immortalized human keratinocyte cell line HaCaT [49], and KH-SV, a human keratinocyte line immortalized by transduction with SV40 large T antigen [50]. In both human skin keratinocyte-derived lines (HaCaT and KH-SV), the cutaneous HPV PsV demonstrated minimal or undetectable signals, whereas mucosal HPV PsV showed more robust infectivity. Similar findings were seen for infection of HeLaT cells, implying that the weaker infectivity of

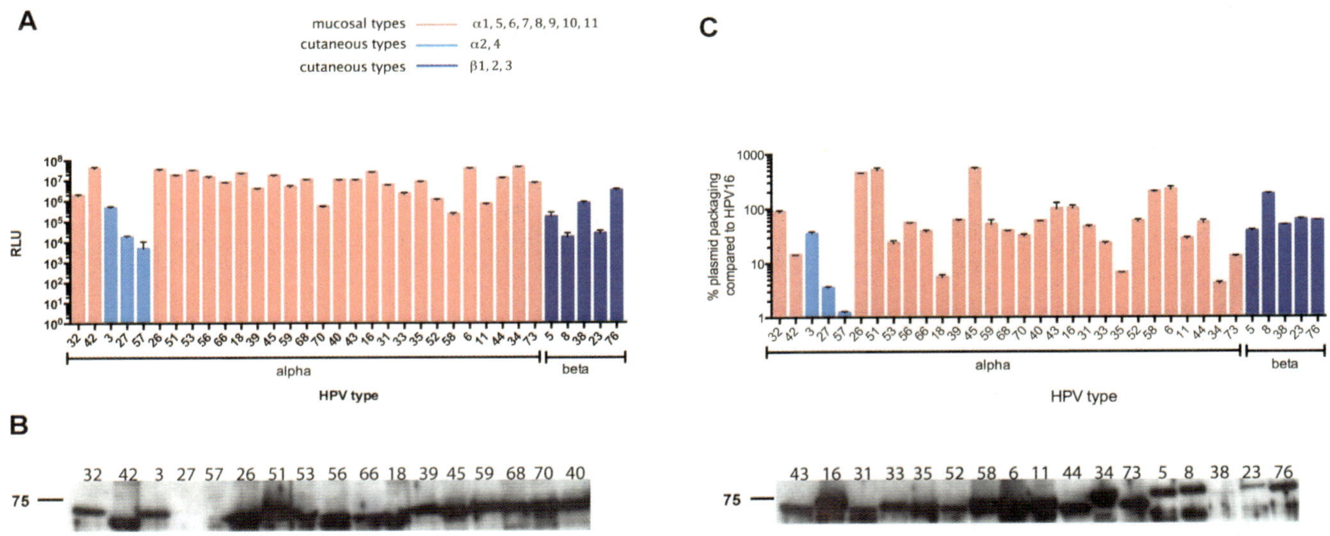

Figure 1. Assessment of infectivity, L2 incorporation, and reporter DNA encapsidation by PsV preparations of 34 HPV types. (A) 250 million particles (as estimated based on L1 concentration) of HPV PsV were transferred to 293TT cells, incubated at 37°C for 72 hours before cell lysis. Luciferase activity was measured in cell lysate (n = 4). (B) Western blot analysis detecting L2 in 100 ng of each HPV PsV preparation using rabbit antiserum to L2 α11-88x8. (C) Reporter plasmid copy number of each PsV preparations for each HPV type sample was measured by quantitative real time PCR. Black and blue bars represent alpha and beta type, respectively, and mean ± standard error plotted.

the cutaneous HPV PsV does not reflect the use of 293TT as target cells or the need to infect a line derived from skin keratinocytes (Figure S2A, B, C).

L2 is known to play several important functions during virion assembly and infection, and therefore differences in the incorporation of L2 may account for the wide range of PsV infectivity by HPV type. Thus, the level of L2 incorporation into the gradient-purified preparations of HPV PsV was analyzed by Western blot (Figure 1B) using a broadly reactive rabbit antiserum to the L2 antigen α11-88x8 [35]. This Western blot analysis suggested that the PsV preparations of several cutaneous HPV types that exhibited low infectivity (Table 1) also contained low levels of L2, notably HPV23, 27, 38 and 57 (Figure 1B). This does reflect the failure of the antiserum to recognize the L2 of these HPV types because this antiserum, but not the pre-immune serum, can neutralize their infection. Furthermore, the L2 band was not apparent on Coomassie-stained SDS-PAGE analysis of these PsV. Rather, this reflects poor expression of L2 and thus low incorporation into the PsV, as Western blot analysis of 293TT cells transfected with these constructs shows low levels of L2 (data not shown).

Differences in the infectivity of each type of HPV PsV might also reflect variable efficiency in reporter plasmid encapsidation. Therefore the number of copies of benzonase-resistant, and therefore presumably encapsidated, reporter plasmid DNA present within 315 ng of each gradient purified HPV PsV preparation was measured by quantitative real time PCR. The lowest levels of reporter DNA encapsidation were observed for PsV of HPV27, 57, and 34 (Figure 1C). Since L2 has been shown to facilitate genomic DNA encapsidation, the low DNA encapsidation by HPV types 27 and 57 may reflect the low levels of L2 incorporated in these PsV. However the amounts of encapsidated plasmid and/or L2 were not always proportional to the relative infectivity (Figure 1A,C), as seen for HPV18 and HPV35 PsV.

Inhibition of HPV infection by Heparin and l-carrageenan

CHO cells deficient in heparan sulfate proteoglycan (HSPG) production are no longer infected by HPV PsV [10], suggesting that HSPG is an important entry factor. Further soluble heparan sulfate can bind to capsids and is an inhibitor of infection for at least some HPV genotypes, but not all [14]. To explore the generalizability of these observations, we tested if heparin universally inhibited infection by PsV of all 34 HPV types within the alpha and beta HPV subfamilies. Ten-fold serial dilutions of heparin (Sigma H-4784), ranging from 10 to 1000 μg/mL, were incubated with the PsV of each HPV type for 1 hour at 37°C prior to transfer to 293TT cells to assess infectivity. Near complete inhibition was observed for PsV of all 29 alpha HPV types at 1000 μg/ml heparin, including HPV 31 (Figure 2A) for which the role of HSPG in infection is controversial [51]. With the exceptions of HPV8 and HPV23, infection by PsV of the beta HPV types was not impeded even at the highest concentration of heparin tested (1000 μg/mL), and paradoxically several demonstrated increased levels of infectivity [52]. Notably, the addition of 10 or 100 μg/mL heparin profoundly increased infectivity of HPV5, HPV57 and HPV76 PsV, slightly increased the infectivity of HPV38 PsV, but inhibited HPV8 and HPV23 PsV (Figures 2A and C). In contrast, even at 10 μg/mL heparin, most alpha HPV type PsVs exhibited significant inhibition.

Carrageenan is also a potent inhibitor of HPV infection via a mechanism resembling that of heparan sulfate [12,13,14,15], although the breadth of its activity has been questioned recently [38]. It is currently being tested as a vaginal microbicide, and may be broadly protective against genital HPV transmission [17]. Therefore, we also tested the impact of carrageenan on in vitro infectivity of PsVs of diverse HPV types. The findings resembled the inhibitory profile of heparin [14,37,53]. PsV of most alpha types were inhibited except HPV27 and HPV57, but carrageenan had limited impact on beta types (Figure 2B, D). Carrageenan was more potent in inhibiting alpha HPV PsV infection than heparin at 10 μg/mL (Figure 2), consistent with earlier findings [12]. Carrageenan also showed some differences in inhibitory efficacy

Table 1. Summary of the phylogeny, tropism, charge and in vitro neutralization by L2 11-88x8 antiserum of the 34 HPV genotypes tested.

Subfamily	HPV type	Mucosal/Cutaneous	Predicted net charge at pH 7.4	Neutralization titer for L2x8 antiserum	95% confidence interval in neutralization titer
α1	32	M	5.2	3,360	2,225 to 5,074
	42	M	3.4	11,450	9,456 to 13,865
α2	3	C	2	11,140	7,314 to 16,967
α4	27	C	−4.2	3,942	350 to 44,402
	57	C	1	3,440	858 to 13,789
α5	26	M	5.2	11,223	7,786 to 16,177
	51	M	5.2	4,420	3,755 to 5,202
α6	53	M	6.3	352	208 to 595
	56	M	5.2	1,536	1,243 to 1,898
	66	M	7.2	870	517 to 1,465
α7	18	M	5.9	12,422	10,780 to 14,312
	39	M	5.1	6,216	3,798 to 10,174
	45	M	5.9	4,913	3,021 to 7,991
	59	M	7.1	8,214	7,255 to 9,300
	68	M	3.1	1,403	980 to 2,008
	70	M	4.1	2,359	1,382 to 4,027
α8	40	M/C	4.2	834	380 to 1,830
	43	M/C	6.2	1,580	1,063 to 2,349
α9	16	M	2	31,266	28,513 to 34,284
	31	M	8	2,212	940 to 5,207
	33	M	4.8	16,207	9,942 to 26,420
	35	M	7	7,458	5,151 to 10,800
	52	M	5.9	927	651 to 1321
	58	M	4.5	14,807	8,904 to 24,622
α10	6	M	7.1	5,553	4,315 to 7,146
	11	M	7.2	27,760	23,455 to 32,855
	44	M	7	5,041	2,716 to 9,358
α11	34	M	5.7	13,140	11,689 to 14,770
	73	M	4.9	8,810	6,853 to 11,325
β1	5	C	−4.7	3,561	492 to 25,770
	8	C	−2.8	17,679	7,256 to 43,073
β2	38	C	−4.8	1709	489 to 5976
	23	C	−3.9	2475	834 to 7347
β3	76	C	−4.9	2110	1154 to 3861

Phylogeny and tropism were taken from de Villiers et al [58], predicted net charge of L1 at pH7.4 was calculated as described in [37]. PsVs of each indicated HPV type carrying a luciferase reporter gene were mixed with titrated rabbit L2 α11-88x8 antiserum for two hours at 37°C, then the mixtures were transferred to 293TT cells and cultured for 72 hours. Cells were then lysed and luciferase activity was measured. Neutralization titer and 95% confidence interval are shown.

against PsV of beta HPV types compared to heparin. For example, carrageenan did not inhibit HPV27 infection whereas heparin did, suggesting subtly distinct mechanisms of inhibition by carrageenan and heparin. Taken together, the results imply that different HPV subfamilies bind HSPG differently during infection, which may contribute to their differing tropism [14]. Further, heparin and carrageenan are broadly inhibitory against PsV of most alpha species of HPV (including all of the high-risk mucosal HPV types tested), but not against PsV infection by beta or certain benign alpha types that can also infect cutaneous sites.

Conservation of furin cleavage as an essential step for infection

After binding to HSPG on extracellular matrix, HPV16 undergoes a conformational change and exposes the previously buried amino terminus of L2 on the capsid surface prior to cell entry [20,21]. The exposed amino-terminus of L2 is sensitive to furin cleavage as it contains a conserved consensus cleavage site, Arg-X-(Arg/Lys)-Arg, and mutation of this site prevents HPV16 PsV infection. The furin inhibitor decanoyl-RVKR-cmk also can prevent HPV16 infection, suggesting cleavage of L2 by furin is a critical step for infection [20]. However, only a few HPV types have been tested and overall significance of furin cleavage among

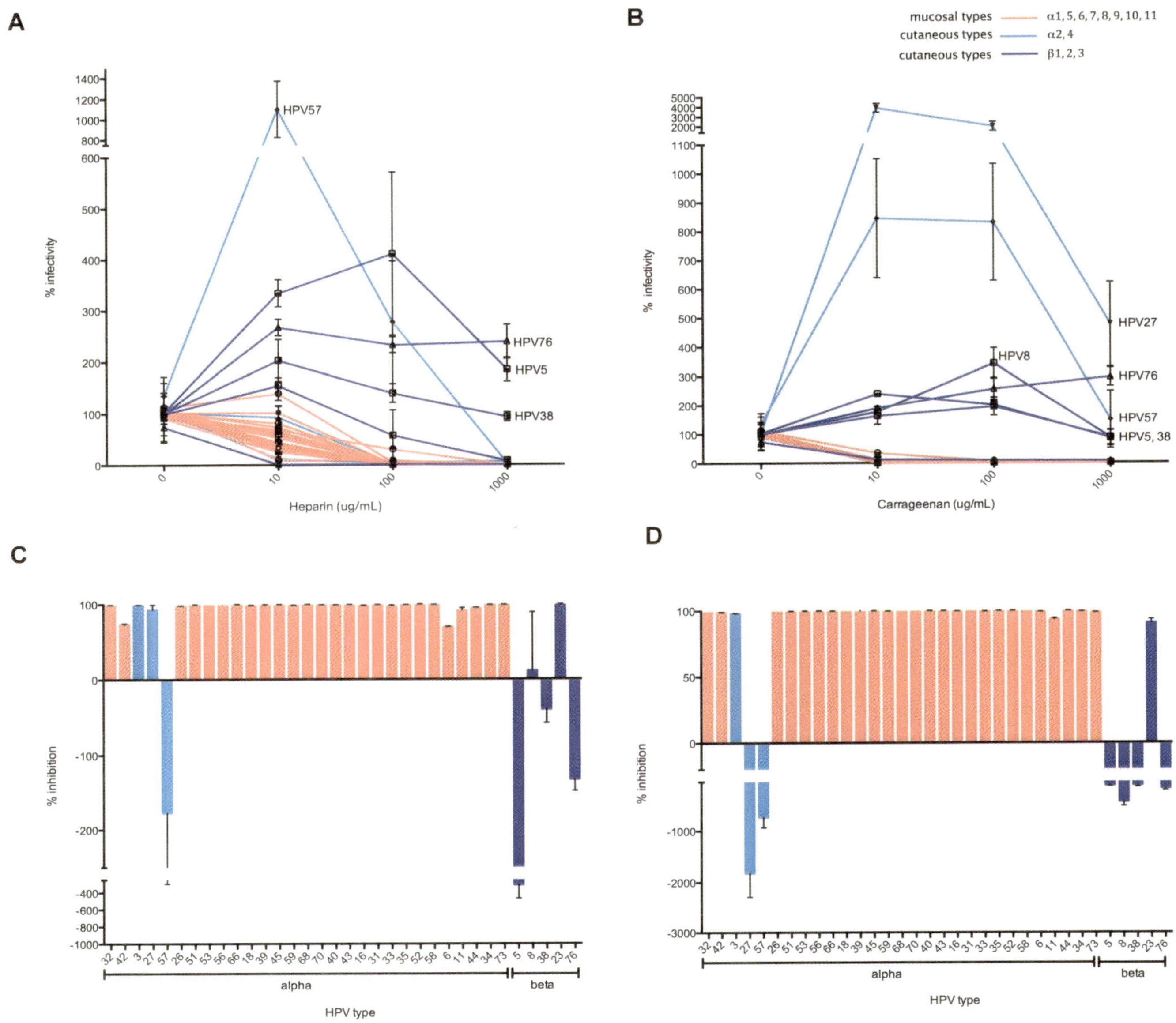

Figure 2. Inhibition of HPV PsV infection by titrations of heparin and carrageenan. PsVs of each HPV type carrying a luciferase reporter gene were incubated with 1000 μg/mL, 100 μg/mL, 10 μg/ml or 0 μg/ml heparin (A) or carrageenan (B) at 37°C for 1 hour. The mixtures were transferred to 293TT cells for 72 h. After incubation cells were lysed and luciferase activity was measured, and percent infection compared to control was calculated (n = 3). The percent inhibition of infection by each HPV PsV in the presence of 100 μg/mL of heparin (C) or carrageenan (D) was also plotted separately. Red and blue bars and lines represent mucosal and cutaneous HPV types, respectively.

diverse HPV types has not been thoroughly addressed so far. Sequence alignment indicated that the furin target sequence, RX(R/K)R, is present in the L2 of all the HPV types for which we developed PsV, suggesting that the function provided by furin cleavage is conserved (data not shown). Therefore we tested whether application of the furin inhibitor at 20 μM (a concentration at which no cell toxicity was observed by XTT assay, data not shown) inhibited infection of 293TT cells by PsV of all 34 HPV types. Infection of 293TT cells by PsV of every alpha HPV was strongly inhibited, although it was less effective against some beta types such as HPV5 (Figure 3). Nevertheless, it is clear that the requirement for furin cleavage during PsV infection is ubiquitous among the 34 diverse HPV types tested.

Conservation of need for cleavage by γ-secretase during infection

The γ-secretase inhibitor XXI potently blocks HPV16 infection, and homozygous deletion of γ-secretase component subunits nicastrin or presenilin-1 also prevents HPV16 infection [27]. To determine whether the need for γ-secretase function during infection is conserved across diverse HPV types, we examined the impact of 500 nM XXI upon infection of 293TT cells by each PsV types. The γ-secretase inhibitor XXI dramatically reduced the infectivity of the PsV of all 34 HPV types tested (Figure 4), implying that γ-secretase is a key cellular factor that diverse genotypes utilize during infection and its inhibition can broadly inhibit HPV infection [27,28].

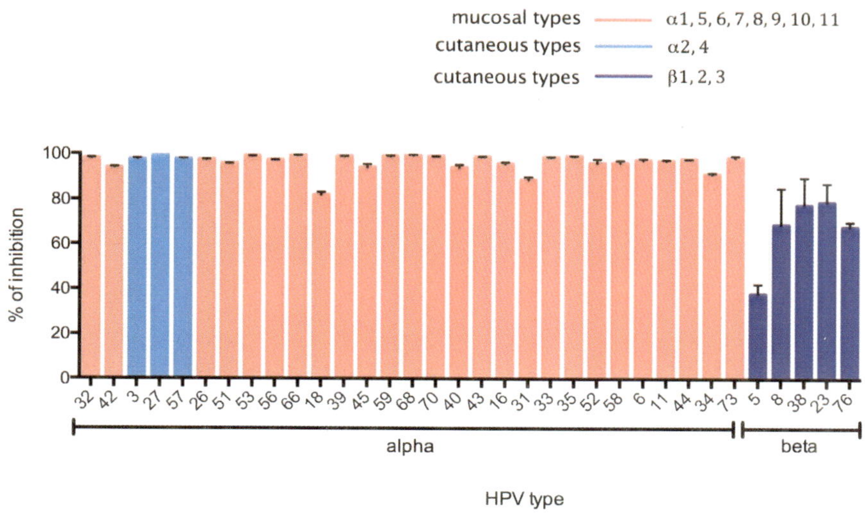

Figure 3. Impact of furin inhibitor on infection by PsV of diverse HPV. PsVs of each indicated HPV type carrying a luciferase reporter gene were transferred to 293TT cells for 72 hours in the presence or absence of 20 μM furin inhibitor. After incubation, cells were lysed, luciferase activity was measured and percent inhibition of infectivity compared to control calculated. Red and blue bars represent mucosal and cutaneous HPV types, respectively.

Neutralization of diverse HPV by antiserum to L2 antigen α11-88x8

The amino terminus of L2 contains a protective epitope and it is also evolutionarily highly conserved between types and even different species. We previously described that rabbit antiserum targeting the L2 antigen α11-88x8 can neutralize a broad spectrum of mucosal HPV types, notably those associated with cervical cancer and benign genital warts, and that passive transfer of this antiserum protects mice from genital HPV PsV challenge [35]. While this candidate vaccine antigen was designed to broadly protect against mucosal HPV that are associated with cervical cancer and genital warts, it may also protect against cutaneous HPV types as there is considerable sequence conservation in the 11-88 region. Cutaneous HPV types have been associated with non-melanoma skin cancers and benign skin warts that are costly to treat or a common nuisance, particularly for immunocompromised patients [6]. To examine the breadth of cross-neutralization against diverse HPV types, we tested antiserum from a rabbit vaccinated with the L2 antigen α11-88x8. PsV from each of the 34 HPV types was incubated with 2-fold serially diluted rabbit serum and the mixture was then transferred to 293TT cells to assess infectivity. The α11-88x8 antiserum detectably neutralized PsV of all alpha and beta HPV types tested (Table 1), whereas the pre-immune serum did not. Likewise, this antiserum reacted with L2 in PsV preprations of all 34 HPV types tested in a Western blot analysis (Figure 1B). These observations suggest the potential of this candidate vaccine antigen to protect against diverse beta types

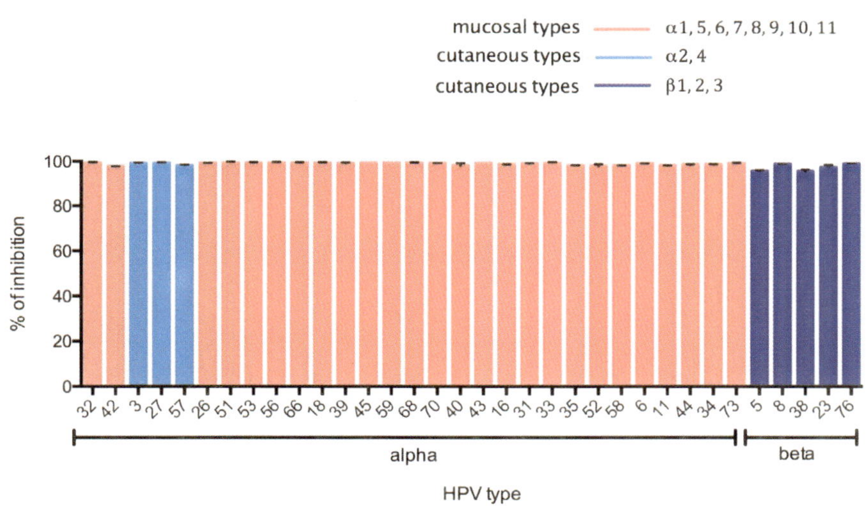

Figure 4. Impact of γ-secretase inhibitor on infection by PsV of diverse HPV. PsVs of each indicated HPV type carrying a luciferase reporter gene were transferred to 293TT cells for 72 hours in the presence or absence of 500 nM γ-secretase inhibitor XXI (n = 3). After incubation, luciferase activity was measured and percent inhibition of infectivity compared to control calculated. Red and blue bars represent mucosal and cutaneous HPV types, respectively.

associated with non-melanoma skin cancer in immunocompromised and EDV patients.

Discussion

The two licensed vaccines safely provide robust protection for men and women against acquiring infections by the two most potent oncogenic types, HPV16 and HPV18, and Gardasil also protects against the two most common types associated with genital warts, HPV6 and HPV11. In spite of their effectiveness, there is still a demand for new approaches for the prevention of HPV infection due to the high cost and type-restricted protection afforded by the licensed vaccines and also the need for immunization [54]. Aside from HPV16 and HPV18, about a dozen other oncogenic alpha HPV types are associated with cervical cancer, although each contributes only a minor fraction. Although the licensed vaccines provide varying degrees of cross-protection against closely related oncogenic HPV types, the extent and duration of cross-protection remain controversial [33]. Consequently, there are ongoing efforts to develop a nonavalent L1 VLP vaccine to target the seven oncogenic HPV types most commonly detected in cervical cancer, as well as HPV6 and HPV11. However, inclusion of 9 HPV VLP types into a single vaccine formulation will most likely increase the cost of vaccine production, which is one of the main limitations to global implementation of HPV immunization. Moreover, there has been little focus on vaccination against cutaneous HPV types, notably the beta species. While the beta HPVs typically have minimal clinical impact among patients with intact immune systems, immunocompromised patients (i.e. HIV-positive patients or those receiving immunosuppressive treatment following solid organ transplantation) and those with the rare hereditary syndrome EDV are vulnerable to non-melanoma skin cancers caused by these beta types, notably HPV5 and HPV8 [6]. It is unlikely that the licensed vaccines or even the new nonavalent vaccine will impact infection by the diverse beta HPV types, and therefore there is interest in alternative approaches to provide coverage against beta HPV.

More than 120 HPV genotypes has been completely characterized so far, but studies of the mechanisms of infection have been focused only on a very limited number of HPV types of the greatest medical significance, mainly due to restricted availability of PsV of a few HPV types. Therefore to assist in understanding the biology of HPV as well as assessing the breadth of protection provided by new vaccine and microbicide candidates, we generated and tested a diverse set of 34 PsV including 29 alpha types and 5 beta types (Table 1). The mechanisms underlying the different tropism of HPV are not understood. The alpha HPV types, with the exception of alpha2 and alpha4 subgroups, preferentially infect the genital mucosa and are sexually transmitted, whereas the beta HPV types infect the keratinizing squamous epithelium of the skin, typically starting during childhood. The distinct tropism may be governed by differences in entry into the cell, or viral transcription or replication, or a combination of these functions. To initially examine whether there are differences in the uptake processes of the predominantly mucosatropic alpha and cutaneotropic beta HPVs we tested the potency of known inhibitors of infection against PsV of the diverse range of HPV types. Use of PsV delivering a luciferase reporter for these studies eliminates any influence of viral tropism that would be conferred by the native viral genome with respect to viral transcription or replication.

The initial studies focused on HSPG because it is the most studied cell surface receptor for HPV, and there is evidence of differential utilization by different genotypes [14,37,38,51]. We verified that the two HSPG mimetics heparin and carrageenan are inhibitors of diverse mucosatropic HPV PsV infection. This is significant because of ongoing efforts to develop carrageenan as a vaginal microbicide and its use as an ingredient in many sexual lubricants. Both compounds completely inhibit infection by most alpha types at high and intermediate concentrations (Figure 2), although most alpha types demonstrated partial inhibition by 10 μg/mL heparin, the lowest concentration tested (Figures 2A and C). However, while infection by HPV27 was blocked by heparin at 1000 μg/mL, carrageenan did not inhibit even at the highest concentration of 1000 μg/mL (Figure 2B), possibly reflecting their different structures and mechanism of particle binding [37,53]. Notably, the alpha4 viruses HPV27 and HPV57 are capable of infecting cutaneous sites. A previous study suggested that cutaneous types tended to have negatively charged L1 at pH 7.4 and lower surface net charge compared to mucosal types [37]. We calculated a net charge for L1 of 34 HPV types at pH 7.4 and beta types (Table 1). Interestingly HPV27 and HPV57 L1 display the lowest net charge at pH 7.4 among the 29 alpha types and they were not inhibited effectively by carrageenan at a concentration of 1000 μg/mL, 100 μg/mL and 10 μg/mL like most beta types and HPV57 was not inhibited by heparin at 100 μg/mL and 10 μg/mL. These net charge differences may contribute to the distinct response of HPV27 and 57 PsV to the HSPG mimetics as compared with the other alpha types [37,53].

When the concentration of heparin or carrageenan was reduced to 10 μg/mL, PsV of some cutaneous HPV types demonstrated enhanced infectivity (Figure 2A, B). This result was unexpected because heparin and carrageenan are inhibitors of mucosatropic HPV infection, although low amounts of heparin increased HPV infectivity in a recent report [52,55,56]. It is possible that when virion surface is partially coated by heparin or carrageenan, it can trigger a conformational change which, in turn, enhances infectivity perhaps by rendering L2 more accessible to furin cleavage [52]. Conversely, if the virion surface is completely coated by heparin or carrageenan due to high affinity, and if the binding groove and charged residues on the capsid surface that interact with the HSPG cellular receptor are masked completely [10], this can potentially prevent cell binding and infection.

Despite efficiently blocking infection by the mucosatropic alpha types, neither heparin nor carrageenan were consistent inhibitors of the cutaneous types, and indeed frequently promoted infection. This failure of heparin to inhibit infection by one beta type was also observed previously for HPV5 [56]. Several studies suggest that key surface exposed positively charged lysine residues in L1 are important for interaction of HPV16 PsV with heparan sulfate, and mutation of these lysine residues resulted in reduced cell binding and infectivity. We aligned L1 of 34 HPV types tested and noted only one of these lysine residues, HPV16 L1 278K, is highly conserved in alpha types but not beta types (data not shown). Differences in interaction with HSPG-like molecules on the cell surface may account in part for the tropism of HPVs for cutaneous versus mucosal epithelia [14]. However, the relationship is not straight forward; heparin inhibited HPV3, HPV23 and HPV27, and carrageenan inhibited HPV3 and HPV23 infection (Figure 2). It is unclear whether heparin and carrageenan fail to inhibit most beta HPVs because they simply cannot bind to the virion, or they do bind but cannot block receptor interaction. A failure to bind beta HPV particles is unlikely since many PsV showed increased infectivity with addition of heparin and carrageenan. A potential concern with these observations is that low numbers of infectious particles in the PsV preparation of the cutaneous HPV types could have led to an artifact, although L2 incorporation and encapsidation of reporter plasmid was similar to the alpha types. It is also important to recognize considerable variability in L2 incorporation, genome encapsidation and infectivity for PsV preparations of different HPV types when using them as a model for native virions assembled in warts [38].

We expected to observe broad spectrum blockade of HPV infection by furin inhibitor because the furin cleavage consensus sequence RX(R/K)R in L2 was conserved for all HPV types examined herein. This sequence and the requirement for furin cleavage is also conserved in bovine (BPV) and other animal papillomaviruses [20]. Furin inhibitor blocked infection by all HPV types tested although not completely for some beta PsV. This may reflect use by the beta types of protein convertases other than furin that are partially inhibited by furin inhibitor [20], or possibly an artifact relating to the lower signal to noise ratio for the less infectious types.

The γ-secretase inhibitor XXI also effectively inhibited PsV infection for all HPV types tested (Figure 4). Beta types, which tend to exhibit somewhat lower sensitivity than alpha types to the furin inhibitor, were strongly inhibited by XXI. The data suggest that all the HPVs follow a common entry pathway dependent upon both furin- and γ-secretase-dependent proteolysis, despite potential differences in interactions with cell surface HSPGs between the mucosal and cutaneous types. However, while several γ-secretase inhibitors that have been tested clinically for prevention of Alzheimer disease might be re-tasked for broad prevention of HPV infection, they have also been associated with squamous cell cancer [57].

Although the amino terminus of L2 is a weaker immunogen compared to L1 VLP, it is considered to provide broader protection [29]. In particular, the concatenated fusion protein L2 α11-88x8 comprising residues ~11-88 of L2 derived from eight alpha HPV types [35] has been shown to induce cross-neutralizing antibodies that broadly protect against the HPV types most commonly found in cervical cancer and benign genital warts. Here we also examined L2 α11-88x8 antiserum for its capacity to cross-neutralize cutaneous beta HPVs that are also associated with cancer, particularly among immunocompromised and EDV patients. Remarkably, the L2 α11-88x8 antiserum neutralized all beta HPV types tested (Table 1). The result implies that the neutralizing epitopes at the amino terminus of L2 are highly conserved and play an important role in both alpha and beta HPV infection, and that an L2 α11-88x8 vaccine might potentially provide broad protection against the diverse alpha and beta HPV family. Serologic studies suggest that beta HPV infections are acquired throughout life, beginning in childhood [6]. Therefore, optimally vaccination against beta HPV would need to begin early.

In conclusion, we have considered agents that block infection via inhibiting receptor interaction, furin cleavage or γ-secretase function as alternative approaches to vaccination to broadly prevent both mucosal and cutaneous HPV infections. At present, carrageenan shows promise as a vaginal microbicide to broadly prevent infection by mucosatropic high-risk papillomaviruses [17]. However our results show that it is unlikely to prevent cutaneous HPV transmission. Further, it would need to be regularly applied at high amounts to ensure full protection. As both furin and γ-secretase contribute to numerous cellular processes, systemic use of their inhibitors are also likely to have significant side effects rendering them impractical despite broad anti-HPV activity, although topical application might be feasible. Nevertheless, our study with 34 medically significant HPV types indicates that there is a conserved infection pathway once the virus enters its host cell, and thus targeting conserved residues of the capsid proteins that interact with the key cellular entry factors has potential for broad protection. Indeed, rabbit antisera to the L2 α11-88x8 antigen provided broad protection against alpha HPV challenge via cross-neutralizing antibodies [35]. Here we find that L2 α11-88x8-specific antibodies also cross-neutralize diverse beta papillomaviruses, suggesting the potential to protect against types associated with non-melanoma skin cancer in immunocompromised or EDV patients (should they mount a sufficient response after vaccination) or the potential of herd immunity in the general population to limit their circulation. Taken together, this study supports the possibility of vaccination with L2 candidate vaccines for pan-prevention of HPV infection.

Supporting Information

Figure S1 Neutralization of PsV by L1 VLP antiserum. PsVs of each indicated HPV type, each carrying a luciferase reporter gene, were mixed with mouse or rabbit L1 VLP antiserum or their respective pre-immune serum (each at 1:50 dilution) for two hours at 37°C, then the mixtures were transferred to 293TT cells and cultured for 72 hours (n = 3). Cells were then lysed and luciferase activity was measured. Percent neutralization by L1 VLP antiserum was plotted. Pre-immune serum was non-neutralizing in all cases. Red and blue bars represent mucosal and cutaneous HPV types, respectively.

Figure S2 Infectivity of diverse HPV on mucosal and skin cell lines. HeLaT (A), HaCaT (B), KH-SV (C) cells were treated with titrations of diverse HPV PsV from alpha and beta subfamilies and incubated at 37°C for 72 hours. Cells were lysed after incubation and luciferase activity was measured. Red and blue bars represent mucosal and cutaneous HPV types, respectively.

Table S1 Sequences of codon modified L1 and L2 genes utilized in expression constructs used to generate new HPV PsV types.

Acknowledgments

We thank Martin Müller and Lutz Gissmann (DKFZ, Heidelberg, Germany), Christopher Buck and John Schiller (NCI, Bethesda, MD), and Helena Faust (Lund University, Malmö, Sweden) and Joakim Dillner (Karolinska Institutet, Stockholm, Sweden) for the provision of L1/L2 expression plasmids.

Author Contributions

Conceived and designed the experiments: RBSR KK. Performed the experiments: KK RJ JWW SJ. Analyzed the data: KK RJ JWW SJ RK RBSR. Contributed reagents/materials/analysis tools: RK RBSR. Wrote the paper: KK RK RBSR.

References

1. Bernard HU, Burk RD, Chen Z, van Doorslaer K, Hausen H, et al. (2010) Classification of papillomaviruses (PVs) based on 189 PV types and proposal of taxonomic amendments. Virology 401: 70–79.

2. zur Hausen H (2002) Papillomaviruses and cancer: from basic studies to clinical application. Nature Rev Cancer 2: 342–350.

3. Munoz N, Bosch FX, de Sanjose S, Herrero R, Castellsague X, et al. (2003) Epidemiologic classification of human papillomavirus types associated with cervical cancer. N Engl J Med 348: 518–527.
4. Munoz N, Bosch FX, Castellsague X, Diaz M, de Sanjose S, et al. (2004) Against which human papillomavirus types shall we vaccinate and screen? The international perspective. Int J Cancer 111: 278–285.
5. Parkin DM, Bray F (2006) Chapter 2: The burden of HPV-related cancers. Vaccine 24 Suppl 3: S11–25.
6. Nindl I, Gottschling M, Stockfleth E (2007) Human papillomaviruses and non-melanoma skin cancer: basic virology and clinical manifestations. Disease markers 23: 247–259.
7. Baker TS, Newcomb WW, Olson NH, Cowsert LM, Olson C, et al. (1991) Structures of bovine and human papillomaviruses. Analysis by cryoelectron microscopy and three-dimensional image reconstruction. Biophys J 60: 1445–1456.
8. Buck CB, Cheng N, Thompson CD, Lowy DR, Steven AC, et al. (2008) Arrangement of L2 within the papillomavirus capsid. J Virol 82: 5190–5197.
9. Chen XS, Garcea RL, Goldberg I, Casini G, Harrison SC (2000) Structure of small virus-like particles assembled from the L1 protein of human papillomavirus 16. Mol Cell 5: 557–567.
10. Joyce JG, Tung JS, Przysiecki CT, Cook JC, Lehman ED, et al. (1999) The L1 major capsid protein of human papillomavirus type 11 recombinant virus-like particles interacts with heparin and cell-surface glycosaminoglycans on human keratinocytes. J Biol Chem 274: 5810–5822.
11. Giroglou T, Florin L, Schafer F, Streeck RE, Sapp M (2001) Human Papillomavirus Infection Requires Cell Surface Heparan Sulfate. J Virol 75: 1565–1570.
12. Buck CB, Thompson CD, Roberts JN, Muller M, Lowy DR, et al. (2006) Carrageenan is a potent inhibitor of papillomavirus infection. PLoS Pathog 2: e69.
13. Roberts JN, Buck CB, Thompson CD, Kines R, Bernardo M, et al. (2007) Genital transmission of HPV in a mouse model is potentiated by nonoxynol-9 and inhibited by carrageenan. Nat Med 13: 857–861.
14. Johnson KM, Kines RC, Roberts JN, Lowy DR, Schiller JT, et al. (2009) Role of heparan sulfate in attachment to and infection of the murine female genital tract by human papillomavirus. J Virol 83: 2067–2074.
15. Roberts JN, Kines RC, Katki HA, Lowy DR, Schiller JT (2011) Effect of Pap smear collection and carrageenan on cervicovaginal human papillomavirus-16 infection in a rhesus macaque model. Journal of the National Cancer Institute 103: 737–743.
16. Knappe M, Bodevin S, Selinka HC, Spillmann D, Streeck RE, et al. (2007) Surface-exposed amino acid residues of HPV16 L1 protein mediating interaction with cell surface heparan sulfate. The Journal of biological chemistry 282: 27913–27922.
17. Marais D, Gawarecki D, Allan B, Ahmed K, Altini L, et al. (2011) The effectiveness of Carraguard, a vaginal microbicide, in protecting women against high-risk human papillomavirus infection. Antiviral therapy 16: 1219–1226.
18. Roden RB, Greenstone HL, Kirnbauer R, Booy FP, Jessie J, et al. (1996) In vitro generation and type-specific neutralization of a human papillomavirus type 16 virion pseudotype. J Virol 70: 5875–5883.
19. Roden RB, Day PM, Bronzo BK, Yutzy WHt, Yang Y, et al. (2001) Positively charged termini of the L2 minor capsid protein are necessary for papillomavirus infection. J Virol 75: 10493–10497.
20. Richards RM, Lowy DR, Schiller JT, Day PM (2006) Cleavage of the papillomavirus minor capsid protein, L2, at a furin consensus site is necessary for infection. Proc Natl Acad Sci U S A 103: 1522–1527.
21. Kines RC, Thompson CD, Lowy DR, Schiller JT, Day PM (2009) The initial steps leading to papillomavirus infection occur on the basement membrane prior to cell surface binding. Proc Natl Acad Sci U S A 106: 20458–20463.
22. Bienkowska-Haba M, Patel HD, Sapp M (2009) Target cell cyclophilins facilitate human papillomavirus type 16 infection. PLoS Pathog 5: e1000524.
23. Woodham AW, Da Silva DM, Skeate JG, Raff AB, Ambroso MR, et al. (2012) The S100A10 subunit of the annexin A2 heterotetramer facilitates L2-mediated human papillomavirus infection. PLoS ONE 7: e43519.
24. Bossis I, Roden RB, Gambhira R, Yang R, Tagaya M, et al. (2005) Interaction of tSNARE syntaxin 18 with the papillomavirus minor capsid protein mediates infection. Journal of virology 79: 6723–6731.
25. Bergant Marusic M, Ozbun MA, Campos SK, Myers MP, Banks L (2012) Human papillomavirus L2 facilitates viral escape from late endosomes via sorting nexin 17. Traffic 13: 455–467.
26. Kamper N, Day PM, Nowak T, Selinka HC, Florin L, et al. (2006) A membrane-destabilizing peptide in capsid protein L2 is required for egress of papillomavirus genomes from endosomes. J Virol 80: 759–768.
27. Karanam B, Peng S, Li T, Buck C, Day PM, et al. (2010) Papillomavirus infection requires gamma secretase. J Virol 84: 10661–10670.
28. Huang HS, Buck CB, Lambert PF (2010) Inhibition of gamma secretase blocks HPV infection. Virology 407: 391–396.
29. Roden R, Wu TC (2006) How will HPV vaccines affect cervical cancer? Nat Rev Cancer 6: 753–763.
30. Brown DR, Kjaer SK, Sigurdsson K, Iversen OE, Hernandez-Avila M, et al. (2009) The impact of quadrivalent human papillomavirus (HPV; types 6, 11, 16, and 18) L1 virus-like particle vaccine on infection and disease due to oncogenic nonvaccine HPV types in generally HPV-naive women aged 16–26 years. J Infect Dis 199: 926–935.
31. Paavonen J, Naud P, Salmeron J, Wheeler CM, Chow SN, et al. (2009) Efficacy of human papillomavirus (HPV)-16/18 AS04-adjuvanted vaccine against cervical infection and precancer caused by oncogenic HPV types (PATRICIA): final analysis of a double-blind, randomised study in young women. Lancet 374: 301–314.
32. Wheeler CM, Castellsague X, Garland SM, Szarewski A, Paavonen J, et al. (2012) Cross-protective efficacy of HPV-16/18 AS04-adjuvanted vaccine against cervical infection and precancer caused by non-vaccine oncogenic HPV types: 4-year end-of-study analysis of the randomised, double-blind PATRICIA trial. The lancet oncology 13: 100–110.
33. Malagon T, Drolet M, Boily MC, Franco EL, Jit M, et al. (2012) Cross-protective efficacy of two human papillomavirus vaccines: a systematic review and meta-analysis. The Lancet infectious diseases 12: 781–789.
34. Jagu S, Karanam B, Gambhira R, Chivukula SV, Chaganti RJ, et al. (2009) Concatenated multitype L2 fusion proteins as candidate prophylactic pan-human papillomavirus vaccines. J Natl Cancer Inst 101: 782–792.
35. Jagu S, Kwak K, Schiller JT, Lowy DR, Kleanthous H, et al. (2013) Phylogenetic considerations in designing a broadly protective multimeric L2 vaccine. J Virol 87: 6127–6136.
36. Jagu S, Kwak K, Karanam B, Huh WK, Damotharan V, et al. (2013) Optimization of Multimeric Human Papillomavirus L2 Vaccines. PLoS ONE 8: e55538.
37. Mistry N, Wibom C, Evander M (2008) Cutaneous and mucosal human papillomaviruses differ in net surface charge, potential impact on tropism. Virology journal 5: 118.
38. Cruz L, Meyers C (2013) Differential Dependence on Host Cell Glycosaminoglycans for Infection of Epithelial Cells by High-Risk HPV Types. PLoS ONE 8: e68379.
39. Buck CB, Pastrana DV, Lowy DR, Schiller JT (2005) Generation of HPV pseudovirions using transfection and their use in neutralization assays. Methods Mol Med 119: 445–462.
40. Zhou J, Liu WJ, Peng SW, Sun XY, Frazer I (1999) Papillomavirus capsid protein expression level depends on the match between codon usage and tRNA availability. J Virol 73: 4972–4982.
41. Leder C, Kleinschmidt JA, Wiethe C, Muller M (2001) Enhancement of capsid gene expression: preparing the human papillomavirus type 16 major structural gene L1 for DNA vaccination purposes. J Virol 75: 9201–9209.
42. Johansson C, Schwartz S (2013) Regulation of human papillomavirus gene expression by splicing and polyadenylation. Nature reviews Microbiology 11: 239–251.
43. Pastrana DV, Buck CB, Pang YY, Thompson CD, Castle PE, et al. (2004) Reactivity of human sera in a sensitive, high-throughput pseudovirus-based papillomavirus neutralization assay for HPV16 and HPV18. Virology 321: 205–216.
44. Kondo K, Ishii Y, Ochi H, Matsumoto T, Yoshikawa H, et al. (2006) Neutralization of HPV16, 18, 31, and 58 pseudovirions with antisera induced by immunizing rabbits with synthetic peptides representing segments of the HPV16 minor capsid protein L2 surface region. Virology.
45. Senger T, Schadlich L, Textor S, Klein C, Michael KM, et al. (2010) Virus-like particles and capsomeres are potent vaccines against cutaneous alpha HPVs. Vaccine 28: 1583–1593.
46. Faust H, Andersson K, Forslund O, Dillner J (2013) Pseudovirion-binding and neutralizing antibodies to cutaneous human papillomaviruses (HPV) correlated with the presence of HPV DNA in skin. The Journal of general virology 94: 1096–1103.
47. Kwak K, Jiang R, Jagu S, Wang JW, Wang C, et al. (2013) Multivalent human papillomavirus L1 DNA vaccination utilizing electroporation. PLoS ONE 8: e60507.
48. Sehr P, Rubio I, Seitz H, Putzker K, Ribeiro-Muller L, et al. (2013) High-throughput pseudovirion-based neutralization assay for analysis of natural and vaccine-induced antibodies against human papillomaviruses. PLoS ONE 8: e75677.
49. Boukamp P, Petrussevska RT, Breitkreutz D, Hornung J, Markham A, et al. (1988) Normal keratinization in a spontaneously immortalized aneuploid human keratinocyte cell line. The Journal of cell biology 106: 761–771.
50. Shafti-Keramat S, Handisurya A, Kriehuber E, Meneguzzi G, Slupetzky K, et al. (2003) Different heparan sulfate proteoglycans serve as cellular receptors for human papillomaviruses. Journal of virology 77: 13125–13135.
51. Patterson NA, Smith JL, Ozbun MA (2005) Human papillomavirus type 31b infection of human keratinocytes does not require heparan sulfate. J Virol 79: 6838–6847.
52. Cerqueira C, Liu Y, Kuhling L, Chai W, Hafezi W, et al. (2013) Heparin increases the infectivity of Human Papillomavirus Type 16 independent of cell surface proteoglycans and induces L1 epitope exposure. Cellular microbiology.
53. Dasgupta J, Bienkowska-Haba M, Ortega ME, Patel HD, Bodevin S, et al. (2011) Structural basis of oligosaccharide receptor recognition by human papillomavirus. The Journal of biological chemistry 286: 2617–2624.
54. Roden R, Monie A, Wu TC (2006) The impact of preventive HPV vaccination. Discov Med 6: 175–181.
55. Surviladze Z, Dziduszko A, Ozbun MA (2012) Essential roles for soluble virion-associated heparan sulfonated proteoglycans and growth factors in human papillomavirus infections. PLoS pathogens 8: e1002519.

Mutations in the Control of Virulence Sensor Gene from *Streptococcus pyogenes* after Infection in Mice Lead to Clonal Bacterial Variants with Altered Gene Regulatory Activity and Virulence

Jeffrey A. Mayfield[1], Zhong Liang[1,2], Garima Agrahari[1,2], Shaun W. Lee[1,3], Deborah L. Donahue[1], Victoria A. Ploplis[1,2], Francis J. Castellino[1,2]*

1 W. M. Keck Center for Transgene Research, University of Notre Dame, Notre Dame, Indiana, United States of America, **2** Department of Chemistry and Biochemistry, University of Notre Dame, Notre Dame, Indiana, United States of America, **3** Department of Biological Sciences, University of Notre Dame, Notre Dame, Indiana, United States of America

Abstract

The cluster of virulence sensor (CovS)/responder (CovR) two-component operon (CovRS) regulates ~15% of the genes of the Group A *Streptococcal pyogenes* (GAS) genome. Bacterial clones containing inactivating mutations in the *covS* gene have been isolated from patients with virulent invasive diseases. We report herein an assessment of the nature and types of *covS* mutations that can occur in both virulent and nonvirulent GAS strains, and assess whether a nonvirulent GAS can attain enhanced virulence through this mechanism. A group of mice were infected with a globally-disseminated clonal M1T1 GAS (isolate 5448), containing wild-type (WT) CovRS (5448/CovR$^+$S$^+$), or less virulent engineered GAS strains AP53/CovR$^+$S$^+$ and Manfredo M5/CovR$^+$S$^+$. SpeB negative GAS clones from wound sites and/or from bacteria disseminated to the spleen were isolated and the *covS* gene was subjected to DNA sequence analysis. Numerous examples of inactivating mutations were found in CovS in all regions of the gene. The mutations found included frame-shift insertions and deletions, and in-frame small and large deletions in the gene. Many of the mutations found resulted in early translation termination of CovS. Thus, the *covS* gene is a genomic mutagenic target that gives GAS enhanced virulence. In cases wherein CovS$^-$ was discovered, these clonal variants exhibited high lethality, further suggesting that randomly mutated *covS* genes occur during the course of infection, and lead to the development of a more invasive infection.

Editor: Adam J. Ratner, Columbia University, United States of America

Funding: Funding provided by HL013423. The funders had no role in study design, data collection and analysis, decision to publish, or preparation of the manuscript.

Competing Interests: The authors have declared that no competing interests exist.

* Email: fcastell@nd.edu

Introduction

Two-component signal-transducing systems (TCS) are found throughout the bacterial world and regulate a number of critical virulence processes, thereby permitting these organisms to survive under the harsh conditions inflicted by the host in its defense. In general, TCS are composed of an extracellular membrane-bound sensor protein and an intracellular nuclear regulatory responder protein [1]. The control of virulence TCS operon (*covRS*) found in the strict human pathogen, *Streptococcus pyogenes* (Group A *Streptococcus*; GAS), is critical for the regulation of ~15% of the GAS genome [2]. Mutations in CovRS that confer phenotypic heterogeneity in the invading bacterial population can assist the bacteria in evading the defense responses of the host, thereby allowing the microorganism to disseminate into deep tissue. Critical GAS virulence genes, *e.g.*, streptokinase (*ska*), streptococcal pyrogenic exotoxin (*spe*)B, and hyaluronic acid capsule biosynthesis genes (*hasABC*), as well as some GAS-adopted prophage genes, *e.g.*, streptodornase (*sda1*), have been shown to be under the control of CovRS [2]. GAS is the causative agent for a number of illnesses, ranging from minor treatable throat and skin infections to more severe diseases, such as streptococcal toxic shock syndrome and necrotizing *fasciitis*. These maladies are growing concerns due to establishment of clonal hypervirulent GAS strains. A better understanding of mechanisms of gene regulation employed by GAS, especially by TCS, such as CovRS, that can serve to rapidly alter bacterial gene expression under host defense pressures, will enable novel approaches to better combat this serious threat to human health.

In contrast to most regulatory systems, CovR, a cytoplasmic transcriptional regulator, represses most of its gene targets. This repression is attenuated when the bacteria are under duress in the host, causing an increase in expression of virulence gene products. The sensor component (CovS) of CovRS is proposed to recognize stress signals, *e.g.*, elevated [Mg^{2+}], temperature, low tissue O_2 tension in tissue, and salinity, upon which CovS autophosphorylates and then transfers this phosphoryl group to CovR, thus altering the affinity of CovR for promoters of its gene targets [3,4]. The complexities in environmental stimuli and specific gene regulation in the CovRS system are not well understood, and remain a topic of some debate [5]. It has been shown that when experiencing environmental pressures during host infection, GAS clones are selected towards those that lack a fully functional CovS component [6]. Several hypervirulent GAS clinical and animal-passaged clones have been isolated with mutations in the *covS* gene that attenuate the activity of its gene product toward CovR [7–11]. One gene under CovRS transcriptional regulation is *speB*, which encodes an extracellular cysteine protease (SpeB) that catalyzes cleavage of a number of host and GAS proteins [12,13]. Several roles for SpeB have been observed in establishing infection, including a role in evading the host autophagy pathway [14] and likely many more will be determined; however, it has been documented that hypervirulent GAS strains with inactivated CovS ($CovR^+S^-$) lack detectable SpeB in culture supernatants [9]. Intact $CovR^+S^+$ greatly enhances *speB* expression, which is necessary for establishing early infectivity, after which downregulation of SpeB expression promotes virulence. This switch in *speB* expression is facilitated by *covS* gene mutations, which then allows CovR to repress *speB* expression and thereby permit other virulence factors, *e.g.*, the products of the *sda1*, streptokinase (*ska*), and streptolysin-O (*slo*) genes, to avoid cleavage by SpeB, thus sustaining their activities as GAS virulence factors. This selection for *covS* mutants suggests that only colonies that are maximally discharging their virulence factors are able to survive in host compartments that are particularly hostile to the microorganism. However, under conditions where host immune surveillance is not present, this sensor protein is likely important for alleviating the energy burden of producing virulence gene products and allows for long-term colonization.

A number of hypervirulent GAS isolates have been characterized by inactivating mutations in CovR or CovS, and it is unclear whether these mutations follow any consistent patterns. The goal of this study was to employ single well-characterized strains of GAS to extensively assess whether consistencies of gene mutations occur in *covS* during host infection that result in hypervirulent strains. Using the invasive globally-disseminated M1T1 GAS strain, *viz.*, 5448/$CovR^+S^+$, and the nonvirulent engineered strain, AP53/$CovR^+S^+$, both of which contain full-length and fully-functional *covS* genes, we performed a number of mouse-passage (MP) studies where the same wild-type (WT) bacteria were used to infect different mice. Infection and dissemination sites were examined for SpeB-negative ($SpeB^-$) clones. These clones were then further characterized to determine the nature of gene mutations in *covS*. A number of such isolates were recovered, further confirmed by increased *sda1* and *ska* expression and activity. The results suggest that many types of mutations can occur in the *covS* gene, leading to the hypothesis that, when establishing infection, the entire *covS* gene is susceptible to mutations, and clones containing CovS-inactivating mutations have the ability to affect numerous end-points that lead to serious invasive disease and resist innate defenses.

Materials and Methods

Bacterial strains and culture

GAS serotype M1T1, strain 5448/*covR*$^+$*S*$^+$/*emm1*$^+$, has been previously isolated from a patient with an invasive GAS infection [15,16]. This GAS strain also contains the lysogenically-inserted prophage-encoded genes, *speA* and *sda1*, which are independent virulence factors. GAS strain Manfredo/*covR*$^+$*S*$^+$/*emm5*, from an GAS avirulent infection [17], was provided by Dr. G. Lindahl (Lund, SW). The clinical GAS isolates, MGAS315/*emm3*$^+$ [18], JRS4/*emm6*$^+$ [19], and MGAS8232/*emm18*$^+$ [20], were provided by Dr. J.R. Scott (Emory University). AP53/*covR*$^+$*S*$^-$/*emm53(pam)*$^+$ has been previously described as a primary isolate from a patient with severe invasive disease. As obtained, we found that this latter isolate has an inactivating mutation in the *covS* gene (ΔT^{1404}), leading to a premature end of translation at amino acid-469 in the CovS protein, and is highly virulent, despite its lack of the particular prophage insertions that provide *sda1* and *speA*. This *covS*$^-$ gene was recomplemented to nonvirulent AP53/*covR*$^+$*S*$^+$/*emm53(pam)*$^+$, through bacterial mutagenesis, in which we reinserted T^{1404} in *covS*$^-$ and restored full $CovR^+S^+$ function to GAS AP53 [21].

All strains were routinely grown on 5% sheep blood agar (SBA) plates (Teknova, Hollister, CA) and cultured at 37°C and 5% CO_2 in Todd-Hewitt broth (BD Biosciences, San Jose, CA), supplemented with 10% yeast (THY). To screen for SpeB proteolytic activity, GAS isolates were plated on THY/milk (3% skim milk) agar plates for ~24 hr at 37°C and 5% CO_2. The strains used in this study are summarized in Table 1.

Subcutaneous infection and organ processing

Overnight cultures of GAS 5448/$CovR^+S^+$, grown from a single colony, were used to inoculate (1:10) 30 ml of pre-warmed THY media. The cells were grown to mid-log phase (LP; A_{600nm} ~0.6), pelleted by centrifugation at 2,500×g for 10 min, then washed 2× in sterile 0.7% saline, followed by resuspension in a final volume sufficient to provide ~$1–2\times10^9$ CFU/ml, as later determined by plating on SBA and counting colonies from serial dilutions. Cohorts of C57Bl/6 mice containing the human plasminogen (hPg) transgene [C57Bl/6(hPg(Tg)] [22], provided by Prof. D. Ginsburg (Ann Arbor, MI), were subcutaneously injected with a dose of ~$1–2\times10^8$ CFU/100 μl. At a time of 3 days post-infection, mice were sacrificed, and the skin wounds, livers, and spleens were harvested and placed into 2 ml of 0.7% saline. Samples were dispersed using a homogenizer (IKA, Wilmington, NC) for ~30 sec at 24,000 rpm on ice. Homogenates were serially diluted and plated for colony counting. Significance of dissemination count differences between organs was determined using an unpaired two-tailed student's t-test. In addition to SBA plating, dilutions were plated on THY milk/agar to detect SpeB proteolytic activity.

SpeB activity assays

Mouse-passaged GAS colonies were visually screened to tentatively identify $SpeB^-$ clones by the lack of a visual lytic (clearing) zone in THY milk/agar after a 24 hr incubation at 37°C in a 5% CO_2 atmosphere. To confirm the presence or absence of SpeB, lytic-negative colonies were cultured in 10 ml of THY media overnight. Following centrifugation at 2,500×g for 10 min, bacterial supernatants were sterile-filtered and concentrated (~10-fold) using centrifugal concentrator devices (Millipore, Billerica, MA) with a 10K molecular weight cutoff. Concentrated supernatants were incubated in activation buffer (1 mM EDTA, 10 mM DTT, 0.1 M acetate, pH 5) for 30 min at 37°C prior to addition of 0.6 mM of the chromogenic substrate, N-benzoyl-proline-phenylalanine-arginine-*p*-nitroanilide-HCl (Sigma, St. Louis, MO). Amidolytic activity was continuously monitored at A_{405nm}. This was repeated at least 2× for each sample with the addition of 28 μM cysteine protease inhibitor, E64, (Sigma-Aldrich, St. Louis, MO) to confirm specificity for SpeB.

Table 1. *Streptococcus pyogenes* strains used in this study.

Strain Name	*emm* Type	Reference
5448/*covR*[+]*S*[+]	1	14
Manfredo/*covR*[+]*S*[+]	5	16
MGAS315	3	17
JRS4	6	13
MGAS8232	18	19
AP53/*covR*[+]*S*[−]	53	20
AP53/*covR*[+]*S*[+]	53	20
AP53/*covR*[+]*S*[+]/(*pam*)[−]	53	20

covS gene sequencing

Genomic DNA (gDNA) was obtained *via* freeze-thaw cell lysis of SpeB$^-$ bacterial isolates. Primers specific for the *covRS* region (876F-GTGCGTGGCATGGGATACGT and 2451R-CCTGT-CACATTAACAATGCCTT) were used to amplify the gene product in all strains by PCR. To identify mutations, nucleotide sequences were obtained using the same primers for all GAS strains. PCR and subsequent sequencing was performed in duplicate or triplicate to confirm the positions and identities of the mutations. Two primers were used to determine the presence or absence of *covS* mutations in inoculum prior to infection (84F-CTGCATTTTCTCTGCCTTTACACTG and 1195R-GTCAA-TCAGAATCATCAAAGCCTGC). These reactions were run using gDNA isolated from overnight cultures of multiple GAS colonies.

DNase activity assays

Sda1-catalyzed DNase activities of the GAS 5448 *covS* mutants were performed as previously described [23]. Strains 5448/CovR$^+$S$^+$ and MP mutants of this strain were grown to LP (A_{600nm} ~0.6) and centrifuged at 2,500×g, after which the supernatants were removed and sterile-filtered. Approximately 1 µl of supernatant was incubated with 1 µg of calf thymus DNA for 5 min at 37°C in 300 mM Tris-Cl/3 mM $MgCl_2$/3 mM $CaCl_2$, pH 8.0. Enzymatic reactions were terminated by addition of 100 mM EDTA. The samples were then subjected to electrophoresis on 1.5% agarose gels and bands were detected *via* ethidium bromide stain.

Polymerase Chain Reaction (PCR) and Reverse Transcription-PCR (RT-PCR)

Total RNA was isolated as described [21] from two independent cultures of WT 5448/*covR*$^+$*S*$^+$ and two of its mouse-passaged *covR*$^+$*S*$^-$ mutants, *viz.*, #12 (skin) and #14 (skin), grown to A_{600nm} ~0.6. The sample was treated twice with DNase to eliminate any contaminating gDNA.

Total genomic DNA (gDNA) was obtained from single GAS colonies of strains that were picked from streaks on sheep blood agar and grown in THY overnight at 37°C. The gDNA was isolated after treatment of the cells with lysozyme/proteinase K and cell lysis buffer (100 mM Tris/5 mM EDTA/0.2% SDS/ 200 mM NaCl, pH 8.5), and extracted with phenol/chloroform/ isoamyl alcohol (25/24/1, v/v/v). The gDNA was precipitated with isopropanol and washed with 70% ethanol.

Primers specific for *sda1* (438F: 5′-GAGAGCCACTGAATCC-GACTAC and 688R: 5′-TACTGCATCCCACCTTTAC-GAT, amplicon size, 251 bp), *ska* (55F: 5′-GGAACAGT-GAAGCCTGTCCAAGCT and 369R: 5′-GTAGCCGTCGT-TACTGTG-AACGTT, amplicon size, 315 bp), and *slo* (2334F: 5′-GCTAGTACAGAAACCAC-AACGAC and 2742R: 5′-GA-TAGGTCC-TATCAGTGACAGAGTC, amplicon size, 409 bp), along with the reference gene, *gapdh* (*plr*) [21], were used for both the RT-PCR of the cDNA and PCR of the gDNA, which was performed as previously described [21].

Plasminogen activation assays

To measure the activity of streptokinase (SK) in conditioned GAS supernatants, hPg activation assays were performed as previously published [24]. Briefly, 0.2 µM Glu^1-hPg, isolated by affinity chromatography [25], was mixed in 96-well plates with 0.25 mM S2251 (*H*-D-Val-Leu-Lys-pNA; Chromogenix, Milan, Italy) in 10 mM Hepes/150 mM NaCl, pH 7.4, at 37°C. The reactions were initiated by addition of 20 µl of supernatants, taken from 30 ml cultures grown to A_{600nm} ~0.6 and A_{600nm} ~1.2 in THY broth that had been concentrated (~10-fold) and resuspended in buffer to remove media components. Human fibrinogen (ERL, South Bend, IN) was added at 1.0 µM to increase activity, since the SK2a produced by this M1 GAS line is stimulated by fibrinogen [24]. After initiation of the activation by conditioned cell supernatants, the reaction was monitored at 405 nm in 1 min intervals for 2 hr at 37°C. The initial velocity (V_i; $mAbs_{405nm}$-min-^{2}) was obtained by taking the slope of the linear portion of the activation curve after squaring the time values.

Mouse survival studies

C57Bl/6(hPg(Tg) male mice (6–10 weeks of age) were injected subcutaneously with ~10^7–10^8 GAS cells. The infected mice were observed for up to 10 days to monitor the occurrence of death. For statistical analysis, Kaplan-Meier survival curves were analyzed by the paired log-rank test using GraphPad PRISM 6 software with p values <0.05 considered significant. These protocols were approved by the Institutional Animal Care and Use Committee (IACUC) of the University of Notre Dame.

Death as an endpoint is used in order to determine survival curves with different strains of bacteria. The survival group was monitored two or more times/day for up to 10 days, after that time any full-term survivors were humanely euthanized as per the procedures established by our local IACUC, *i.e.*, mice were euthanized by a automated CO_2 system. The criterion used in this study for early euthanasia was placing a mouse on its side and if unable to right itself, or stand on all four legs, the mouse was euthanized by cervical dislocation. Otherwise, mice in this group must progress to death to mimic terminal disease states in patients.

Mice continue to eat, drink, and remain in motion even as the disease progresses.

No analgesics were employed in this work. Inflammation is a key experimental component, and any compounds that might alter the inflammatory process would be counterproductive. Great care was taken to use agents that would not interfere with the experimental outcome. A variety of analgesics were considered and it was concluded that: 1) non-steroidal anti-inflammatory agents or opiods cannot be used due to interference with the inflammatory process [26]; 2) butorphanol cannot be used due to seeming interference with inflammation [27]; and 3) buprenorphine cannot be used because it interferes with the inflammatory process [28].

The mice in these experiments were housed with enrichment, such as extra bedding materials. Some feed was placed on the bottom of the cages to enable mice to eat without standing (in case the hind limb is sore from the wound). The water bottle in the cages was very low and mice only needed to extend their neck to drink. Mice were not housed individually since this would induce stress in the mice.

Results

Bacterial dissemination readily occurs with GAS 5448/CovR$^+$S$^+$

Using the highly virulent GAS, 5448/CovR$^+$S$^+$, to infect mice, bacterial dissemination from skin to deep tissue occurs within a three day period, yielding measureable levels of GAS colony forming units (CFU) in liver and spleen tissue. Representative plots of the bacterial counts taken from all tissues are shown in Figure 1, with each point representing a different mouse. On average, significantly more bacteria were recovered from the skin lesion ($\sim 2\times10^5$ CFU) than from the deeper tissues, *viz*., liver and spleen, which yielded $\sim 9\times10^4$ and $\sim 1\times10^4$ CFU, respectively ($P<0.001$ for each). In the case of the less virulent AP53/CovR$^+$S$^+$, Manfredo M5/CovR$^+$S$^+$ and AP53/CovR$^+$S$^+$/ΔM53 strains, little dissemination was observed (data not shown), relative to the WT M1T1 5448 strain, but, nonetheless, bacteria were recovered from the skin to assess whether CovS switching could occur at the wound sites in these strains.

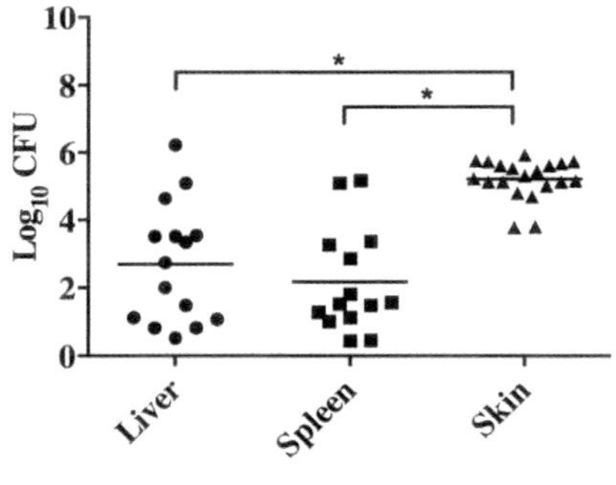

Figure 1. GAS strain 5448 dissemination from skin to deep tissue. Analysis of bacterial loads in liver, spleen, and skin wound tissue. C57Bl/6[hPg(Tg)] mice were injected with a dose of $\sim$1–2×10^8 CFU/100 µl of 5448 WT-5448/CovR$^+$S$^+$. At 3 days post-infection, organs were harvested and bacterial counts obtained from serial dilutions of homogenized tissues. Asterisks indicate statistical significance determined by unpaired two-tailed students t-test, $P<0.001$.

CovS mutants were identified in GAS 5448/CovR$^+$S$^+$ infections

Strains with SpeB$^-$ phenotypes are typically characterized by mutations in the *covR* or *covS* gene, with a preponderance of alterations in the latter gene [29,30]. In order to determine whether the *in vivo* mutations in the *covS* gene reveal a pattern, several SpeB$^-$ isolates were recovered from separately infected mice and their *covS* genes were sequenced. Samples were obtained not only from wound sites, but also from spleens, since we hypothesized that deeper tissue isolates would contain more virulent mutants. Plating tissue homogenates on THY-milk/agar plates allowed the ability to rapidly screen for SpeB activity by visually observing the switch from the lytic zone found around the SpeB$^+$ colonies to the lack of such zones in SpeB$^-$ colonies. Random colonies that appeared to be SpeB$^-$ (no clearing) and β-hemolytic on blood agar (not shown), were further analyzed for SpeB proteolytic activity in concentrated culture supernatants using a spectrophotometric assay. Each infected mouse yielded several GAS clonal isolates, yet only a small percentage were SpeB$^-$, with the remaining being SpeB$^+$, similar to the injected sample (Table 2).

The great majority of CovS$^-$ mutations in recovered SpeB$^-$ colonies were either deletions or insertions of 1 to 612 base pairs (bp) of DNA (Table 2). These changes occurred within the putative functional CovS protein domains (see footnote of Table 2 [8,11]). The regions were established based on sequence comparison to similar histidine kinase sensor proteins and include two transmembrane regions (TMI and TMII), an extracellular sensor loop (EC Loop), a histidine kinases/adenylyl cyclases/methyl-binding proteins/phosphatases (HAMP) region, a histidine kinase or phosphoacceptor (HisKA) region, and a histidine kinase-like ATPase (HATPase) region [8,11]. Of the 17 different mutations identified in spleen, and/or skin isolates, 6 occurred solely in the HATPase domain and a single isolate contained a mutation in the HisKA portion of the protein. The remaining isolates possessed mutations in multiple domains or in regions between the assigned domains. A total of 11 mutations resulted in premature truncation, either from in-frame or out-of-frame deletions or insertions, which led to the occurrence of premature translation stop codons. However, one of the mutations, identified from strains recovered from six different mice (#7-11 and #13), as well as a distinct mutation in another mouse (#1), represented large deletions within the gene that still terminated with the original stop codon. Only one of the mutants, 5448/#4, had two in-frame nucleotide point mutations. While many other mutations are likely to be present in the CovS$^-$ strains that were not tested, our aim was to examine whether commonality existed in the types of mutants that were randomly isolated.

From these results, we conclude that there does not appear to be a particular motif or region of the *covS* gene that is not susceptible to mutation, but it is of interest that the same large DNA deletion occurred in multiple mice (#7–11 and #13), suggesting that this was a more susceptible mutagenic region of the gene. Six identical *covS* mutations appeared in GAS isolates from multiple mice. Strikingly, mutant strains #12 (skin) and #14 (spleen) have the same 31 bp insertion, which is located at different positions of the DNA, *viz*., bp-140 and bp-160, respectively. Thus, the overall distribution of mutations encompasses most of the *covS* gene.

CovS mutations were not identified in the GAS 5448/covR$^+$S$^+$ inoculum prior to infection

Since several covS mutations resulted in significantly smaller covS genes, *e.g.*, Mouse 1 Spleen (167 bp deletion) and Mouse 7

Table 2. Mutations found in *covS* gene of GAS strain 5448/*covS*$^+$ during infection in mice.[a]

Mouse	Tissue[b]	Gene Mutation	NT[c]	# bp[d]	# clones[e]	Protein Mutation[f]
1	Spleen	Deletion	974–1140	167	1	Delete 325–380
	Spleen	Deletion	1243	1	2	Stop-458
2	Spleen	Deletion	1243	1	2	Stop-458
3	Spleen	Deletion	279–297	19	10	Stop-156
4	Spleen	Deletion	279–297	19	3	Stop-156
	Spleen	Insertion	96	11	2	Stop-39
	Spleen	Mutation	404–405, 845	3	2	S135F, L282S
5	Spleen	Insertion	468	1	7	Stop-165
6	Spleen	Insertion	1357	1	7	Stop-478
	Spleen	Deletion	83	1	3	Stop-36
7	Spleen	Deletion	229–840	612	2	Delete 77-280
	Skin	Deletion	229–840	612	4	Delete 77-280
8	Spleen	Deletion	229–840	612	6	Delete 77-280
	Skin	Deletion	229–840	612	3	Delete 77-280
9	Spleen	Deletion	229–840	612	5	Delete 77-280
	Skin	Deletion	229–840	612	1	Delete 77-280
10	Spleen	Deletion	229–840	612	5	Delete 77-280
	Skin	Deletion	229–840	612	1	Delete 77-280
11	Spleen	Deletion	229–840	612	2	Delete 77-280
12	Spleen	Deletion	1104–1140	37	6	Stop-377
	Skin	Insertion	140	31	1	Stop-71
13	Spleen	Deletion	229-840	612	1	Delete 77-280
	Spleen	Insertion	160	31	1	Stop-71
	Skin	Insertion	998	4	1	Stop-339
14	Spleen	Insertion	160	31	1	Stop-71
	Spleen	Deletion	1104–1140	37	1	Stop-377
	Skin	Deletion	1211–1215	5	1	Stop-407
15	Spleen	Deletion	1104–1140	37	1	Stop-377
	Skin	Insertion	96	11	1	Stop-39
16	Skin	Insertion	140	31	2	Stop-71
17	Skin	Deletion	1376–1382	7	1	Stop-466

[a]Putative domains of CovS as defined elsewhere [8,11], where mutations occur: CovS: TMI (22–33); EC Loop (34–180); TMII (181–205); HAMP (208–266); HisKA (269–333); HATPase (386–492).
[b]Tissue from which clones were obtained.
[c]Nucleotide (NT) position of change, or range of change, based on position of the *covS* start codon.
[d]Number of nucleotides of WT-*covS* replaced, inserted, or deleted.
[e]Number of clones sequenced.
[f]Effect on CovS protein.

Spleen (612 bp deletion), the possibility that these mutations were present in the inoculum prior to infection was determined. A set of primers was designed such that the full-length covS gene would generate a ~1102 bp band and the deletion mutants would generate bands corresponding to loss of 612 bp or 167 bp. Figure 2 shows the results of the extended PCR analysis on genomic DNA isolated from overnight cultures. It is clear that each lane contains a single PCR product that corresponds to the size of *covS* gene, suggesting that the initial inoculum contains bacteria with only full-length *covS* and that mutations arise and are selected for during the onset of infection.

Identification of covS mutants in GAS AP53/CovR$^+$S$^+$ infections

Since GAS 5448/CovR$^+$S$^+$ is highly virulent and has prophage genes lysogenically inserted, it is possible, and has indeed been proposed, that the acquisition of separate prophage regions encoding the streptodornase gene, *sda1*, and/or the superantigen *speA* gene, in synergy with the genetic scaffold of the clonal 5448/CovR$^+$S$^+$, stimulates CovS switching [31]. According to our DNA analysis of multiple strains of GAS, we find clear evidence for genomic full-length *sda1* in the *emm1* strain, 5448, along with other GAS strains with different M-protein serotypes, *e.g.*, *emm6* (D471) and *emm18* (MGAS8232) (Fig. 3A). We did not identify *sda1* in our clonal *emm3* strain (Fig. 3A), suggesting that this particular GAS strain had not acquired the *sda1*-containing prophage. Also, we

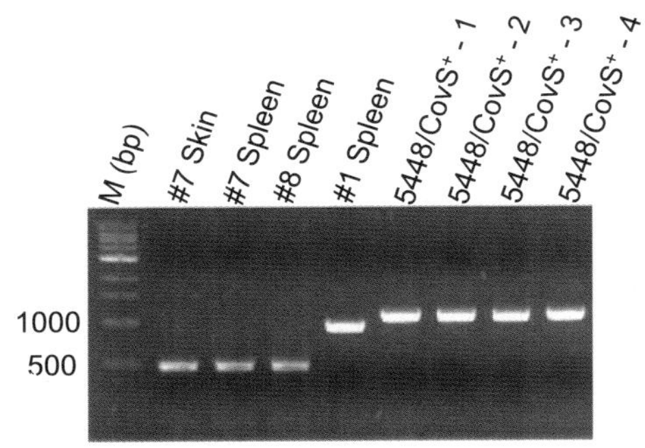

Figure 2. PCR of GAS 5448/covR⁺S⁺ inoculum prior to infection. Primers specific for regions of the *covS* gene that did not undergo mutations, but whose products would reveal the presence of a mutation, were used for PCR analysis. Genomic DNA isolated from overnight cultures of four different colonies of 5448/CovR⁺S⁺ was tested to determine if any mutations were present prior to injection. Mutant strains identified in this study were used as controls in lanes 2–5.
doi:10.1371/journal.pone.0100698.g002

found that the phage displayed a full-length *speA* gene in GAS *emm1* (5448), *emm3* (MGAS315), *emm6* (D471), and *emm18* (MGAS8232) (Fig. 3B). Other GAS strains, *e.g.*, *emm1* (SF370) and *emm5* (Manfredo), as well as the two closely related *emm53* serotype strains, AP53 and NS88.2, do not contain either of these particular prophage DNA inserts (Fig. 3B). The parent nonclonal *emm1* strain of 5448, *viz.*, SF370, also did not express *sda1* or *speA* (Fig. 3A,B). Thus, the genes, *sda1* and *speA*, originate from different phage insertions [32], of which 0, 1, or both can exist in other GAS strains, along with other types of prophage acquisitions.

We next sought to determine whether the virulence incorporated into the clonal GAS 5448 by the prophage encoded genes, and/or the particular M1 protein, was responsible for CovS⁺ switching. Both possibilities have been brought forward [33,34]. Therefore, a variant of the human isolate, AP53/*covS*⁻, was employed which was generated by reinsertion of the deleted T[1404]

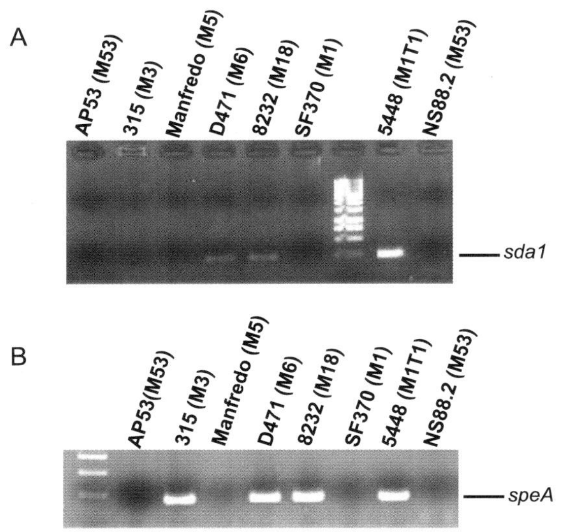

Figure 3. PCR of gDNA. Primers specific for the (A) *sda1* gene and (B) *speA* gene were used for PCR analysis of genomic DNA. The GAS strains employed are indicated in the figure along with the *emm* serotype for each of these strains (in parenthesis). M refers to the molecular size marker.

into this *covS*⁻ to restore WT CovS⁺ and provide AP53/CovR⁺S⁺ [21], which is not virulent in the mouse model used [35], to assess whether *covS* switching can reoccur in a nonvirulent GAS strain. This variant not only possesses an intact *covS*⁺ gene, but also does not contain the prophage-inserted genes, *sda1* and *speA* [35], and has a very different functional M-protein, *emm53*, than the M-protein, *emm1*, found in GAS 5448. In the case of AP53/CovS⁺ infections, we only examined GAS clones within the wound, using the same methodology described for study of 5448/CovR⁺S⁺. While, qualitatively, far fewer SpeB⁻ clones were observed *via* screening (~5–10% of the total), five different CovS⁻ variants in five different mouse wounds, initiated through subcutaneous administration AP53/CovR⁺S⁺, were randomly identified. These mutants were positioned in a narrow range of the C-terminal translated sequence of CovS (Table 3), thus showing some mutagenic preference for this area of the gene, at least in this GAS strain. These mouse mutants are in addition to the original patient isolate, AP53/*covS*⁻, which contains a sixth known *covS* inactivating mutation, specifically an in-frame deletion of T[1404] in *covS*, generating a premature stop codon in *covS* at amino acid sequence position-469 [21]. Thus, CovS switching occurs with variable frequencies independent of the nature of the M-proteins and independent of the presence of the prophage genes, *sda1* and *speA*. While switching in these latter types of GAS may represent more rare events, it nonetheless explains the appearance of *covS*⁻ genes, and the appearance of clonal virulent strains that have emerged from different types of nonvirulent strains of GAS. However, while the type of M-protein may not govern phase switching, a M-protein is required for CovS switching, since we found no SpeB⁻ isolates after several AP53/CovS⁺/ΔM53 infections.

Identification of covS mutants in GAS Mandfredo/CovR⁺S⁺/emm5 infections

The possibility of phase switching was also assessed in the more avirulent GAS Mandfredo/CovR⁺S⁺ strain that contains a fibrinogen binding M5 protein, and did not incorporate phage-encoded SpeA or Sda1 (Fig. 3). After infection, no lethality or deep tissue dissemination was observed. Thus, we screened GAS at the wound site and found a low percentage (<3%) of SpeB⁻ clones, which were randomly sequenced. The data show (Table 4) that switching to CovS⁻ strains did occur at the wound site. In one mouse, a SpeB⁻ clone (#1) with a truncation mutation was found near the amino-terminus. In a second mouse three SpeB⁻ clones were found with an in-frame deletion of Lys-263. Of interest, this single amino acid deletion abrogated SpeB production. In this same mouse, another SpeB⁻ clone was found with a five nucleotide deletion that was translated to a stop codon at amino acid 407. Comparison of survival of Manfredo/CovR⁺S⁺ with Manfredo CovR⁺S⁻ (clone #3, Table 4) did not show a significant difference (Fig. 4C), suggesting that in this low virulence strain, the inactivation of CovS is insufficient in itself to generate a hypervirulent strain of GAS.

Mouse survival is diminished in covS⁻ switched strains of GAS

To prove that these CovS⁻ mutants were capable of high virulence, some of the isolated strains were examined for lethality in C57Bl/6[hPg(Tg)] mice. It has been shown that a WT *covS* gene (CovS⁺) indirectly represses expression of a number of virulence factors, including SK, HasABC, and SLO [36,37], and ineffective CovS regulation of CovR leads to an increase in virulence and death [21]. In the case of GAS 5448/CovR⁺S⁺, the two mouse-

Table 3. Mutations found in *covS* gene of GAS strain AP53/*covS*$^+$ during infection.

AP53 Clone	Tissue	#Mice or Humans with Mutation	Gene Mutation	NT[a]	# bp[b]	Protein Mutation[c]
1[d]	Mouse Skin	1	In-frame replacement	1205	12	Stop-406
2[d]	Mouse Skin	1	Frame-shift replacement (1 bp insert)	1205	20	Stop-410
3	Mouse Skin	1	Single bp replacement	1162	1	Stop-388
4	Mouse Skin	1	Frame-shift deletion	1432-1453	22	Stop-497
5	Mouse Skin	1	In-frame replacement	1399	1	Stop-467
6	Human Invasive Wound	1	Deletion	1404	1	Stop-469

[a]Nucleotide (NT) position of change based on position of *covS* start codon, ATG.
[b]Number of nucleotides of WT-*covS* replaced, inserted, or deleted.
[c]Effect on CovS protein.
[d]1 and 2 were isolated from wounds in the same mouse.

passaged CovS$^-$ mutant strains tested here showed a small, but clear ($p<0.05$), decrease in mouse survival relative to the 5448/CovS$^+$ strain (Fig. 4A). This is not unexpected, as this strain contains the inserted prophage virulence enhancer genes, *speA* and *sdaI*, rendering 5448/CovR$^+$S$^+$ a highly virulent strain. Nonetheless, the lack of a WT *covS*$^+$ gene appears to provide an increased ability of GAS to infect and kill their host, with all 5448/CovR$^+$S$^+$ injected mice expiring within five days and all 5448/CovR$^+$S$^-$ injected mice, infected with clones #12 (skin) or #14 (skin), expiring within three days.

Since the 5448/CovR$^+$S$^+$ strain was already highly lethal prior to mouse passage, another GAS strain, AP53/CovR$^+$S$^+$, was examined, which does not show lethality in this model [35], and does not possess prophage-expressed SdaI or SpeA, to assess the effects of MP CovS$^-$ isolates on its virulence. The example MP GAS chosen for virulence studies was clone #4 of Table 3. The survival data show that clone #4 was as virulent as the human-passaged AP53/CovR$^+$S$^-$, with all mice expiring within 2 days (Fig. 4B). AP53/CovR$^+$S$^+$-infected mice remained viable in this model, as shown earlier. These data demonstrate that after

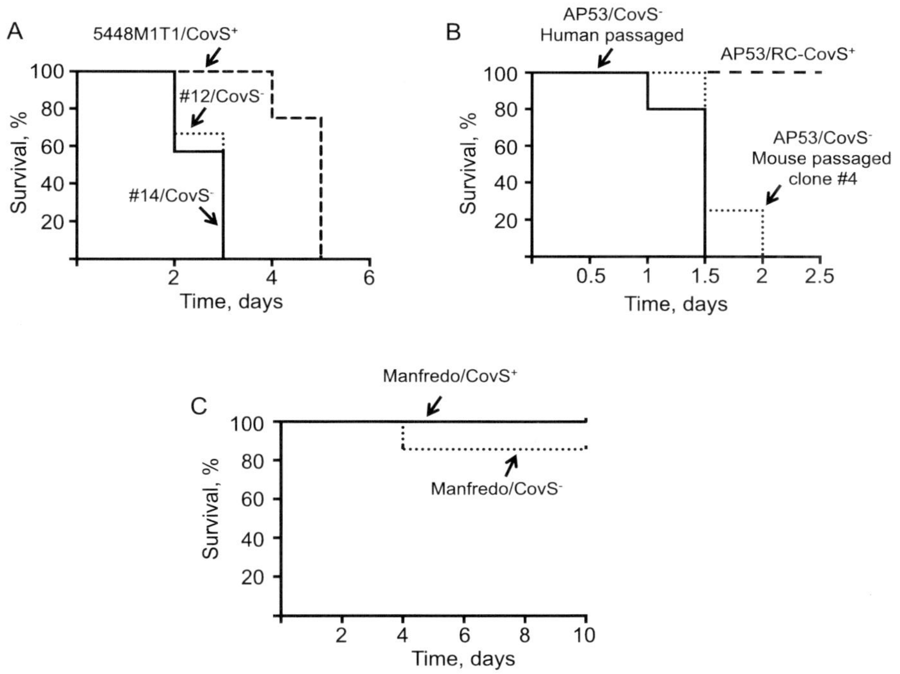

Figure 4. Survival of hPg-transgenic mice after infection with mouse-passaged GAS strains. C57Bl/6[hPg(Tg)] male mice (6–10 weeks of age) containing the hPg transgene were injected subcutaneously with GAS cells and the mice were monitored for death as an end-point. (A) 5448/CovR$^+$S$^+$/M1$^+$, and mouse-passaged 5448/CovR$^+$S$^-$/M1$^+$ strains #12 (skin) and #14 (skin). A total of 1.2×10^7 cells were injected. $P<0.05$ when comparing the wild-type strain to the two MP strains. (B) AP53/CovR$^+$S$^-$/M53$^+$ (human passaged) and AP53/CovR$^+$S$^-$/M53$^+$ clonal strain #4 (Table 3) obtained after mouse passaging of AP53/CovR$^+$S$^+$/M53$^+$. A dose of 1×10^8 cells was injected. $P<0.05$ when comparing the covS$^+$ strain to the human passaged or mouse passaged covS mutants. (C) Manfredo/CovR$^+$S$^+$/M5$^+$ and Manfredo/CovR$^+$S$^-$/M5$^+$ clonal strain #3 (Table 4) obtained after mouse passaging of Manfredo/CovR$^+$S$^+$/M5$^+$. A total of 1.4×10^7 cells were injected. These two curves were not statistically different. N = 4–8 mice for each tested strain.

Table 4. Mutations found in *covS* gene of GAS strain Manfredo M5/*covS*$^{+}$ during infection.

Mouse #	Tissue	Gene Mutation	NT[a]	# bp[b]	Protein Mutation[c]
1	Mouse Skin	Truncation	83	1	Stop-36
2	Mouse Skin	In-frame deletion	787–789	3	Delete K263
3	Mouse Skin	In-frame deletion	787–789	3	Delete K263
4	Mouse Skin	In-frame deletion	787–789	3	Delete K263
5	Mouse Skin	Deletion	1215–1219	5	Stop-407

[a]Nucleotide (NT) position of change based on position of *covS* start codon, ATG.
[b]Number of nucleotides of WT-*covS* replaced, inserted, or deleted.
[c]Effect on CovS protein.

infection, nonvirulent GAS can undergo switching, *via* transcriptional regulatory gene alterations, to provide hypervirulent strains, and that this mechanism is a critical evolutionary adaptation of GAS for survival in the human host.

DNase activity and transcription are enhanced in phase switched GAS

Extracellular DNase activity has been shown to be essential for degradation of neutrophil extracellular DNA traps (NETs), and CovS^{-} mutants of 5448 displayed an increased amount of DNase activity in their supernatants [34]. Upon examination of the DNase activity of the LP growth supernatants of MP clonal isolates #12 (skin) and #14 (skin), it is clear that calf thymus DNA was much more efficiently degraded in these strains than the supernatants from the WT CovR^{+}S^{+} strain (Fig. 5A), the latter of which is near the negative control (THY media only). These results demonstrate that the increased DNase activity exhibited by CovS^{-} mutants of 5448 contribute significantly to this end-point of the host immune response.

To show that the increased DNase activity, shown in Figure 5A, of MP mutants #12 and #14, was consistent with increased DNase activity of the specific nuclease, Sda1, mRNA levels of the *sda1* gene were measured using RT-PCR. Total RNA was isolated from 5448/CovR^{+}S^{+}, and the two representative 5448/CovR^{+}S^{-} MP mutants, #12 and #14, and assayed with primers specific for *sda1*, along with a reference gene, *gapdh* (*plr*). It is clear from Figure 5B that the expression ratios of *sda1* in the two mutant strains are much higher, by ~6-fold, when compared to the level of *sda1* in 5448/CovR^{+}S^{+} cultures. Increased expression of *sda1* correlates with increased enzymatic DNase activity observed in Figure 5A, and confirms the role of CovS in *sda1* gene regulation.

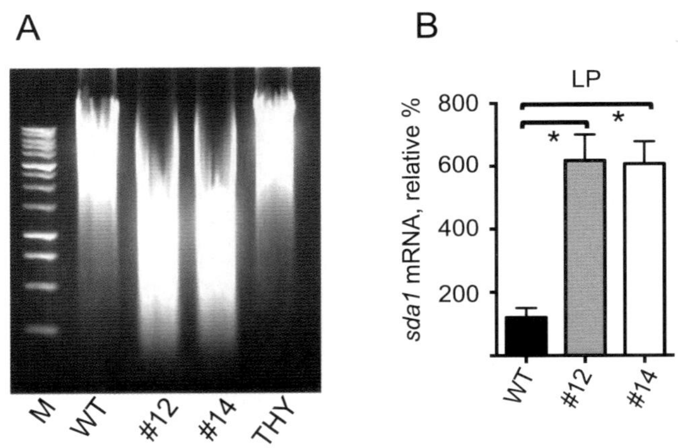

Figure 5. DNase activity and transcript levels in WT-5448/CovR^{+}S^{+} and mouse-passaged clones of 5448/CovR^{+}S^{-} in culture supernatants. (A) Cultures of WT-5448/CovR^{+}S^{+} and clonal mouse-passaged 5448/CovR^{+}S^{-} isolates #12 (skin) and #14 (skin) were grown to mid-log phase (LP; A_{600nm} ~0.6) and their supernatants monitored for DNase activity. Supernatants were incubated with 1 µg of calf thymus DNA for 5 min at 37°C. DNase activity was confirmed by visualizing DNA fragmentation by ethidium bromide staining and UV-light detection. THY in lane 5 represents the negative control. *B*, The effect of mouse-passaged GAS 5448 on *sda1* gene expression is shown using mRNA isolated from washed cells harvested at mid-log phase (LP; A_{600nm} ~0.6) and early stationary phase (SP; A_{600nm} ~1.2) growth. WT-5448/CovR^{+}S^{+} and mouse-passaged isolates (5448/CovR^{+}S^{-}) #12 (skin) and #14 (skin) were employed. The relative % gene expression levels of the mouse-passaged strains are relative to those in WT-5448/CovR^{+}S^{+}.

CovS inactivating mutations diminish SpeB expression and enhance SK activity

The levels of SpeB and SK activities were determined in both WT 5448/CovR^{+}S^{+} and mouse-passaged strain #12 (5448/CovR^{+}S^{-}) at various stages of cell growth that spanned early log-phase (LP; A_{600nm} = 0.6) through stationary phase (SP; A_{600nm} = 1.2). Figure 6A shows that SpeB activity is only observed in the WT 5448 CovR^{+}S^{+} strain grown to SP. SpeB is not observed to any great extent at any time during cell growth of the MP strain, 5448/CovR^{+}S^{-} clone #12.

Figure 6B shows the amounts of SK activity present in the culture supernatants of the M1T1, determined as initial rates of hPg activation by conditioned GAS culture supernatants removed at various stages of growth. SK levels in supernatants of 5448/CovR^{+}S^{-} clone #12 are higher at all growth stages than WT-5448/CovR^{+}S^{+} in conditioned media and is primarily produced during log-phase (LP) growth. While *ska* mRNA levels increase ~5-fold in two separate clones of MP strains 5448/CovR^{+}S^{-} #12 and #14 in cells extracted at mid-LP, little detectable *ska* mRNA is present in 5448/CovR^{+}S^{-} cell extracts at early-SP (Fig. 6C). Thus, little new SK expression occurs during SP growth of 5448/CovR^{+}S^{-}. The fact that SK protein levels are high at SP growth of 5448/CovR^{+}S^{-} (Fig. 6B) is due to a combination of the accumulated SK during growth and the fact that SpeB, which is known to degrade active SK [38], is greatly reduced in 5448/CovR^{+}S^{-} at all growth times. Thus, downregulation of SpeB in culture supernatants of 5448/CovR^{+}S^{-}, allows SK to persist during the SP in these latter supernatants.

To ascertain that control of other virulence genes is sustained during MP of the WT-5448 strain, and to provide credible evidence, to the extent practicable, that only *covS* is undergoing *in*

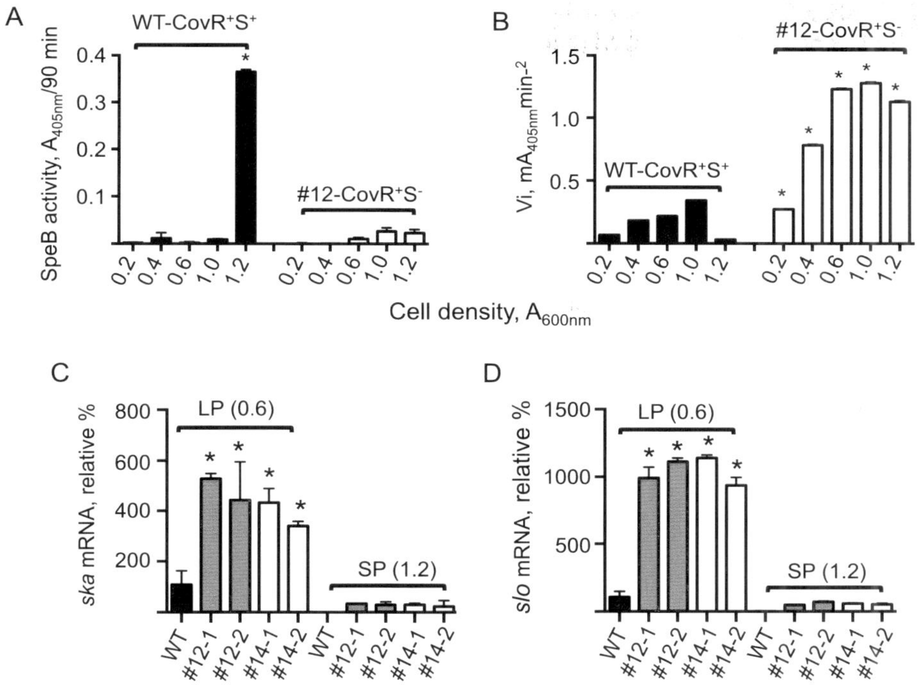

Figure 6. Gene expression in WT-5448/CovR$^+$S$^+$ and mouse-passaged clones of 5448/CovR$^+$S$^-$ in cells and in culture supernatants. (A) Levels of SpeB enzymatic activity measured spectrophotometrically in conditioned culture supernatants of WT-5448/CovR$^+$S$^+$ and mouse-passaged 5448-CovR$^+$S$^-$ strain #12 (skin) from Table 2. Aliquots of the supernatants were sampled at various cell densities, measured as A_{600nm}. 5448/CovR$^+$S$^+$ shows the highest amount of SpeB activity when grown to early-SP (A_{600nm} = 1.2). Very little SpeB is measured during LP (A_{600nm} = 0.2–1.0). The data are expressed as A_{405nm}, reflecting hydrolysis of the chromogenic substrate, after 90 min incubation. (B) Initial rates (V_i) of hPg activation by culture supernatants sampled at various cell densities, reflecting SK activity in WT-5448/CovR$^+$S$^+$ and mouse-passaged 5448/CovR$^+$S$^-$ strain #12 (skin). Higher amounts of SK are present in conditioned culture media of 5448/CovR$^+$S$^-$ strain #12 than in that obtained from growth of WT-5448/CovR$^+$S$^+$. *$P<0.01$ in a two-tailed comparison of each measurement between WT-5448/CovR$^+$S$^+$ and 5448/CovR$^+$S$^-$ strain #12 at the same cell densities. (C-D) The effect of mouse-passaged GAS 5448 on (C) *ska* and (D) *slo* gene transcription. Total RNA was isolated from washed cells harvested at mid-LP (A_{600nm} ~0.6) and early-SP (A_{600nm} ~1.2) growth. WT-5448/CovR$^+$S$^+$ and 2 independent clones from mouse-passaged 5448/CovR$^+$S$^-$ #12 (#12-1 and #12-2) and #14 (#14-1 and #14-2) were employed for the RT-PCR assays. The % gene expression levels the mouse-passaged strains are relative to those in WT-5448/CovR$^+$S$^+$.

vivo mutagenesis, the levels of an additional extracellular virulence-determinant, *viz.*, the toxin gene, *slo*, were determined in the MP strains. The *slo* gene encodes its product, streptolysin-O (SLO), an extracellular membrane pore-forming cytolysin that enhances another end-point of GAS virulence, *viz.*, the killing of host immune cells [39]. It is expected that this gene would be upregulated in GAS strains with enhanced virulence. As predicted, the data of Figure 6D show that the *slo* mRNA levels of two separate clones of MP GAS 5448/CovR$^+$S$^-$ #12 and 5448/CovR$^+$S$^-$ #14, grown to mid-LP (A_{600nm} ~0.6), are highly upregulated, by ~10 fold, as compared to WT-5448/CovR$^+$S$^+$ at the same growth stage. These data further show that *slo* mRNA is severely downregulated in each of these cell lines as growth proceeds to SP (A_{600nm} ~1.2). At this latter point of growth, the mRNA levels of *slo* are severely depressed in both WT 5448/CovR$^+$S$^+$ and clones #12 and #14 of 5448/CovR$^+$S$^-$.

Discussion and Conclusions

Many of the genes critical for GAS adherence, attachment, and invasion of its host are regulated by the CovRS system. In addition, this regulatory system affects genes involved in eliciting and evading immune responses [2,35]. Hyperinvasive clinical isolates have been found to contain mutations in the *covS* gene, primarily causing a truncation in the protein with resulting loss of activity and, thus, regulatory function. Under non-stress conditions, CovR represses many virulence genes, and, with CovS inactivating mutants, CovR repression is shifted to a different set of targets, important among these is the extracellular cysteine protease, SpeB. SpeB has been associated with the degradation of a number of protein targets, originating from the host and from GAS, such as complement proteins, SK, and M-protein [38,40,41]. This combination of up-regulation of bacterial virulence, *e.g.*, assisting the bacteria with penetration of the host extracellular matrix, and reduction of SpeB mediated degradation of GAS virulence determinants increases persistence of many virulence-associated gene products and also suggests that this protease must be upregulated and downregulated at different times of infection in some strains. Clearly an additional advantage of SpeB expression would occur during an invasive phase since SpeB has been shown to degrade epithelial tight junction proteins [42]. Thus, selection for SpeB$^-$, *via* CovS inactivating mutations, is a result of the bacterial evolution that assists its survival [33]. These types of mechanisms have allowed clonal variants of invasive GAS to develop and persist, accounting for the numerous hypervirulent strains that continue to be identified.

The majority of *covS* mutants thus far isolated have resulted in premature truncations in CovS that are contained in the HisKA or HATPase regionsat the C-terminal domains of CovS [8,10,33,34]. Even if such truncated versions of CovS are expressed, this sensor would not have the ability to be phosphorylated, and thus could not regulate transcription *via* CovR. In addition, mutations in the *covR* gene have also been observed, the majority of which are point mutations that are believed to have no effects on DNA binding, but CovS phosphorylation is seemingly influenced [29,43]. Differences have also been observed between full *covS* gene inactivations and animal-passaged generated *covS* mutants [44], suggesting that perhaps the remaining *covS* has retained some function, or the possibility that other gene changes take place during passage. Regardless, the goal of this work was to determine whether particular mutations in *covS* are favored after animal passage, and if a mechanism for such SpeB switching could be established.

In the case of hypervirulent M1T1 strain 5448/CovS$^+$, mutations observed in our controlled study consisted primarily of either insertions or deletions of nucleotides. Deletions of single nucleotides or up to as many as 612 were observed. The insertions ranged from 1 to 31 nucleotides, and the larger insertions appear to be repeated sequences from the gene itself. For example, in mouse-passage strain #4, a clone is found with an 11 bp insertion at position 96, with the sequence GCATTTTCTCT. This sequence is a repeat of the full-length sequence immediately upstream. Previous studies have shown very similar mutations occurring in this same region, such as a reported 11 bp insert at position 103 from a CovS-deficient strain isolated from the blood of a patient with an infection [45]. A similar CovS mutant GAS strain was isolated from an animal-passage study that contained an 11 bp insert at position 99 [10]. In both cases, the inserts create repeated sequences that result in frame-shifts and premature truncation of the *covS* gene. GAS 5448 mutant clones #13 and #14 from this study contain a 31-nucleotide insertion, that, while not identical, are very similar to the sequence around the insertion location.

In addition to the large insertions, a number of mutants have been isolated with deleted regions of *covS*. The most common mutants represented in the literature involve deletion of 1–2 bp, although a number of others have been found with 5–10 bp deletions. In this work, mutants were recovered with deletions of > 600 bp. This type of deletion allows for the possibility that during replication, strand separation and re-annealing of *covS* leads to some secondary structure formation resulting in misalignment. This type of slipped-strand mismatching is a common mechanism of phase variation in other bacterial species, and often arises in areas rich in simple sequence repeats (SSRs) or variable-nucleotide tandem repeats (VNTRs) [46]. Slipped-strand mismatching could explain both large and small insertions and deletions. It was recently shown that GAS strains that lack a 12 bp tandem repeat in the multiple gene regulator of GAS, *viz*., the *mga* promoter region, were asymptomatic carrier strains, whereas strains with a 12 bp tandem repeat were much more virulent. This suggests a means to regulate the degree of infection via such a mechanism [47]. Here, we observe that 5448/*covS* mutants #12, #13, and #14 contain these VNTRs. In contrast to the *mga* inserts that result in modified regulation upstream of the coding sequence, *covS* coding region insertions and deletions result in truncation of the transcript and a non-functional protein, thus allowing for another type of phase variation mechanism in GAS.

It has been shown that SpeB switching can occur in a number of GAS strains and appears to occur independently of the M-protein-type [9]. Our studies are in accord with this and show that 5448/CovR$^+$S$^+$/M1, AP53/CovR$^+$S$^+$/M53, as well as Manfredo/M5, three diverse M proteins, generate CovS$^-$ mutants. Also, neither AP53/CovR$^+$S$^+$ nor Manfredo M5/CovR$^+$S$^+$ contain the prophage lysogenic inserts that express Sda1 or SpeA, two widely accepted virulence factors that have been implicated in CovS$^+$ phase switching. Since CovS switching occurs in AP53/CovR$^+$S$^+$ and Manfredo M5/CovR$^+$S$^+$, albeit at much lower rates than 5448/CovR$^+$S$^+$, it is obvious that these particular prophage genes are not absolute requirements for phase switching, although these genes may facilitate such events by being more inherently virulent and evading host defenses more effectively, thus exposing the bacteria to different compartments of the host and longer survival times in infected tissue. Also, considering the fact that AP53/CovR$^+$S$^-$ displays an invasive phenotype in a human CovS$^-$ isolate, and in mice, it is clear that the virulent strain of AP53 is derived from the nonvirulent parent strain through CovS inactivating mutations. This conclusion is consistent with that of a previous study [7]. However, when the skin was infected with AP53/CovR$^+$S$^+$/ΔPAM, no evidence for SpeB$^-$ clones in the skin wounds was found. Thus, M-protein, directly or indirectly, is necessary for this switching, but its exact nature may be less important.

Of the CovS$^+$ strains examined, the M1T1 strain has a high propensity to phase switch from CovS$^+$ to CovS$^-$. While it was initially thought that the *sda1* gene, present in virulent *emm1* M1T1 strains, was critical for this switching mechanism to occur [8], insertion of the same gene into another non-virulent *emm1* strain, SF370, did not enhance its ability to switch to SpeB$^-$, at least not at a high rate [31]. In addition to *sda1* and M-protein (*emm*), hyaluronic acid synthesis genes (*hasABC*) are believed to be important for the SpeB-switch to take place [34], likely by a more encapsulated GAS subverting host killing. Overall, the mechanism of how such genes enable the switching to occur more readily is unclear, although the ability to evade neutrophil phagocytosis and the host immune system seem to be critical. It is also unclear as to the properties of the M1T1 that confer a higher propensity to switch compared to other GAS strains, other than a possible role for enhanced virulence in a CovS$^+$ strain.

In the MP CovS$^-$ mutants, it was also determined whether other virulence genes were susceptible to mutation. Although a genome-wide analysis of GAS indicated that a 7 bp frameshift in CovS was sufficient to enhance survival during phagocytosis and to evade killing by polymorphonuclear cells [7] nonetheless, we assessed CovRS-responsive genes, *sda1*, *ska*, and *slo*, and indirectly *emm* and *hasABC*. None of these important GAS virulence genes underwent mutagenesis during MP, as determined by RT-PCR and/or protein analyses, and their expressions were controlled by CovRS. While, of course other genes that were not examined could undergo mutagenesis, it was felt that a good sampling was obtained by these choices of genes. However, since highly virulent GAS is either a laboratory-engineered strain generated from less virulent animal isolates, which are usually CovR$^+$S$^+$, or obtained as highly virulent isolates, which are usually CovR$^+$S$^-$, or are derived from isolates that contain virulent prophage inserts, *e.g.*, Sda1$^+$/SpeA$^+$, many gene changes have occurred in the animal host that are highly varied. Despite this, one general change that does occur in animal passage is CovS$^+$ switching to many types of CovS$^-$, and mechanisms that illuminate this point are of particular value.

While the AP53 strain showed a very large effect of CovS$^-$ gene switching on virulence, as defined by death, the Manfredo strain did not show such an effect. This latter low virulence strain did not gain in this property as a result of CovS switching. There are many stages involved between infection and death that could require gene interactions between the host and microbe, and which may depend upon the total genetic architecture of the particular GAS strain. This fertile area requires study to reveal the mechanisms involved in overall virulence of the GAS.

In conclusion, the *covRS* operon appears to be a particular mutagenic target within the bacterial genome, and all regions of the *covS* gene are susceptible to mutations that inactivate this sensor component of this operon and thus assist GAS virulence. In addition to *covRS*, other such genomic mutagenesis targets exist in regulatory TCS genes [48], *e.g.*, *fasBCAX* and *ihk/irr*, and one-component gene regulators, *e.g.*, *rgg* [49], *ralp* [50], and *mga* [51]. While exceptions exist, overall, it is generally agreed that mutations found in such regulatory systems result in hypervirulent strains of GAS, and that these mutations arise under the selective pressures of survival in a host. The ability of GAS and other Gram+ pathogens to undergo selection *in vivo* leading to altered phenotypes is of high clinical significance. Bacteria are able to colonize human hosts for long periods of time. Thus, a greater understanding of the triggers and mechanisms that allow them to become more virulent is of significance to global health and to vaccine development.

Author Contributions

Conceived and designed the experiments: FC VP ZL. Performed the experiments: JM GA DD SL ZL. Analyzed the data: ZL JM GA DD SL FC. Contributed to the writing of the manuscript: JM VP FC.

References

1. Gao R, Stock AM (2009) Biological insights from structures of two-component proteins. Annu Rev Microbiol 63: 133–154.
2. Graham MR, Smoot LM, Migliaccio CA, Virtaneva K, Sturdevant DE, et al. (2002) Virulence control in group A Streptococcus by a two-component gene regulatory system: global expression profiling and in vivo infection modeling. Proc Natl Acad Sci USA 99: 13855–13860.
3. Dalton TL, Scott JR (2004) CovS inactivates CovR and is required for growth under conditions of general stress in Streptococcus pyogenes. J Bacteriol 186: 3928–3937.
4. Tran-Winkler HJ, Love JF, Gryllos I, Wessels MR (2011) Signal transduction through CsrRS confers an invasive phenotype in group A Streptococcus. PLoS Pathog 7: e1002361.
5. Churchward G (2007) The two faces of Janus: virulence gene regulation by CovR/S in group A streptococci. Mol Microbiol 64: 34–41.
6. Cole JN, Barnett TC, Nizet V, Walker MJ (2011) Molecular insight into invasive group A streptococcal disease. Nat Rev Microbiol 9: 724–736.
7. Sumby P, Whitney AR, Graviss EA, DeLeo FR, Musser JM (2006) Genome-wide analysis of group a streptococci reveals a mutation that modulates global phenotype and disease specificity. PLoS Pathog 2: e5.
8. Walker MJ, Hollands A, Sanderson-Smith ML, Cole JN, Kirk JK, et al. (2007) DNase Sda1 provides selection pressure for a switch to invasive group A streptococcal infection. Nat Med 13: 981–985.
9. Maamary PG, Sanderson-Smith ML, Aziz RK, Hollands A, Cole JN, et al. (2010) Parameters governing invasive disease propensity of non-M1 serotype group A streptococci. J Innate Immun 2: 596–606.
10. Maamary PG, Ben-Zakour NL, Cole JN, Hollands A, Aziz RK, et al. (2012) Tracing the evolutionary history of the pandemic group A streptococcal M1T1 clone. FASEB J 26: 4675–4684.
11. Tatsuno I, Okada R, Zhang Y, Isaka M, Hasegawa T (2013) Partial loss of CovS function in Streptococcus pyogenes causes severe invasive disease. BMC Res Notes 6: 126.
12. Nomizu M, Pietrzynski G, Kato T, Lachance P, Menard R, et al. (2001) Substrate specificity of the streptococcal cysteine protease. J Biol Chem 276: 44551–44556.
13. Carroll RK, Shelburne SA, Olsen RJ, Suber B, Sahasrabhojane P, et al. (2011) Naturally occurring single amino acid replacements in a regulatory protein alter streptococcal gene expression and virulence in mice. J Clin Invest 121: 1956–1968.
14. Barnett TC, Liebl D, Seymour LM, Gillen CM, Lim JY, et al. (2013) The globally disseminated M1T1 clone of group A Streptococcus evades autophagy for intracellular replication. Cell Host Microbe 14: 675–682.
15. Aziz RK, Pabst MJ, Jeng A, Kansal R, Low DE, et al. (2004) Invasive M1T1 group A Streptococcus undergoes a phase-shift in vivo to prevent proteolytic degradation of multiple virulence factors by SpeB. Mol Microbiol 51: 123–134.
16. Chatellier S, Ihendyane N, Kansal RG, Khambaty F, Basma H, et al. (2000) Genetic relatedness and superantigen expression in group A streptococcus serotype M1 isolates from patients with severe and nonsevere invasive diseases. Infect Immun 68: 3523–3534.
17. Miller L, Gray L, Beachey E, Kehoe M (1988) Antigenic variation among group A streptococcal M proteins. Nucleotide sequence of the serotype 5 M protein gene and its relationship with genes encoding types 6 and 24 M proteins. J Biol Chem 263: 5668–5673.
18. Musser JM, Hauser AR, Kim MH, Schlievert PM, Nelson K, et al. (1991) Streptococcus pyogenes causing toxic-shock-like syndrome and other invasive diseases: clonal diversity and pyrogenic exotoxin expression. Proc Natl Acad Sci, USA 88: 2668–2672.
19. Scott JR, Guenthner PC, Malone LM, Fischetti VA (1986) Conversion of an M-group A streptococcus to M+ by transfer of a plasmid containing an M6 gene. J Exp Med 164: 1641–1651.
20. Smoot JC, Barbian KD, Van Gompel JJ, Smoot LM, Chaussee MS, et al. (2002) Genome sequence and comparative microarray analysis of serotype M18 group A Streptococcus strains associated with acute rheumatic fever outbreaks. Proc Natl Acad Sci USA 99: 4668–4673.
21. Liang Z, Zhang Y, Agrahari G, Chandrahas V, Glinton K, et al. (2013) A natural inactivating mutation in the CovS component of the CovRS regulatory operon in a pattern D Streptococcal pyogenes strain influences virulence-associated genes. J Biol Chem 288: 6561–6573.
22. Sun H, Ringdahl U, Homeister JW, Fay WP, Engelberg NC, et al. (2004) Plasminogen is a critical host pathogenicity factor for Group A streptococcal infection. Science 305: 1283–1286.
23. Hollands A, Aziz RK, Kansal R, Kotb M, Nizet V, et al. (2008) A naturally occurring mutation in ropB suppresses SpeB expression and reduces M1T1 group A streptococcal systemic virulence. PLoS One 3: e4102.
24. Zhang Y, Liang Z, Hsueh HT, Ploplis VA, Castellino FJ (2012) Characterization of streptokinases from Group A streptococci reveals a strong functional relationship that supports the coinheritance of plasminogen-binding M-Protein and cluster 2b streptokinase. J Biol Chem 287: 42093–42103.
25. Brockway WJ, Castellino FJ (1972) Measurement of the binding of antifibrinolytic amino acids to various plasminogens. Arch Biochem Biophys 151: 194–199.
26. Walker JS (2003) Anti-inflammatory effects of opioids. Adv Exp Med Biol 521: 148–160.
27. Vachon P, Moreau JP (2002) Butorphanol decreases edema following carrageenan-induced paw inflammation in rats. Contemp Top Lab Anim Sci 41: 15–17.
28. Walker JS, Chandler AK, Wilson JL, Binder W, Day RO (1996) Effect of mu-opioids morphine and buprenorphine on the development of adjuvant arthritis in rats. Inflamm Res 45: 557–563.
29. Engleberg NC, Heath A, Miller A, Rivera C, DiRita VJ (2001) Spontaneous mutations in the CsrRS two-component regulatory system of Streptococcus pyogenes result in enhanced virulence in a murine model of skin and soft tissue infection. J Infect Dis 183: 1043–1054.
30. Ikebe T, Ato M, Matsumura T, Hasegawa H, Sata T, et al. (2010) Highly frequent mutations in negative regulators of multiple virulence genes in group A streptococcal toxic shock syndrome isolates. PLoS Pathog 6: e1000832.
31. Venturini C, Ong CL, Gillen CM, Ben-Zakour NL, Maamary PG, et al. (2013) Acquisition of the Sda1-encoding bacteriophage does not enhance virulence of the M1 Streptococcus pyogenes strain SF370. Infect Immun 81: 2062–2069.
32. Aziz RK, Edwards RA, Taylor WW, Low DE, McGeer A, et al. (2005) Mosaic prophages with horizontally acquired genes account for the emergence and diversification of the globally disseminated M1T1 clone of Streptococcus pyogenes. J Bacteriol 187: 3311–3318.
33. Aziz RK, Kansal R, Aronow BJ, Taylor WL, Rowe SL, et al. (2010) Microevolution of group A streptococci in vivo: capturing regulatory networks engaged in sociomicrobiology, niche adaptation, and hypervirulence. PLoS One 5: e9798.
34. Cole JN, Pence MA, von Köckritz-Blickwede M, Hollands A, Gallo RL, et al. (2010) M protein and hyaluronic acid capsule are essential for in vivo selection of covRS mutations characteristic of invasive serotype M1T1 group A Streptococcus. MBio 1: e00191–e00210.
35. Agrahari G, Liang Z, Mayfield JA, Balsara RD, Ploplis VA, et al. (2013) Complement-mediated opsonization of invasive Group A Streptococcus pyogenes strain AP53 is regulated by the bacterial two-component cluster of virulence responder/sensor (CovRS) system. J Biol Chem 288: 27494–27504.
36. Federle MJ, McIver KS, Scott JR (1999) A response regulator that represses transcription of several virulence operons in the group A streptococcus. J Bacteriol 181: 3649–3657.
37. Treviño J, Perez N, Ramirez-Peña E, Liu Z, Shelburne SA, et al. (2009) CovS simultaneously activates and inhibits the CovR-mediated repression of distinct subsets of group A Streptococcus virulence factor-encoding genes. Infect Immun 77: 3141–3149.
38. Rezcallah MS, Boyle MD, Sledjeski DD (2004) Mouse skin passage of Streptococcus pyogenes results in increased streptokinase expression and activity. Microbiology 150: 365–371.
39. Wannamaker LW (1983) Streptococcal toxins. Rev Infect Dis 5: S723–S732.
40. Raeder R, Woischnik M, Podbielski A, Boyle MD (1998) A secreted streptococcal cysteine protease can cleave a surface-expressed M1 protein and alter the immunoglobulin binding properties. Res Microbiol 149: 539–548.
41. Honda-Ogawa M, Ogawa T, Terao Y, Sumitomo T, Nakata M, et al. (2013) Cysteine proteinase from Streptococcus pyogenes enables evasion of innate

immunity via degradation of complement factors. J Biol Chem 288: 15854–15864.
42. Sumitomo T, Nakata M, Higashino M, Terao Y, Kawabata S (2013) Group A streptococcal cysteine protease cleaves epithelial junctions and contributes to bacterial translocation. J Biol Chem 288: 13317–13324.
43. Horstmann N, Sahasrabhojane P, Suber B, Kumaraswami M, Olsen RJ, et al. (2011) Distinct single amino acid replacements in the control of virulence regulator protein differentially impact streptococcal pathogenesis. PLoS Pathog 7: e1002311.
44. Kansal RG, Datta V, Aziz RK, Abdeltawab NF, Rowe S, et al. (2010) Dissection of the molecular basis for hypervirulence of an in vivo-selected phenotype of the widely disseminated M1T1 strain of group A Streptococcus bacteria. J Infect Dis 201: 855–865.
45. Garcia AF, Abe LM, Erdem G, Cortez CL, Kurahara D, et al. (2010) An insert in the covS gene distinguishes a pharyngeal and a blood isolate of Streptococcus pyogenes found in the same individual. Microbiology 156: 3085–3095.
46. Moxon R, Bayliss C, Hood D (2006) Bacterial contingency loci: the role of simple sequence DNA repeats in bacterial adaptation. Annu Rev Genet 40: 307–333.
47. Flores AR, Olsen RJ, Wunsche A, Kumaraswami M, Shelburne SA, et al. (2013) Natural variation in the promoter of the gene encoding the Mga regulator alters host-pathogen interactions in group a Streptococcus carrier strains. Infect Immun 81: 4128–4138.
48. Smoot LM, Smoot JC, Graham MR, Somerville GA, Sturdevant DE, et al. (2001) Global differential gene expression in response to growth temperature alteration in group A Streptococcus. Proc Natl Acad Sci USA 98: 10416–10421.
49. Kappeler KV, Anbalagan S, Dmitriev AV, McDowell EJ, Neely MN, et al. (2009) A naturally occurring Rgg variant in serotype M3 Streptococcus pyogenes does not activate speB expression due to altered specificity of DNA binding. Infect Immun 77: 5411–5417.
50. Le Breton Y, Mistry P, Valdes KM, Quigley J, Kumar N, et al. (2013) Genome-wide identification of genes required for fitness of group A Streptococcus in human blood. Infect Immun 81: 862–875.
51. McIver KS, Scott JR (1997) Role of mga in growth phase regulation of virulence genes of the group A streptococcus. J Bacteriol 179: 5178–5187.

Permissions

All chapters in this book were first published in PLOS ONE, by The Public Library of Science; hereby published with permission under the Creative Commons Attribution License or equivalent. Every chapter published in this book has been scrutinized by our experts. Their significance has been extensively debated. The topics covered herein carry significant findings which will fuel the growth of the discipline. They may even be implemented as practical applications or may be referred to as a beginning point for another development.

The contributors of this book come from diverse backgrounds, making this book a truly international effort. This book will bring forth new frontiers with its revolutionizing research information and detailed analysis of the nascent developments around the world.

We would like to thank all the contributing authors for lending their expertise to make the book truly unique. They have played a crucial role in the development of this book. Without their invaluable contributions this book wouldn't have been possible. They have made vital efforts to compile up to date information on the varied aspects of this subject to make this book a valuable addition to the collection of many professionals and students.

This book was conceptualized with the vision of imparting up-to-date information and advanced data in this field. To ensure the same, a matchless editorial board was set up. Every individual on the board went through rigorous rounds of assessment to prove their worth. After which they invested a large part of their time researching and compiling the most relevant data for our readers.

The editorial board has been involved in producing this book since its inception. They have spent rigorous hours researching and exploring the diverse topics which have resulted in the successful publishing of this book. They have passed on their knowledge of decades through this book. To expedite this challenging task, the publisher supported the team at every step. A small team of assistant editors was also appointed to further simplify the editing procedure and attain best results for the readers.

Apart from the editorial board, the designing team has also invested a significant amount of their time in understanding the subject and creating the most relevant covers. They scrutinized every image to scout for the most suitable representation of the subject and create an appropriate cover for the book.

The publishing team has been an ardent support to the editorial, designing and production team. Their endless efforts to recruit the best for this project, has resulted in the accomplishment of this book. They are a veteran in the field of academics and their pool of knowledge is as vast as their experience in printing. Their expertise and guidance has proved useful at every step. Their uncompromising quality standards have made this book an exceptional effort. Their encouragement from time to time has been an inspiration for everyone.

The publisher and the editorial board hope that this book will prove to be a valuable piece of knowledge for researchers, students, practitioners and scholars across the globe.

Contributors

Ching Wen Tseng, Pierre A. Kyme, Andrea Arruda and George Y. Liu
Division of Pediatric Infectious Diseases, Cedars-Sinai Medical Center, Los Angeles, California, United States of America
Department of Pediatrics, David Geffen School of Medicine, University of California Los Angeles, Los Angeles, California, United States of America
The Immunobiology Research Institute, Cedars-Sinai Medical Center, Los Angeles, California, United States of America

V. Krishnan Ramanujan and Wafa Tawackoli
Department of Surgery and Department of Biomedical Sciences, Cedars-Sinai Medical Center, Los Angeles, California, United States of America

Moez Berrich, Martine Monteil, Henri Jean Boulouis and Nadia Haddad
Unité Mixte de Recherche de Biologie Moléculaire et Immunologie Parasitaires et Fongiques, Ecole Nationale Vétérinaire d'Alfort, Université Paris-Est, Maisons-Alfort, France

Claudine Kieda, Catherine Grillon and Nathalie Lamerant
Unité Propre de Recherche 4301, Centre de Biophysique Molé culaire, Centre National de la Recherche Scientifique, Orléans, France

Julie Gavard
Unité 1016 Inserm, Institut Cochin, CNRS, Université Paris Descartes, Paris, France

John K. Davies
Department of Microbiology, Monash University, Clayton, Australia

Timothy P. Stinear
Department of Microbiology, Monash University, Clayton, Australia
Department of Microbiology and Immunology, University of Melbourne, Parkville, Australia

Kyra Y. L. Chua
Department of Microbiology, Monash University, Clayton, Australia,
Department of Microbiology and Immunology, University of Melbourne, Parkville, Australia
Department of Infectious Diseases, Austin Centre for Infection Research, Austin Health, Heidelberg, Australia

Benjamin P. Howden
Department of Microbiology, Monash University, Clayton, Australia,
Department of Microbiology and Immunology, University of Melbourne, Parkville, Australia
Department of Infectious Diseases, Austin Centre for Infection Research, Austin Health, Heidelberg, Australia
Department of Microbiology, Austin Health, Heidelberg, Australia

Torsten Seemann and Paul F. Harrison
Victorian Bioinformatics Consortium, Monash University, Clayton, Australia

Paul D. R. Johnson
Department of Infectious Diseases, Austin Centre for Infection Research, Austin Health, Heidelberg, Australia

Shaun Monagle
Department of Anatomical Pathology, Eastern Health, Box Hill, Australia

Tony M. Korman
Department of Infectious Diseases, Monash Medical Centre, Clayton, Australia

Geoffrey W. Coombs
Department of Microbiology and Infectious Diseases, PathWest Laboratory Medicine WA, Royal Perth Hospital, Perth, Australia

Brian O. Howden
Microsurgical Consultants, Blackburn, Australia

Luyang Cao, Chao Dai, Zhongjie Li, Zheng Fan, Yu Song, Yingliang Wu, Zhijian Cao and Wenxin Li
State Key Laboratory of Virology, College of Life Sciences, Wuhan University, Wuhan, P. R. China

Jann-Tay Wang, Yee-Chun Chen and Shan-Chwen Chang
Department of Internal Medicine, National Taiwan University Hospital, National Taiwan University, Taipei, Taiwan

Jiun-Ling Wang
Department of Internal Medicine, National Taiwan University Hospital, National Taiwan University, Taipei, Taiwan
Department of Internal Medicine, E-Da Hospital/IShou University, Kaohsiung County, Taiwan

Shey-Ying Chen
Department of Emergency Medicine, National Taiwan University Hospital, National Taiwan University, Taipei, Taiwan

Tamar Lasky
MIE Resources, Kingston, Rhode Island, United States of America

Jay Greenspan
Thomas Jefferson University, Nemours Children's Clinics, Wilmington, Delaware, United States of America

Frank R. Ernst
Clinical and Outcomes Research, Premier Research Services, Premier Healthcare Alliance, Charlotte, North Carolina, United States of America

Liliana Gonzalez
Computer Science and Statistics, University of Rhode Island, Kingston, Rhode Island, United States of America

Yurong Zhang, Amy Tong, Batu K. Sharma-Kuinkel, Thomas Rude, Sun Hee Ahn and Felicia Ruffin
Division of Infectious Diseases, Department of Medicine, Duke University Medical Center, Durham, North Carolina, United States of America

Vance G. Fowler Jr
Division of Infectious Diseases, Department of Medicine, Duke University Medical Center, Durham, North Carolina, United States of America
Duke Clinical Research Institute, Durham, North Carolina, United States of America

Supaporn Lamlertthon
Division of Infectious Diseases, Department of Medicine, Duke University Medical Center, Durham, North Carolina, United States of America
Naresuan University, Phitsanulok, Phitsanulok Province, Thailand

Steven Y. C. Tong
Division of Infectious Diseases, Department of Medicine, Duke University Medical Center, Durham, North Carolina, United States of America
Menzies School of Health Research, Darwin, Northern Territory, Australia

Lily Llorens, Ganesh Tamarana, Donald Biek and Ian Critchley
Cerexa, Inc., Oakland, California, United States of America

Janine Arnott, Hannah Hesselgreaves and Bridget Young
Institute of Psychology, Health and Society, University of Liverpool, Liverpool, United Kingdom

Anthony J. Nunn and Matthew Peak
Alder Hey Children's National Health Service Foundation Trust, Liverpool, United Kingdom

Munir Pirmohamed and Rosalind L. Smyth
Institute of Translational Medicine, University of Liverpool, Liverpool, United Kingdom

Mark A. Turner
Institute of Translational Medicine, Liverpool Women's National Health Service Foundation Trust and University of Liverpool, Liverpool, United Kingdom

Urszula Lipinska, Katleen Hermans, Lieve Meulemans and Freddy Haesebrouck
Department of Pathology, Bacteriology and Avian Diseases, Faculty of Veterinary Medicine, Ghent University, Merelbeke, Belgium

Luc Duchateau
Department of Physiology and Biometry, Faculty of Veterinary Medicine, Ghent University, Merelbeke, Belgium

Cedric Badiou
Centre National de Référence des Staphylocoques, Université Lyon 1, Lyon, France
INSERM U851, IFR128, Lyon, France

Oana Dumitrescu, Jerome Etienne and Gerard Lina
Centre National de Référence des Staphylocoques, Université Lyon 1, Lyon, France
INSERM U851, IFR128, Lyon, France
Hospices Civils de Lyon, Lyon, France

Philipp Warnke, Liesa Warning and Andreas Podbielski
Institute of Medical Microbiology, Virology, and Hygiene, Rostock University Hospital, Rostock, Germany

Muya Shu, Yanhan Wang, Sherwin Kuo, Alvin Coda and Richard L. Gallo
Division of Dermatology, Department of Medicine, University of California San Diego, La Jolla, California, United States of America

Jinghua Yu
Sanford-Burnham Institute for Medical Research, La Jolla, California, United States of America

Yong Jiang
Surface Bioadvances Inc., San Diego, California, United States of America

Chun-Ming Huang
Division of Dermatology, Department of Medicine, University of California San Diego, La Jolla, California, United States of America
Moores Cancer Center, University of California San Diego, La Jolla, California, United States of America

Lamine Baba-Moussa and Haziz Sina
Département de Biochimie et de Biologie Cellulaire, Université d'Abomey-Calavi, Cotonou, Benin

Jean-Michel Scheftel and Gilles Prévost
Institut de Bactériologie, Unite´ EA-4438 Physiopathologie et Médecine, Strasbourg, France

Brigitte Moreau
Service de Biologie Polyvalente, Centre Hospitalier de Cayenne, Cayenne, Guyane Française

Dominique Sainte-Marie
Service de Dermatologie, Centre Hospitalier de Cayenne et Institut Guyanais de Dermatologie Tropicale, Cayenne, Guyane Française

Simeon O. Kotchoni
Department of Biology, Rutgers University, Camden, New Jersey, United States of America

Christopher Weidenmaier, Rachel M. McLoughlin and Jean C. Lee
Channing Laboratory, Department of Medicine, Brigham and Women's Hospital and Harvard Medical School, Boston, Massachusetts, United States of America

Hsieh-Shong Leu and Ching-Tai Huang
Division of Infectious Diseases, Department of Internal Medicine, Chang Gung Memorial Hospital, Chang Gung University College of Medicine, Taoyuan, Taiwan

Ting-Shu Wu
Division of Infectious Diseases, Department of Internal Medicine, Chang Gung Memorial Hospital, Chang Gung University College of Medicine, Taoyuan, Taiwan
Graduate Institute of Clinical Medical Sciences, Chang Gung University, Taoyuan, Taiwan

Cheng-Hsun Chiu
Division of Infectious Diseases, Department of Pediatrics, Chang Gung Children's Hospital, Chang Gung Memorial Hospital, Chang Gung University College of Medicine, Taoyuan, Taiwan

Chih-Hsun Yang
Department of Dermatology, Chang Gung Memorial Hospital, Chang Gung, Taoyuan, Taiwan

Yi-Chieh Chen
Department of Plastic and Reconstructive Surgery, Chang Gung Memorial Hospital, Chang Gung University College of Medicine, Taoyuan, Taiwan

Tsu-Lan Wu, Lin-Hui Su and An-Jing Kuo
Department of Laboratory Medicine, Chang Gung Memorial Hospital, Chang Gung University College of Medicine, Taoyuan, Taiwan
Department of Medical Biotechnology and Laboratory Sciences, Chang Gung University, Taoyuan, Taiwan

Pi-Yueh Chang and Ju-Hsin Chia
Department of Laboratory Medicine, Chang Gung Memorial Hospital, Chang Gung University College of Medicine, Taoyuan, Taiwan
Department of Medical Biotechnology and Laboratory Sciences, Chang Gung University, Taoyuan, Taiwan
Graduate Institute of Medical Biotechnology and Laboratory Sciences, Chang
Gung University, Taoyuan, Taiwan

Chia-Chen Lu
Department of Respiratory Therapy, Fu-Jen Catholic University, New Taipei, Taiwan

Hsin-Chih Lai
Department of Medical Biotechnology and Laboratory Sciences, Chang Gung University, Taoyuan, Taiwan
Graduate Institute of Medical Biotechnology and Laboratory Sciences, Chang
Gung University, Taoyuan, Taiwan
Research Center for Pathogenic Bacteria, Chang Gung University, Taoyuan, Taiwan

Wen-Tsung Lo, Chih-Chien Wang, Wei-Jen Lin, Ching-Shen Teng, Ching-Feng Huang and Shyi-Jou Chen
Department of Pediatrics, Tri-Service General Hospital, National Defense Medical Center, Taipei, Taiwan,

Sheng-Ru Wang
Department of Pediatrics, Wan Fang Hospital, Taipei, Taiwan

Dongqing Li, Hu Lei, Zhiheng Li, Hongquan Li, Yue Wang and Yuping Lai
Shanghai Key Laboratory of Regulatory Biology, School of Life Sciences, East China Normal University, Shanghai, People's Republic of China

Shalaka S. Hampras, Anna R. Giuliano, Martha E. Abrahamsen, Bradley A. Sirak and Dana E. Rollison
Department of Cancer Epidemiology, Moffitt Cancer Center, Tampa, Florida, United States of America

Hui-Yi Lin and Kate J. Fisher
Department of Biostatistics, Moffitt Cancer Center, Tampa, Florida, United States of America

Michelle R. Iannacone
QIMR Berghofer Medical Research Institute, Cancer and Population Studies, Royal Brisbane Hospital, Brisbane, Queensland, Australia

Tarik Gheit and Massimo Tommasino
Infections and Cancer Biology Group, International Agency for Research on Cancer-World Health Organization, Lyon, France

Rebecca A. Brady, Christopher P. Mocca, Ranjani Prabhakara, Roger D. Plaut, Tod J. Merkel and Drusilla L. Burns
Center for Biologics Evaluation and Research, Food and Drug Administration, Bethesda, Maryland, United States of America

Mark E. Shirtliff
Department of Microbial Pathogenesis, University of Maryland School of Dentistry, Baltimore, Maryland, United States of America
Department of Microbiology and Immunology, University of Maryland School of Medicine, Baltimore, Maryland, United States of America

Fabiana Venegas Pires, Lígia Maria Abraão and Carlos Magno Castelo Branco Fortaleza
Departamento de Doenças Tropicais, Faculdade de Medicina de Botucatu, Universidade Estadual Paulista, Botucatu, Brazil
Maria de Lourdes Ribeiro de Souza da Cunha, Patrícia Y. F. Martins and Carlos Henrique Camargo
Departamento de Microbiologia e Imunologia, Instituto de Biociências de Botucatu, Universidade Estadual Paulista, Botucatu, Brazil

Hannelore Brandt, Simone Baumgartner, Leyla R. Davis, Christian Bel and Sandro Hodel
Institute of Evolutionary Biology and Environmental Studies, University of Zurich, Zurich, Switzerland

Douglas C. Woodhams
Institute of Evolutionary Biology and Environmental Studies, University of Zurich, Zurich, Switzerland
Department of Ecology and Evolutionary Biology, University of Colorado, Boulder, Colorado, United States of America

Valerie McKenzie
Department of Ecology and Evolutionary Biology, University of Colorado, Boulder, Colorado, United States of America

Jos Kielgast
Section for Freshwater Biology, Department of Biology, University of Copenhagen, Copenhagen, Denmark

Eliane Küpfer
Institute of Evolutionary Biology and Environmental Studies, University of Zurich, Zurich, Switzerland
Department of Evolutionary Biology, Technical University of Braunschweig, Braunschweig, Germany

Ursina Tobler and Benedikt R. Schmidt
Institute of Evolutionary Biology and Environmental Studies, University of Zurich, Zurich, Switzerland
KARCH, Neuchâtel, Switzerland

Rob Knight
Howard Hughes Medical Institute and Department of Chemistry and Biochemistry, BioFrontiers Institute, University of Colorado, Boulder, Colorado, United States of America

Jose A. Suaya
Glaxo Smith Kline Vaccines, Philadelphia, Pennsylvania, United States of America

Debra F. Eisenberg and Christy Fang
Health Core, Inc., Wilmington, Delaware, United States of America

Loren G. Miller
Los Angeles BioMedical Research Center at Harbor-UCLA, Division of Infectious Diseases, Harbor-UCLA Medical Center, Torrance, California, United States of America
David Geffen School of Medicine at UCLA, Los Angeles, California, United States of America

Andrew M. Edwards and Ruth C. Massey
Department of Biology and Biochemistry, University of Bath, Bath, United Kingdom

Ursula Potter
Microscopic Analysis Suite, University of Bath, Bath, United Kingdom

Nicola A. G. Meenan
Department of Biology, University of York, York, United Kingdom

Jennifer R. Potts
Department of Biology, University of York, York, United Kingdom
Department of Chemistry, University of York, York, United Kingdom

Kihyuck Kwak, Rosie Jiang, Joshua W. Wang and Subhashini Jagu
Department of Pathology, The Johns Hopkins University, Baltimore, Maryland, United States of America

Reinhard Kirnbauer
Laboratory of Viral Oncology, Division of Immunology, Allergy and Infectious Diseases, Department of Dermatology, Medical University Vienna (MUW), Vienna, Austria

Richard B. S. Roden
Department of Pathology, The Johns Hopkins University, Baltimore, Maryland, United States of America
Department of Gynecology and Obstetrics, The Johns Hopkins University, Baltimore, Maryland, United States of America
Department of Oncology, The Johns Hopkins University, Baltimore, Maryland, United States of America

Jeffrey A. Mayfield and Deborah L. Donahue
W. M. Keck Center for Transgene Research, University of Notre Dame, Notre Dame, Indiana, United States of America

Zhong Liang, Garima Agrahari, Victoria A. Ploplis and Francis J. Castellino
W. M. Keck Center for Transgene Research, University of Notre Dame, Notre Dame, Indiana, United States of America
Department of Chemistry and Biochemistry, University of Notre Dame, Notre Dame, Indiana, United States of America

Shaun W. Lee
W. M. Keck Center for Transgene Research, University of Notre Dame, Notre Dame, Indiana, United States of America
Department of Biological Sciences, University of Notre Dame, Notre Dame, Indiana, United States of America

Index